# MANAGEMENT OF ACUTE HAND INJURIES
## A BIOLOGICAL APPROACH

# MANAGEMENT OF
# ACUTE HAND INJURIES
## A BIOLOGICAL APPROACH

**PAUL M. WEEKS, M.D.**

Professor of Surgery (Plastic and Reconstructive Surgery), Washington University School of Medicine; Plastic Surgeon-in-Chief, Barnes Hospital; Director, Milliken Hand Rehabilitation Center, Irene Walter Johnson Institute of Rehabilitation, St. Louis, Missouri

**R. CHRISTIE WRAY, M.D.**

Associate Professor of Surgery (Plastic and Reconstructive Surgery), Washington University School of Medicine, St. Louis, Missouri

**In collaboration with**

**BARBEL HOLTMANN, M.D.**

Assistant Professor of Surgery (Plastic and Reconstructive Surgery), Washington University School of Medicine; Plastic Surgeon-in-Chief, St. Louis County Hospital, St. Louis, Missouri

**With Chapter 7 contributed by**

**STEPHEN J. MATHES, M.D.**

Assistant Professor of Surgery (Plastic and Reconstructive Surgery), Washington University School of Medicine; Director of Microsurgery Service, St. Louis, Missouri

SECOND EDITION
with 496 illustrations

**THE C. V. MOSBY COMPANY**

Saint Louis 1978

SECOND EDITION

Previous edition copyrighted 1973

Printed in the United States of America

The C. V. Mosby Company
11830 Westline Industrial Drive, St. Louis, Missouri 63141


Library of Congress Cataloging in Publication Data

    Weeks, Paul M.
    Management of acute hand injuries.

    Includes bibliographies and index.
    1.   Hand—Wounds and injuries.   I.   Wray,
Robert Christie, joint author.   II.   Title.
[DNLM:   1.   Hand injuries—Therapy.   WE830 W396m]
RD559.W4    1978       617.1        78-5718
ISBN   0-8016-5371-1


CB/CB/B   9  8  7  6  5  4  3  2  1

# PREFACE

Injury of the hand may involve skin, bone, nerve, tendon, or joint, either singly or in combination. Accomplishments through surgical techniques are limited by the biological processes of tissue repair and regeneration that come into play after the technical feats of the surgeon have been completed. These biological processes can produce either a favorable environment that permits complete functional recovery or an unfavorable environment that compromises functional recovery. The object of this second edition is to provide current concepts regarding tissue healing, surgical techniques, and postoperative management; hence the division of the book into three sections. The first section presents the biological processes involved in the healing of tissues in the hand, that is, skin, tendon, and cartilage repair, bone and nerve regeneration, and the structure and function of digital joints. The second section presents methods for managing injury to these tissues. Recent perfection of the techniques for reestablishment of circulation in devascularized parts has led to the inclusion of a chapter on these techniques.

The third section presents methods of postoperative management. Further, this final section presents alternate methods of management when primary care has failed to produce a satisfactory result.

In this edition careful documentation of the results of treatment by each method of management is included when available. In addition, our experience gathered in the Milliken Hand Rehabilitation Center during the past 7 years is presented. Each patient was carefully evaluated and extensively documented. The opportunity to obtain documentation and provide rehabilitative care of our patients has been made possible through the support of Mr. Thomas Moore, whose generosity led to the establishment and continued operation of the Milliken Hand Rehabilitation Center.

With admiration and gratitude we recognize the enthusiastic work of our therapists in the Hand Rehabilitation Center: Patty Phelps, Virginia Woods, Elizabeth Walker, Mary Kuxhaus, Ramona Lanka, and Pattie Paynter.

*Paul M. Weeks*
*R. Christie Wray*

# CONTENTS

# THE BIOLOGICAL BASIS
# FOR MANAGEMENT

# CHAPTER 1

# Wound healing and tissue coverage

The incurrence of a wound initiates acceleration of normal physiological processes toward the restoration of tissue integrity. As a result of this acceleration, a new phenomenon is introduced—contraction—which aids in wound closure but which by its very nature is most detrimental functionally. The only major difference in the healing of perfectly coapted wounds and open wounds is the time required for healing to be completed and the degree of tissue contraction associated with open wounds. We will limit our discussion to the healing of an open wound since it manifests the physiological principles more clearly. All surgery is based on the premise of obtaining adequate healing of the operative wound; thus a thorough understanding of this fundamental biological process is mandatory.

## CELLULAR PHENOMENON

A wound may be inflicted by blunt trauma, laceration, or avulsion, or may result from tissue coagulation by thermal, electrical, or chemical agents.

Initially, vasodilatation in the traumatized area, thrombosis of damaged vessels, and contraction of muscular vessels are observed. In the area immediately surrounding the wound, protein and fluid are exuded from the intact but injured vessels. An outpouring of vascular fluids rich in fibrin occurs (Fig. 1-1). Albumin, which is of smaller molecular size than globulin, readily passes between the vascular endothelial cell junctions and into the extracellular spaces. The resulting fluid shift renders the damaged area edematous and produces a relative vascular insufficiency in the wound as evidenced by a very low tissue $Po_2$. Polymorphonuclear cells and mononuclear cells of vascular origin migrate into the wound. Macrophages that appear in the wound matrix originate from the bone marrow.

Utilizing viscose cellulose sponges to induce a matrix of granulation tissue, Hunt and associates (1975) studied the oxygen and carbon dioxide tensions in these sponges during the first 30 days of wound healing. At the moment of implantation of the sponge, the $Po_2$ dropped sharply (Fig. 1-2). This was followed by a more gradual decline during the succeeding 2 days until a minimum value was reached at 5 days after wounding. Between the fifth and thirtieth days, there was a progressive and almost linear increase in $Po_2$. Two hours after sponge implantation, the mean $Pco_2$ was 37 mm Hg. It rose to a plateau of 112 to 119 mm Hg between 2

**3**

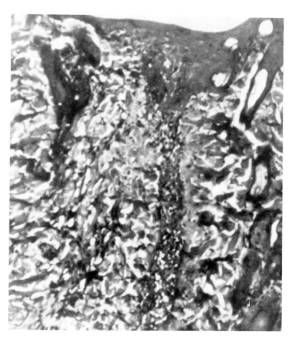

**Fig. 1-1.** The incised wound at 48 hours exhibits cellular debris between the dermal edges and complete repair of the surface epithelium.

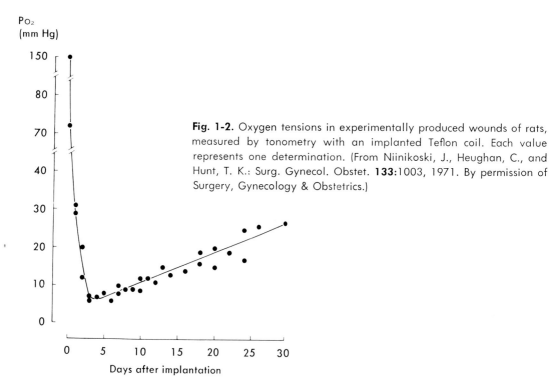

**Fig. 1-2.** Oxygen tensions in experimentally produced wounds of rats, measured by tonometry with an implanted Teflon coil. Each value represents one determination. (From Niinikoski, J., Heughan, C., and Hunt, T. K.: Surg. Gynecol. Obstet. **133:**1003, 1971. By permission of Surgery, Gynecology & Obstetrics.)

and 4 days after wounding (Fig. 1-3). It then dropped abruptly to 93 to 99 mm Hg until the eighth day, at which time it again increased rapidly until day 10, when there began a rapid fall from the tenth to the fifteenth day, with a plateau from the fifteenth to the twenty-fifth day, and a gradual decline until the thirtieth day. Measurement of the pH 2 hours after implantation revealed the mean level to be 7.32. It fell rapidly for the next 2 days to about 6.9, where it remained until the ninth day. The pH then gradually rose to 7.13 by the thirtieth day.

Within 48 to 72 hours after the wound is incurred, the quantity of lymphocytes and mononuclear cells has peaked and begins declining. The neutrophilic leukocytes, which exhibit minimal direct phagocytic activity, undergo cell lysis and degranulation to prepare the extracellular matrix for removal by the macrophages. Alexander and co-workers have suggested from their studies that the biological mediators of cellular proliferation in wounds are located in lysosomal granules of cells and are released by death or injury of the involved cells. Because of their crucial role in in-flammatory processes and a short biological half-life, neutrophils that enter wounds during the first 2 or 3 days and then disintegrate probably supply the majority of these mediators. The active factions appear to have a molecular weight of less than 50,000. Monocytes, whose role is primarily one of phagocytosis, actively ingest both neutrophilic granules and fibrin. During the first 3 to 4 days, devitalized tissues and fibrin are phagocytized to prepare the wound for the ingrowth of new capillaries. Ross investigated the role of macrophages in wound repair by studying the healing processes in wounds depleted of this cell. Hydrocortisone administration to guinea pigs produced a prolonged monocytopenia, and antimacrophage serum was used to eliminate tissue macrophages. The macrophage level in the wounds of those monocytopenic animals was reduced to approximately one-third of the level of the control group. Fibrosis in the wounds was virtually unaffected. Collagen synthesis was similar to that of control wounds in all stages of repair. The appearance of fibroblasts in the treated animals was delayed until 5 days after wounding, and the subsequent rate of proliferation was slower than that of the control group. Débridement and fibrosis of these wounds was delayed. These studies

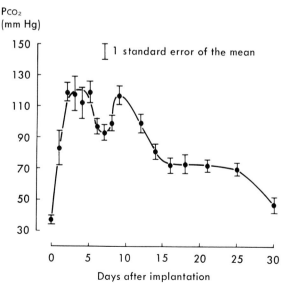

Fig. 1-3. Carbon dioxide tensions in experimentally produced wounds of rats, measured by aspiration of fluid from the dead space. Each value represents the mean of 4 to 13 determinations. (From Niinikoski, J., Heughan, C., and Hunt, T. K.: Surg. Gynecol. Obstet. 133:1003, 1971. By permission of Surgery, Gynecology & Obstetrics.)

indicate that in the repair process the principal cell responsible for wound débridement is the macrophage. Furthermore, the macrophage may be required to stimulate fibroblast proliferation. Obviously the burn wound that exhibits extensive tissue destruction requires an extended period of autogenous wound débridement before granulation tissue can begin forming. Surgical removal (débridement) of as much devitalized tissue as feasible at the time of initial wounding will aid in shortening this period of phagocytosis.

Myers and Wolf observed that the earliest vascular crossing of a skin wound occurred 3 days after wounding. Capillary buds are formed continuously behind the advancing syncytium of fibroblasts that have made their appearance in the wound by the third day. Wound fibroblasts are probably derived from resident fibrocytes, that is, fibrocytes normally present in the tissue before injury. However, evidence suggests that blood-borne mononuclear cells can give rise to some of the fibrocytic cells participating in wound repair. Sumrall and Johnson made multiple skin incisions on the backs of rats and gave a single injection of tritiated thymidine at varying periods of time after incision. Serial biopsies up to 15½ hours after injury taken from animals injected at 4, 7, 8, and 11½ hours after injury did not show labelling of monocytes, fibrocytes, or endothelial cells. Biopsies taken from these same animals at varying intervals after 16 hours showed labelling of these cells. This has been interpreted to indicate that new labelled fibrocytes that appeared in the wound were labelled at a distant site, since labelling did not occur locally 1 hour after a pulse injection of tritiated thymidine. Fibroblasts exhibit motion only when proliferating or actively secreting collagen and glycosaminoglycans. The fibroblasts migrate on a fibrin network oriented in the open wound by contraction of the blood clot, thus centrally aligning the fibrin network attached to the wound margins and base. Migrating fibroblasts act as a leading edge for the capillary buds and deposit collagen and glycosaminoglycans to provide a framework upon which the immature capillaries can build. Cell migration is gained by the action of the ruffled undulating membrane of the fibroblast. When this membrane contacts a second fibroblast, migration in that particular direction is inhibited (contact inhibition) and redirected to areas clear of fibroblasts. Thus, all cell migration is subsequently directed toward the center of the fibrin coagulum of the wound.

Three factors have been shown to have significant influence on fibroblastic activity: (1) the migration-promoting factor, (2) the survival factor, and (3) the serum growth factor.

Wolf and Lipton demonstrated the presence of a factor in rat serum that promotes the migration of mouse fibroblasts. Magnesium and calcium are essential for maximum activity of this promoting factor. Once cells are exposed to the serum, there is an 8- to 10-hour lag period before cell migration can be detected. The serum must be constantly present to have continued cell movement. The growth of fibroblasts in tissue culture ceases when the population reaches a characteristic cell density. If a wound is made by scratching a line across the sheet of cells, the cells will migrate into the denuded area, synthesize DNA, and undergo mitosis. The serum migration-promoting factor is stable for up to 6 months at 4° C. The migration-promoting activity in human serum is due to the presence of a high molecular weight molecule. The mouse cells will not migrate into a denuded area in the absence of serum. Serum alone is, however, not sufficient to achieve migration of mouse fibroblasts. The migration of the mouse cells depends on the presence of amino acids, calcium, and magnesium in the media. The presence of contractile microfilaments has previously been shown to be necessary for cell motility.

The migration-promoting factor has been

shown to be distinct from the growth and survival factors. Neither the serum migration-promoting activity nor the survival factor is depleted by growing or resting cells, but serum growth factors are. The migration-promoting activity and growth factors are present in human urine; serum is another ready source of migration-promoting factor activity.

Meanwhile, marked changes have occurred in the epithelial cells at the wound margins during the first 24 hours of the injury. The epidermis must be damaged before the epithelial cells can respond since damage to the dermis alone will produce no response in the overlying epidermis. Mitotic response of epidermal cells to an open wound is limited to those cells positioned within 1 or 2 mm of the wound edge. Vertically, the epidermal mitotic activity is confined to the basal layer. After the wound is incurred, the basal layer and the cells in the distal stratum spinosum begin mitosis. Cells in the outer layers, such as the stratum granulosum, cannot revert to the mitotic process. A mitotic inhibitor, which has been isolated from the epidermis and identified as a glycoprotein with a molecular weight of approximately 30,000, is synthesized within the epidermis to control its mitotic activity. The concentration of this inhibitor is greatest in the distal keratinizing cells and lowest in the basal cells. This substance, chalone, is present in a number of tissues throughout the body. Yamaguchi and colleagues have suggested that the epidermal chalones inhibit the epidermal cell proliferation in at least three different processes of the cell cycle. One is the DNA synthesis in S phase, the second is the transition from $G_1$ to S phase, and the third is the transition from $G_2$ to M phase. The high epidermal mitotic activity associated with wound healing is facilitated by the local loss of this tissue-specific hormone. Stress hormones inhibit mitosis in normal epidermis but progressively lose this ability in the epidermis adjacent to the wound. Within 12 to 24

hours the epidermal cells are actively synthesizing DNA and by 24 to 36 hours have undergone active mitosis. The cells that undergo mitosis do not migrate. The cells that migrate develop a high mitotic rate only after they have reached their final positions in the wound matrix. The advancing epidermal cells move as a sheet onto the wound matrix, ever maintaining their attachments with adjacent epidermal cells. Because a basal lamina has not developed at this time, the cells are migrating directly upon the wound matrix. As the cells migrate, they become flattened and appear less differentiated, as evidenced by a quantitative increase in the number of free ribosomes and a decrease in rough endoplasmic reticulum and number of tonofilaments. Some of the epidermal cells ingest fibrin strains and serum protein as they migrate, degenerate, and undergo necrosis. By the third day, basal lamina and hemidesmosomes become evident attached to the cells behind the advancing edge. As formation of the basal lamina and hemidesmosomes is completed, the attached cells become more differentiated.

The underlying granulation tissue continues to exhibit a low $Po_2$ during the first week. Increasing inspired oxygen, as suggested clinically, is effective only when blood volume and local nutritive flow to the wound are adequate. Thus, these factors control the efficacy of supplemental oxygen administration. If the supply of oxygen in the wound is inadequate, healing is limited. Highly vascularized tissues heal more rapidly than do poorly vascularized tissues. Collagen synthesis and tensile strength gain in rat wounds increase as ambient oxygen concentrations increase. The administration of 70% oxygen results in a gain of tensile strength of approximately 30% above control levels.

Distant trauma, for example, muscle trauma, significantly interferes with wound tensile strength gain. The wound $Po_2$ is slightly lowered and the wound $Pco_2$ is significantly elevated. A concomitant inhibition of collagen synthesis is observed. Dextran administration reverses this inhibition, suggesting that oxygen supply depends more on blood volume and local nutritive flow than on oxygen-carrying capacity.

Activator substances may play a role in initiating and regulating the progression of the inflammatory process from the exudative to the reparative (proliferative) phase. Current data indicate the existence of a connective tissue activating substance which is a water- and saline-soluble polypeptide and has a molecular weight between 4,000 and 10,000. This substance possesses one or more labile sulfhydryl groups per molecule that are essential to its biological activity. The substance is widely distributed; the absolute amount in a tissue is related to cell density. When this activator is exposed to synovial fibroblasts, the fibroblasts promptly exhibit a hypermetabolic state characterized by a 3- to 40-fold increase in hyaluronic acid formation, glucose uptake, lactate formation, and hydrogen ion liberation. Concomitantly, the formation of soluble and fibrous collagen is depressed. Within 7 to 9 days, the rate of hyaluronic acid synthesis levels off and decelerates, allowing the cells to shift to a state that favors the production of collagen. Thereafter, collagen synthesis is the dominant activity of these cells. The need for a signal is readily apparent, and it is suggested that the connective-tissue activator is at least in part responsible.

Studies comparing the effect of this connective-tissue activator on synovial fibroblasts and dermal fibroblasts revealed that the latter are less sensitive to the connective-tissue activator and apparently have metabolic requirements best met by the extracts of dermal cells. These studies reinforce the concept of the differences in fibroblasts of diverse origins.

## FIBROUS TISSUE AND GLYCOSAMINOGLYCAN SYNTHESIS

The primary metabolic function of migrating fibroblasts is synthesis of collagen.

What evokes synthesis of this protein? Messenger RNA extracted from *E coli* initiates, in cell-free systems, protein synthesis with formyl (CHO) methionine, alanine, or serine in the lead position. In the production of these proteins, the cells remove the formyl group from methionine or split off the entire formyl methionine unit after synthesis of the protein chain has been initiated. Further studies reveal that messenger RNA uses a special codon, AUG GUG, at the beginning of a strand to order the initiation of protein synthesis with formylated methionine in the lead position. Thus, only the formylatable variety of methionine transfer RNA can initiate synthesis, suggesting that this variety of transfer RNA has a special configuration that fits into a particular site on the ribosome.

Substantiation of this point is provided by the addition of puromycin to the medium. Puromycin has a structure similar to that of the end of a transfer RNA molecule that attaches to an amino acid through its $NH_2$ group and subsequently forms a peptide bond with the adjacent amino acid. However, because puromycin lacks the free carboxyl (COOH) group of an amino acid and cannot form a second peptide bond, chain elongation is prevented and the aberrant polypeptide chain is immediately expelled from the cell. Thus, the formyl group may be utilized to initiate formation of the first peptide bond that activates nascent polypeptide production.

The initial step in collagen synthesis is the formation of a polypeptide chain whose amino acid sequence is formed in response to messenger RNA (Fig. 1-4). In such a polypeptide chain of 1,000 amino acid residues, approximately 330 are glycine, 130 proline, 100 hydroxyproline, 110 alanine, and the remaining residues distributed among fourteen other amino acids. The amino acids may be arranged on the polypeptide chain in a variety of configurations, but the sequences glycine-proline-hydroxyproline and glycine-proline-

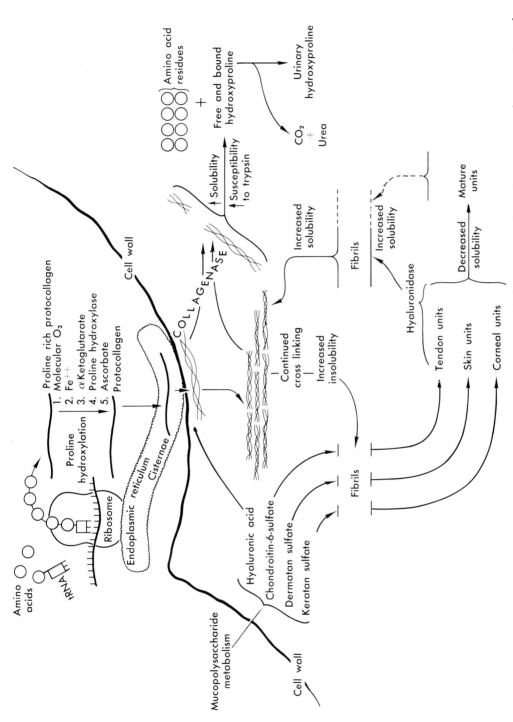

**Fig. 1-4.** A schematic representation of the synthesis and degradation of collagen. Note the ultimate structural organization of collagen and the glycosaminoglycan involved.

alanine are the most frequent. Hydroxy-proline and hydroxylysine are obtained by hydroxylation of proline and lysine after the amino acids are incorporated into the polypeptide chain but before the chain can be extruded from the cell. Proline hydroxylation is accomplished in the presence of molecular oxygen, iron ($Fe^{++}$), alpha ketoglutarate, ascorbate, and proline hydroxylase. A similar environment is necessary for lysine hydroxylation except that the enzyme responsible is a different hydroxylase. Proline hydroxylase preferentially hydroxylates prolines in the position immediately preceding glycine and proto-collagen proline.

Inhibition of collagen formation at this level could result from anaerobic conditions, or the presence of chelating agents that would bind the $Fe^{++}$ cofactor, or a dietary deficiency of vitamin C. Of these three, vitamin C deficiency has historically been of greater interest to investigators. Studies suggest that the role of ascorbic acid is in microsomal electron transport leading to proline hydroxylation.

A deficiency of L-ascorbic acid markedly impairs the cells' ability to synthesize collagen in response to wounding. Yet, under these same conditions some collagen is formed. Evidence suggests that an ascorbic acid–dependent and an ascorbic acid–independent system are available within the cell for collagen production. Ascorbic acid is required in the maintenance of rapidly formed labile wound collagen but not in the maintenance of structural collagen. Thus, the scorbutic individual exhibits marked impairment of wound tensile strength gain.

Normal collagen synthesis requires the production of polypeptide chains that are released from the ribosomes along the endoplasmic reticulum and deposited extracellularly at points where the cisternae of the endoplasmic reticulum and the external cell membrane are in close apposition. The extruded polypeptide chains aggregate on the surface of the cell to form the basic collagen unit—tropocollagen.

Three polypeptide chains, approximately 1,000 amino acid residues in length, wrap around each other to form a superhelix. These three chains are bound together by hydrogen bonds between the oxygen atoms that are located where amino acids are joined by peptide linkages in an adjacent chain. Subsequent structural organization is based on the development of intramolecular and intermolecular crosslinks. Such linkages result in the tensile strength gain of the nascent collagen fibers. As the number of intermolecular crosslinks increases, the collagen fibrils become increasingly insoluble, as evidenced by the fibrils' resistance to solubility in increasing concentrations of saline. An optimal number of linkages exists for maximum collagen fiber stability.

Niinikoski and associates analyzed wound fluid at 7, 11, 16, and 17 days after wounding to determine the effects of various oxygen concentrations on enzymatic activity in the wound. Animals were exposed to either room air, 12% oxygen, or 55% oxygen. Measurement of respiratory gas tensions revealed significant portions of the wound tissue existing in extremely low oxygen tension. Earlier studies have shown that the accumulation of collagen and the amount of ribonucleic acid produced in cellulose sponges are decreased by hypoxia and increased by hyperoxia to reach a peak at 70% ambient oxygen at one atmosphere, thereafter decreasing again during constant exposure to higher oxygen tensions. The wound tensile strength also varied according to the ambient oxygen tension up to a point where 70% oxygen increased the tensile strength gain by 30%.

In normal wounds glycolysis dominates during the synthesis of collagen. In glycolysis no oxygen is consumed during the conversion of glucose to lactate. Niinikoski and colleagues showed that the consumption of glucose in a wound increases as the oxygen tension is increased. In this work, enzyme activities in the limiting step of glycolysis, citric acid cycle, and pentophosphatase cycle were determined in cellulose sponge implants of rats chronically breathing 12% oxygen, air, or 55% oxygen. Respiratory gas tensions and concentration of pyruvate and lactate were measured, and wound fluid was aspirated from the implants. Significant portions of the repaired tissue existed in conditions of extreme low oxygen tension. The wound $Pco_2$ increased and paralleled the inspired $Pco_2$ probably because of enhanced production of carbon dioxide. Thus, hyperoxia shifted the wound metabolism from anaerobic to aerobic glycolysis. This occurred concurrently with activation of the citric acid cycle.

Oxygen delivery to the cells requires diffusion of oxygen across the capillary endothelium, the extracellular matrix, cell membrane, and cytoplasm to the mitochondrium. It has been shown that under normal conditions, diffusion limits the availability of oxygen to wound tissue cells.

Often anemia is implicated as determining wound healing by interfering with the transfer of oxygen to the cells. Hunt and colleagues (1974) studied the effects of anemia on wound oxygen tension in anemic and control animals. The wound oxygen tensions were identical in both groups. It was concluded that there was no significant change in the oxygen economy in the experimental wounds of normal rabbits made anemic by bleeding and retransfusing plasma. Thus, mild or moderate, uncomplicated, normovolemic anemia in otherwise healthy individuals does not impair delivery of oxygen to the wound and is of no consequence to wound healing.

Seifter and associates reasoned that collagen synthesis, which is one of the critical steps of wound repair, might be accelerated at early stages by the addition of exogenous collagen-producing cells to the healing wound. The effect of reimplantation of rat fibroblasts grown in culture on the rate of collagen synthesis in subcutaneously implanted Ivalon polyvinyl alcohol sponges was studied. The hydroxyproline content of sponges inoculated with fibroblasts at the time of subcutaneous implantation and removed 4 days later was significantly more than the control level. At 7 days, the collagen content of the fibroblast-inoculated sponges was more than twice that of the control sponges. The fibroblasts in the inoculum were sufficient to provide a significant acceleration of collagen synthesis during early stages of wound repair. This suggests the possibility of accelerating the healing process in man by introducing collagen-forming fibroblasts into the wound.

Collagen synthesis can be stimulated by vitamin A, a lysosomal labilizing compound. Of the labilizing compounds, testosterone and vitamin A have been shown to reverse the retarding effects of glucocorticoids on wound repair. Glucocorticoids and aspirin, which are anti-inflammatory agents, are known to be lysosomal stabilizers. Vitamin E has also been shown to be a lysosomal stabilizer. Hunt and associates (1971) studied the effects of anti-inflammatory agents (which stabilize lysosomes) on the inhibition of collagen synthesis. This study revealed that corticoids and vitamin E significantly retarded both collagen synthesis and tensile strength of the wounds at 7 days after wounding. Vitamin E did not alter the effects of the glucocorticoids. Vitamin A reversed the retarding effect of vitamin E. The animals that received vitamin A plus vitamin E healed significantly faster than did the control group. Vitamin E can act as either a lysosomal labilizer in vitro or a lysosomal stabilizer in vivo. Furthermore, vitamin E protects lysosomal membranes from the labilizing effects of excessive vitamin A.

Sandberg has demonstrated that cortisone administration after the second day following injury did not retard healing as measured by collagen accumulation and wound strength. Thus, the effects of gluco-corticoids are diminished after inflammation has become established. Therefore, the action of glucocorticoids apparently depends more on its anti-inflammatory than its antisynthetic action. These findings lend further support to the idea that lysosomal stabilizers inhibit collagen synthesis and repair, whereas lysosomal labilizers reverse this retardation.

During this early period the fibroblasts are also synthesizing glycosaminoglycans (mucopolysaccharides). The importance of these substances must not be overlooked. Seven distinct mucopolysaccharides have been described. All except keratan sulfate are composed of repeating units of hexosamine (galactosamine or glucosamine) and uronic acid. Keratan sulfate is composed of a repeating unit containing galactose and 6-sulfoglucosamine. Hyaluronic acid is composed of repeating units of glucosamine and glucuronic acids which form a polymer associated with a small amount of protein. The other mucopolysaccharides occur in tissues in the form of protein-polysaccharide complexes.

In granulating wounds, the isolation and identification of each mucopolysaccharide has shown the presence of hyaluronic acid, chondroitin-4-sulfate, and dermatan sulfate. Chondroitin-4-sulfate and dermatan sulfate increase progressively from the fifth to the seventeenth day (Fig. 1-5). No chondroitin-6-sulfate is present. Following an initial fall from the fifth to the tenth day, the hyaluronic acid fraction remains relatively constant. What is the significance of the mucopolysaccharides present? Extracts of wounds up to 3 days stimulate fibroblasts in tissue culture whereas 4- to 15-day wound extracts inhibit fibroblastic activity. Furthermore, mucopolysaccharide determines, in vitro, the diameter of collagen fibril formation. When dermatan sulfate is added to a collagen solution, larger fibers can be observed aggregating than when chondroitin-4-sulfate is added. In vivo the

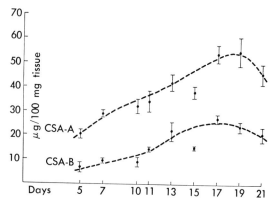

**Fig. 1-5.** Chondroitin-4-Sulfate (CSA-A) and dermatan-sulfate (CSA-B) content of skin wound granulation tissue. Results expressed as mean ± 1 SD. (Reproduced from Bentley, J. P.: Ann. Surg. **165:**186, 1967.)

fine collagen fibrils of the cornea are associated with keratan sulfate, whereas the heavier fibers of skin are complexed with a high content of dermatan sulfate, and the thick fibers in tendons are associated with chondroitin sulfate. Thus, the mucopolysaccharides aid in orientation of the collagen subunits during aggregation to form fibrils and contribute to determining ultimate fiber size and functional capacity. This difference in function is particularly striking when one compares the cornea, exhibiting impeccable clarity, with the Achilles tendon.

**FIBROUS TISSUE ORGANIZATION**

The levels of collagen organization are represented in Fig. 1-6. At the molecular level, polypeptide chains form the triple helix characteristic of tropocollagen. End-to-end attachment of the tropocollagen units produces a filament that is 140 to 200 angstroms in diameter and of unlimited length. These filaments are longitudinally organized into fibrils measuring approximately 2,000 A in diameter. The primitive fibers formed are 100,000 A in diameter and visible with the light microscope.

Of particular importance are the dimensions of the spaces between the longi-

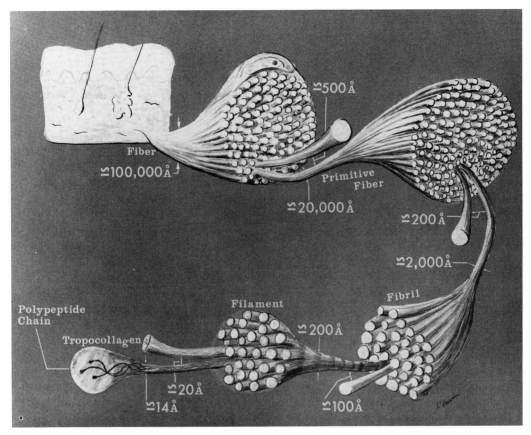

**Fig. 1-6.** Organization of the components of the collagen fiber. (From Bryant, W. M., Greenwell, J. E., and Weeks, P. M.: Surg. Gynecol. Obstet. **126:**27, 1968.)

tudinally oriented components. The following approximate spacings between components have been suggested: polypeptide chains, 10 to 16 A; filaments, 100 A; fibrils, 200 A; primitive fibers, 500 A; and fibers, 1,000 A. Study of the effects of tanning agents on collagen offers further support of the existence of large gaps between collagen components. The introduction of crosslinks—5 A in length—during tanning fails to bridge the gaps between the larger components.

The state of organization of collagen at any component level depends on the balance of cohesive and dispersive forces between components (Fig. 1-7). An imbalance of these forces will be reflected by a change in the tissue's compliance. Progressive increase in cohesive forces accounts for the progressive insolubility of nascent collagen in solutions exhibiting increased dispersive forces. If the solution's dispersive forces exceed the cohesiveness of the collagen, the collagen becomes soluble. The forces contributing to cohesiveness include hydrostatic forces, electrovalent bonds, covalent bonds, and the mucopolysaccharide milieu. The hydrostatic forces exerted by the solution are relatively insignificant. Electrovalent bonding permits variation in distance between polypeptide chains from 10 to 16 A without disruption of the bond. However, a covalent bond such as hydrogen spans only 2.8 A. In view

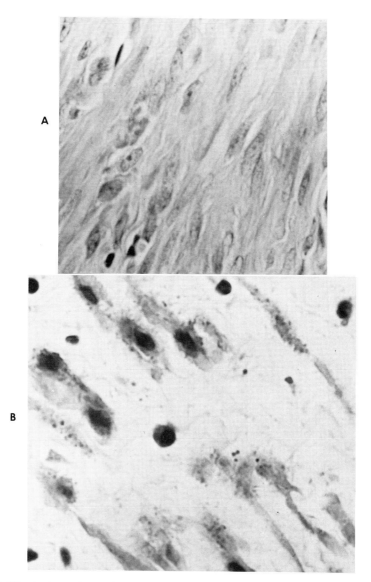

**Fig. 1-7.** Histologic sections of cervix (×638). **A,** The fibrous tissue in the normal cervix is tightly bound, presenting a rigid structure. **B,** No changes occurred in the total collagen content; however, the dispersive forces have exceeded the cohesive forces and result in the collagen becoming more compliant. (From Bryant, W. M., Greenwell, J. E., and Weeks, P. M.: Surg. Gynecol. Obstet. **126:**27, 1968.)

of the spatial organization of collagen components, it is evident that the cohesive forces contributed by electrovalent and covalent bonds are operative only at the polypeptide chain and tropocollagen levels. The distances between filaments, fibrils, primitive fibers, and fibers preclude such bonding. This, coupled with evidence from earlier discussion, suggests a limit to which collagen molecules can interact with each other to form fibrils, thereby limiting the diameter of the fibrils. To form the larger fibers, fibrils interact with a spacer. The precise contributions of the glycoproteins and mucopolysaccharides to the organization of collagen are unknown. The interaction of these two groups of substances with collagen has been inferred from the experimental data available. Further aggregation to form bundles would require electrostatic interaction between larger fibers and the glycosaminoglycans or glycoproteins. Apparently an optimal quantitative and qualitative relationship exists. When the fiber systems are overloaded with the spacer, a decrease in fiber tensile strength occurs.

The dispersive forces include mechanical deforming force, osmotic swelling, and the mucopolysaccharide milieu. In a system of isolated fibers, extrinsic stress will be applied as a shearing force between longitudinally oriented collagen fibers. Initially, however, when extrinsic force is applied to a segment of skin, the resiliency of the fiber weave accounts for the lengthening. All subsequent stress acts as a shearing force and aids in longitudinal cleavage of the fibers.

The dispersive forces associated with the inflow of water are limited by the strong cohesive forces of the fibrous structure; that is, the constrictive effect of fiber weave demonstrably influences the swelling of collagen. Whole skin absorbs only 3 to 4 times its weight in water. The hydrated fiber demonstrates a marked decrease in tensile strength as compared with its dry counterpart.

In considering the mucopolysaccharide milieu, the characteristics and contributions of each particular mucopolysaccharide must be affirmed. Chondroitin sulfate has been associated with increased tissue rigidity and hyaluronic acid with increased tissue compliance. The dissociation of chondroitin sulfate from collagen in the auricular cartilage of the rabbit results in marked decrease in cartilage rigidity. Conversely, the hydrophilic property of hy-aluronic acid is held responsible for various physiological phenomena including tissue edema, production of the graafian follicle cavity by local water binding, and ovulation that is accomplished by increased colloidal osmotic pressure. These observations suggest that when hyaluronic acid increases above a critical level, the resulting influx of water creates an imbalance between the cohesive and dispersive forces; this imbalance is reflected by change in the tissue's compliance.

## FIBROUS TISSUE DEGRADATION

For the healing wound to undergo constant remodelling, mechanisms must be operative for collagen and mucopolysaccharide degradation. The presence of collagenolytic activity was first demonstrated in the tadpole undergoing rapid resorption of its tail. Isolating the enzyme had been difficult because such a minute quantity of collagenase is contained in the tissues at a given time. A tissue culture system was devised that utilized reconstituted collagen gel for the substrate. The cells were cultured on this substrate, and collagenase activity was identified by the zone of liquefaction of the gel substrate (Fig. 1-8). With this model, granulating wounds in guinea pigs have revealed intense collagenolytic activity in the whole edge of the wound containing both epithelium and new mesenchyme (100% produce lysis). The central granulation tissue, which had no epithelium, produced lysis in 23% of the tissues. In tissue taken from the wound edges, separation of epithelium and marginal granulation tissue revealed that 80% of the epithelial samples were active and 45% of the mesenchymal tissues were active.

Control granulation tissue that had not produced lytic activity became highly active after exposure to epithelium for 24 to 48 hours. This suggests that the epithelium plays an induction role on the central granulation tissue. Marked collagenase

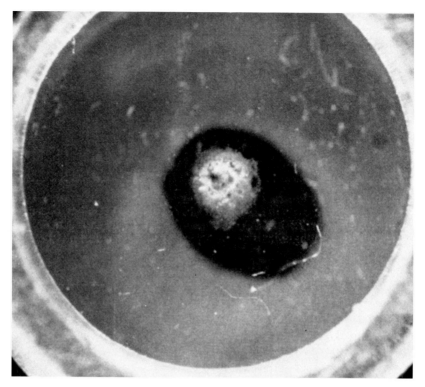

**Fig. 1-8.** Tadpole fin implant on reconstituted calf-skin collagen gel after incubation for 24 hours at 37° C. (From Lapiere, C. M., and Gross, J.: Mechanisms of heart tissue destruction, American Association for the Advancement of Science, Publication No. 75, Washington, D.C., 1963.)

activity is detectable on the second day and continues long after the wound has healed clinically. This activity, which was produced by the epithelium and not the underlying mesenchymal cells, may continue even in the absence of collagen synthesis. Both epithelial and mesenchymal wound tissue cultures from fully scorbutic guinea pigs have demonstrated marked amounts of collagenase activity. Granulation tissue loses its collagenolytic activity rapidly after coverage of the wound by skin grafting.

In man, cultures of wound edges that contain proliferating epithelium and new mesenchymal tissues show 100% lysis. Granulation tissue is also markedly active (99% lysis). When the marginal tissues of the wound are separated into epithelium and granulation tissue, the edge of granulation tissue demonstrates a high degree of activity (93%) whereas the epithelium is active in only 28% of cases.

Collagenase produces cleavage of the tropocollagen molecule (TC) into two units, a larger fragment (TC$^A$) and a smaller fragment (TC$^B$). These two fragments represent three fourths and one fourth of the length of the intact collagen molecule respectively. Once these fragments are produced, there is no further attack on the two fragments by collagenase. But the tropocollagen fragments exhibit marked solubility in physiological saline at room temperature (TC$^B$ is soluble even in distilled water) and a much greater susceptibility to degradation by trypsin. These observations are in sharp contrast to the characteristics of native tropocollagen under similar conditions.

But what renders the larger collagen bundles and fibers accessible to the action of collagenase? Earlier discussion suggested that the mucopolysaccharides in the interstitial spaces control the size and orientation of collagen fiber fabrication and that when an optimal size fiber is prepared, larger units are constructed by interspersing a mucopolysaccharide or glycoprotein between the fibers, allowing collagen bundle formation. Examination of the physical characteristics of large collagen fibers reveals that if the fibers are subjected to a force, they extend approximately 20% and after maximum extension break. If the breakage occurred because of disruption of the intramolecular covalent bonds, a force of 300 $kg/mm^2$ would be required. Yet the average tensile strength of these collagen fibers is only 10 to 12 $kg/mm^2$. Thus breakage occurs by the slippage of microfibrils over each other. This slippage can be accounted for by either breakage of weak bonds between the ends of tropocollagen molecules or by breakage of the cohesive forces between the fibrils.

Cohesive forces between fibrils are affected by interaction between a glycoprotein and collagen fibrils of limited diameter. In skin, the diameter of these fibrils is 500 to 800 A. If the interfibrillar glycoprotein is removed by amylase or the chelating agent EDTA, the tensile strength of the collagen fiber is reduced. Conversely, a marked increase in collagen tensile strength can be gained by treating collagen with $10^{-3}$M KCN. The KCN alters the organization of the interfibrillar material without affecting the collagen fibrils per se.

During resorption of macroscopic bundles of collagen, hyaluronidase produced by mesenchymal cells appears early and breaks down the mucopolysaccharides within the collagen bundles, dispersing the ground substance and releasing a large amount of water. The collagen bundles become less tightly bound and ultimately disperse. Concomitantly, the epithelial cells produce collagenase, initiating the ultimate solubilization of collagen as outlined earlier.

Elastic fibers, interspersed among the collagen bundles, provide the skin with its elasticity. These fibers consist of two components: microfibrils approximately 110 A in diameter and an amorphous material —elastin. If one follows the teleological development of elastin, embryonic elastic fibers devoid of the amorphous component are seen initially. The microfibrils accumulate on the cell surface, and as development proceeds, the amorphous material becomes increasingly evident. In fact, by adulthood these fibers consist predominantly of the amorphous material.

Chemical analysis reveals that the microfibrillar protein is markedly different from elastin. It is concluded that the protein of the microfibrils in elastic fibers is not a precursor of elastin. Tropoelastin, elastin's precursor, is synthesized by the ribosomes. Tropoelastin is composed predominantly of amino acids (such as, valine, alanine, glycine, and proline) that are hydrophobic or uncharged, so that the molecule tends to be insoluble in water. After its synthesis tropoelastin is transported outside the cell and arrives at the surface of a growing elastic fiber. Here lysine of the tropoelastin unit undergoes enzymatic alteration to form an aldehyde group. The enzyme lysyl oxidase converts most of the lysines in the tropoelastin molecule into aldehydes, which condense to form desmosomes by cross linkages (Fig. 1-9). The resulting elastin molecule is insoluble. Aggregation of these subunits produces a fiber that behaves like an array of small interconnected springs. Apparently the function of the microfibril is to shape elas-

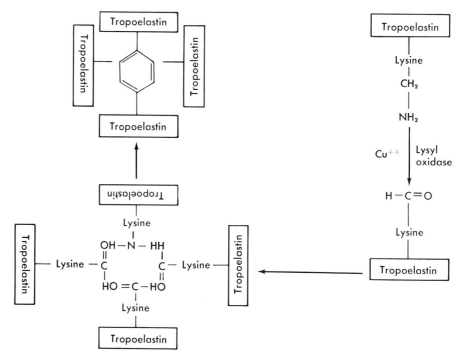

**Fig. 1-9.** The enzyme lysyl oxidase in the presence of copper converts the terminal lysine of tropoelastin into an aldehyde. Three aldehydes and a lysine react to form desmosine.

tin subunits into a fibrous configuration. Inhibition of the enzyme lysyl oxidase, as in osteolathyrism, produces inhibition of these aldehyde cross-links in elastin and collagen.

## WOUND CONTRACTION

As collagen, elastin, and mucopolysaccharide deposition and remodelling, and fibroblastic and epithelial cell migration continue, the overall shape of the wound begins to change. A wound that was round initially becomes elliptical and finally linear, whereas a rectangular wound eventually assumes a stellate shape. The forces responsible for this change in wound shape have been grouped into a phenomenon called contraction.

Luccioli divides normal wound contraction into the following five phases: (1) immediate retraction of the wound edge caused by the elasticity of the surrounding skin; (2) early decrease in wound size beginning within hours of wounding and extending to day 3 (possibly due to dehydration of eschar); (3) a latent period up to day 6; (4) wound contraction from day 6 to day 17; and (5) scar maturation from day 17 onward associated with the gradual expansion and molding of the wound related to the pull of the surrounding tissues on the maturing scar.

Contraction is a major component in the healing of open wounds. It is beneficial to the healing wound but functionally detrimental when it occurs across flexion creases or involves mobile tissues, for example, the dorsum of the hand (Fig. 1-10). Steroids reduce tensile strength gain of closed wounds only if given within 3 days after wounding, while the inflammatory response is developing. Yet steroids administered 5 days after an open wound occurs significantly inhibit wound contrac-

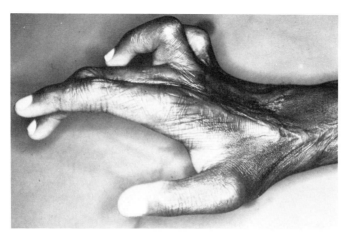

**Fig. 1-10.** Contraction of healing wound on the dorsum of the hand has resulted in marked hyperextension of the metacarpophalangeal joints of the ring and little fingers and impairment in flexion of all fingers.

tion even after the process is well established. Even steroid administration 16 days after the wound is incurred immediately reduces the rate of contraction. The initial process in contraction is the formation of granulation tissue. If this tissue is prevented from forming, then contraction will not occur. Thus, cortisone, which impairs granulation tissue formation, will inhibit wound contraction.

Two systems have been primarily implicated in the production of contraction: the cellular system and the fluid-fiber system. The fluid-fiber system consists of collagen and elastic fibers in a milieu of interstitial fluid. The cellular system (fibroblasts) is interspersed in this milieu. The process of contraction in the healing wound can be accomplished by physicochemical changes in the fluid-fiber system, by fibroblastic proliferation and central migration pulling the wound edges together, or by fibroblastic migration initially exerting tension of the skin edges. This tension is maintained by the fluid-fiber component while the fibroblasts migrate further centrally, thereby creating renewed tension on the skin edges.

The following evidence has been presented in questioning the contribution of the fluid-fiber system to wound contraction. In scorbutic animals, which exhibit marked impairment of collagen synthesis and wound tensile strength gain, wound contraction occurs at a normal rate. In lathyrism the cross-linking of collagen subunits is inhibited, yet collagen production is not altered. Thus, wound tensile strength gain in the lathyritic animal is markedly depressed, but the rate of wound contraction is unimpaired. More precisely, the interrelationships of the fluid-fiber system necessary for wound tensile strength gain are not responsible for wound contraction. Furthermore, the rate of tensile strength gain in a closed wound parallels the net accumulation of collagen more closely than any other measurable process. However, contraction cannot be correlated with production of collagen or other substances yet measured.

Study of the cellular system reveals that centrally migrating fibroblasts can exert significant tension on wound margins. These fibroblasts reside both in the central granulation tissue and at the advancing skin edge. Repeated removal of the central cell mass does not affect contraction, but if the skin edge is removed the tension of contraction is released. This suggests that the peripheral fibroblasts exert tension on the wound edges as the cells migrate centrally.

In vitro, fibroblasts, cultured upon fibrin frameworks, migrate along these fibrin strands. Central orientation of fibrin in the open wound is accomplished by the contracting blood clot that pulls on the fibrin network attached to the wound margins and base. As noted earlier, contact inhibition also has a role in directing fibroblasts toward the central defect.

Migrating fibroblasts, in vitro, exert a tension of $3.38 \times 10^4$ dynes/cm$^2$ of cross-sectional area. In vivo the force of contraction, of large skin wounds in rabbits, was found to be $3.2 \times 10^4$ dynes/cm$^2$—a striking similarity! Irradiation of the skin area 24 to 48 hours prior to wounding inhibits wound contraction. Because some of the fibroblasts involved in healing wounds are derived from the immediate wound area, it is concluded that the inhibition of contraction results from the inactivation of these fibroblasts. Furthermore, poisoning the granulation tissue with potassium cyanide markedly limits contraction; this fact suggests that a cytochrome-dependent mechanism is involved. Therefore, the contraction would appear to be of intracellular origin.

The contribution of the fibroblasts to wound contraction may be due to contraction of smooth muscle within the fibroblasts. Gabbiani and associates demonstrated that contracting granulation tissue contains fibroblasts that have developed characteristics typical of smooth muscle. Furthermore, strips of contracting granulation tissue, when tested pharmacologically in vitro, behave similarly to smooth muscle. Thus, these authors suggest that fibroblasts can differentiate into a cell structurally and functionally similar to smooth muscle and that this cell, the myofibroblast, plays an important role in connective tissue contraction.

Topical application of a smooth muscle antagonist in two animals whose wounds were undergoing active contraction revealed a significant inhibition in the rate of contraction. The clinical implications are obvious but as yet unproved.

The use of dynamic hand splints—as championed by the Galveston Shriner's group—is directed toward overcoming the force of contraction to permit tissue coverage and maintenance of mobile joints (Fig. 1-11).

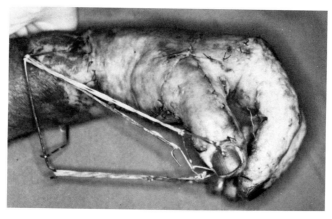

**Fig. 1-11.** The dynamic splint is utilized to overcome the forces of contraction generated in the healing wound. In this case, the dorsal skin of the hand, fingers, and thumb sustained third-degree thermal burns that will heal by marked contraction if not splinted.

Contraction can be lessened by skin grafts containing a portion of the dermis but cannot be lessened by grafts of epithelium alone. Recruitment of granulation tissue beneath the split-thickness graft will render the graft only partially effective in controlling contraction. Contraction may be terminated by reduction of the fibroblastic population because fibroblasts are no longer present in sufficient number to overcome the opposing tension of skin. However, the process may be reactivated by applying a skin graft to the wound center. The mechanism responsible is the introduction of new fibroblasts present in the graft.

After contraction has been completed and the wound margins have been coapted, tensile strength of the wound is gained primarily through the collagen system. Collagen production and degradation continue for months, even years, after the initial wounding. Skin wounds reach approximately 75% of the tensile strength of unwounded skin at 150 days after the wound is incurred. Extracts (0.14M to 0.45M saline) of these wounds reveal a higher soluble collagen content in wounded skin than in unwounded skin. This soluble fraction reaches a maximum at 40 to 60 days and diminishes to control values by 150 days. The continued rise in wound tensile strength suggests that either continued introduction of collagen production is providing additional structural strength or that continued introduction of chemical bonds is strengthening the individual collagen fibers.

## CLINICAL IMPLICATIONS OF BIOLOGICAL PRINCIPLES
### Débridement, immunization

Since the progress of healing a wound is influenced markedly by the initial phase of autogenous débridement, it is evident that surgical débridement is of particular importance in the initial management. This minimizes cellular débridement necessary, reduces the probability of infection, and

allows rapid progression to the healing phase. Surgical débridement requires as complete removal of devitalized tissues as feasible. In extensive wounds, such as burns, the gain of extensive débridement must be weighed against its deleterious effects, especially massive blood loss. Electrical burns that exhibit a progressive devitalization of tissue may require multiple stages of débridement. If infection can be controlled in these two instances, the devitalized areas may be allowed to demarcate completely before débridement is accomplished. In such cases the surgeon accepts delayed healing as inevitable.

The control of bacterial colonization is of particular importance. Often a contaminated wound can be converted to a clean wound by extensive wound irrigations and débridement and can permit primary closure in areas with abundant blood supply, such as the hands and face.

Hamer has noted that all open wounds contain bacteria and remain contaminated with varying levels of bacteria until successful wound closure has been accomplished. In a standardized experimental model three methods of irrigation were compared employing quantitative bacteriology of the tissues to evaluate their effectiveness in decreasing bacterial levels and reducing wound infection. The pulsating jet lavage was found to be significantly better than the gravitational flow irrigation or wound irrigation with a bulb syringe. In any traumatic wound, the ability of the host to combat infection is greatly influenced by the level of the bacteria, foreign body contamination, necrotic tissue, and blood clots. Meticulous mechanical and surgical removal of debris in contused or compromised tissue remains the single most important step in managing a contaminated wound. However, contaminated abdominal wounds are different. Here the thicker layer of subcutaneous fat with its poor blood supply provides a perfect medium for bacterial colonization. Such wounds are better managed by secondary closure, that is, initial closure of the musculofascial layers and later (3 to 4 days) approximation of the skin edges. This delay allows the wound area to mobilize its defenses adequately and begin granulation tissue formation.

Gruber determined the effects of commonly used antiseptics on wound healing. He applied acetic acid, hydrogen peroxide, and providone-iodine solutions to experimental wounds in rats and to human donor sites to test their effects on wound healing. Controlled donor sites were treated with saline or dry Owens gauze. The acetic acid and providone-iodine solutions had no significant gross or microscopic effect on the wound. The hydrogen peroxide solution seemed to hasten the separation of the scab and to shorten the healing time. Bullae and ulceration appeared if hydrogen peroxide treatment was applied after the wound crust had separated. Gruber suggests that the use of hydrogen peroxide should be avoided after crust separation. When only dry Owens gauze was used to treat split skin graft donor areas, scab separation was prolonged 3 days, and greater subepidermal reaction and inflammatory changes were noted.

Of particular importance is the proper tetanus immunization of the wounded patient. When the patient has been actively immunized within the past 10 years, he will probably need only 0.5 ml of adsorbed tetanus toxoid as a booster unless it is certain that he has received a booster within the previous 12 months. Those with severe, neglected, and old (more than 24 hours) tetanus-prone wounds will need 0.5 ml of adsorbed toxoid unless it is certain that a booster was received within the previous 6 months. For the patients who have received active immunization more than 10 years previously and have not received a booster within the past 10 years, most will require only 0.5 ml of adsorbed tetanus toxoid. However, if the wound indicates a

possibility that tetanus might develop, the following should be administered: adsorbed tetanus toxoid, 0.5 ml; tetanus immune globulin (human), 250 units; and oxytetracycline or penicillin prophylactically. If individuals not previously immunized sustain clean minor wounds in which tetanus is most unlikely, 0.5 ml of adsorbed tetanus toxoid (initial immunizing dose) should be given. With all other wounds 0.5 ml of adsorbed tetanus toxoid (initial immunizing dose), 250 to 500 units of tetanus immune globulin (human), and oxytetracycline or penicillin prophylactically should be administered.

Methods for control of contraction become obvious in view of the earlier discussion. If the forces contributing to contraction—fibroblastic migration—are counteracted with an equal or greater force, then contraction with its deforming features will be prevented. This has been accomplished clinically by the use of countertraction to prevent flexion contraction of the upper and lower extremities and the cervical area. Countertraction is usually transmitted to the involved flexion crease by way of Steinmann pins inserted into appropriate bony structures. This traction must be maintained until the fibroblasts "give up." Furthermore, remember that skin grafting introduces a new recruitment of fibroblasts, so that traction must be maintained until healing of the graft is complete.

Clinically and experimentally, full-thickness skin grafts have been shown to inhibit wound contraction to a greater extent than do split-thickness skin grafts. This is true even if the full-thickness grafts are thinner than the split grafts. Full-thickness grafts are obtained by sharp dissection, whereas split-thickness grafts are obtained with dermatone glue or mineral oil. Because stripping the epithelium with glue or oil results in epithelial hyperplasia, Rudolph studied the effects of the various methods of obtaining skin grafts on wound contraction. His studies revealed that both skin graft contraction and epithelial hyperplasia occur independently of the way the grafts are obtained. He suggests that the reason full- and split-thickness skin grafts inhibit wound contraction differently must be intrinsic to the skin graft rather than the recipient site.

### Wound closure not requiring grafting

The goals of primary wound closure are (1) to obliterate "dead space" and provide tensile strength until the wound has healed adequately, (2) to reestablish tissue continuity with minimal tension on the wound edges, (3) to prevent embarrassment of blood supply at the wound margins, and (4) to preserve contour and anticipate functional implications of wound contraction.

Closure of fascia in areas of stress, such as the abdominal wall, usually requires the use of nonabsorbable sutures of great tensile strength. This suture will restore the resistant forces of the fascial layer until collagen deposition and remodelling are adequate. Any dead space in the subcutaneous fatty tissues must be obliterated to discourage the collection of seromas or hematomas that provide perfect culture media for bacteria. This may be accomplished with absorbable or nonabsorbable sutures.

The break in skin integrity by wounding results in retraction of the wound edges. Reapproximation of the dermal layer is of prime importance since this is the fibrous tissue layer that provides great tensile strength. Failure to obtain and maintain accurate coaptation of the dermal edges results in broad unsightly scars. For this, nonabsorbable or chromatized absorbable sutures are used to maintain perfect coaptation. Once this is obtained, the epithelial edges are usually perfectly aligned. However, fine sutures may be used to permit precise "levelling" of the epithelial edges. Since the epithelium response to wounding is so rapid and effective, these superficial sutures may be removed in 2 to 3 days. As a precaution, however, application of an external splint, such as tape, minimizes the retraction forces on the wound edges.

Blood supply at the wound edges may be embarrassed by the suture technique. The use of widely spaced horizontal mattress stitches is to be discouraged. More accurate tissue positioning that minimizes vascular impairment can be obtained by vertical mattress stitches with interspersed superficial levelling stitches.

Functional impairment by contraction can be anticipated when the wound crosses a flexion crease, such as those on a joint; involves very mobile tissues, such as eyelids; or extends across areas of changing body contour, such as the lower neck region. The decision concerning the potential significance of contraction requires a basic knowledge of wound healing tempered by experience.

It is in anticipation of contraction that procedures such as the Z-plasty, W-plasty, and modifications of these, have been used to interrupt straight line closures. That such procedures are effective certainly reinforces the concept that contraction is a function of the dermis and not the underlying subcutaneous tissues. Thus the Z-plasty's effectiveness is in its ability to confuse the dermis.

### Wound closure requiring grafting

The tissues available to replace lost tissue can be classified as either free grafts or pedicle grafts (Table 1-1). The free graft maintains no attachments to the donor area whereas the pedicle flap is attached at its base to maintain the flap's viability. The qualities of each of the types of tissues available for skin coverage will be discussed briefly.

Before we use free grafts for wound coverage, it is essential to review the healing of skin grafts. Of prime importance is the establishment of circulation in the

**Table 1-1.** Components of tissue type and indications for use in wound coverage*

| Type | Components | Indication for use |
| --- | --- | --- |
| Free | | |
| Split-thickness | Epidermis, partial thickness dermis | Exposed subcutaneous tissue or muscle |
| Full-thickness | Epidermis, full thickness dermis | |
| Composite | Double skin fold and interposed cartilage | Not in acute cases |
| Pedicle | | |
| Simple | Epidermis, dermis, and subcutaneous tissue | Exposed tendon, joint, bone, major vessels and through-and-through losses of oral, thoracic, or abdominal cavities |
| Compound | Epidermis, dermis, subcutaneous tissue, bone, tendon, joint, and associated structures as functional units | Usually not in acute cases but for later restorative procedures |

*Graft selection to replace tissue loss is determined by the tissues in the bed of the wound and the function of these tissues.

graft. It was believed that the initial nourishment of a skin graft was through plasmatic circulation, but it has been shown that there is no true plasmatic circulation in grafted vessels. Furthermore, it is suggested that plasma is absorbed into the graft vessels rather than circulated. After a graft is obtained and transplanted, it soon becomes edematous and can gain as much as 40% in weight. Within 48 hours there is communication between the host and graft vessels. However, there is disagreement on whether the intrinsic vessels of the graft are reused or whether new vessels grow into the graft and replace the old vessels. The lymphatic circulation of a graft is restored by the fifth or sixth day after grafting.

The marked changes in the epidermis and dermis of a free graft deserve comment. After the application of a split-thickness skin graft, mitosis of the follicular and granular epithelial cells occurs (the epithelial cells migrate toward the surface), and there is marked swelling of the surface epithelium. This produces a doubling in thickness of the epithelium during the first 4 days after grafting. The mitotic activity observed in the epidermis of split-

thickness skin grafts is much more marked than that in full-thickness skin grafts. From the fourth to the eighth day, there is marked proliferation and thickening of the epithelial layer of the graft. Desquamation of the epithelium occurs and is accompanied by upward migration of the follicular epithelium. Thereafter the epithelial hypertrophy begins to subside. At 24 days, the epithelium has returned to the thickness of normal skin.

The ribonucleic acid content of the graft epithelium remains unchanged until the fourth day, when there is a marked increase in ribonucleic acid content in the basal layers of the epithelium. This suggests an acceleration of protein synthesis. Within 10 days the ribonucleic acid content begins diminishing. Enzymatic activity in the epithelium parallels changes observed in the ribonucleic acid content.

To regain the sweating function in grafted skin, the grafted skin must undergo adequate sympathetic reinnervation, and adequate amounts of glandular tissue must be transplanted in the graft. The sweating function in a skin graft follows the pattern of the recipient site. Hair growth from grafted skin depends on the presence and survival of hair follicles in the graft. The original hair shafts become entrapped in the desquamating superficial layer and are lost from the graft. The generation of hair from the transplanted follicles begins soon thereafter, and new hair can be detected by the fourteenth day after grafting. In a full-thickness graft where there is less epithelial desquamation, hair may remain present from the time of grafting. Split grafts are less likely to result in hair growth than are full-thickness grafts.

In the dermis of the free graft, the population of fibroblasts decreases during the first 3 days after graft transplantation. Even the surviving cells demonstrate some changes due to hypoxia. Within 3 days fibroblastlike cells appear in the graft bed and in the graft itself. Within 7 to 8 days both the cell population and the enzymatic activity exceed that of normal skin. The source of the fibroblasts found in healing grafts may be either large blood-borne mononuclear cells or local cells that have survived transplantation.

Collagen is the primary structural component of the dermis. Randolph and Klein have demonstrated through the use of skin grafts from animals repeatedly labelled with $H^3$ proline that at least 85% of the original graft collagen undergoes metabolic turnover within 5 months after grafting. Such turnover is 2 to 40 times greater than the turnover of collagen in unwounded skin.

Contraction in skin grafts occurs in two stages. When a split graft is obtained it may contract 22%. (Very thin split-thickness skin grafts may contract 9%.) Full-thickness skin grafts may be reduced 44%. After the initial contraction associated with obtaining a graft, there is subsequent contraction associated with the healing process; the amount of subsequent contraction is determined by the thickness of the graft. Full-thickness skin grafts tend to remain the same size; whereas the thinner a split-thickness skin graft, the more it will contract. The graft is not actually contracting but is following the lead of the contracting recipient site. Little information is available as to how or why skin grafts alter wound contraction.

*Free grafts.* Since the free graft derives its nourishment by osmosis from the recipient site, the thinner the dermis transferred, the more osmosis is facilitated and the greater the chance for take of the graft. The split graft is the most versatile type of tissue coverage the surgeon can employ. Extensive coverage may be gained with a single sheet of free graft that has been meshed. The application of a split graft to an infected wound markedly reduces the bacterial count within the first 24 hours. Furthermore, the application of split grafts to blood agar cultures containing a uniform distribution of beta hemolytic streptococci results in complete inhibition of red cell lysis in the area beneath and immediately surrounding the graft. These observations, coupled with clinical experience, have led to the practice of repeated applications of split grafts to infected wounds to control infection and permit definitive grafting in a relatively clean bed. The full-thickness graft includes the entire thickness of the dermis. This provides better wound coverage because the full graft will contract much less and the additional dermis provides greater resiliency to the graft.

Composite grafts are a specialized form of free grafts. Typically the graft is obtained from the ear and transferred to a nasal defect. The double fold of auricular skin containing the enclosed auricular cartilage is cleanly detached from the ear and placed in a freshly excised defect in the nose. The abundant vasculature of both structures permits extensive inosculation, thereby reestablishing circulation within the graft in a matter of hours. There is a limit to the size of composite graft transferable. These grafts have not been utilized in reconstructive hand surgery.

*Pedicle grafts.* Because of the loose subcutaneous tissue or fat in its base and the presence of dermal edges at its periphery, the pedicle flap heals primarily about its periphery, thereby minimizing scar formation between its base and the recipient site. Furthermore, the flap experiences minimal contraction when placed over freshly excised wounds. The pedicle flap tissue maintains its original resiliency and resistance to trauma. These factors make it the most desirable tissue for coverage in an area subject to repeated trauma or over flexion creases subjected to severe stress.

There are two basic types of pedicle flaps: simple and compound. Simple pedicle flaps contain epidermis, dermis, and subcutaneous tissues supported by a vascular pedicle. The vascular pedicle may be broad-based, containing many fine vessels or only an isolated artery and accompanying vein. These flaps are of particular value when coverage is required in areas not subjected to trauma or not participating in functional acts requiring fine stereognosis and proprioception, such as the dorsum of the hand, and through-and-through losses of oral, thoracic, or abdominal cavities (Fig. 1-12). When stereognosis and proprioception are required, the compound pedicle flap is unexcelled.

The compound pedicle flap may incorporate bony tissues, neural tissues, tendon units, and joints if necessary. This is the most sophisticated flap developed, both technically and functionally. Examples in-

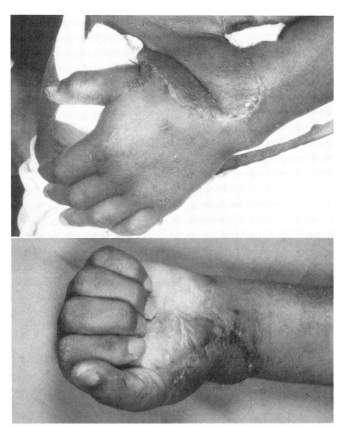

**Fig. 1-12.** The abdominal pedicle flap has been set into the wrist defect. After detachment the flap provides coverage that permits joint motion.

clude: transfer of sensory islands of tissue to provide stereognosis and proprioception in fine touch; transfer of joints from damaged digits to render an adjacent damaged digit functional; and transfer of entire digits to replace an avulsed or congenitally absent thumb (Fig. 1-13).

*Indication for selection of graft.* Since only free and pedicle grafts are available to obtain coverage, establishment of the indications for use of each renders decision making simple. The composite graft is almost never used in acute injuries and will be omitted from this discussion.

*Free graft utilization.* Split- and full-thickness grafts heal primarily between the dermis of the graft and the recipient site by new collagen deposition; consequently these grafts must be placed over vascular beds where movement, such as gliding of tendon and joint tissues, is not of prime consideration. Thus, when subcutaneous tissues, muscle, or granulation tissue form the recipient site, the use of free grafts is indicated. The choice between split- and full-thickness grafts depends on how much contraction the recipient site can tolerate and still retain its function. Areas such as the trunk, extremities, and scalp are most often closed with split grafts. Full-thick-

ness grafts are excellent in the lower eyelids, face, and flexion creases. Of course the size of the graft required may dictate use of a thick split-thickness graft to permit healing of the donor site without requiring overgrafting. Thick split grafts placed on muscle impose minimal restrictions on muscle contraction.

*Simple pedicle flap utilization.* The pedicle flap heals primarily about its periphery because this is the only area where the fibroblasts of the dermis come into contact with recipient dermal areas. This flap is most useful in covering areas where joint or tendons are exposed. Furthermore, bone stripped of its periosteum requires flap coverage to maintain the bone's viability. Even if bone is exposed with its periosteum intact, for example, the dorsum of the hand, the ultimate need for reestablishing tendon continuity across the area requires tissue coverage which will permit tendon gliding.

*Compound pedicle flap utilization.* Because of the possibility of loss by infection, kinking of the pedicle, and unrecognized trauma to the intended pedicle, compound flaps are usually employed after wound closure and healing have been obtained by other methods. When the healed tissues

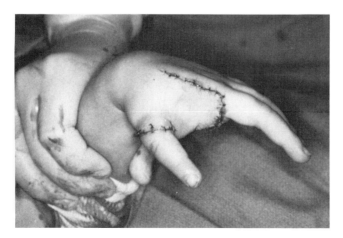

**Fig. 1-13.** All components of the index finger have been transferred as an island flap to reconstruct an absent thumb.

have matured, as evidenced in the scar by loss of redness, thickness and immobility, then compound flaps can be utilized.

It should be quite clear that the day-to-day management of wounds is steeped in a basic understanding of the biological principles involved in the healing wound. Management based on these principles provides a springboard for careful, accurate evaluation of clinical and laboratory observations. As the biological principles become further elucidated, so will the advancement of our methods of clinical practice.

## BIBLIOGRAPHY

Alexander, W. J., Bossert, J. E., McClellan, M. A., and Altemeir, W. A.: Stimulants of cellular proliferation in wounds, Arch. Surg. **130:**167, 1971.

Bentley, J. P.: The chondroitin sulfates of healing skin wounds, Acta Chem. Scand. **19:**2235, 1965.

Bentley, J. P.: Rate of chondroitin sulfate formation in wound healing, Ann. Surg. **165:**186, 1967.

Bryant, W. M., Greenwell, J. D., and Weeks, P. M.: Alterations in collagen organization during dilatation of the cervix uteri, Surg. Gynecol. Obstet. **126:**27, 1968.

Bullough, W. S.: Epithelial repair in repair and regeneration. In Dunphy, J. E., and Van Winkle, H. W., Jr., editors: Repair and regeneration; the scientific basis for surgical practice, New York, 1968, McGraw-Hill Book Co.

Clark, B. F. C., and Marcker, K. A.: How proteins start, Sci. Am. **218:**36, 1968.

Ehrlich, H. P., Tarver, H., and Hunt, T. K.: Inhibitory effects of vitamin E on collagen synthesis and wound repair, Ann. Surg. **175:**235, 1972.

Forrester, J. C., Zederfeldt, B. H., Hayes, T. L., and Hunt, T. R.: Mechanical, biochemical and architectural features of repair. In Dunphy, J. E., and Van Winkle, H. W., Jr., editors: Repair and regeneration; the scientific basis for surgical practice, New York, 1968, McGraw-Hill Book Co.

Furste, W., Skudder, P. A., and Hampton, O. P.: A guide to prophylaxis against tetanus in wound management, American College of Surgeons Bulletin, 1967, p. 23

Gabbiani, G., Hirschel, B. J., Ryan, G. B., and others: Granulation tissue as a contractile organ, J. Exp. Med. **135:**719, 1972.

Gould, B. S.: Collagen biosynthesis. In Gould, B. S., editor: Treatise on collagen, New York, 1968, Academic Press, Inc.

Grillo, H. C., and Gross, J.: Studies in wound healing; contraction in vitamin C deficiency, Proc. Soc. Exp. Biol. Med. **101:**268, 1959.

Grillo, H. C.: Origin of fibroblasts in wound healing; an autoradiographic study of inhibition of cellular proliferation by local X-irradiation, Ann. Surg. **157:**453, 1963.

Grillo, H. C., and Potsaid, M. S.: Studies in wound healing, 4. Retardation of contraction by local X-irradiation and observations relating to the origin of fibroblasts in repair, Ann. Surg. **154:**741, 1961.

Gross, J., and Lapiere, C. M.: Collagenolytic activity in amphibian tissues; a tissue culture assay, Proc. Natl. Acad. Sci. USA **48:**1014, 1962.

Gruber, R. P., Vistnes, L., and Pardoe, R.: The effect of commonly used antiseptics on wound healing, Plas. Reconstr. Surg. **55:**472, 1975.

Hamer, M. L., Robson, M. C., Krizek, T. J., and Southwick, W. O.: Quantitative bacterial analysis of comparative wound irrigations, Ann. Surg. **181:**819, 1975.

Harrington, D. B., and Meyer, R., Jr.: Effects of small amounts of electric current at the cellular level, Ann. N.Y. Acad. Sci. **238:**300, 1974.

Heughan, C., Chir. B., Grislis, G., and Hunt, T. K.: The effect of anemia on wound healing, Ann. Surg. **179:**163, 1974.

Higton, D. I. R., and James, D. W.: The force of contraction of full-thickness wounds of rabbit skin, Br. J. Surg. **51:**462, 1964.

Hunt, T. K., Linsey, M., Grislis, G., and others: The effect of differing ambient oxygen tensions on wound infection, Ann. of Surg. **181:**35, 1975.

Hunt, T. K., and Pai, M. P.: The effect of varying ambient oxygen tensions on wound metabolism and collagen synthesis, Surg. Gynecol. Obstet. **135:**561, 1972.

Hunt, T. K., Twomey, P., Zederfeldt, B., and others: Respiratory gas tension and pH in healing wounds, Am. J. Surg. **114:**302, 1967.

Kulonen, E., Niinikoski, J., and Pentinen, R.: Effect of the supply of oxygen on the tensile strength of healing skin wound and granulation tissue, Acta Physiol. Scand. **70:**112, 1967.

Lane, J. M., Bora, F. W., Jr., and Black, J.: cis-Hydroxyproline limits work necessary to flex a digit after tendon injury, Clin. Orthop. **109:**193, 1975.

Lane, J. M., Bora, F. W., Jr., Prockop, D. J., and others: Inhibition of scar formation by the proline analog cis-hydroxyproline, J. Surg. Res. **13:**135, 1972.

Leibovich, S. J., and Ross, R.: The role of the

macrophage in wound repair, Am. J. Pathol. **78:**71, 1975.

Luccioli, G. M., Kahn, D. S., and Robertson, H. R.: Histologic study of wound contraction in the rabbit, Ann. Surg. **160:**1030, 1964.

Morton, D., Madden, J. W., and Peacock, E. E.: Effect of a local smooth muscle antagonist on wound contraction, Surg. Forum **23:**511, 1972.

Myers, B., and Wolf, M.: Vascularization of the healing wound, Am. Surg. **40:**716, 1974.

Niinikoski, J., Heughan, C., and Hunt, T. K.: Oxygen and carbon dioxide tensions in experimental wounds, Surg. Gynecol. Obstet. **133:** 1003, 1971.

Peacock, E. E., Jr.: Some aspects of fibrogenesis during healing of primary and secondary wounds, Surg. Gynecol. Obstet. **115:**408, 1962.

Prockop, D. J., and Kivirikko, K. I.: Hydroxyproline and the metabolism of collagen. In Gould, B. S., editor: Treatise on collagen, New York, 1968, Academic Press, Inc.

Ross, R.: The fibroblast and wound repair, Biol. Rev. **43:**51, 1968.

Rudolph, R.: The effect of skin graft preparation in wound contraction, Surg. Gynecol. Obstet. **142:**49, 1976.

Rudolph, R., and Klein, L.: Healing processes in skin grafts, Surg. Gynecol. Obstet. **136:**641, 1973.

Sandberg, N.: Time relationship between administration of cortisone and wound healing in rats, Acta Chir. Scand. **127:**446, 1964.

Seifter, E., Manner, G., Crowley, L. V., and Levenson, S. M.: Enhancement by cultured fibroblasts of reparative collagen synthesis in rats, Proc. Soc. Exp. Biol. Med. **146:**8, 1974.

Speer, D. P., Peacock, E. E., Jr., and Milos, C.: The use of large molecular weight compounds to produce local lathyrism in healing wounds, J. Surg. Res. **19:**169, 1975.

Stephens, F. O., Dunphy, J. E., and Hunt, T. K.: Effect of delayed administration of corticosteroids on wound contraction, Ann. Surg. **173:** 214, 1971.

Sumrall, A. J., and Johnson, W. C.: The origin of dermal fibrocytes in wound repair, Dermatologica **146:**107, 1973.

Van Winkle, W., Jr.: The fibroblasts in wound healing, Surg. Gynecol. Obstet. **124:**369, 1967.

Van Winkle, W., Jr.: Wound contraction, Surg. Gynecol. Obstet. **125:**131, 1967.

Van Winkle, W., Jr.: The epithelium in wound healing, Surg. Gynecol. Obstet. **127:**1089, 1968.

Van Winkle, W., Jr.: The tensile strength of wounds and factors that influence it, Surg. Gynecol. Obstet. **129:**819, 1969.

Vihersaari, T., Kivisaari, J., and Niinikoski, J.: Effect of changes in inspired oxygen tension on wound metabolism, Ann. Surg. **179:**889, 1973.

Wolf, L., and Lipton, A.: Studies on serum stimulation of mouse fibroblast migration, Exp. Cell Res. **88:**499, 1973.

Yamaguchi, T., Hirobe, T., Kinjo, Y., and Manaka, K.: The effect of chalone on the cell cycle in the epidermis during wound healing, Exp. Cell Res. **89:**247, 1974.

Zederfeldt, B.: Studies on wound healing and trauma with special reference to intravascular aggregation of erythrocytes, Acta Chir. Scand. **224**(Suppl.):1, 1957.

# CHAPTER 2

# Bone regeneration and articular cartilage repair

## BONE DEVELOPMENT

There are two basic methods of bone formation, intramembranous and endochondral.

Intramembranous bone formation is initiated by the condensation of embryonic connective tissues in well-vascularized areas. The connective tissue cells (osteoblasts) metabolize collagen and glycosaminoglycan, which form in the matrix prior to the appearance of hydroxyapatite crystals. These crystals form interlacing bony lamellae, which by progressive growth surround the osteoblasts and convert these cells into osteocytes. Orderly growth is followed by development of bone in surrounding connective tissues and formation of a central marrow cavity. The outermost layer of the connective tissues forms the periosteum.

Endochondral bone formation requires conversion of the condensations of connective tissue to hyaline cartilage and subsequent transformation of the hyaline cartilage into bone. The bones of the extremities are among those that develop from hyaline cartilage. These bones develop a primary ossification center within the cartilage (Fig. 2-1). This ossification center evolves by the death of cartilage cells and the accumulation of chondromucoprotein and collagen prior to the deposition of hydroxyapatite crystals. As the area calcifies, vascularization and connective tissue cell invasion are prominent. Osteoblasts derived from these connective tissues secrete a bony matrix on the calcified cartilaginous matrix. With entrapment by concretions, the osteoblasts assume the function of osteocytes. At this stage basically intramembranous ossification is occurring.

Bony growth is primarily by intramembranous ossification that forms the cortical layer of the diaphysis and the appearance of a second ossification center within the cartilage at the ends of each bone. The layer of unossified cartilage between the primary and secondary ossification centers persists as the epiphyseal growth plate. Subsequent growth in length occurs through proliferation and ossification of the cartilage of epiphyseal plate on its diaphyseal side. Epiphyseal cartilage cells undergo mitosis and hypertrophy prior to cell death and calcification of the cartilaginous matrix (Fig. 2-2). These lacunae become vascularized and transformed into bone. Thus, growth in bone length is primarily through endochondral ossification, whereas increase in circumference is by intramembranous bone formation.

The two fundamental processes in bone

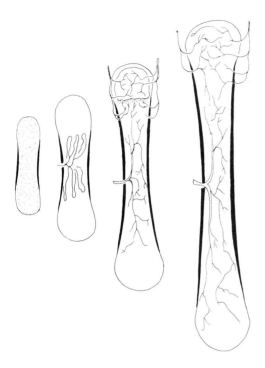

**Fig. 2-1.** The cartilage model for a bone develops a periosteal sleeve in its central portion. Blood vessels invade the central zone of ossification and the distal end of the cartilage form to initiate a second zone of ossification. Cartilage persists between the two zones as the epiphyseal plate. Growth continues until the epiphyseal plate is obliterated. (From Maximow, A. A., and Bloom, W.: A textbook of histology, Philadelphia, 1952, W. B. Saunders Co.)

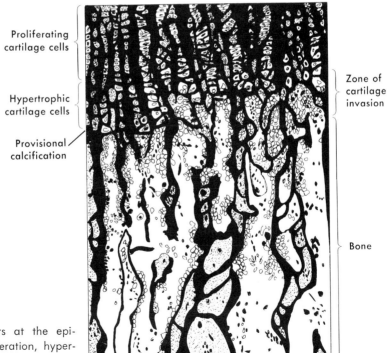

Proliferating cartilage cells

Hypertrophic cartilage cells

Provisional calcification

Zone of cartilage invasion

Bone

**Fig. 2-2.** Growth occurs at the epiphyseal plate by proliferation, hypertrophy, and invasion of the cartilage cells with ultimate calcification.

remodelling are bony resorption and deposition. Both can occur simultaneously and are responsible, in conjunction with other factors, for the final shape and size of each bone. The involved cells in bone resorption and deposition include: (1) the osteoblasts that lay down the matrix of new bone, (2) the osteoclasts that resorb bone, and (3) the osteocytes, which are situated within the bony matrix, and whose function is not entirely known. The osteoblast synthesizes collagen and glycosaminoglycans to form the matrix and may be involved in the transfer of calcium from the extracellular fluid to the matrix. The osteoblast can retain this synthetic function or can become embedded in the matrix to become an osteocyte.

An osteocyte is considered to control directly or indirectly the migration of metabolites along the lacunar-canalicular systems. This osteocyte is an essential constituent of bone because when this cell dies, the surrounding matrix dies, is resorbed, and eventually replaced by living bone. The typical osteoclast is a large multinucleated cell whose function is to remove bony matrix and mineral, a function facilitated by the presence of collagenase in the cell. The cell has a striated or ruffled brushed border where it abuts bone. This cell is apparently under the control of parathyroid hormone. Through the activities of these cells the biological half-life of a unit of bone (osteon) is about 7 years in a middle-aged man and about 1 year in a child.

Mature bone consists of an outer shell of cortical bone surrounding a medullary cavity composed of cancellous bone (Fig. 2-3). Cortical bone provides strength to the skeletal system and increases in those

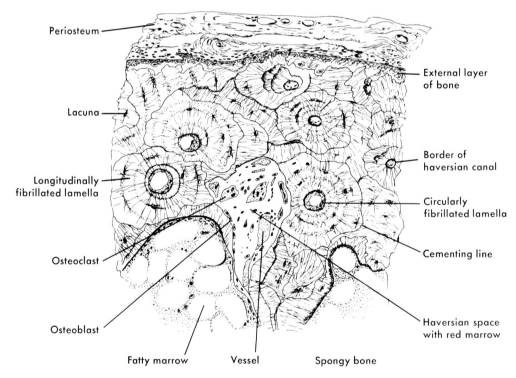

**Fig. 2-3.** Cortical bone that comprises the shaft of the long bones is composed of haversian canal systems and sheets of bone running parallel to the periosteum (×110). (From Maximow, A. A., and Bloom, W.: A textbook of histology, Philadelphia, 1952, W. B. Saunders Co.)

areas where great strength is required. Compact bone is composed of sheets of bone that parallel the bony surface in the cortex. Some sheets are concentrically oriented around a vascular channel. Osteocytes are situated in lacunae between these concentric layers. This concentric arrangement—the haversian system—is frequently separated from neighboring haversian systems by sheets of bone not participating in haversian system formation. Cortical bone is lined externally by the periosteum which, among its functions, serves as a source of osteoblasts when bone is fractured. Fibrous strands of periosteum penetrate the underlying cortical bone to provide a rigid attachment between the two structures. The periosteum has a rich vascular and nerve supply. Internally, endosteum lines the medullary cavity and can also significantly participate in fracture healing.

Cancellous bone consists of a spongy network of trabeculae concerned primarily with bone formation and hematopoiesis. Cancellous bone is found predominantly under synovial joints and areas in which forces are applied over large areas.

The density of cortical bone is about 2.0, whereas the density of cancellous bone including the marrow spaces varies from 0.025 to 0.80. Cortical bone is about 30 times stronger weight per weight than is cancellous bone.

## SOME MECHANICAL PROPERTIES OF BONE

Bone provides the support for the body and, as such, has peculiar mechanical properties. A knowledge of the properties requires definition of the measurements used to describe these properties. Strain reflects the change in bone length when a load is applied to a bone. If the load results in an increase in bone length, this is termed tensile strain. Conversely, a decrease in bone length in response to a load is termed compressive strain.

Stress forms within a bone in response to a force acting upon the bone, and this stress is expressed as force per unit area. A stress-strain curve for bone can be obtained by calculation of the stresses and strains in a simple loading system (Fig. 2-4). If the strain returns to zero immediately after removal of a load, then this strain is an elastic strain. As a load increases, a point is reached where the stress developing in response to the load is no longer proportional to the strain. When the load is removed and the bone does not lose all of its strain, the residual strain is termed plastic strain. The point between elastic strain and plastic strain is the elastic limit—a point where smaller increments of load produce disproportionate strain and the bone ultimately breaks.

The less the deformation is in response to a given load, the stiffer the bone. Stiffness can be expressed by dividing stress by strain for any part of the stress-strain curve where the curve is straight. This measure

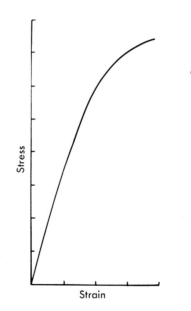

**Fig. 2-4.** Plotting a stress-strain curve for bone reveals that as the load increases, a point is reached where the resultant stress is no longer proportional to the strain.

of stiffness is the modulus of elasticity. The amount of energy a bone can absorb (and still behave linearly) is directly related to the square of the stress and inversely proportional to the bone's elasticity. Thus, the greater the modulus of elasticity, the less energy the bone can absorb before fracture occurs and vice versa. With age, the modulus of elasticity increases, and consequently, young bones require more force to fracture than those in elderly persons. We must not overlook the significance of rate of loading; that is, a bone loaded quickly absorbs more energy than if loaded slowly. This implies that strain is more important in fracture production than stress. Since fatigue is associated with frequency of loading, a bone may fracture if loaded repeatedly to stresses that it could normally tolerate if loaded to these stresses less frequently. The frequency required to produce failure increases as the maximum stress decreases.

The tensile strength of bone is less than its compressive strength. Consequently, when a bone is bent, the convex side is under tension and the concave side subjected to compression. The bone fractures on the convex side first. Interestingly, with compression on the concave side and tension on the convex side, a middle zone or neutral plane must exist.

A direct relationship exists between the static strength of bone and its ash content. As the ash content increases from 63% to 70%, the breaking stress increases threefold. Further elevation of bone ash content results in increased strength but reduces the ability of bone to withstand dynamic loads. Bone apatite acts as a hardener. In the presence of an ash content of 63% to 68%, the collagen matrix is saturated with apatite crystals. When the ash content is elevated, cracks may develop in the solid mineral phase, reducing both the impact and the static strength of the bone. Interestingly, the incus and petrosal bone of the ox and the tympanic bulla and mal-leus of the whale have very high ash contents, approaching 86% for the tympanic bulla of the whale. As a consequence, these bones are very hard and very brittle but perfectly designed for their function.

## BONE REGENERATION
### Fracture repair

The cellular response is the sine qua non of tissue repair and regeneration. In some tissues, such as skin and tendon, fibroblasts proliferate and repair the wound through fibrous tissue production and organization into scar. In bone, healing is accomplished by the regeneration of bone. For regeneration to occur, undifferentiated cells must arise from existing cell lines or by dedifferentiation of mature cells. It is from these cells that the callus develops in the healing fracture.

After fracture, bleeding occurs between the bone ends and into the surrounding soft tissues. A clot forms which then retracts, exuding serum about the fracture site. During the first 24 hours the pH of the hematoma is 6.9, and it rises to 7.6 by the tenth day. After clot formation polymorphonuclear leukocytes containing cellular debris migrate into the clot. This inflammatory exudate contains a leukoglobulin that produces swelling of the collagen bundles, lymphatic blockage, and destruction of endothelial lining of vessels. Thereafter fibroblastic proliferation and migration of endothelial buds into the fibrin clot herald the regenerative phase.

Osteoblasts and chondroblasts appear simultaneously. These cells, whose origin is debated, arise from existing cells in the deeper layers of the periosteum, endosteum, trabecular tissues, or from primitive connective tissue cells. Osteogenesis occurs either by the initial formation of cartilage like that which predominates in avascular areas around the ends of cortical bone or by intramembranous ossification like that which occurs at the periosteal-cortex junction and in the endosteal areas (Fig. 2-5).

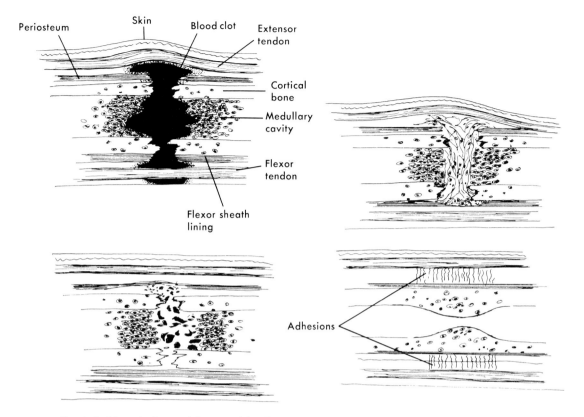

**Fig. 2-5.** After phalangeal fracture, blood extravasates into the flexor sheath if the posterior wall of the fibro-osseous tunnel has been violated. After clot retraction, fibroblasts and endothelial cells migrate between the fracture ends, and osteoblasts appear with the subsequent regeneration of bone. In this case the ensuing scar can inhibit gliding of the flexor and extensor tendons.

The osteoblasts form trabeculae about the central canals leading to the formation of osteogenic tissue in which calcium salts are deposited. This proliferation of osteoblasts can be observed in studies using bone-localizing isotopes, which are metabolized in the same manner as calcium. Johannsen administered $^{87m}$Sr (half-life 2.8 hours) to 30 patients with fractures and made repeated observations regarding radioisotope localization both prior to weight bearing and after weight bearing. The activity over the fracture site varied during the healing process, displaying two distinct activity peaks. The first peak occurred between 8 to 32 days after injury, corresponding to initial proliferation of osteoblasts in response to the injury. A second peak occurred over the fracture site within 8 to 45 days following weight bearing without cast immobilization. The application of stress to the fracture site produced a functional reorganization of the bone that was reflected by an increase in osteoblastic activity; this activity over the fracture was higher than in the normal extremity for more than 6 months after the fracture was clinically healed.

The constituents of bone may be classified as either inorganic or organic. The inorganic material primarily consists of calcium hydroxyapatite, proteins, citrate, water, and other trace substances. The major portion of the organic materials is contributed by collagen and the glycosaminoglycans. Mineralization can occur precipitously where the masses of crystals obscure the structure of the underlying cartilage, or the process may occur by a more orderly deposition of small crystals between the bands of collagen fibrils. Both patterns have been observed in tissue cultures, and as yet it is uncertain why there are two distinct patterns. The total concentration of glycosaminoglycans as well as the concentration of the individual glycosaminoglycans decreases as the callus becomes highly mineralized.

A marked local variation exists in the mineral salt content of the callus. The uptake of radiophosphorus arises abruptly to a maximum at 10 to 15 days after fracture. Collagen, which is demonstrable within a week after fracture, reaches its maximum content before the callus becomes highly mineralized. The main component of the glycosaminoglycans in callus during all stages of fracture repair is chondroitin-4-sulfate. Its greatest concentration is noted in the 2-week-old callus. The synthesis of chondroitin sulfate in callus is most intense immediately before mineralization of the callus reaches its peak.

### Control mechanisms

The experiments of Becker and associates have produced exciting insight into bone regeneration. These will be discussed later and will be related to clinical observations. After producing fractures in experimental animals, Becker and colleagues made the following observations. Within 2 hours after fracture, red cells were attached to the bone edges by a fibrin clot. These red cells within the clot underwent morphological changes as the fibrin strands assumed the staining characteristics of collagen. During the first weeks the initial step in the healing process was the formation of a hematoma and organization of

the cellular elements in the hematoma. Serial electron micrographs of the red cells in the fracture hematoma revealed a gradual change in cell morphology until these red cells assumed the characteristics of metabolically active osteoblasts, usually within 3 weeks after fracture. Thus, the blastema responsible for healing in these experimental animals is not derived primarily from periosteum but is a direct product of the fracture hematoma. As these cells gradually assumed a uniform appearance, they became embedded in the developing fibrocartilaginous matrix. From 3 to 6 weeks after fracture, osteoid appeared in the fracture callus. During this stage vascular channels were relatively sparse. The appearance of bony spicules heralded union of the bony fragments. Thickening and maturation of the bony trabeculae accompanied bridging of the fracture site by bone. Histologically, the healed fractures in the frog's bone were not significantly different from those seen in mammals.

These observations led Becker and co-workers to speculate that the red cell is fundamental in the formation of the fracture callus. They suggest that bone regeneration can be divided into four phases. First, hematoma rich in fibrin forms about the fractured bone ends; second, dedifferentiation of the cells within the hematoma occurs; third, these cells undergo redifferentiation into cells capable of synthesizing collagen and glycosaminoglycans; and fourth, endochondral ossification within the matrix of the mature fracture callus occurs directly adjacent to the fracture surfaces. Since these phases may proceed at different rates, a mixed picture of cartilage fibrous tissue and osseous tissue may be seen within the callus. The relative contributions of periosteum and osteogenic cells within the bone and marrow are unknown.

What provides the stimulus for dedifferentiation of these cells? An electrical potential is measurable in normal intact bone

(Fig. 2-6). Immediately after fracture the periosteum directly over a fracture site becomes negative. Positive potentials on the fractured ends of the bones with respect to the remainder of the shaft produce a dipole within the fracture hematoma. The periosteal potential at the fracture site returns to normal levels at 7 days after fracture, and the longitudinal electrical gradient of the bone is restored.

Fukada and Yasuda demonstrated that mechanical loading of a bone resulted in the development of electrical potentials within the bony tissues. These potentials were proportional to the amount of loading. When the tissues were compressed, the potentials were negative, and when the tissues were placed under tension, the potentials became positive. This has subsequently been described as the piezoelectric potential in the crystalline substance of bony tissues. However, Bassett (1962) has suggested that these potentials are not due to the piezoelectric effect only, because the potentials were delayed and retained during loading. He introduced the concept of electrical semiconductors. The presence of these electrical potentials in living tissues

could influence the ionic migration of calcium and phosphate ions toward the cathode and sodium and chloride ions toward an anode. Friedenberg and Brighton measured the electrical potential pattern in rabbit bones and noted that the metaphysis was negative in relation to the epiphysis, which in relation to the diaphysis was isoelectric or slightly negative. In potential measurements on the skin overlying diaphyseal fractures in human tibias, it was found that the diaphysis was negative in relation to the epiphysis. Shortly after the occurrence of the diaphyseal fracture, the metaphyseal potential was strongly negative.

When bone is stressed to fracture, the residual stresses within the bone gradually dissipate after fracture. If all nerve pathways to a limb are interrupted, there is a prompt alteration in these potentials, which indicates that the potentials are neurally related. Thus, the origin of the stress-generated potentials in bone is probably not derived solely from the piezoelectric effect of collagen. Singer has demonstrated the requirement for the presence of neural elements in regenerating tissues. Electron micrographs of fully mineralized compact bone have revealed that the cortical channels in human femurs are extensively innervated, yet no nerve endings have been identified. Becker and associates suggest that the periosteal potentials serve a regulatory function over the local cellular electrical process of fracture healing. In the absence of this periosteal function, one would expect an unregulated callus formation like that observed in paraplegics and lepers.

To transfer the preceding observations to mammals, one need only postulate that similar electrical factors at the fracture site stimulate the target cells. In man's case, the periosteal and endosteal stem cells, as well as possibly the associate hematopoietic marrow, are the target cells. Previous work by Becker has demonstrated

**Recordings in vivo and after bone excision**

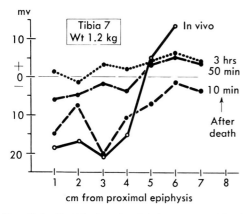

**Fig. 2-6.** Electrical potential is measurable in normal bone. (From Friedenberg, Z. B., and Brighton, C. T.: J. Bone Joint Surg. **48A:**915, 1966.)

in vivo that the administration of small continuous electric currents from implanted devices stimulates endosteal mitotic activity and results in subsequent formation of bony callus in mammals. In 1963 Cieszynski noted that in experimental animals it is possible to influence the healing of the fractured leg either by negative or positive potentials. Application of a positive potential on the fractured leg increased the breaking strength of the fracture callus. Application of a negative potential did not improve healing. Jorgensen examined experimentally the stability of fractures after treatment with a slow-pulsating asymmetrical direct current in humans. His results were as follows: (1) the average time for obtaining stability of the fracture was 30% lower in the electrically stimulated group than in the control group; (2) a greater incidence of skin infection with secretion around the Hoffmann screws was noted in the stimulated group; (3) an increase of skin temperature occurred above the fracture down onto the foot shortly after the stimulation was initiated; and (4) in one patient where the poles were not reversed in the electrodes for 3 weeks, there was a localized osteitis in the bone at the positive pole.

It is proposed that fracture healing in all vertebrates is governed by basically the same control mechanism. The stimulus for the initial cellular response, be it dedifferentiation of nucleated red cells from the hematoma or mitotic activity in periosteal or endosteal stem cells, is electric in nature and derived from the bone matrix and periosteum. Exposure of cells to electric forces activates some unit of the cell, which results in cell dedifferentiation. Yet this electric phenomenon has been shown to be responsible only for the dedifferentiation process. The nature of the signal producing redifferentiation into fibrocartilaginous cell is unknown.

Mature mammalian circulating monocytes can dedifferentiate into fibroblasts in wounded tissue. It is speculated that immature cells of the erythroid series in mammalian hematopoietic tissue may also be capable of dedifferentiation, provided they have not matured to the extent of losing their nuclei. Thus, one would expect that fractures in bones having an active hematopoietic marrow would heal at a more rapid rate than similar bones containing an inactive fatty marrow. Clinically, long bones fractured in infancy exhibit a rapid rate of healing like that observed in rib and sternal fractures of adults.

Other studies have utilized tritiated thymidine, which specifically labels DNA during the period of chromosomal replication and allows identification of the cells mitotically active during fracture healing. No increase in cell proliferation was detectable within 8 hours of injury; yet at 16 hours cellular proliferation was evident throughout the entire length of the diaphysis. This activity was observed in cells of the periosteum, the fracture site, and the mesenchymal cells outside the periosteum. The maximum proliferative response was seen in the periosteum at 32 hours after fracture. Minimal labelling of the endosteal cells was observed; the peak occurred 24 hours after fracture. This permits us to question the contribution of the subcortical endosteum to internal callus formation. However, osteogenic cells within the intertrabecular spaces and the osteoblasts lining the trabeculae were heavily labeled with tritium. These cells may contribute to the formation of the internal callus.

### Environmental effects at fracture site

The differentiation of fibrous tissue, fibrocartilage, and hyaline cartilage from periosteum and endosteum in the formation of fibrocartilage and callus is influenced by local conditions existing in the gap between the bone ends. Blood supply markedly influences the local environment at a fracture site. A brief review of the vascular supply of bone is indicated.

Before closure of the epiphysis, the vascular supply of the diaphysis is distinct from that of the epiphysis. The epiphysis is supplied by one or more nutrient arteries that pierce its external surface. When the epiphysis is completely covered by articular cartilage, the blood vessels enter the epiphysis by piercing the perichondrium at the periphery of the epiphyseal plate. When articular cartilage does not completely cover the epiphysis, the vessels enter distal to the epiphyseal plate and dislocation of the epiphysis can occur without vascular injury. With closure of the epiphyseal growth plate, there is no barrier between the epiphysis and diaphysis. The periosteal circulation, which contributes capillaries to the newly formed haversian systems during apposition growth, is particularly important in the event of bony fracture. Brookes considers the entire blood supply to reach bone from the endosteal surface. The cortical capillary network communicates not only with the capillaries outside the bone but also internally with the marrow. Usually the blood flow is from the endosteum to the periosteum; but if medullary arterial pressure should fall, the flow may be reversed. This reversal of blood flow through the cortex is described by Rhinelander as occurring in the healing of experimental fractures in dogs, and he emphasized the importance of the medulloperiosteal vascular anastomosis. Interruption of the local periosteal circulation by tight application of a bone plate suppresses even the medullary blood supply to the cortex beneath the plate. If the plate is loosened, new periosteal vessels are formed, leading to perfusion of the cortex at all levels.

Three main sources of blood supply to the tibia of the dog have been demonstrated: the nutrient artery, the metaphyseal vessels, and the periosteal vessels. The nutrient vessels communicate freely with the metaphyseal vessels but not with the periosteal vessels in the resting adult bone.

Thus it is concluded that in the adult dog, at least 90% of the cortex is perfused by the endosteal blood supply and probably the same is true in adult humans. In children, the periosteal vessels perfuse the outer one third of the cortex. When a long bone is fractured, the nutrient vessels are ruptured. The distal fragment must derive its blood supply from the periosteal vessels. These vessels enter the bone perpendicular to its long axis and remain intact after a fracture to provide blood supply to the periosteum on both sides of the fracture line. The viable periosteum on either side of the fracture site hypertrophies and rapidly seals the fracture gap. Macnab and De Haas noted that if this periosteum is destroyed, it is impossible for a periosteal seal to form about the fracture site. Fibrous tissue will invade the fracture site, and a fibrous union will result (Fig. 2-7). If a portion of a bone is resected

Periosteal seal

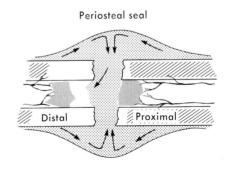

Fibrous tissue infiltration

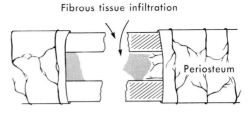

Denuded cortex

**Fig. 2-7.** Removal of periosteum from the fracture site is associated with fibrous tissue ingrowth, predisposing to pseudarthrosis formation. (From Macnab, I., and De Haas, W. G.: Clin. Orthop. **105:**27, 1974.)

including the periosteum, there is no attempt by the bone to bridge the gap with new bone formation. However, if the bone ends are connected by a polyethylene tube, bone will grow down the tube to bridge the gap. If the polyethylene tube is perforated, fibrous tissue will infiltrate through the perforations, and the bone ends will be connected by a fibrous tissue scar. The important role played by the periosteum and periosteal vessels in preventing a fibrous union and accelerating fracture healing has been demonstrated in the following experiment: When a fracture is produced experimentally and great care is taken to preserve the continuity of the periosteum, the vessels are seen to penetrate the cortex and thereby help to reestablish the endosteal circulation right up to the fracture site. When this occurs, the endosteal callus in the distal fragment can form at the fracture site instead of some distance from it. Thus, the integrity of the periosteum is of vital importance to the rate of healing of a fracture.

Culture of endosteal cells in vitro reveals the variability of response of the cells to change in environmental oxygen (Fig. 2-8). If oxygenation is adequate, a transient phase of calcification is observed. However, if oxygenation is inadequate, osteogenesis is blocked and hyaline cartilage formation becomes prominent. When the concentration of oxygen is lowered to 35% oxygen and 5% carbon dioxide, fewer cultures become calcified. A further reduction in oxygen concentration to 5% while maintaining the carbon dioxide concentration at 5% results in complete blockage of calcification. Collagen fiber production is scanty and the tissues resemble hyaline cartilage. Thus, osteogenic cells appear capable of forming either bone or cartilage in response to the degree of vascularization and subsequent oxygenation. In a low oxygen environment the cells behave as chondroblasts. In higher oxygen tensions the same cells behave as osteoblasts.

The effect of stresses within the cell masses has been delineated. Cortical cells

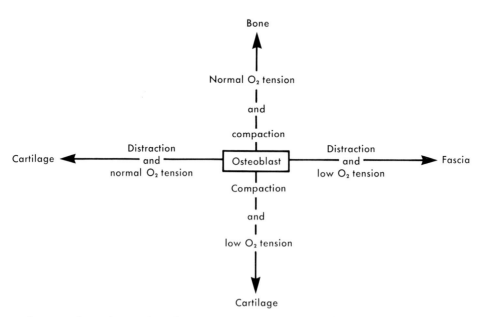

**Fig. 2-8.** The pathway of synthesis of osteoblasts in tissue culture is determined by oxygen tension and the forces acting on the cells.

cultured in an environment of 35% oxygen, 60% nitrogen, and 5% carbon dioxide contracted into a compact cell mass, and new bone formation was evident within 14 days. In those cultures in which contraction of cell masses had been uneven, the new bone formed was distorted. In the presence of 5% oxygen and 5% carbon dioxide, the cortical bone cells proliferated and migrated, yet bone formation did not occur. Instead, hyaline and fibrocartilage were found at the periphery of the cell mass with bundles of collagen and small chondrocytes evident in the fibrocartilage. When these cells were prevented from contracting by being stretched over progressively larger silicone rods during the growth period, no cartilage, bone, or calcification was observed in the cultures that had been subjected to uniform stretch. The tissue formed resembled developing tendon or fascia. In some cultures where uniform tension in the cell mass was not maintained, contraction occurred and bony and cartilaginous deposits were observed.

These studies demostrate the influence of mechanical forces, in combination with environmental factors, on the type of connective tissue that differentiates in a culture of cells arising from bone. Furthermore, oxygen concentration can significantly alter collagen synthesis. When oxygen in the gas phase is raised from 10% to 20% and reaches a maximum value of 30%, collagen synthesis increases markedly. The increased collagen synthesis associated with an increasing oxygen concentration is accompanied by a progressive increase in collagen degradation. At 30% oxygen, the ratio of collagen synthesis to collagen degradation for both new and old collagen is approximately 2:1. At an oxygen concentration of 50%, the ratio of collagen synthesis to accompanying collagen degradation is approximately 3:2 for the new collagen pool and 1:1 for the total collagen. Bone collagen present in the specimen at the time of explantation is more susceptible to

resorption than the collagen synthesized during culture. This implies that more mature collagen is degraded in preference to nascent collagen. However, a portion of the nascent collagen is rapidly degraded and does not participate in the formation of mature collagen. If 20% to 30% of the newly synthesized collagen does not participate in the ordinary tissue maturation process during the period of active synthesis and degradation, then the difference between the rate of degradation of old collagen and that of newly synthesized collagen that does enter into the normal maturation process is even more pronounced. It should be noted that morphologically much of the collagen synthesized in culture is uncalcified and, although susceptible to osteoclast resorption, it is not attacked to the same degree as calcified bone. In summary, at low oxygen tensions the rate of collagen synthesis exceeds that of degradation. At higher oxygen tensions the rates of both synthesis and degradation increase; the rate of synthesis and degradation is approximately equal until an oxygen tension of 50% is reached.

Brighton and Krebs studied the oxygen tension in vivo of healing fibula fractures in the rabbit at 4, 7, 10, 14, 17, 21, 25, 30, and 35 days after fracture. At each sitting animals were anesthetized and the muscles reflected to expose the fracture callus without disturbing the periosteum. An oxygen electrode was inserted into the fracture callus with micromanipulators. The oxygen tensions ranged from a very low level in fracture hematoma to a very high level in the diaphyseal bone. Cartilage and newly formed fiber bone exhibited a low oxygen tension through the twenty-fifth day after fracture. However, by the thirtieth day, the oxygen tension within the fiber bone had increased significantly, and by the thirty-fifth day, it was essentially identical to that of diaphyseal bone (Fig. 2-9). Measurements of the strength of the fracture callus reveal that from the seventeenth

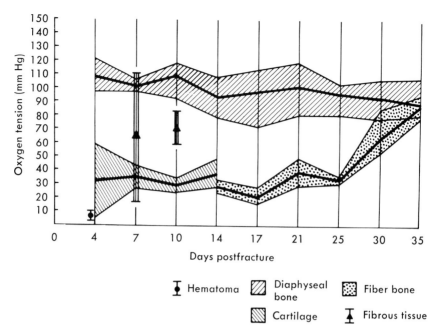

**Fig. 2-9.** Chart depicting oxygen tensions in the various tissues comprising the fracture callus at different postfracture days. (From Brighton, C. T., and Krebs, A. G.: J. Bone Joint Surg. **54A**:323, 1972.)

day after fracture, the fracture callus was essentially healed. The results of these experiments differ from those observed in the in vitro studies of Bassett and Herrmann in which the presence of compaction and high oxygen concentration favored bone formation, and low oxygen concentrations favored cartilage formation. In their experiments the compression forces generated by cells crowding together in the center of the plasma clot may account for this difference.

The low oxygen tensions observed by Brighton and Krebs could be due to either an increased oxygen consumption by the bone and cartilage cells or to a decreased delivery of oxygen to the fracture site. The associated increase in vascularity and blood flow about a fracture site does not necessarily mean that tissue profusion at the cellular level is concomitantly increased. It is possible that the increase in cellularity

produces a state of relative anoxia throughout the callus. Once the fracture is healed, the medullary cavity is reconstituted, and vascularity may assume a more even balance with cellularity, resulting in an increase in the oxygen tension at the fracture area compared with that of normal diaphyseal levels.

Thus, low oxygen tension in the fracture callus persists throughout and beyond the period of mechanical restoration of bone continuity and well into the stage of callus reorganization and medullary canal reconstitution. These observers suggest that the physiological role that oxygen plays in fracture healing may be as follows: (1) The low oxygen tension present in callus early after fracture may serve as a stimulus in the formation of osteoblasts and chondroblasts; (2) the low oxygen tension may result in release of calcium from the mitochondria in cartilage cells, which serves as

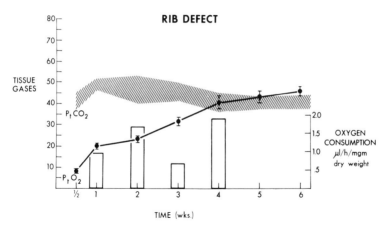

**Fig. 2-10.** This tissue oxygen ($P_t o_2$), carbon dioxide ($P_t co_2$), and oxygen consumption values obtained in healing rib defects as a function of time. The shaded area represents the average and standard deviation values for $P_t co_2$ in mm Hg. The single line is the average and standard deviation for $P_t o_2$ in mm Hg. The top of the bar graph represents the average value obtained for oxygen consumption. (From Heppenstall, R., Grislis, G., and Hunt, T. K.: Clin. Orthop. **106:**357, 1975.)

a nidus for the beginning of ossification of the callus; (3) molecular oxygen is required for the hydroxylation of proline, but the absolute requirement for oxygen might be small and adequately provided even at the low oxygen tensions measured; and (4) even though the electron transport system in mitochondria requires molecular oxygen, cartilage and bone cells participate predominantly in anaerobic metabolism. Thus, the absolute amount of oxygen required for mitochondria is low.

The studies of Brighton and Krebs did not measure oxygen consumption nor determine whether the low oxygen tensions were due to an increased oxygen consumption or to a decreased oxygen supply to the area. Heppenstall and associates undertook a study to demonstrate the altered blood flow, the oxygen–carbon dioxide content, and the oxygen consumption in the fracture callus and to correlate these findings with the histology. These studies revealed that the tissue oxygen level was very low at 3 days (8.0 mm Hg) after fracture and gradually rose by 3 weeks ($32 \pm 2$ mm Hg) with a further rise at 6 weeks ($46 \pm$

2 mm Hg). The tissue carbon dioxide level was $42 \pm 4$ mm Hg at 3 days and gradually rose to $47 \pm 7$ mm Hg at 2 weeks with a gradual decline to $42 \pm 3$ mm Hg at 6 weeks (Fig. 2-10). Histologically, new bone was present at 2 weeks and was abundant by 4 weeks. Oxygen consumption of tissue slices from the healing defect was not elevated above values reported for normal bone. The most significant finding of this experiment was that new bone is formed under hypoxic conditions that are not associated with an increase in oxygen consumption. This observation suggests that the hypoxic environment during bone deposition is not related to increased utilization but to a decrease in oxygen supply at a cellular level. The tissues remain hypoxic even though vascularity is increasing, probably because of an apparent increase in cellularity, as suggested earlier.

Previous in vitro studies have demonstrated that bone formation increased in association with low oxygen tensions and decreased with high oxygen tensions. Biochemical studies have also revealed that bone cells follow predominantly anaerobic pathways. In the study performed by Hunt and colleagues, the low oxygen tension combined with low oxygen consumption reflects a state of anaerobic metabolism as new bone is being formed by the healing tissue. Heppenstall and associates suggest that the physiological role that oxygen plays in osseous repair may be as follows. First, it may act as a stimulus for repair through the existing large gradient in oxygen tension between the terminal arteriole, capillary, and wound margin. Once the vascular pattern has reconstituted, the gradient will diminish and abolish the stimulus for vascular ingrowth and repair. Second, the oxygen may provide the initial stimulus for differentiation of mesenchymal cells in an area of injured osseous tissue. Third, perhaps the physiological role of oxygen in repair is different in soft and hard tissues. Previous soft tissue studies have demonstrated that the hypoxia itself limits the rate of repair.

### Effects of mobilization

As noted previously, mechanical stresses influence the differentiation of primitive connective tissue cells. The function of cartilage in fracture healing is unclear since fractures can heal without cartilage formation, that is, by intramembranous bone formation. When fracture sites are not immobilized, hyaline cartilage is noted in the peripheral callus within 48 hours. The medullary space at the bony ends becomes filled with immature bone capped by a mass of hyaline cartilage. Further accumulations of hyaline cartilage appear at the edge of the fracture cleft, where motion would induce maximal stress, and not within the medullary canals of the fragments. At 12 to 16 weeks, the fibrocartilage covering the fracture ends produces a typical pseudarthrosis (Fig. 2-11). If the fracture site is rigidly immobilized, for example by internal fixation, no cartilage is evident at 48 hours, and at 1 week after fracture only an occasional chondrocyte is

evident. If, however, rotatory motion is allowed to occur in this fracture, even at 2 to 3 weeks after injury, a marked accumulation of hyaline cartilage occurs. Thus, cartilage formation and persistence of cartilage is related to mechanical factors. Hypoxia, as noted in the tissue culture data previously mentioned, may induce cartilage formation. Hypoxia can result either from inadequate vascular perfusion or from rapid growth of a fracture callus, which produces a relative ischemia.

When a bony fracture is rigidly fixed and held, radiography shows no visible bony callus formation. It may be difficult to determine when the fracture has consolidated. This process of primary bone healing is morphologically different from that of fractures treated by less rigid forms of immobilization. Muheim undertook to establish a normal uptake curve of strontium 87m (half-life 2.8 hours) for lower leg fractures in patients treated by conservative and operative means. With con-

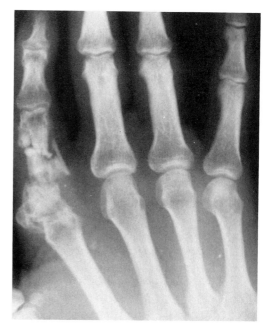

**Fig. 2-11.** Movement at a fracture site induces cartilage formation and possible pseudarthrosis.

servative treatment, the uptake ratios increased over a 28-week observation period. This increase was particularly marked at the beginning of weight bearing, which is usually from the eleventh to the seventeenth week. With rigid fracture immobilization, uptake ratios decreased slightly over a 30-week observation period, except for a slight rise at the beginning of weight bearing.

Clinically, compression has been noted to stimulate osteogenic activity. However, excessive compression results in bone resorption and delays osteogenesis. The beneficial effect of compression appears to be promotion of osseous union in cancellous bone but not in cortical bone. This benefit may be due simply to better immobilization of the fracture site. Certainly the experimental results reported earlier on the effects of compression on osteogenesis revealed that compaction and high oxygen tension stimulated bone formation. The ideal pressure has been assumed to be within the physiological limits of force exerted by the muscles and gravity.

### Effect of iron deficiency anemia

Animals rendered anemic by repeated bloodletting and maintenance on a low-iron diet exhibit a high incidence (33%) of nonunion in experimentally induced fractures. Furthermore, tensile strength gain at the fracture site is significantly depressed. Histologically, the medullary canal is closed by fibrous tissue and fibrocartilage formation. No osseous trabeculae bridging the fracture site are evident. At 3 weeks the cartilage plate has widened and exhibits a depression of osteogenesis on both sides. Anemia may depress fracture healing by interfering with tissue oxygenation. Since tissue oxygenation is sensitive to circulating blood volume, anemia may reduce the quantity of oxygen available at the fracture site. As discussed earlier, collagen synthesis and degradation depend on adequate oxygen tension.

Cellular differentiation, a prime factor in fracture healing, is markedly affected by changes in oxygen tension. In tissue culture, the oxygen available determines the cell's metabolic response; osteogenesis occurs when adequate quantities of oxygen are available, and chondrogenesis occurs when the oxygen concentration is severely reduced. In support of the effects of oxygen tension on fracture healing, Makley and colleagues demonstrated that reduced barometric pressure in unacclimated animals resulted in a significant retardation of fracture healing.

Studies in man and animals have revealed the presence of five molecular forms of lactic dehydrogenase (LDH) isoenzymes in bone. These enzymes function in the reversal reaction of pyruvate to lactate in which a pair of electrons is transferred to a coenzyme, nicotinamide adenine dinucleotide (NAD). The dehydrogenase enzymes initiate energy-yielding reactions resulting in the eventual production of adenosine triphosphate (ATP).

The LDH isoenzymes consist of polypeptide subunits H and M, four of which are combined in various proportions to form tetramers of the five various isoenzymes. The concentration of H or M subunits in a tissue corresponds to the presence of aerobic or anaerobic metabolism, respectively. Tissues that are well oxygenated and function under aerobic conditions have a high concentration of $LDH_1$, whereas those that function under anaerobic conditions have a higher concentration of the $LDH_5$ form. At 6 days after fracture, the callus contains $LDH_{1,2,3}$ with $LDH_1$ being present in the greatest quantity and $LDH_{4,5}$ present in very small quantities. At 9 days $LDH_3$ was present in greatest concentration, but by 12 days $LDH_1$ had become predominant, and by 15 days there was a marked increase in $LDH_1$. This reveals a change in the fracture callus from a predominantly aerobic metabolism at 6 days to a predominance

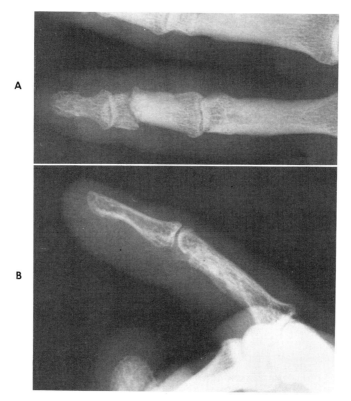

**Fig. 2-12. A,** Failure to adequately reduce and immobilize a middle phalanx fracture can result in delayed union. **B,** Proper reduction and immobilization have permitted healing.

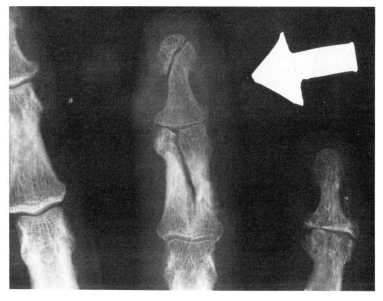

**Fig. 2-13.** Failure to obtain complete reduction results in the interposition of soft tissues and the development of nonunion.

of the anaerobic type of metabolism at 9 days with a subsequent return to aerobic metabolism thereafter.

This suggests that cellular hypoxia caused by local vascular insufficiency in the fracture callus necessitates the change to an anaerobic type of metabolism if osteogenesis is to occur. Subsequent vascular invasion permits a shift to an aerobic type of metabolism.

**Failure to achieve union**

Nonunion of a fractured bone denotes cessation of the regenerative processes at the fracture site. Clinically, this is evidenced by local edema, an increase in skin temperature in the area of the fracture, and the presence of a pseudarthrosis that produces pain on movement. Roentgeno-grams reveal a break in the continuity of the bone, sclerosis, rounding of the fracture ends, and occlusion of the medullary canal by newly formed compact bone (Fig. 2-12). Osteoporosis may be prominent. Histologically, nonunion is characterized by dense avascular fibrous tissue between the fragments, the absence of bony trabeculae bridging the fracture site, and the presence of fibrocartilage covering the ends of the fracture forming a pseudarthrosis.

The classic causes for delay of fracture healing with or without pseudarthrosis formation include: inadequate reduction of the fracture with or without soft interposition between the fracture ends (Fig. 2-13); distraction of the bone ends by excessive traction or during application of internal fixation devices; loss of bone, for example, by gunshot injury (Fig. 2-14); improper operative techniques (Fig. 2-15); and inadequate immobilization (Fig. 2-16). Other causes include inadequate blood supply, infection, metabolic disturbances, and local pathological conditions.

The importance of soft tissue interposition was demonstrated by Altner and colleagues, who removed a cylindrical segment of bone in dogs and interposed muscle between the bone ends. At 5 months, there was 60% bony union in the control animals, whereas in the experimental animals with muscle interposition, 100% presented with nonunion.

Jacobs and Ray showed that fracture healing is markedly impaired when a surgeon transects a bone with power tools. Bone union occurred much faster when the bone was cut with hand tools. Temperature elevations of at least 5° C occurred in the bone when a power tool was used. The use of a coolant resulted in limiting the rise in bone temperature to 3° C. Heat damage to the bone may be an important factor in causing nonunions as a result of the use of power tools.

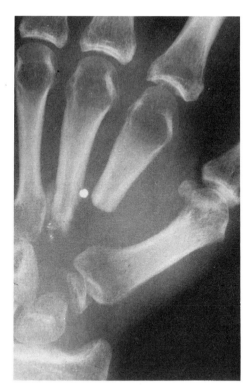

**Fig. 2-14.** Loss of bony substance after a shotgun wound results in loss of stability of the involved digits.

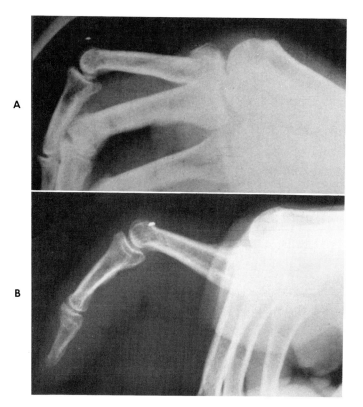

**Fig. 2-15. A,** Fracture of the base of the proximal phalanx with volar displacement. **B,** Failure to control the base of the proximal phalanx through the use of an external apparatus or internal fixation resulted in a severe deformity.

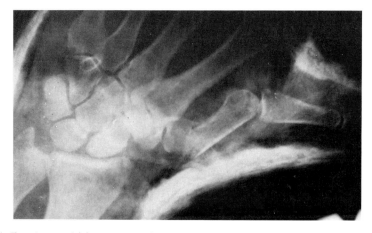

**Fig. 2-16.** Traction could have assisted in counteracting the proximal pull of the abductor pollicis longus.

## Metaphyseal and diaphyseal healing

The roentgenological and histological characteristics of metaphyseal and diaphyseal fractures have been reported in experimental studies. The nondisplaced stable metaphyseal fracture heals without any roentgenographic evidence of periosteal callus formation (Fig. 2-17). Microscopic examination reveals a predominance of fibrous tissue in the fracture site and periosteum. Bone regeneration is accomplished through intramembranous bone formation. Since metaphyseal fractures heal primarily without periosteal callus and without roentgenographic evidence of callus formation, assessment of the stability of the fracture is primarily empirical. If, instead of clinical stability, the histological aspect is taken as a criterion of union, osteoid maturation of the uniting callus of a stable metaphyseal fracture extends from the seventeenth to the fortieth day. The displaced or unstable metaphyseal fracture exhibits periosteal callus formation on roentgenogram. Cartilage and dense fibrous tissue are evident on microscopic examination of the fracture callus. During the healing of metaphyseal fractures, an endosteal callus forms. This callus ultimately bridges the fracture gap and appears as a single radiopaque band. Once union is initiated, this band is no longer evident on roentgenogram. Metaphyseal fractures heal more rapidly than do diaphyseal fractures, probably because of the greater diameter of bone presenting a larger exposure of cancellous bone to the fracture site.

Diaphyseal fractures heal by periosteal callus formation that can be assessed by roentgenograms. Osteoid maturation of the uniting callus extends from the twenty-fifth

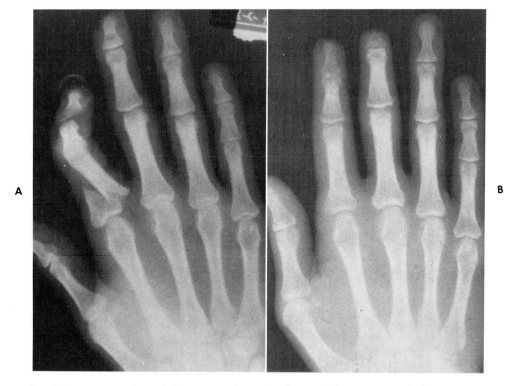

**Fig. 2-17. A,** Metaphyseal fracture involving the base of the proximal phalanx. **B,** At 6 weeks the base of the minimal callus formation is evident.

to the fifty-fifth day. The periosteal reaction produces an anchoring callus (Fig. 2-18, *A*). A sealing callus is formed by the reaction of the endosteum, and the callus that bridges the fracture site is formed by endochondral ossification. Yet if rigid internal fixation of diaphyseal fractures is obtained, healing may occur by intramembranous bone formation without periosteal callus (Fig. 2-18, *B*). Consequently, evaluation of fracture stability must include all of the above factors.

Factors that determine the rate of fracture healing include the type of fracture (spiral, oblique, transverse, or comminuted), associated soft tissue injury, the presence of comminution, whether or not the fracture is compounded, the local blood supply, and the patient's age and general condition. Neither diathermy nor ultrasound has any appreciable effect on bone growth or frac-

ture healing. The effect of arteriovenous fistulas on fracture healing is not known; however, such a fistula does cause overgrowth of the involved limb.

Use of a venous tourniquet proximal to a fracture site will stimulate bone formation. Kruse and Kelly attempted to define quantitatively the effect of a venous tourniquet on bone remodelling at the site of a fracture. If the increase in venous pressure is maintained, a marked increase in periosteal appositional bone will occur. Periosteal appositional bone formation may be of prime importance in fracture healing. Kruse and Kelly demonstrated that the application of a tourniquet proximal to the site of a fracture resulted in accelerated fracture healing. The effect of the tourniquet was to stimulate the periosteum of the fracture bone to produce more new periosteal appositional bone.

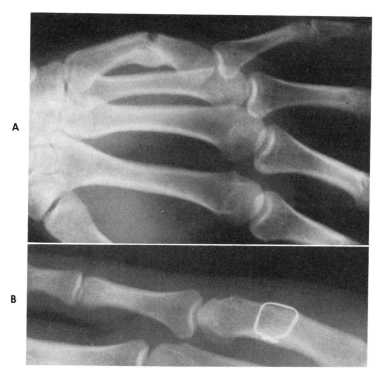

**Fig. 2-18. A,** Diaphyseal fracture of the fifth metacarpal demonstrates marked callus formation. **B,** Diaphyseal fracture of the fifth metacarpal rigidly immobilized by internal fixation demonstrates minimal callus formation.

The internal callus, or new endosteal bone after 6 weeks of healing, was increased on the side of the tourniquet. Later there was more internal callus on the control side. At the healed stage, longitudinal sections showed more endosteal bone at the fracture defect on the tourniquet side. The endosteal new bone first formed proximal and distal to the fracture defect and later filled the fracture defect. There are several hypotheses—based on blood flow, pH, and respiratory gas tensions in the blood—to explain the increase in periosteal and endosteal bone deposition observed distal to a venous tourniquet.

Brookes and Singh have observed a decrease in pH and $Po_2$ and an increase in $Pco_2$ in blood obtained through drill holes made in the diaphysis distal to a venous ligation. They believe flow changes account for the increased bone formation.

## ARTICULAR CARTILAGE REPAIR
### Organization and constituents

Articular cartilage, which is avascular, aneural, and alymphatic, may be divided into four distinct zones. The outer zone consists of flattened cells immediately adjacent to the surface, with the long axis of the cells parallel to the articular surface. In the second zone, the cells become more ovoid and less organized. In the third zone, the cells have become small and rounded and are arranged in short irregular columns perpendicular to the joint surface. The fourth zone consists of small irregular cells located in lacunae of the calcified matrix. Interposed between the third and fourth zones is a thin wavy line—designated the tide mark by Collins—that is evident on hematoxylin and eosin stain. Electromicrographs have revealed a zone of tightly packed collagen bundles running parallel and slightly subjacent to the surface. This zone, originally thought to be collagen-free, consists of a dense network of collagen fibers 40 to 120 A in diameter. This zone, which is deficient in polysac-charide as compared with deeper zones, is believed to serve a protective function by its increased compliance.

Gross examination of articular cartilage suggested that the surface is smooth; yet on histological and electromicrographic examination, pitting and irregularities of the surface are evident. The scanning electron micrograph has revealed an irregular corrugated pattern believed significant in joint lubrication. The stiffness of the cartilaginous matrix is the result of the collagen fibers. The arcades described by Benninghoff and Timmer have not been verified by electromicrographs. A more random orientation of the fibers, virtual absence of the continuous arcade, and the lack of a unit type of organization have been demonstrated. Chondrocytes are surrounded by a milieu rich in polysaccharide but poor in collagen. Mitotic figures have been observed in immature cartilage, but after epiphyseal closure the chondrocytes in articular cartilage show no evidence of mitotic activity.

The organic constituents of cartilage include collagen and the glycosaminoglycan-protein complexes. These high molecular weight complexes have exceptional viscous and hydrophilic properties. In fact, the water content of fresh articular cartilage approaches 80%. Most of this water is not tightly bound but forms a gel in combination with the glycosaminoglycans and can be removed by drying or heating. With aging, the water content of cartilage decreases only slightly. These protein polysaccharides are heterogenous and can be separated into three major groups. In articular cartilage only three glycosaminoglycan units have been found—chondroitin-4-sulfate, chondroitin-6-sulfate, and keratan sulfate. As a consequence, the sulfate concentration in cartilage is marked. Protein polysaccharides are not distributed diffusely throughout the collagen but are found to occur in highest concentrations in immediately surrounding cells. Protein polysaccharide concentration is decreased in the more superficial portion of the gliding zones and is also significantly less in the interterritorial zones. However, keratan sulfate is located primarily between zones. The most prevalent glycosaminoglycan in articular cartilage is chondroitin-6-sulfate. Keratan sulfate occurs in low concentrations in children but gradually increases with age and never contributes more than a small percentage of the total glycosaminoglycan. The water-binding capacity and polyelectrolytic resiliency of the articular surface aid in providing water for surface lubrication.

Electrolytes traverse the cartilaginous matrix rapidly; the equal diffusion rate between live and cadaveric cartilage indicates that the process is passive. Thus, the concentration of electrolytes in cartilage is essentially the same as in the intracellular and extracellular fluids of the tissues with the exception of sulfate and sodium. Diffusion of larger molecules across cartilage is slowed. Cationic dyes traverse cartilage more rapidly than anionic ones, indicating affinity for the polyanionic matrix and the importance of charge in predicting the rate of diffusion.

## Metabolism

Adult cartilage nutrients are supplied primarily from the synovial fluid. Minimal diffusion occurs through the underlying bone and plate, but this route may be more significant before closure of the epiphysis; however, after epiphyseal closure, the appearance of the tide mark and the deposition of apatite must limit this route of diffusion.

Anaerobic metabolic pathways are well developed in articular cartilage, as evidenced by its high concentration of lactic acid. Cartilage has a low oxygen consumption, a high aerobic production of lactate from glucose, a high concentration of lactate, and an anaerobic character as evidenced by its constituent enzymes, the lac-

tate dehydrogenases. Cartilage cells can synthesize collagen, glycosaminoglycans, and protein, which form complexes with one another. These metabolic functions may occur simultaneously or consecutively. In fact, the entire protein polysaccharide molecule may be synthesized almost simultaneously by a single cell.

The half-life of radiolabelled glycine and sulfate in articular cartilage is 8 days. The rapidity of this turnover suggests the presence of an active remodelling system. This "fast fraction" is limited to approximately one fourth of the total glycosaminoglycan-protein complex in articular cartilage. The rate of synthesis, established by utilizing radiolabelled sulfate, acetate, and glucosamine, is rapid and linear. Thus, articular cartilage is capable of rapid degradation and synthesis. It is suggested that as the mature protein polysaccharide complex becomes more extensively crosslinked, it becomes less hydrophilic than the nascent macromolecules. Since this protein polysaccharide complex must maintain a high affinity for water, a rapid turnover is necessary.

## Lubrication

The development of wear changes in joints is related in part to the joint's ability to withstand compressive forces. The marked compliance of articular cartilage has been established experimentally, and it has been assumed that the compressive forces to which a joint is subjected are altered primarily by the cartilage and to a lesser extent by the viscous synovial fluid. Although synovial fluid is markedly viscoelastic, the fluid film between two joints has been shown to have no significant dynamic force-attenuating qualities when subjected to impact tests. The viscoelastic nature of articular cartilage has been well established, and its compliance has been shown to be a result of the flow of the interstitial water.

Friction occurs between the articular

surfaces during joint movement. In ordinary dry sliding friction, for example, two metals sliding on each other, the friction force is that force necessary to overcome the points of contact between the two sheets of metal. The actual area of contact is much smaller than the apparent area of the sheet because of the surface irregularities in the material. Electron micrographs of articular cartilage have revealed an irregular surface composed of valleys and peaks. If a lubricant is introduced between the two articular surfaces to reduce the number of actual contact points, the lubrication is called boundary layer. The friction force depends on the characteristics of the film and the irregular surfaces.

Boundary lubrication can be an important factor in producing surface damage, because it imposes relatively high shear forces along the surface. Zarek has shown that even in normal use, tensile stresses are set up along the articular surface because of cartilage deformation. The addition of a large shear stress may be sufficient to rupture the cartilaginous surface.

When synovial fluid completely separates the articular surfaces so that no irregularities are in contact, it is providing hydrodynamic lubrication. In this circumstance the frictional forces are dependent on the characteristics of the fluid film per se. Synovial fluid is an excellent lubricant when the load carried is light; but as the load increases, very high shear rates of friction are produced in the synovial fluid. Increasing the viscosity of fluid does not improve its lubricating ability. Similarly, lowering its viscosity by digestion with hyaluronidase does not make it a worse lubricant. The lubricating component of synovial fluid is the mucin. If mucin is filtered from synovial fluid, the mucin-free fluid fails to lubricate. As a consequence, synovial fluid acts as a boundary lubricant. Articular surfaces exhibit such a low coefficient of friction that hydrodynamic lubrication alone cannot account for these

low levels. When two cartilage surfaces are placed in close proximity, contact takes place between the peaks of the opposing surfaces. Increasing the opposing forces brings more of the surface peaks into contact and traps synovial fluid in the valleys. Water diffuses from the trapped synovial fluid into the cartilage, yielding concentrated hyaluronic acid–protein complexes scattered over the cartilage surface. This phenomenon of synovial fluid—thixotropy—is the ability of the fluid to increase its viscosity when the velocity gradient across the fluid decreases as two surfaces glide over one another. An additional aid in reducing the coefficient of friction is the ability of the superficial layer of articular cartilage to deform laterally during joint movement. This maintains a lower velocity gradient across the synovial fluid than would occur in the absence of this phenomenon.

In rheumatoid arthritis this peculiar property—thixotropy—is lost, and the elastic properties of the fluid are reduced as a result of the dissociation of the hyaluronic acid–protein complex. In degenerative joint disease the synovial fluid is less thixotropic, and cartilage is less able to deform elastically. In both conditions, therefore, cartilage surfaces are more likely to be in contact when loaded during movement and to undergo thinning, fibrillation, and erosion.

### Repair

In discussing the healing of cartilage injuries, distinction must be made between injury of cartilage alone and injury that involves cartilage and the underlying bone. Healing in the following injuries will be compared: (1) injury limited to a partial thickness of the cartilage, (2) injuries penetrating completely through the full thickness of cartilage and extending to the subjacent bone, and (3) injuries produced by removal of a plug tissue that includes cartilage and a portion of the underlying bone.

In all three types of injury the cartilage margins showed identical response. On the first day after injury the area of cartilage immediately adjacent to the site of injury underwent necrosis. Chondrocyte proliferation began on the first day, reaching a maximum at 48 hours and gradually subsiding over the next 14 days. However, this cell proliferation contributed nothing to the eventual healing of the wound except perhaps to reconstitute the narrow zone of necrosis that was observed adjacent to the wound edges. This reaction has been termed chondrodegeneration. When the wound violated the subjacent bone, the inflammatory response from the base of the wound was marked; but no inflammatory response occurred in the substance of the articular cartilage. Even when complete healing by fibrocartilaginous proliferation has occurred from the base, the cartilaginous margins of the defect remain clearly separated from the newly formed cartilage.

When the defect includes cartilage and subjacent bone, a marked variation in healing has been observed. Excellent healing of the defect by fibrocartilage formation may occur, or healing may result in a slightly depressed area covered by firm connective tissue containing islands of cartilage. In other instances, the defect may remain, increase in size, and expose eburnated bone in the base of the defect.

The Ghadiallys have demonstrated the flow of cartilage into articular cartilage defects. They produced full-thickness defects in the articular cartilage of a weight-bearing joint that extended into the subchondral bone. The reaction that followed consisted of two components: (1) a sliding and flowing of cartilage over the edge of the defect, and (2) a filling of the defect by repaired tissue arising from the marrow space. When a scan and electron microscopic study of the deep defects was utilized, it was possible to demonstrate the flow of cartilage cells from the edge of the defect. In most cases, the cartilage flowed

downward to the core defect. The repaired tissue grew in, along, and over the reflected cartilage. In some cases, the flowing cartilage extended over the repaired tissue and, as a result of load bearing and joint movement, became fragmented.

The most satisfactory healing occurs when the defect extends through the subchondral bone. Granulation tissue from the marrow spaces gradually fills the defect and progresses through the stages of fibrous tissue and fibrocartilage formation to form hyaline cartilage (Fig. 2-19). In such defects the calcified zone of cartilage may be reformed.

This chondrofibrosis has been classified as epichondral, intrinsic, and subchondral. In the traumatized joint, epicondylar pannus formation may unite the bones at several points and the adhesions restrict joint motion. A comparison of the effects of immobilization versus mobilization after injury to articular cartilage and subjacent bone revealed that on the mobilized side, the crater filled rapidly and no pannus formation extended to the crater or elsewhere. The synovial membrane and the articular cartilages appeared normal except for the crater. On the immobilized side, a heavy pannus extended from the synovial membrane to the crater floor. Pannus formations appeared in the periphery of the joint, well removed from the crater. The crater base became covered by granulation tissue, and the synovial membrane appeared dull. There was a quantitative increase in synovial fluid.

Clinical experience has shown that an intra-articular fracture subjected to prolonged immobilization can be accompanied by a disabling degree of chondrofibrosis. In severe intra-articular fractures, accurate reduction and early mobilization reduces the degree of chondrofibrosis and the threat of fibrous ankylosis. If the joint is appropriately mobilized, certain types of pannus formations are reversible. Reversibility means that the pannus formation

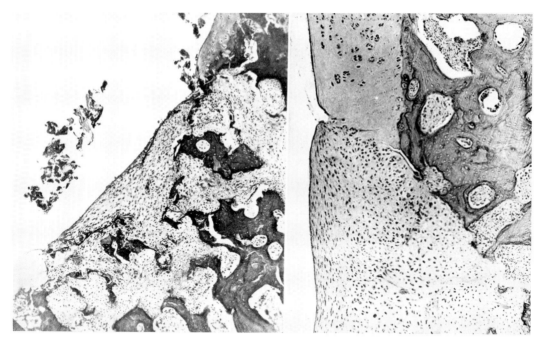

**Fig. 2-19.** A loss of articular cartilage and violation of the underlying bone results in a fibrous tissue reaction that gradually fills the defect and may be converted to cartilage. (From Key, J. A.: J. Bone Joint Surg. **13:**725, 1931.)

extending between the articular surfaces either is destroyed or becomes so thin as to be insignificant when the joint is again mobilized. There is marked variation in the degree of chondrofibrosis that develops. The destructiveness of this pannus may well determine the ultimate functional result.

In the presence of vasomotor dysfunction, that is, reflex sympathetic dystrophy, chondrofibrosis is much more destructive. A pannus overlying a normal area of articular cartilage may invade and destroy the underlying cartilage, or relatively little or no cartilage may be destroyed. A pannus that tightly unites the articular surfaces may destroy only the tangential layer of the cartilage and then become quiescent. The attachment of the pannus to the surface of the articular cartilage can vary from extreme looseness to extreme tightness.

### Changes in immobilized joints

In humans, articular cartilage undergoes changes when the digital joints are immobilized for extended periods of time for extracapsular diseases, for example, collateral ligament shortening, skin contracture, tendon shortening, or palmar fibrosis. Long-standing interphalangeal joint flexion associated with Dupuytren's contracture can result in eventual loss of cartilage from the unopposed surfaces of the articular cartilage. Yet the cartilage remains normal in those parts of each joint where there is contact between the opposing articular surfaces. On direct examination the unused areas of cartilage exhibit a loss of sheen and an irregularity of the joint surface that had become pitted and eroded at its margins. In the longer-term cases, cartilage is completely lost from the unused area on the dorsum of the proximal phalanx (Fig. 2-20). The overlying extensor tendons may become adherent to the exposed bone.

Microscopically, the cartilaginous changes include irregularity of the surface of the unopposed cartilage, fissuring of the superficial zone and an alteration in the staining characteristics of the chondrocytes. The cartilage is thin and covered by an overgrowth of small vessels that extend into the surface defects in the cartilage matrix. At the margin of the zone of altered cartilage there is increased cellularity in the periosteum, and a vascular proliferation appears to invade beneath the overhanging edge of cartilage. This vascular tissue erodes the subchondral bone and extends between its trabeculae. A thin layer of capillaries extends across the unused portion of the joint surface.

Hall's experimental studies in rats reveal similar changes in the areas where articular cartilage was not in contact with the opposing cartilage. After only 23 days of immobilization, changes appeared and progressed over the following months in a pattern similar to those reported previously in humans.

Apparently, mechanical limitation of joint motion may bring about these changes by interfering with cartilage nutrition. Diffusion of the nutrients through cartilage is assisted by intermittent compression of the

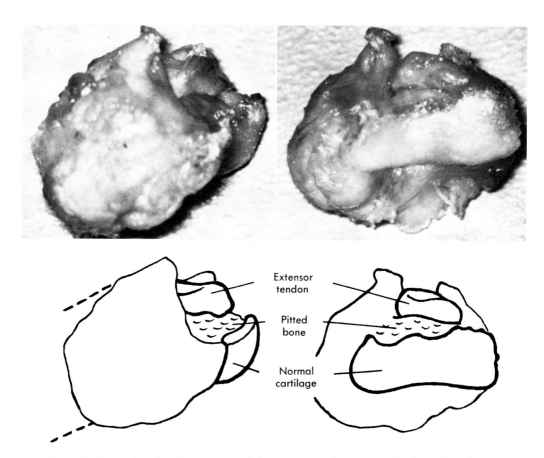

**Fig. 2-20.** Sagittal section through interphalangeal joint showing tendon fixed by adhesions to the eroded bone matrix of the proximal phalanx (×10). (From Field, P. L., and Hueston, J. T.: Br. J. Plast. Surg. **12:**186, 1969.)

cartilage as the joint moves. Consequently, restriction of motion may impair nutrition of the noncompressed cartilage and result in eventual atrophy. Yet compression must be intermittent and within physiological limits. Compression beyond these limits is an effective means of reducing chondrocyte nutrition, thereby leading to cell death. After 4 days of compression the underlying cartilaginous matrix and cells exhibit altered staining characteristics. The cartilage becomes fibrillar, involved chondrocytes die, and the underlying bone becomes eburnated and sclerotic. The eburnated bone may undergo further degeneration to give the radiographic appearance of a bone cyst. The clinical implications of these observations are obvious.

## BIBLIOGRAPHY

Altner, P. C., Grana, L., and Gordon, M.: An experimental study on the significance of muscle tissue interposition on fracture healing, Clin. Orthop. 111:269, 1975.

Bassett, C. A. L., and Herrmann, I.: Influence of oxygen concentration and mechanical factors on differentiation of connective tissue in vitro, Nature 190:460, 1961.

Bassett, C. A. L.: Current concepts of bone formation, J. Bone Joint Surg. 44A:1217, 1962.

Becker, R. L., Bassett, C. A. L., and Bachmann, C. H.: Bioelectrical factors controlling bone structure. In Frost, H., editor: Bone biodynamics, New York, 1963, Little Brown and Co.

Becker, R. O., and Murray, D. G.: The electrical control system regulating fracture healing in amphibians, Clin. Orthop. 73:169, 1970.

Bennett, G. A., and Bauer, W.: Further studies concerning the repair of articular cartilage in dog joints, J. Bone Joint Surg. 17:141, 1935.

Benninghoff, A., and Timmer, G. J.: Über Die Kompakt-Architektur Der Grossen Rohren Knochen, Klin. Wochenschr. 26:126, 1948.

Bohr, H.: Studies on fracture healing, J. Bone Joint Surg. 37A:326, 1955.

Brighton, C. T., Krebs, A. G.: Oxygen tension of healing fractures in the rabbit, J. Bone Joint Surg. 54A:323, 1972.

Brookes, M.: The blood supply of bone, London, 1971, Butterworth & Co. Ltd.

Brookes, M., and Singh, M.: Bone blood pH and gas tensions after femoral vein ligation, Surg. Gynecol. Obstet. 135:873, 1972.

Bruce, R., and Straclan, S.: Lactate dehydrogenase isozymes in healing bone, J. Oral Surg. 25:542, 1967.

Calandruccis, R., and Gilmer, W. S.: Proliferation, regeneration, and repair of articular cartilage of immature animals, J. Bone Joint Surg. 44A:431, 1962.

Cieszynski, T.: Studies on the regeneration of ossal tissue, 2. Treatment of bone fractures in experimental animal with electric energy, Arch. Immunol. Ther. Exp. (Warsz.) 11:199-217, 1963.

Cooper, R.: Nerves in cortical bone, Science 160:327, 1968.

Currey, J. D.: The mechanical consequences of variation in the mineral content of bone, J. Biomech. 2:1, 1969.

Field, P. L., and Hueston, J. T.: Articular cartilage loss in long-standing flexion deformity of the proximal interphalangeal joints, Aust. N.Z. J. Surg. 40:70, 1970.

Friedenburg, Z. B., and Brighton, C. T.: Bioelectric potentials in bone, J. Bone Joint Surg. 48A:915, 1966.

Fritz, P. J., and Jacobson, K. B.: Lactic dehydrogenase subfractionation of isozymes, Science 140:64, 1963.

Fukada, E., and Yasuda, J.: On the piezoelectric effect of bone, Jap. J. Physiol. 12:1158, 1957.

Ghadially, J. A., and Ghadially, F. N.: Evidence of cartilage flow in deep defects in articular cartilage, Virchows Archiv. (Cell Path.) 18:193, 1975.

Hall, M. C.: Articular changes in the knee of the adult rat after prolonged immobilization in extension, Clin. Orthop. 34:184, 1964.

Heppenstall, R. B., Grislis, G., and Hunt, T. K.: Tissue gas tensions and oxygen consumption in healing bone defects, Clin. Orthop. 106:357, 1975.

Jacobs, R. L., and Ray, R. D.: The effect of heat on bone healing, Arch. Surg. 104:687, 1972.

Jarry, L., and Uhthoff, H. K.: Differences in healing of metaphyseal and diaphyseal fractures, Can. J. Surg. 14:127, 1971.

Johannsen, A.: Fracture healing controlled by 87mSr uptake, Acta Orthop. Scand. 44:628, 1973.

Jorgensen, T. E.: The effect of electric current on the healing time of crural fractures, Acta Orthop. Scand. 43:421, 1972.

Key, A.: Experimental arthritis; the changes in joints produced by creating defects in the articular cartilage, J. Bone Joint Surg. 13:725, 1931.

Kruse, R. L., and Kelly, P. J.: Acceleration of fracture healing distal to a venous tourniquet, J. Bone Joint Surg. 56A:730, 1974.

Lindholm, R. V., and Lindholm, T. S.: Mast cells in endosteal and periosteal bone repair, Acta Orthop. Scand. **41**:129, 1970.

Macnab, I., and De Haas, W. G.: The role of periosteal blood supply in the healing of fractures of the tibia, Clin. Orthop. **105**:27, 1974.

Makley, J. T., Heiple, K. G., Chase, S. W., and others: The effect of reduced barometric pressure on fracture healing in rats, J. Bone Joint Surg. **49A**:903, 1967.

Mankin, H. J.: Localization of tritiated thymidine in articular cartilage of rabbits, J. Bone Joint Surg. **44A**:688, 1962.

Mankin, H. J.: The articular cartilages; a review, Am. Acad. Orthop. Surg. **19**:204, 1970.

Meachim, G.: The effect of scarification on articular cartilage in the rabbit, J. Bone Joint Surg. **45B**:150, 1963.

Muheim, G.: Assessment of fracture healing in man by serial $87^m$ strontium-scintimetry, Acta Orthop. Scand. **44**:621, 1973.

Radin, E. L., Paul, I. L., Lowy, M.: A comparison of the dynamic force-transmitting properties of subchondral bone and articular cartilage, J. Bone Joint Surg. **52A**:444, 1970.

Rhinelander, F. W., and Baragry, R. A.: Microangiography in bone healing, J. Bone Joint Surg. **44A**:1273, 1962.

Singer, M.: The influence of the nerve in regeneration of the amphibian extremity, Quart. Rev. Biol. **27**:169, 1952.

Stern, B., Glimacher, M. J., and Goldhaber, P.: The effect of various oxygen tensions on the synthesis and degradation of bone collagen in tissue culture, Proc. Soc. Exp. Biol. Med. **121**:869, 1966.

Tonna, E. A., and Cronkite, E. P.: Cellular response to fracture studied with tritiated thymidine, J. Bone Joint Surg. **43A**:352, 1961.

Urist, M. R., Wallace, T. H., and Adams, T.: The function of fibrocartilaginous fracture callus, J. Bone Joint Surg. **47B**:304, 1965.

Walker, P. S., Dowson, D., Longfield, M. D., and others: "Boosted lubrication" in synovial joints by fluid entrapment and enrichment, Ann. Rheum. Dis. **27**:512, 1968.

Walker, P. S., Sikorski, J., Dowson, D., and others: Behaviour of synovial fluid on surfaces of articular cartilage, Ann. Rheum. Dis. **28**:1, 1969.

Zarek, J. M.: Dynamic consideration in load-bearing bones with special reference to osteosynthesis and articular cartilage studies on the anatomy and function of bone and joints. In Evans, F. G., editor: Studies on the anatomy and function of bone and joints, New York, 1966, Springer-Verlag New York Inc.

# CHAPTER 3
# Nerve regeneration

The anatomy and physiology of peripheral nerves in response to injury are presented here to prepare for later discussions concerning clinical management of injured nerves.

## NERVE TRUNKS

Nerve fibers are the structural units of peripheral nerve trunks. At the core of a nerve fiber is the axon, a cytoplasmic extension of a centrally located nerve cell body (neuron), often several feet in length (Fig. 3-1). Axoplasm is that cytoplasmic extension of the neuron that constitutes the axon. It is a viscous fluid that appears to stream peripherally. Streams of axoplasm have an affinity for and adhere to the surfaces of Schwann cells. The survival and function of the axon depend on its continuity with the parent cell body. The axon is surrounded by a sheath composed of single-layered Schwann cells and an outer connective tissue covering, the endoneurium. One or more axons may be present within one nerve fiber. If the axon degenerates, it leaves behind the Schwann tube, or endoneurial tube, which serves as a conduit for regenerating axons.

The functional unit of peripheral nerve trunks consists of a neuron with its axonal process and the end organ or receptor where the axon terminates. Impulses or stimuli to or from the central nervous system (CNS) are conveyed via this functional unit.

Motor nerve fibers originate from anterior horn cells in the spinal cord. They carry efferent impulses from the CNS, terminating in the motor end-plates of skeletal muscle. Sensory nerve fibers originate from cell bodies in the dorsal root ganglia. These fibers carry afferent impulses to the CNS from their peripheral terminations, which are free or include a variety of specialized end organs, or receptors, such as Meissner's corpuscles. Sympathetic fibers are the postganglionic extensions of neurons of the ganglionated sympathetic nerve trunk. They terminate peripherally in such organs as vessel walls, hair muscles, and glandular structures of skin.

Morphologically, peripheral nerve fibers are characterized as being myelinated or unmyelinated. Myelin is a complex lipoprotein system whose origin is thought to be the Schwann cell. It has a characteristic laminated structure believed to result from compression of several layers of Schwann cell cytoplasm wrapped around a single axon. Longitudinally, myelin is broken into segments that outline the nodes and internodes of nerve fibers. The nodes of Ranvier

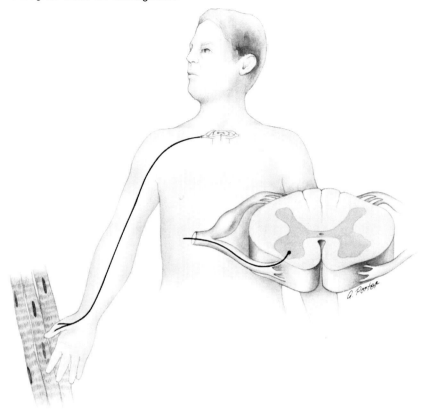

**Fig. 3-1.** The motor cell body is located in the anterior horn of the spinal cord. The cell's cytoplasm continues distally in its axon process.

represent the junctions between adjacent Schwann cells. In myelinated fibers there is one Schwann cell to each myelin segment; by contrast, in unmyelinated nerve fibers several axons are usually ensheathed by the cytoplasm of one Schwann cell. Myelination of a nerve fiber is controlled by the parent cell.

The significance of myelination is related to the rate of conduction of action potentials across the two types of fibers. The spread of current is continuous, and conduction appears to be a uniform process in unmyelinated fibers. In myelinated fibers, conduction is discontinuous, or saltatory. The impulse skips from one node of Ranvier to the next because the insulating nature of the myelin sheath allows currents to pass through the membrane only at the nodes. Conduction velocity is therefore greater in myelinated fibers.

Nerve fibers are arranged in distinct bundles within peripheral nerve trunks. Each bundle, or funiculus, is encircled by a thin, firm connective tissue sheath, the perineurium. Each funiculus usually contains a mixture of motor, sensory, and sympathetic fibers. Most nerve trunks contain more than one funiculus. Funiculi branch and anastomose every few millimeters, forming a plexus along the entire length of the nerve (Fig. 3-2). Therefore, serial cross-sections of a single nerve trunk show a variation in the size, number, and location of funiculi. This rapid change in funicular anatomy makes correct approximation of correspond-

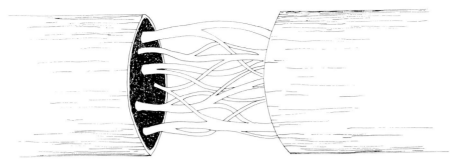

**Fig. 3-2.** There is a marked variation in the composition of a funiculus from one level to another as a result of the frequent crossover of axons.

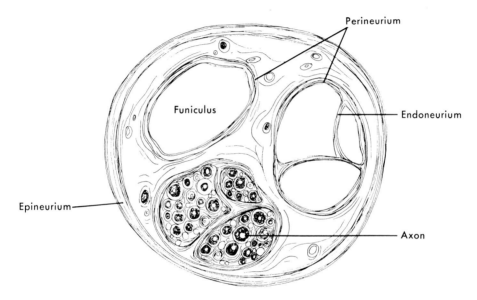

**Fig. 3-3.** The peripheral nerve trunks contain funiculi and a variable amount of connective tissue.

ing funiculi difficult or impossible even when only a short segment of nerve is missing. Component nerve fibers within funiculi are also redistributed as a result of funicular plexus formation.

Several funiculi are held together by a loose, areolar connective tissue framework, the epineurium, which also forms the outer sheath of a peripheral nerve trunk. The epineurium comprises 30% to 75% of the cross-sectional area of a nerve trunk.

Three distinct layers of connective tissue have thus been described as parts of a peripheral nerve (Fig. 3-3). The epineurium provides a protective function for the nerve trunk by means of its loose matrix, which cushions funiculi against compression. Epineurium consists of collagen and elastic fibers, most of which are longitudinally oriented; and fibrocytes and adipose tissue, present primarily in interfunicular areas.

The thin, dense perineurium that surrounds funiculi provides tensile strength for the nerve trunk and acts as a diffusion barrier for the nerve fibers within it. It is composed primarily of collagen fibrils and mesothelial cells (fibroblasts). The longitudinal, circular, and oblique arrangement of perineurial collagen fibers is responsible for providing the tensile strength of a nerve trunk. As a diffusion barrier, it provides homeostasis for the enclosed nerve fibers.

Endoneurium also provides strength and elasticity, but to a lesser extent. This is demonstrated by the fact that spinal nerve roots are more susceptible to stretch and compression injuries than peripheral nerve trunks because they lack perineurium and have only small amounts of epineurial tissue. A denervated distal segment of nerve has the same strength and elasticity and can carry the same load as the remaining normal proximal segment.

The elasticity of fibers in the epineurium contributes to the tortuous course of a peripheral nerve in its bed. Funiculi lie slack within the epineurium, which results in a pouring out of funiculi when a nerve trunk is transected. Nerve fibers also run an undulating course within the funiculus. These factors permit some stretching of peripheral nerve trunks during normal limb movements. When tension is applied to the end of a transected nerve, the nerve elongates by taking up the slack of the funiculi within epineurial tissues. When taut, the perineurium resists further elongation, thus protecting nerve fibers within the funiculus. As tension increases, the normal undulations of the nerve fibers disappear. If tension is further increased, the cross-sectional area of the funiculus is reduced. This causes compression of the funiculus and reduction of the blood supply to the nerve fibers. Subsequent increases in tension result in rupture of nerve fibers within the funiculus.

The elastic limit of a nerve trunk ranges from 20% to as low as 6%. This elastic limit depends on the rate and amount of loading. When loaded in small increments at low rates, nerve trunks can be stretched beyond their normal range of elasticity without altering function. Conversely, abrupt loading may produce early alteration of function within nerve trunks. This may be of clinical significance in the postoperative mobilization of joints acutely flexed to reduce tension on a nerve repair.

## NERVE VASCULATURE

Each peripheral nerve is abundantly vascularized throughout its entire length by a network of intercommunicating intrinsic vessels, augmented at irregular intervals by extrinsic nutrient arteries. The extrinsic nutrient vessels reach the peripheral nerve through its mesoneurium, which is similar to the mesentery of the intestine (Fig. 3-4). Coiled arteries within the mesoneurium permit vascular supply from relatively immobile major vessels to reach nerves, which may undergo considerable changes in position in response to joint motion. The nutrient vessels traverse the mesoneurium to reach and enter the nerve trunk only on the mesoneurial side. The mesoneurium varies with the anatomical location of the nerve in order to accommodate movement or lack of movement. Where greater mobility is required, such as across joint flexion creases, the mesoneurium is longer and more complex. The coiled vessels within the mesoneurium uncoil to accommodate movement of the nerve during joint motion. For example, in the proximal forearm the mesoneurium of the ulnar nerve lies on the medial aspect of the nerve but assumes a more lateral position in the mid and distal forearm. In the proximal forearm the mesoneurium is lateral to the median nerve. At the wrist, the mesoneurium enters the medial aspect of the nerve. In the carpal tunnel, the intrinsic blood supply of the median nerve is augmented by vessels entering the nerve proximal and distal to the transverse carpal ligament. The distal vessels arise from the superficial palmar arch.

The intrinsic blood supply of a peripheral nerve is arranged in four longitudinally oriented systems of vessels located on the surface of the nerve, in interfunicular tissue,

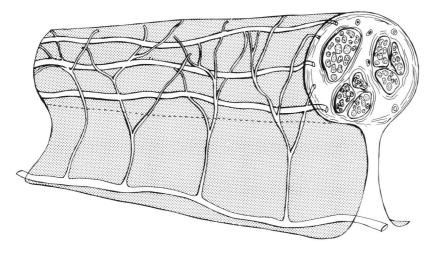

**Fig. 3-4.** The blood supply of a peripheral nerve is provided by its longitudinal plexus and the nutrient arteries.

in perineurium, and within funiculi. These systems anastomose freely with each other.

Lundborg and Branemark described in vivo intraneural microvascular blood flow patterns using intravital microscopic technique. They found no one direction of blood flow seeming to predominate in any segment of the tibial nerve of rabbits. The direction of flow in a single longitudinal vessel often varied, changing direction at almost every anastomosis along its course. The direction of blood flow appeared to change suddenly when a nearby area of nerve was crushed or divided. Under normal conditions only a part of the intraneural microvascular bed was functioning at any one time. So-called reserve vessels began to function immediately when the nerve was traumatized.

Maintenance of normal peripheral nerve fiber structure and function depends on an adequate blood supply, in addition to continuity between the axon and its parent cell body. Division of nutrient arteries to a nerve trunk is generally well tolerated provided the intrinsic longitudinal system of the vessels remains intact. Examination of functional and histological changes in nerves after ligation of nutrient arteries shows no differences in the conduction capacities but does show histological changes of ischemia 2 weeks after vessel interruption. If only the intrinsic system of vessels is interrupted, as in nerve transection, there is minimal reduction in the intraneural circulation. When both the longitudinal intrinsic vessel system and the regional nutrient arteries are interrupted (nerve transection with mobilization of the nerve ends), circulation in the nerve may be compromised, particularly if tension (suture) is applied at the same time.

The importance of blood supply for function of peripheral nerves remains somewhat controversial, particularly as it relates to mobilization of transected nerve ends during neurorrhaphy. Kline and associates clearly showed no difference in postinjury conduction velocities or nerve action potential amplitudes in monkeys after division of only the nutrient arteries and after division of both the nutrient arteries plus the longitudinal intrinsic vessels. They concluded that functional recovery therefore did not depend on initial preservation of collateral blood supply in injured nerve trunks. Yet others have reported retarded nerve regeneration following extensive mobilization of severed human nerves. Most authors recommend against extensive mobilization. Alteration in the microvascular circulation of the nerve and histological changes such as decreased axon counts have been demonstrated after interruption of the extrinsic and intrinsic blood supply of a nerve. No controlled studies are available, however, demonstrating decreased functional recovery.

## AXOPLASM SYNTHESIS AND MIGRATION

Protein synthesis in the neuron appears limited to the cell body. Both sedentary and mobile proteins are synthesized; the former are metabolized more slowly than the latter. The mobile proteins are presumed to migrate into the cell processes. Tracer studies have demonstrated movement of newly synthesized proteins from the cell body to the axon hillock, then peripherally into the axon process. When these nascent proteins are labelled with radioisotopes, the rate of their migration into uninjured peripheral nerves approaches 1.5 mm per day. Proteins migrating from the cell body into the axon replace proteins that are being degraded. Continuous delivery of new protein components is necessary to maintain normal axon function.

Continuous and peristaltic centrifugal movement of axoplasm from the perikaryon to the nerve ending is a traditional concept. More recent studies concerning the migration of proteins labeled with radioactive tracers suggest the continual migration of neuronal cytoplasm in both directions. Biochemical information from the cell body to the axon and back again may be provided by this bidirectional streaming. The cell body can thus obtain information regarding the metabolic state of its long cytoplasmic process. The bidirectional flow theory was supported by a study involving axonal acetylcholinesterase, an enzyme located exclusively in the axon. After transection of a peripheral nerve, acetylcholinesterase ac-

tivity increased rapidly at both proximal and distal nerve stumps, presumably due to the bidirectional flow of the enzyme within the axoplasm and its subsequent arrest near the cut ends of the nerve.

## NERVE INJURY

Three fundamental types of nerve injury have been defined. The least severe is that which produces a temporary interruption of conduction without loss of axonal continuity between neurons and end organs. The basis of this type of injury is thought to be a disruption of normal biochemical functions of the axoplasm, localized at the site of injury. A second type of nerve injury is that involving loss of continuity of the axon or severe disorganization of axonal mechanisms so that the axon distal to and, for a variable distance, proximal to the site of injury fails to survive. The endoneurial sheath remains intact, however, ensuring that the regenerating axon will reach its original end organ. Unless proximal degeneration results in cell death, recovery should be complete. The third type of nerve injury involves disruption of both axon and the endoneurial tube. The chances of the regenerating axon regrowing into its original endoneurial tube distal to the injury are no longer 100%. This type of injury can be subdivided into further categories, based on the degree of injury to other components of the nerve trunk: disruption of the axon and endoneurial tube alone; disruption of the axon and endoneurial tube, plus the structure of the entire funiculus; and disruption of the entire nerve trunk. With increasing damage to the component structures of the nerve trunk, the chance that an axon will regenerate along its original endoneurial tube becomes increasingly less. At the site of the injury, more scar forms, which obstructs the growth of regenerating axon branches. The degree and amount of degeneration proximal to the injury become greater; complete cell death becomes more common. Spontaneous recovery of function after this type of injury is poor or nonexistent.

The changes that occur after interruption of the continuity of a peripheral nerve involve the whole functional unit, composed of the cell body, the axon proximal and distal to the injury, and the peripherally innervated end organ.

### Reaction to injury in the cell body

For largely unknown reasons, the degree of injury sustained by the centrally located neurons varies greatly after injury. Two fairly constant factors related to neuronal disturbance are intensity and level of axonal injury. The greater the violence to the axon (avulsion injury as opposed to transection), the more intense the retrograde reaction. The more proximal the axon division, the greater the cell damage.

Enlargement of the neuron is evident during the first week after injury. Thereafter, the cell body remains enlarged throughout the period of axon regeneration (Fig. 3-5), if axon regeneration occurs. Neuron hypertrophy is presumably due to an anabolic state within the cell associated with axon regeneration. If regeneration is prevented by capping the proximal nerve stump, the neuron atrophies.

Additional histological changes occur to varying degrees in the parent cell after axonal injury. These include alterations in the size of the nucleus and nucleolus; alteration in the staining qualities of Nissl granules, which proceed to dissolution in more severe reactions; fragmentation of the Golgi apparatus; vacuolization of protoplasm; and displacement of the nucleus from the center of the cell. These histological changes all reflect changes in the biochemistry of the cell.

The most sensitive histological indicator of degenerative change in the neuron is a decrease in the amount of stainable basophilic material (Nissl granules) and its dispersal through the cell in finer particles. This process is termed chromatolysis and is the optical manifestation of physiochemical changes resulting in the breaking up of aggregates of RNA into smaller particles. The reorganization and migration of these RNA particles represent their conversion into a more active form. An elevation in enzymatic activity and amino acid synthesis accompanies this structural change. Such activity is necessary for cell survival and axon regeneration. The morphological changes of chromatolysis appear within 24 hours after axon division and progress until a maximum is reached about 18 days after injury. If the neuron recovers, these nucleoproteins eventually reaccumulate until there is complete restoration of the size and shape of the cell and its characteristic pattern of Nissl granules. The recovery period varies greatly but may extend over several months. The end result can be full recovery or persistence of a residual defect that reduces the efficiency of the unit. If the neuron does not recover, cell necrosis ensues. Estimates of the number of cells failing to survive after nerve division or compression range from 16% to 85%.

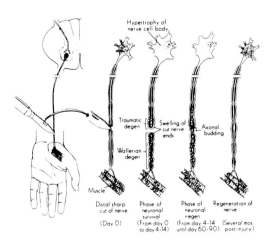

**Fig. 3-5.** After section of a peripheral nerve trunk, the distal and proximal stumps undergo degeneration. The anterior horn cell hypertrophies in preparation for axoplasm regeneration. (From Grabb, W. C.: Orthop. Clin. North Am. **1:**421, 1970.)

Following injury to anterior horn cells in the spinal cord, astrocytes and small glial cells in the vicinity of the neuron proliferate within 24 hours of nerve injury and contact the nerve cells. There is a progressive increase in these microglia until each cell body has been contacted. These glial cells also undergo morphological and biochemical changes. Various elements of the glial cells show increased enzymatic activity, protein synthesis, cell enlargement, and proliferation. The simultaneous neuronal and perineuronal glial reactions suggest a close interaction between neurons and glial cells. It has been postulated that axon regeneration may not begin until this entire system is activated. In neurons that fail to survive, the glial cells lift off their synaptic ending and penetrate the neuronal cytoplasm. The neuron is then phagocytosed by the glial cell.

## Reaction to injury in the proximal nerve stump

Shortly after nerve laceration, both free ends of the nerve become edematous, resulting in a threefold increase in the cross-sectional area of the nerve. The edema forms in response to the accumulation of a gel-like amorphous substance containing a large quantity of acidic mucopolysaccharides. The edema subsides very slowly, usually requiring several weeks to disappear completely. Within the severed nerve end, the axon undergoes wallerian degeneration for a variable distance proximal to the site of injury (see following section). This degeneration may or may not extend to involve the neuron itself. Schwann cells begin proliferating 48 to 72 hours after injury. Axon sprouting begins by 96 hours after injury if the injury has been sharp

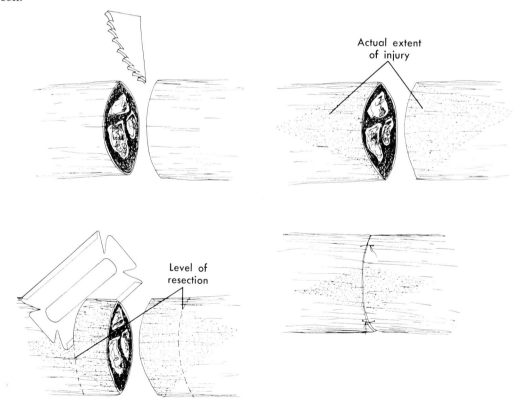

**Fig. 3-6.** If the extent of nerve injury is not appreciated at the time of primary suture, less than an optimal result will be produced.

and if minimal concomitant injury has occurred. Yet the typical nerve laceration is seldom well controlled, and significant injury extends for many millimeters on each side of the cut (Fig. 3-6). Thus, an accurate demarcation of the level of retrograde degeneration cannot be made for several days after injury. During this time, the Schwann cells have proliferated and assumed a phagocytic role. Concomitant proliferation of fibroblasts originating from the endoneurium, perineurium, and epineurium of the injured nerve trunk occurs prior to the onset of collagen synthesis. The newly synthesized fibrous tissue lacks longitudinal alignment, and the regenerating axons become entangled in a disorganized clump, the neuroma. Production of collagen by the fibroblasts is the dominant activity in the nerve ends early after injury. Axon regeneration may be minimal or negligible during this period. Within 3 weeks after injury, axonal regeneration becomes prominent. This time period has been interpreted as the anabolic phase of the parent cell body.

### Reaction to injury in the distal nerve stump

Some of the changes in the distal stump immediately after injury reflect those seen in the proximal stump. There is early and distinct edema formation and extensive connective tissue proliferation. Schwann cells and fibroblasts proliferate and, together with the newly synthesized fibrous tissue, form a glioma. Since the distal stump after transection does not contain any axonal elements capable of long-term survival, the glioma lacks the neural elements present in the proximal neuroma.

The entire length of axon distal to the injury undergoes wallerian degeneration. This is characterized by axonal enlargement into an amorphous mass that includes fragmentation of neural filaments, appearance of irregularities in contour and staining, and separation from the myelin sheath. Axon degeneration is probably precipitated by an accumulation of metabolic breakdown products, which causes disruption of lysosomes. Release of enzymes within the lysosomes leads to metabolic degradation of the axoplasm. The axon fragments at 48 to 72 hours after injury, and all traces of axon are usually lost by the second week.

Following division of the axon, nerve conduction capability of the distal segment continues for variable periods. Muscles respond to nerve stimulation for 4 to 5 days following axon division. Ascending nerve action potentials can be recorded for 6 to 8 days. Degeneration is more marked in those portions of the axon that first lose ability to conduct impulses.

Changes in myelin become evident at 28 to 96 hours after injury, when axon disintegration is already well advanced. Myelin fragments into droplets surrounding axon debris. Myelin globules have been reported in Schwann cell cytoplasm at 2 to 3 days. Chemical disintegration of myelin, consisting of the breakdown of complex lipids into simpler fats, commences on approximately the eighth day. The entire amorphous mass of axon and myelin debris is removed by phagocytosis, a process usually completed by the end of the second week.

Degeneration of axon and myelin is accompanied by increased activity in the Schwann cells, evident within 24 hours after injury. Schwann cell proliferation after nerve injury in mice has been shown to be almost eight times higher around myelinated nerves than around unmyelinated nerves. Schwann cell nuclei enlarge and the amount of cytoplasm increases, becomes vacuolated, and contains many granules. These changes represent an increase in the protein-synthesizing apparatus of the Schwann cell. Schwann cell activity peaks at the same time that wallerian degeneration and removal of debris peak. Schwann cells may provide enzymes that destroy the myelin sheath. Since myelin debris has been reported within their cytoplasm, Schwann cells are believed to function as macrophages, emptying the endoneurial sheath of debris. The events of wallerian degeneration have been shown by most investigators to occur simultaneously along the entire length of the nerve fiber distal to the site of injury. At the fifth to eighth week after injury, the distal endoneurial tube with its inner lining of Schwan cells has been entirely emptied of debris.

The empty endoneurial tube collapses and shrinks. This is a reversible process owing to the elastic properties of endoneurium. Shrinkage of the endoneurial tube is progressive, however, as the duration of the period of denervation increases. It has been shown to reach a maximum at approximately 3 months after injury. To what extent the endoneurial tube can expand in response to ingrowing axons after this time is unknown. Collapse of the empty endoneurial tubes results in atrophy of the funiculus. But there is little change in the epineurium as a result of wallerian degeneration. Therefore, the degree of shrinkage of the entire nerve trunk distal to the site of injury depends on what percentage of its cross-sectional area is occupied by funiculi.

The events of wallerian degeneration can be summarized as follows:

1. During the first week after injury, physical disintegration of axon and myelin occurs. There is intense Schwann cell proliferation and activity. This is followed by entry of macrophages into the interior of the nerve fiber.

2. During the second and third weeks after injury, chemical disintegration of axon and myelin is followed by phagocytic removal of debris. Schwann cell and fibroblastic activities decrease with the removal of debris.

3. During the fifth to eighth week, the endoneurial tube is emptied of debris, leaving a core of Schwann cells enclosed in endoneurium (the endoneurial sheath), which collapses.

## Changes in human muscle after denervation

A series of well-defined changes occurs in human skeletal muscle following denervation. The muscle fibers undergo a progressive but irregular shrinkage. There is disruption of the internal longitudinal arrangement of the muscle fiber. This is followed by the splitting of fibers into fibrils, which undergo fragmentation. Fibroblasts surround and ultimately phagocytose the fragments. Muscle nuclei undergo degenerative changes soon after denervation, gradually fragment and disappear in later stages. The motor end-plates exhibit a progressive depletion of their cytoplasm, which becomes granular. Proliferating connective tissue is evident around larger vessels and between muscle fibers. A progressive increase in connective tissue and fat occurs. Yet even up to 3 years after denervation, very few muscle fibers have undergone complete disintegration. The greatest changes during this period are shrinkage of muscle fibers and an increase in connective tissue. After 3 years, irregular areas of muscle fiber destruction become evident, eventually leading to ultimate loss of all muscle tissue and its replacement by connective tissue and fat. Reinnervation at this stage cannot reverse these changes. To what extent functional recovery can occur after reinnervation in the presence of less severe muscle changes depends on the duration of denervation; that is, longer periods of denervation produce less return of function after reinnervation because of irreversible changes in the muscle. The changes in skeletal muscle resulting from denervation are reversible only by reinnervation by motor nerve fibers. Attempts at reinnervation by sensory or sympathetic nerve fibers have proved uniformly unsuccessful.

The regenerating motor axon grows into the region of the original end-plate and terminates there. It is directed there by the endoneurium. A number of investigators have demonstrated the formation of new end-plates by ingrowing motor nerve fibers.

No nerve terminals exhibiting cholinesterase activity outside the zone of original end-plates have been demonstrated, however. Neuromuscular junctions have been observed to contain well-developed secondary synaptic clefts, which may persist for an extended period of time after denervation. A scarcity of secondary synaptic clefts in the neuromuscular junctions of regenerated nerve fibers has also been observed. This suggests that regenerating nerve fibers may terminate in the vicinity, but not necessarily at the exact site of the original end-plates.

The changes occurring in human skeletal muscles following denervation have been documented in a series describing muscle biopsies in 86 cases in which the period of denervation ranged from 42 days to 30 years. The following conclusions were reached:

1. Denervation leads to progressive shrinkage and ultimate destruction of the muscle fibers.
2. Up to 3 years after denervation, no destruction was demonstrated in the muscle fibers, but muscle atrophy and connective tissue proliferation precluded functional recovery after re-innervation.
3. From 3 years onward, destructive changes are evident.
4. Up to 3 months after denervation, the morphology of the distal nerve is intact, and individual Schwann tubes can be followed by their end-plates. After 3 months, these end-plates become increasingly distorted by proliferating connective tissue.
5. In the early stages of denervation, there is progressive thickening of vessel walls.
6. In the later stages of denervation, muscle is replaced by connective tissue and fat.

## Changes in sensory end organs after denervation

Sensory disturbances following denervation may be classified as follows: (1) ab-normal sensations, or paresthesias, (2) increased or decreased sensitivity, (3) partial or total absence of sensation, and (4) referred sensation, including false localization. Two areas of sensory change can be identified in the cutaneous distribution of a peripheral nerve after denervation. One area is insensitive to all forms of sensation, representing the autonomous zone supplied exclusively by the severed nerve. The second area is peripheral to this, where some sensation is retained, but in modified form. The changes occurring in this peripheral area are reduction in the number of functional receptor systems and reduction in the density of innervation resulting in sensory deficit for all types of sensation, including defective localization.

In contrast to the well-defined changes occurring in motor fiber end organs following denervation, changes in sensory end organs have not been extensively studied. Dellon and co-workers addressed themselves to this problem by studying the sequential morphological effects of denervation upon the corpuscular sensory endings in the hands of rhesus monkeys. Their study showed temporally progressive alterations in the Meissner corpuscle structure. As early as 72 hours after sensory nerve division, the denervated Meissner corpuscle appeared to have decreased slightly in size. Nerve terminals within the corpuscle degenerated within 72 hours and were no longer demonstrable by 2 weeks after denervation. Concurrent with axonal degeneration, there was loss of normally pink-staining material and loss of the normal lobular pattern of the corpuscle. This progressed to formation of an ovoid, containing interlaced blue-staining fibrils. A reduction in corpuscular size was presumably due to loss of content. The loss of content was thought to represent loss of axon terminals in the corpuscle due to axon degeneration. These authors postulated that because of progressive changes and shrinkage in the Meissner corpuscle, a certain time limit after denervation would be reached when the end organ would be incapable of responding fully to a regenerating axon. Based on their work and the reports of others claiming decreased functional recovery after delayed nerve repair, they felt this time factor was probably 4 months after nerve injury.

Sensory recovery depends on reinnervation of persisting corpuscles, rather than on growth of new corpuscles in response to a regenerating axon. This concept is supported by a study that failed to identify Meissner corpuscles but did demonstrate regenerating nerve fibers in forearm skin transplanted to the volar surface of the fingertip.

Jabaley and co-workers, by means of tissue biopsies and objective and subjective tests of sensory function (see Chapter 12), compared histological and functional recovery in patients with 26 peripheral nerve repairs. Histological evaluation of tissue biopsies included presence or absence of identifiable nerve terminals within various sensory end organs. They found no correlation whatsoever between degree and level of histological reinnervation and functional return of sensation. They concluded that factors additional to axonal regrowth alone were responsible for producing return of sensation following peripheral nerve repair.

## NERVE REGENERATION

Following division of a nerve trunk, the period of nerve regeneration can be characterized as consisting of four separate phases. The first is the initial delay while the neuron recovers so that axon growth can occur and the axon tip can reach the site of injury. The duration of this delay is determined by the severity of the nerve injury and its proximity to the cell body. The second phase is the delay associated with growth of the axon tip across the abundant scar tissue at the site of injury. This is followed by the period of growth of the axon tip distal to the site of injury to reach its peripheral termination. The last phase is that of func-

tional recovery after the axon tip has reached its termination.

The anabolic state of the parent cell body associated with a regeneration axon has already been described. Protein synthesis required for axon regeneration is believed to occur primarily in the neuron. Migration of poteins has been shown by radioactive tracer techniques to occur at a rate of 0.8 mm per day in the adult rat and 1.5 mm per day in the young animal. Though this process is accelerated during regeneration, there is a delay before the required metabolites are available for growth at the axon tip.

Of interest is the discovery of nerve growth factor (NGF) in mouse tumors over 30 years ago. It is a protein that since then has also been isolated from certain snake venoms and in male mouse submandibular glands. NGF has been shown to stimulate rapid in vivo and in vitro neurite outgrowth from embryonic sensory and sympathetic ganglia. Its mechanisms of action and application to nerve regeneration in humans remains unknown, however.

Growth of the axon tip commences at the site where proximal wallerian degeneration ceased. A growth cone at the axon tip leads to elongation of the axoplasm. Marked branching of the axon tip occurs. These axon sprouts reach the area of scar composed of proliferating Schwann cells, fibroblasts, and connective tissue. The number of axons attempting to cross the site of nerve division may be several times the number of axons 2 cm proximal to the division. Although the proliferating Schwann cells within the endonuerial tubes extend from the distal face of the severed nerve proximally across the scar, there is little chance of their uniting with the tubes to which they once belonged. As the axon sprouts grow across the junctional scar tissue, some will enter empty endoneurial tubes of the distal trunk because of the affinity of axoplasm for the surface of the Schwann cells. The rest will be misdirected to escape into surrounding tissues, or they will double back into the proximal part of the nerve.

The empty endoneurial tubes with their Schwann cell columns are collapsed. This tends to somewhat impede the progress of the axon tip, which is being propelled distally by anabolic forces in the cell body. In general, the smaller unmyelinated fibers are most successful in crossing the site of nerve division. Eventually, the axons migrate distally toward the motor and sensory end organs.

Myelination of axon branches proceeds centrifugally down nerve fibers and is determined by the parent cell. The first signs of myelination have been observed from 7 to 21 days after the appearance of axon sprouts. With the segmentation of myelin there is a reorientation of the Schwann cells so that there is one Schwann cell per myelin segment. The nodal arrangement is restored with one exception: The nodal pattern is more regular than that of uninjured nerve fibers. If end organ connections are made by the advancing axon tip, axon diameter enlarges, and the original dimensions of the axon-myelin relationship are restored.

Even when satisfactory reinnervation of an end organ occurs, histological and neurophysiological evidence indicates that the regenerated axons are considerably reduced in diameter in comparison to normal axons. Nerve conduction velocities in humans are only 20% to 60% of normal values even with satisfactory return of nerve function.

### Rate of nerve regeneration

It is generally difficult to measure rates of nerve regeneration. Most observations in humans are based on the advance of functional recovery, which includes many variables. Tinel's sign (Fig. 3-7) is used as a clinical guide to detect the progress of sensory nerve regeneration. This sign is accepted as evidence of the presence of young, highly sensitive, regenerating sensory nerve processes, which result in a radiating tingling sensation that is felt in the cutaneous distribution of an injured nerve when the nerve trunk is lightly percussed.

Many factors influence the rate of regeneration. Because the rate of nerve regeneration has been shown to be the same after immediate versus delayed nerve suture, these factors probably operate at and proximal to the site of injury. This evidence also suggests that shrinkage of the distal endoneurial tube is a reversible process and does not influence the rate of regeneration adversely.

The nature of the injury in part determines the severity of retrograde neuronal changes. Residual neuronal disturbances can reduce the capacity of the neuron to propel the axon tip. The level of the injury also determines the degree of retrograde changes, with more proximal injuries causing greater disturbances. The level of

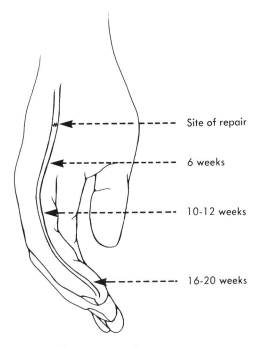

**Fig. 3-7.** The progress of sensory nerve regeneration is detected by an advancing Tinel sign.

the lesion determines the initial velocity of regeneration. The closer the axon tip is to the cell body, the faster the rate of regeneration. The rate gradually slows as the distance from the cell body increases. The rate of regeneration over a given nerve segment, as measured by a constant distance from the cell body, is always the same, however, regardless of the level of the nerve injury. The increased velocity of regeneration closer to the cell body probably results from greater neuronal growth forces propelling the axon tip distally against lesser degrees of peripheral resistance. This relationship is reversed with increasing distance between the axon tip and cell body.

Scar tissue at the site of injury also causes some delay in the rate of nerve regeneration because it acts as an obstacle to regenerating axon tips.

The duration of the period of denervation appears to have no perceptible adverse effect on axon regeneration. The capacity of the axon stump for sprouting has been demonstrated to be retained for at least 2 years after injury in humans.

Generally, rates of growth are maximal in early life. There is no evidence, however, indicating that the rate of nerve regeneration in children is faster than in adults.

Certain chemical agents have been shown to exert an effect on the rate of nerve regeneration. Steroids administered to rabbits decrease the rate of growth of regenerating axons. Triiodothyronine will double the rate of axonal outgrowth distal to a crush lesion in rats. Triiodothyronine has been given to at least 1 patient in an attempt to stimulate axonal regeneration. The author claimed beneficial effects from the triiodothyronine. A controlled clinical trial would be necessary, however, to define the usefulness of this hormone.

Because of the multiplicity and complexity of factors known to influence the rate of nerve regeneration and functional recovery, no specific data regarding the rate of axon tip advance will be presented here. The generalization can be made, however, that after repair of a divided peripheral nerve trunk, a 3- to 4-week latent period is followed by axon advance of approximately 1 mm per day distal to the repair.

## Problems associated with nerve regeneration

The problems associated with nerve regeneration are multiple. The net effect is impaired functional recovery of varying degrees following all types of nerve injury that include at least disruption of the axon. The more additional nerve trunk structures that are injured, the more impaired the ultimate functional recovery will be.

The various factors operating to produce impaired functional recovery have been described. Retrograde neuronal effects can result in impaired recovery of the cell body or failure of the neuron to survive. This reduces the number of regenerating axons available for reinnervation. Most regenerating axons fail to reach the endoneurial tubes in the funiculi of the distal nerve segment for reasons such as the gap that exists between the severed nerve ends, discrepancy in cross-sectional morphology of the two nerve ends, and the scar tissue between the nerve ends that obstructs and misdirects the axons. The discrepancy in cross-sectional morphology between the nerve ends is a result of shrinkage of the distal endoneurial tubes following denervation. It is also the result of plexus formation of funiculi, which alters the cross-sectional appearance of the nerve every few millimeters. The crossover and branching of nerve fibers within funiculi create a further discrepancy in the cross-sectional pattern of the nerve. For a regenerating axon to reach its original endoneurial tube is relatively impossible in injuries involving division of a peripheral nerve trunk.

Changes in end organs due to denervation must also be considered a factor in the production of impaired functional recovery even after reinnervation has occurred. Reinnervation of an end organ by a nerve fiber functionally different from the original, that is, a sensory axon entering an endoneurial tube that terminates in a muscle end-plate, results in failure of functional recovery. Functionally alike fibers entering other than their own endoneurial tubes result in altered functional recovery. The chances for either are great because of nerve fiber crossover and funicular plexus formation.

The surgeon can theoretically modify some of these factors by providing a better environment for healing at the site of injury. Sutures placed in the epineurium to repair a divided nerve decrease the gap over which regenerating axons must travel. Suture approximation of individual funiculi (Fig. 3-8) has been advocated by many, although others have found no advantage with this method over epineurial repair, and controlled clinical trials are lacking.

In experimental animals, nerve crushing prior and proximal to nerve division has been shown to lead to more rapid axon regrowth. On this basis, secondary nerve repair has been recommended by a number of investigators. There are, however, no

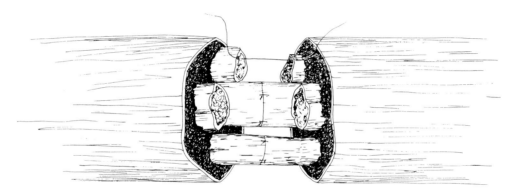

**Fig. 3-8.** Reapproximation of the individual funiculi ensures proper orientation of the nerve and minimizes corrective tissue interposition.

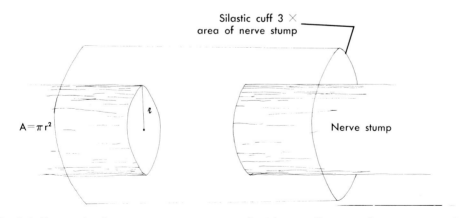

Silastic cuff 3 ×
area of nerve stump

$A = \pi r^2$

$r$

Nerve stump

**Fig. 3-9.** The proximal nerve stump requires use of a Silastic cuff 3 times the cross-sectional area of the nerve.

controlled studies in experimental animals or patients showing that secondary nerve repair is more beneficial than primary nerve repair.

Protection of the suture line after nerve repair by wrapping a cuff around the suture line may modify the scar at and between the nerve ends. It does not prevent proliferation of fibroblasts and connective tissue formation, because the fibroblasts probably originate solely from within the nerve trunk, as previously described, and not from surrounding tissues. Wrapping some type of inert material around the suture line may, however, decrease the amount of edema seen in nerve ends after injury, which distorts the stroma and aggravates the irregularity in the pattern of regeneration. Of the various materials used for this purpose, silicone rubber is probably the most acceptable because it is the most inert. Studies have shown that the internal diameter of a cuff wrapped around the suture line must have a cross-sectional area three times that of the proximal nerve stump as measured at surgery (Fig. 3-9) in order to prevent later compression of the suture line by the cuff. There are no controlled studies, however, showing improved axonal regeneration and/or functional recovery with the shielding of nerve suture lines.

**BIBLIOGRAPHY**

Benech, C. R., Saá, E. A., and Franchi, C. M.: Short-term lysine uptake in partially injured and in sectional nerves, Exp. Neurol. **23**:465, 1969.

Bowden, R. E. M., and Gutmann, E.: Denervation and re-innervation of human voluntary muscle, Brain **64**:273, 1944.

Bradshaw, R., and Young, M.: Nerve growth factor—recent developments and perspectives, Biochem. Pharmacol. **25**:1445, 1976.

Brown, P. W.: The time factor in surgery of upper extremity peripheral nerve injury, Clin. Orthop. **68**:15, 1970.

Dellon, A. L., Witebsky, F. G., and Terrill, R. E.: The denervated Meissner corpuscle; a sequential histological study after nerve division in the rhesus monkey, Plast. Reconstr. Surg. **56**:182, 1975.

Droz, B., and Leblond, C. P.: Axonal migration of proteins in the central nervous system and peripheral nerves as shown by radioautography, J. Comp. Neurol. **121**:325, 1963.

Fischer, E., and Turano, A.: Schwann cells in wallerian degeneration, Arch. Pathol. **75**:517, 1963.

Gamble, H. J.: Comparative electron microscopic observation on the connective tissue of a peripheral nerve and a spinal nerve root in the cat, J. Anat. **98**:17, 1964.

Gamble, H. J., and Eames, R. A.: An electron microscope study of the connective tissues of human peripheral nerve, J. Anat. **98**:655, 1964.

Gaster, R., and others: Comparison of nerve regeneration rates following controlled freezing of crushing, Arch. Surg. **103**:378, 1971.

Gilliatt, R. W., and Hjorth, R. J.: Nerve conduction during Wallerian degeneration in the baboon, J. Neurol. Neurosurg. Psychiatry **35**:335, 1972.

Gray, E. G.: The fine structures of nerves, Comp. Biochem. Physiol. **36**:419, 1970.

Gutmann, E., and others: The rate of regeneration of nerve, J. Exp. Biol. **19**:14, 1942.

Gutmann, E., and Sanders, F. K.: Recovery of fibre numbers and diameters in the regeneration of peripheral nerves, J. Physiol. **101**:489, 1943.

Guth, L.: Neuromuscular function after regeneration of interrupted nerve fibers into partially denervated muscle, Exp. Neurol. **6**:129, 1962.

Haftek, J., and Thomas, P. K.: Electron-microscope observations on the effects of localized crush injuries on the connective tissues of peripheral nerve, J. Anat. **103**:233, 1968.

Hubbard, J. H.: The quality of nerve regeneration, Surg. Clin. North Am. **52**:1099, 1972.

Iwayama, T.: Relation of regenerating nerve terminals to original endplates, Nature **224**:81, 1969.

Jabaley, M. E., Burns, J. E., Orcutt, B. S., and Bryant, W. M.: Comparison of histologic and functional recovery after peripheral nerve repair, J. Hand Surg. **1**:119, 1976.

Jacobs, J. M., and Cavanagh, J. B.: Species differences in internode formation following two types of peripheral nerve injury, J. Anat. **105**:295, 1969.

Joseph, B. S.: Somatofugal events in wallerian degeneration; a conceptual overview, Brain Res. **59**:1, 1973.

Kline, D. G., and Hackett, E. R.: Reappraisal of timing for exploration of civilian peripheral nerve injuries, Surgery **78**:54, 1975.

Korr, I. M., Wilkinson, P. N., and Chornock, F. W.: Axonal delivery of neuroplasmic components to muscle cells, Science **155**:342, 1967.

Lasek, R. J.: Biodirectional transport of radioactively labeled axonplasmic components, Nature **216:**1212, 1967.

Lehman, R. A., and Hayer, G. J.: Degeneration and regeneration in peripheral nerve, Brain **90:** 285, 1967.

Lubinska, L., and Niemierko, S.: Velocity and intensity of bidirectional migration of acetylcholinesterase in transected nerves, Brain Res. **27:**329, 1971.

Lundborg, G., and Branemark, P. I.: Microvascular structure and function of peripheral nerves, Adv. Microcirc. **1:**66, 1968.

McQuarrie, I. G.: Nerve regeneration and thyroid hormone treatment, J. Neurol. Sci. **26:**499, 1975.

McQuarrie, I. G., and Grafstein, B.: Axon outgrowth enhanced by a previous nerve injury, Arch. Neurol. **29:**53, 1973.

Miani, N.: Proximo-distal movement along the axon of protein synthesized in the perikaryon of regenerating neurons, Nature **185:**541, 1960.

Millesi, H., Meissl, G., and Berger, A.: The interfascicular nerve-grafting of the median and ulnar nerves, J. Bone Joint Surg. **54-A:**727, 1972.

Ochs, S.: Fast axoplasmic transport in the fibres of chromatolysed neurones, J. Physiol. **255:**249, 1976.

Pinner, B., and Campbell, J. B.: Alkaline phosphatase activity of incisures and nodes during degeneration and regeneration of peripheral nerve fibers, Exp. Neurol. **12:**159, 1965.

Remensnyder, J. P.: Physiology of nerve healing and nerve grafts. In Krizek, T. J., and Hoopes, J. E., editors: Symposium on basic science in plastic surgery, St. Louis, 1976, The C. V. Mosby Co.

Ridley, A.: A biopsy study of the innervation of forearm skin grafted to the fingertip, Brain **93:** 547, 1970.

Rix, R.: Combined nerve and tendon injury in the palm, J.A.M.A. **217:**480, 1971.

Romine, J. S., Bray, G. M., and Aguayo, A. J.: Schwann cell multiplication after crush injury of unmyelinated fibers, Arch. Neurol. **33:**49, 1976.

Rotshenker, S., and Rahamimoff, R.: Neuromuscular synapse: stochastic properties of spontaneous release of transmitter, Science **170:**648, 1970.

Seddon, H.: Surgical disorders of the peripheral nerves, ed. 2, London, 1975, Churchill Livingstone.

Seddon, H. J.: Three types of nerve injury, Brain **66:**237, 1943.

Shanthaveerappa, T. R., and Bourne, G. H.: Perineural epithelium; a new concept of its role in the integrity of the peripheral nervous system, Science **154:**1464, 1966.

Smith, J. W.: Factors influencing nerve repair, Arch. Surg. **93:**335, 1966.

Spencer, P. S., and Thomas, P. K.: The examination of isolated nerve fibers by light and electron microscopy with observations on demyelination proximal to neuromas, Acta Neuropathol. **16:**177, 1970.

Sunderland, S.: Nerves and nerve injuries, London, 1972, Churchill Livingstone.

Sunderland, S., and Bradley, K. C.: Denervation atrophy of the distal stump of a severed nerve, J. Comp. Neurol. **93:**401, 1950.

Takahashi, Y., Nomura, M., and Furusawa, S.: In vitro incorporation of $C_{14}$-amino acids into proteins of peripheral nerve during wallerian degeneration, J. Neurochem. **7:**97, 1961.

Terzis, J. K., Dykes, R. W., and Hackstian, R. W.: Electrophysiological recordings in peripheral nerve surgery; a review, J. Hand Surg. **1:** 52, 1976.

Thomas, P. K.: Changes in the endoneurial sheaths of peripheral myelinated nerve fibers during wallerian degeneration, J. Anat. **98:**175, 1964.

Thomas, P. K.: The connective tissue of peripheral nerve; an electron microscopic study, J. Anat. **97:**35, 1963.

Thomas, P. K.: The influence of repeated crush injuries on the nuclear population of peripheral nerve, J. Physiol. **201:**69, 1969.

Torvik, A., and Skjorten, F.: Electron microscopic observations on nerve cell regeneration and degeneration after axon lesions, Acta Neuropathol. **17:**248, 1971.

Torvik, A., and Skjorten, F.: Glial changes in retrograde nerve cell reaction II, Acta Neuropathol. **17:**265, 1971.

Waller, A.: On the sensory, motory and vasomotory symptoms resulting from refrigeration and compression of the ulnar and other nerves in man, Proc. R. Soc. Lond. **12:**89, 1862.

Young, J. Z.: Factors influencing the regeneration of nerves, Adv. Surg. **1:**215, 1949.

Young, J. Z.: Narrowing of nerve fibers at the nodes of Ranvier, J. Anat. **83:**55, 1949.

Young, J. Z.: The history of the shape of a nerve fibre. In Le Gros Clark, W. E., and Medawar, P. B., editors: Essays on growth and form, Oxford, 1945, Clarendon Press.

Zalequski, A.: Effects of reinnervation on denervated skeletal muscle by axons of motor, sensory, and sympathetic neurons, Am. J. Physiol. **219:**1675, 1970.

# CHAPTER 4
# Tendon gliding and repair

## FUNCTIONAL ANATOMY OF TENDON GLIDING
### Structural and mechanical properties of tendon

Tendon serves the following functions: (1) force transmitter, (2) dynamic amplifier during rapid muscle contraction, (3) elastic energy store, and (4) force attenuator during rapid and unexpected movement. Structurally, tendon consists of primary tendon bundles, which are also called fibers. These fibers may demonstrate considerable lateral adhesion, for example, the palmaris or plantaris tendon, or may be independent, as in the prime wrist extensors. Alternating light and dark transverse bands approximately 70 mm wide are visible with the naked eye. As tension is applied to the tendon, these bands disappear, only to reappear during relaxation. If human tendon is subjected to hyaluronidase until its surfaces are partially disrupted, the presence of helical coiling of the fibers is evident, as is the structural arrangement that produces a planar surface wave.

The mechanical properties are generally defined according to the response to tensile tests when loading occurs along the long axis of the tendon. The load deformation characteristics of tendon are nonlinear. Initial loading indicates a lax response with

gradual stiffening, leading to a quasi-linear relationship. At higher stresses the tissue ruptures, and the entire curve becomes sigmoidal. As the stress-strain curve begins to rise, the wave form on the surface of the tendon disappears as stress continues to increase. Under constant load, tendon extends progressively with time (creep); and when tendon is held at constant elongation, it exhibits stress relaxation (Fig. 4-1). The glycosaminoglycans are thought to be responsible for the time-dependent characteristics of tendon. Treatment of tendon with hyaluronidase markedly reduces tendon's resistance to extension. The tensile strength of fresh tendon is approximately 5 to 10 kg/mm$^2$.

Tendons transmit muscle action across the appropriate joints. For this function to occur most efficiently, the tendons are retained by pulley systems at the wrist and in the digits. Gliding is facilitated by the formation of sheaths that contain a lubricant—synovial fluid. The functional anatomy of these structures will be reviewed prior to considering their reactions to injury and its surgical implications.

### Extensor tendons

The extensor tendons are invested in synovial sheaths located primarily over the radiocarpometacarpal area (Fig. 4-2).

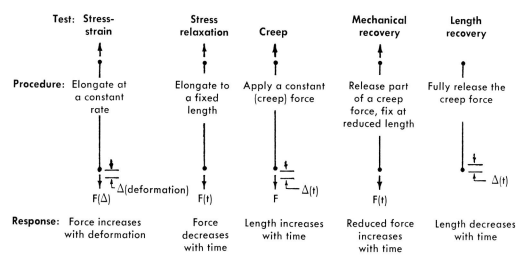

**Fig. 4-1.** Tests used to define mechanical properties of tendon.

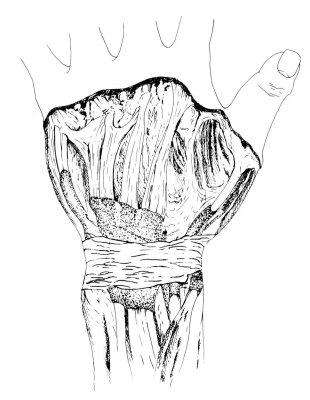

**Fig. 4-2.** The synovial sheaths of the extensor tendons extend beyond the confines of the fibro-osseous tunnels that are limited to a narrow band across the wrist.

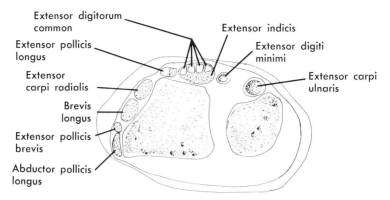

**Fig. 4-3.** A cross-section at the wrist reveals the positioning of the extensor tendons within the fibro-osseous sheaths.

These synovial sheaths are enclosed by the dense dorsal retinacular ligament that forms the pulley system for the extensor tendons. The tendons of the extensor digitorum communis and the extensor indicis propius are enclosed in a single synovial sheath that extends 10 to 15 mm proximal to the dorsal retinacular ligament.

The synovial sheath of the abductor pollicis longus and the extensor pollicis brevis extends from the intersection of these muscles with the tendons of the radial wrist extensors to the metacarpal phalangeal joint of the thumb. Individual sheaths exist for the extensor digiti quinti, the extensor carpi ulnaris, and the extensor pollicis longus, whereas the extensor carpi radialis longus and brevis share a synovial sheath.

The fibro-osseous tunnels of the extensor tendons are limited to the wrist area, with the fibrous portion composed of the dorsal retinacular ligament and the volar surface formed from the ligaments interconnecting the bony radius, carpals, and metacarpals (Fig. 4-3).

**Flexor tendons**

The fibro-osseous tunnels of the flexor tendons consist of conduits that begin at the level of the distal palmar crease and extend to the distal phalanx. The posterior

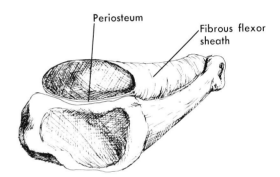

**Fig. 4-4.** A portion of the posterior wall of the flexor fibro-osseous tunnel in the phalanges is formed by the periosteum of the phalanx.

wall of each tunnel is formed by the volar plates of the metacarpophalangeal and interphalangeal joints, and the periosteum of the intervening phalanges (Fig. 4-4). This tunnel terminates at the insertion of the profundus tendon into the distal phalanx.

The anterior wall consists of a fibrous tissue covering that encircles the flexor tendons and attaches to the lateral edges of the volar plates of the previously mentioned joints and the anterolateral edge of the phalanges.

Doyle and Blythe have described the gross and microscopic anatomy of the flexor

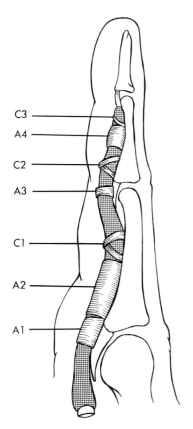

C3

A4

C2

A3

C1

A2

A1

**Fig. 4-5.** Four annular bands and three cruciate ligaments are present in the digital sheath within a finger.

sheath and pulley of the finger. The flexor synovial sheath is covered by a series of annular and cruciform fibers that vary in length from 2 mm to 20 mm. Four distinct annular bands have been identified (Fig. 4-5). The first annular band (A1) begins just proximal to the level of the metacarpophalangeal joint. This band is 8 to 10 mm long, arising primarily from the volar plate and to a lesser extent from the proximal phalanx. The second annular band (A2) arises entirely from the proximal phalanx and is separated from A1 by 1 to 3 mm. A2 is the longest band, extending 8 to 20 mm. It is of maximum thickness in its distal half. The first cruciform band is just distal to A2 and attaches entirely to the proximal phalanx.

A3 is located at the level of the proximal interphalangeal joint and arises primarily from the volar plate. This band is much shorter than A1 or A2. Just distal to A3 is the second cruciform band (C2), which is located over the base of the middle phalanx. A4 overlies the central part of the middle phalanx and is approximately 10 to 12 mm long. Just distal to A4 is C3, a thin band.

Doyle and Blythe determined the function of the pulleys by serial excision and measured the effects of resection on the ability to flex the fingertip, the force required, and the distance of tendon excursion for the digit to touch the palm (Table 4-1). It is evident that A2 and A4 are required for normal tendon function. When A4 was absent, the fingertip failed to touch the palm by 2 to 5 mm. When A2 was absent, there was marked increase in the distance to the palm.

Doyle and Blythe have described the anatomy of the thumb flexor synovial sheath and pulleys. They observed that the thumb flexor synovial sheath is similar to that of the finger. It begins about 2 cm proximal to the radial styloid and ends at the insertion of the flexor pollicis tendon. Three constant pulleys were identified (Fig. 4-6). One is oblique and the other two are annular. A1 is located at the level of the metacarpophalangeal joint and is 7 to 9 mm long and $\simeq$ 0.5 mm thick. It arises from the volar plate at the metacarpophalangeal joint and the base of the proximal phalanx. A2 is centered over the volar plate of the proximal interphalangeal joint where it is 8 to 10 mm long and $\simeq$ 0.25 mm thick. The oblique pulley extends obliquely across the center portion of the proximal phalanx. It is 9 to 11 mm long and 0.5 mm thick. The ulnar side of the pulley appears to be in continuity with one portion of the insertion of the adductor pollicis tendon.

The influence of these pulleys on joint flexion at 2.5 cm of tendon excursion was

**Table 4-1.** Serial resection determination of the relative functional importance of the various pulleys*

| Pulleys | | | | | | | Failure to touch palm (mm) |
|---|---|---|---|---|---|---|---|
| A1 | A2 | C1 | A3 | C2 | A4 | | 0 |
| | A2 | C1 | A3 | C2 | A4 | C3 | 0 |
| | A2 | | | | A4 | C3 | 0 |
| | A2 | | | | A4 | | 0 |
| A1 | A2 | C1 | A3 | C2 | | | 2-5 |
| A1 | A2 | C1 | A3 | | | | 5-8 |
| A1 | A2 | C1 | | | | | 10-12 |
| | A2 | | | | | | 12-15 |
| | | C1 | A3 | C2 | | C3 | 12-15 |
| | | | | | A4 | | 20-25 |
| | | | | | A4 | | 25-30 |

From Doyle, J. R., and Blythe, W.: The finger flexon tendon sheath and pulleys; anatomy and reconstruction. In American Academy of Orthopaedic Surgeons: Symposium on tendon surgery in the hand, St. Louis, 1975, The C. V. Mosby Co.
*A2 and A4 were required for normal tendon function. If A4 was absent, the fingertip failed to touch the palm by 2 to 5 mm when a predetermined force and excursion were applied to the profundus tendon. Of the two critical pulleys, A2 was noted to be the most important, since the fingertip more closely approximated the palm (12 to 15 mm) when only A2 was intact in contrast to a 20 to 25 mm loss of flexion when only A4 was present.

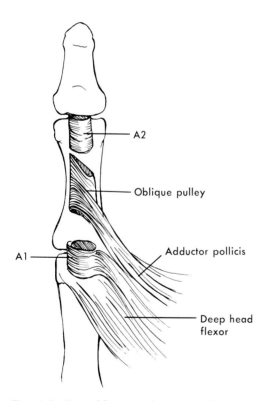

**Fig. 4-6.** One oblique and two annular ligaments are present in the digital sheath of the thumb.

**Table 4-2.** Joint flexion at 2.5 cm tendon excursion*

| Pulleys intact | | | Metacarpo-phalangeal | Interphalan-geal |
|---|---|---|---|---|
| A1 | ObL | A2 | 48° | 31° |
| | ObL | A2 | 49° | 31° |
| | | A2 | 57° | 22° |
| A1 | | A2 | 51° | 26° |

*Excision of the first annular pulley results in no significant change in joint motion with 2.5 cm flexor pollicis longus tendon excursion. However, significant loss of interphalangeal joint flexion occurs with release of the annular and oblique pulleys, although the total arc of motion remains nearly the same. Absence of the oblique pulley results in only slight loss of motion if the first and second annular pulleys are intact.

determined (Table 4-2). It is evident that resection of A1 is associated with no significant loss of flexion at the metacarpophalangeal or interphalangeal joints. When A1 and the oblique ligament are excised, significant changes occur. Movement is decreased at the interphalangeal joint but increased at the metacarpophalangeal joint. It is concluded that the oblique pulley in the proximal phalanx is the most important pulley for maintaining normal flexor pollicis longus action, and A2 is the least important.

Synovial sheaths line the fibro-osseous tunnels of all digits. But in the index, long, and ring fingers, the synovial sheaths envelop the flexor tendons from a point about 10 mm proximal to the proximal border of the deep transverse ligament to the pro-

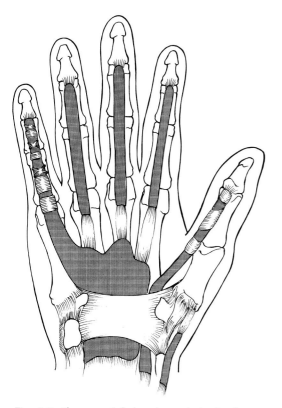

**Fig. 4-7.** The synovial sheaths encircle the flexor tendons from the level of the wrist to their insertions, except for the index, long, and ring fingers in the midpalmar area.

fundus insertion. The thumb and little finger have separate synovial sheaths that extend proximally from the insertion of the profundus through the carpal tunnel and into the distal forearm, where large proximal synovial sacs are formed (Fig. 4-7). The ulnar synovial sac enlarges to invest the flexor tendons of the index, long, ring, and little finger tendons in the proximal palm, carpal tunnel, and distal forearm. This leaves the index, long, and ring finger flexor tendons free of synovial sheath covering for 1 to 3 cm in the palm. At the wrist the ulnar synovial sheath is arranged into three superimposed compartments which maintain a common communication along its ulnar aspect. The most superficial compartment is positioned anterior to the flexor sublimis tendons; the middle compartment is interposed between the flexor sublimis and profundus tendons; and the deep compartment lies between the profundus tendons and the posterior aspect of the carpal tunnel and the pronator quadratus fascia. Thus, the lumbrical muscles are completely outside the ulnar sac. This synovial sheath arrangement occurs in 71% of the population.

The synovial membranes form a parietal and visceral layer around the flexor tendons, which is most evident within the fibro-osseous tunnels (Fig. 4-8). The parietal synovial layer lines the fibro-osseous portion of the tunnel, whereas the visceral layer is intimately applied to the tendon surface. The parietal synovial sheath layer is reflected from the fibro-osseous tunnel onto the flexor tendons at the distal insertion of the tendons and again at the proximal extent of the synovial membrane as outlined previously. This forms a closed sac in which the tendons glide. At the proximal reflection there is an accordion-like fold in the synovial membrane to allow unimpeded excursion of the flexor tendons. After reflection of the parietal synovial membrane onto the tendon, it is termed the "visceral synovium." At the

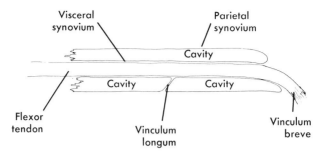

**Fig. 4-8.** The synovial sheath forms a visceral and parietal layer; the space between contains synovial fluid.

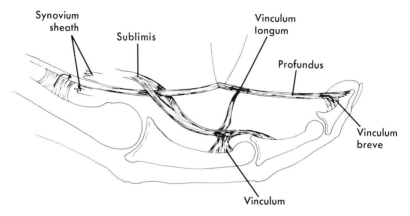

**Fig. 4-9.** Within the fibro-osseous tunnel, the profundus tendon receives its blood supply through its vinculum breve, vinculum longum, and the proximal attachments in the palm.

level of the sublimis tendon decussations, the visceral synovium of the profundus tendon is reflected volarward, forming a thin process to join the sublimis at the proximal extent of its decussations.

The segmental sources of the extrinsic vasculature of flexor tendons are: (1) musculotendinous junction, (2) paratenon vessels, (3) plical and vincular vessels (meso-tenon) in sheathed areas, and (4) tendino-osseous junction. Of particular interest is the circulation within the digital sheath.

Arterial branches arise from the digital arteries at the level of the two vincula brevia. The branches penetrate the fibrous tendon sheath and anastomose beneath the dorsal synovial lining. The vessels enter the vinculum breve to the sublimis tendon and

continue into the vinculum longum (Fig. 4-9). Thus if the neurovascular bundle is mobilized anteriorly along with the volar skin and subcutaneous tissue through a midaxial approach, the vascular branches to the vinculum on that side will be divided. If the opposite neurovascular bundle has been injured, the blood supply of the flexor tendon will be compromised.

The vincula brevia are constant, triangular, midline condensations of the synovial sheath. The distal vinculum extends approximately 1 cm along the termination of the profundus tendon into the distal phalanx. The vinculum breve of the sublimis tendon is reflected from both slips of the tendon to attach to the proximal interphalangeal joints.

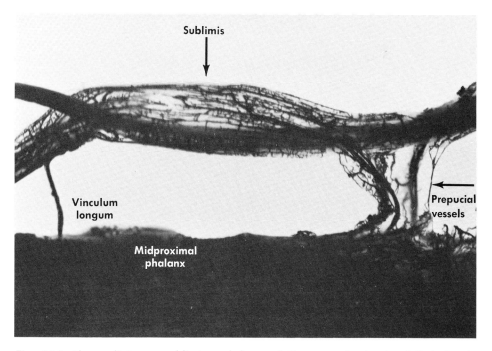

**Sublimis**

**Vinculum longum**

**Prepucial vessels**

**Midproximal phalanx**

**Fig. 4-10.** Flexor digitorum sublimis and flexor digitorum profundus in digital sheath. Prepucial fold with termination of palmer vessels is on the right. The termination of the vinculum longum coursing across inferior surface of flexor digitorum sublimis onto the flexor digitorum profundus is at the left. Note the lack of communication of longitudinal vessels in crossover area at the midproximal phalanx level. (From Caplan, H. S., Hunter, J. M., and Merklin, R. J.: Intrinsic vascularization of flexor tendons. In American Academy of Orthopaedic Surgeons: Symposium on tendon surgery in the hand, St. Louis, 1975, The C. V. Mosby Co.)

Three anatomical variants of the vincula longa have been identified: (1) a single or bifid vinculum longum that appears to be a continuation of the vincula brevia through the slips of the sublimis tendon; (2) a slender vinculum longum extending between the profundus and sublimis tendons into the area between the two vincula brevia; and (3) a thin vinculum longum extending from the tendon sheath overlying the proximal phalanx. Since the vinculum longum arises as a continuation of the vinculum breve to the sublimis tendon, removal of the sublimis tendon and interference with its vinculum breve will compromise the blood supply to the profundus tendon.

Caplan and associates studied the intrinsic blood supply of tendons in 20 fetal upper extremities and described two vascular patterns: the paratenon and the vincular. Within the tendon, longitudinally oriented vessels are present in the hilum of the tendon, in the epitenon, and in the endotenon. Within the endotenon are a single arteriole and one or two venules. There is frequent communication between the intratendinous vessels and between the segmental vessels of the paratenon. This system terminates proximally at the level of the base of the proximal phalanx where the vessels become intratendinous, forming the prepucial fold (Fig. 4-10).

The vincular system is dorsally placed in respect to the tendons and forms a single longitudinal system on the dorsal surface of the flexor sublimis and flexor profundus tendons. The intratendinous vasculature is predominantly dorsal. The intratendinous vessels in the sublimis are concentrated in the central portion of the tendinous slips, whereas the more peripheral fasciculi are virtually avascular. The main vascular channel of the flexor profundus tendon is on the dorsal surface of the tendon (Fig. 4-11). In cross section, the intrinsic system is limited to the central portion of each half of the flexor profundus tendon. The volar and lateral surfaces of the flexor profundus tendon are virtually avascular. This implies that any suture technique that keeps the actual suture on the volar surface of the tunnel will interfere with the blood supply to a lesser extent than those sutures placed on the dorsal surface of the tendon. All

vessels and capillary loops thus far demonstrated are interfascicular, and none penetrate the collagen bundles.

As a result of these arrangements, the blood supply of the flexor profundus within the digital sheath is derived from three sources: the proximal palmar vessels, the vinculum longum, and the bony tendinous insertion (vinculum breve). The sublimis tendon derives its blood supply from the proximal palmar vessels and its vinculum breve. The relative contributions of these vascular attachments to the tendon have been studied in the monkey, since the vascular supply of the profundus tendon in the monkey hand is anatomically identical to that in humans. Since the profundus tendon has three sources of blood supply,

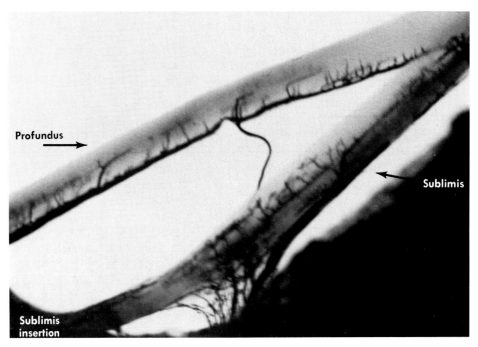

**Fig. 4-11.** Vinculum longum to the flexor digitorum profundus arising from the vinculum breve of the flexor digitorum sublimis and passing through Camper's chiasm (insertion of the flexor digitorum profundus is on the left; decussation of the flexor digitorum sublimis is on the right). Note the perpendicular vascular connections (vascular loops) on both the flexor digitorum sublimis and the flexor digitorum profundus. (From Caplan, H. S., Hunter, J. M., and Merklin, R. J.: Intrinsic vascularization of flexor tendons. In American Academy of Orthopaedic Surgeons: Symposium on tendon surgery in the hand, St. Louis, 1975, The C. V. Mosby Co.)

the blood supply of the tendons was selectively interrupted according to computations of the supply sources (eight including controls). Technetium-99 localization in the tendon was determined and charted per unit weight for the length of the tendon. It was evident that, in controls, the proximal portion of the profundus was less well perfused than the distal portion (Fig. 4-12). This distal portion was perfused primarily through the vinculum breve, while the proximal portion was perfused primarily by palmar vessels. The vinculum longum as such did not maintain the normal levels of perfusion in any portion of the tendon. Hunter has demonstrated that interruption of the vinculum longum leaves the tendon ends in this area without adequate perfusion from the intrinsic vasculature. The importance of these observations will be emphasized when we discuss healing within the fibro-osseous tunnel.

Recall that tendon gliding is facilitated by the physical arrangement of the structures immediately surrounding the tendon. This paratenon is a loose areolar tissue con-

taining long elastic fibers running between the tendon and the surrounding tissues. As the tendon glides, the curled elastic fibers straighten out to permit an unimpeded excursion. All tendons have some form of mesotenon or mesentery. In the fibro-osseous tunnels the mesotenon is represented by the vinculum longum and the vinculum breve. Outside the synovial sheath where the tendon lies in its paratenon, a mesotenon is present that is transversed by the vascular supply of the tendon.

## REACTION OF TENDONS TO INJURY

Most studies of tendon healing have been concerned with healing within the fibro-osseous tunnels. It would be pertinent at this point to make the qualification that such studies deal with healing within synovial sheaths located within the fibro-osseous tunnels. Of course, the same synovial reaction to injury would be expected in the synovial sheaths that extend around the flexor tendons into the forearm. Consequently, the primary difference in the digit is the presence of the rigid, nonyielding fibro-osseous tunnel that encircles the tendons. Therefore, any discussion of tendon healing in the digit must deal with the reaction to injury by the individual structures and finally the interaction of the individual structures when one structure is injured. Thus, we will discuss the effects of trauma in the perisheath area, trauma to the fibro-osseous tunnel and underlying parietal synovium, and trauma to the visceral synovium and tendon. The role of the endotenon and tendon cell as well as the role of the vinculum will be considered.

Trauma to the perisheath structures that does not violate the parietal or visceral synovium has no adverse effects on tendon gliding. Even when the anterior aspect of the fibro-osseous tunnel (including parietal synovium) is excised, a new sheath forms with the development of only light filmy adhesions between the underlying tendon and the new sheath. It should

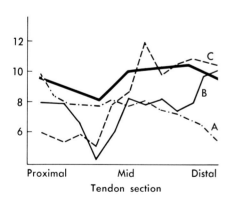

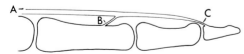

**Fig. 4-12.** Study of the blood supply, as indicated by radioactivity, reveals the relative contributions of the three vascular sources to the profundus tendon.

be emphasized that the visceral synovium was not violated. However, when the parietal and visceral synovium are lacerated, that is, laceration of the sheath and the tendon at the same level, the stage is set for rigid scar formation between the cut tendon ends and the free edge of the fibroosseous tunnel (Fig. 4-13). If the free end of the tendon retracts into an area of intact parietal synovium, the tendon end rounds off, and no adhesions are formed with the lateral walls (Fig. 4-14). The need for violation of both visceral and parietal synovium to produce adhesion formation is evidenced by simple placement of a fine wire suture into an intact digital flexor tendon. This causes a significant tendinous and peritendinous reaction.

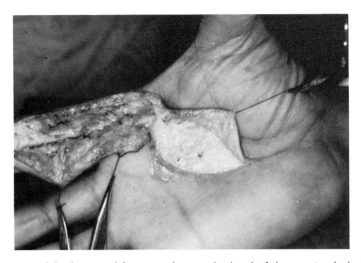

**Fig. 4-13.** Repair of the lacerated flexor tendons at the level of the proximal phalanx without proper suture technique or management of the digital sheath has resulted in extensive unyielding adhesion formation.

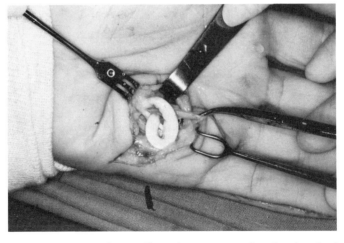

**Fig. 4-14.** When a lacerated tendon is allowed to retract within the sheath, the end of the tendon rounds off and does not form adhesions to the surrounding structures.

Since the scar that forms in the fibro-osseous tunnel can be so dense and can completely restrict tendon gliding, we must be concerned with how the reacting cells (fibroblasts) arrive at the site of injury. The fibroblasts required for tendon healing may originate from the tendon, the surrounding fibrous tissue, or both.

The flexor profundus tendon in the fibro-osseous tunnel is covered with an outer lining of visceral synovium that becomes extremely thin in the area of the decussations of the sublimis, where intimate gliding contact between the sublimis and profundus occurs. The tendon is subdivided into compartments containing longitudinally oriented collagen bundles by the endotenon and epitenon.

Observations on the derivation of the fibroblasts in tendon healing have resulted in basically three theories concerning the origin of the fibroblasts that participate in healing. One theory proposes that the tendon ends provide the fibroblasts responsible for repair. A second theory suggests that the peritendinous tissues provide the initial fibroblastic ingrowth followed later by the appearance of fibroblasts from the free tendon ends. And a third theory proposes that only the peritendinous tissue can provide the fibroblasts necessary for tendon healing.

Extensive studies of tendon ends displaced from the site of sheath laceration support the concept that the connective tissue cells comprising a tendon are capable of producing immature cells. After tendon injury, the cells within the epitenon and endotenon react earliest and account for the greatest amount of proliferating tissue. The more differentiated and specialized connective tissue cells in the tendon bundles react later. This is based on observation that soon after injury there is a proliferation of the epitenon (visceral synovium) that covers the end of the tendon and that only after 2 to 3 weeks does cellularity develop between the bundles within the tendon.

Lundborg and Rank utilized an ingenious technique to study tendon healing. Short lengths of rabbit tendon were transected and repaired. The repaired segments were placed in the knee joint and examined at intervals from 2 to 42 days. Within the first week there was detectable rounding of the free ends, and by 2 weeks this was complete. Within 3 weeks, the suture line was completely smooth.

Microscopic examination revealed fibroblasts covering the tendon ends and participating in the healing process at the site of repair. Necrosis occurred within the central part of the tendons, usually evident within 1 week, and by 6 weeks these areas were extensive.

At the tendon repair site, the suture gap was covered with a thin layer of cells, and the superficial gap became filled with proliferating fibroblasts. In the depths of the repair, no detectable fibroplasia was evident until 2 weeks after repair. It was thought that these represented tendon cells from the interspaces between collagen bundles.

It is concluded from the studies that tendon healing can occur without participation from surrounding tissues; yet the cells covering the surfaces and ends of the tendon may have originated by implantation from the synovial joint lining. However, the experiment presented above is the strongest evidence available that a tendon can heal itself.

If one concedes that a tendon can heal by intrinsic factors, the next and most important question is whether or not this healing is adequate. Certainly the rate of tensile strength gain would be much less than in those instances where the peritendinous tissues participated in the healing process. These observations, coupled with the observation that maintenance of the integrity of either the visceral or parietal synovium minimizes adhesion formation, have practical clinical implications. Verdan reported repair of lacerated flexor tendons within the fibro-osseous tunnels by using a proximal blocking needle to trap the proximal end of the tendon in the fibro-osseous tunnel (where the parietal synovium was intact). When the proximal and distal phalanges were flexed, the tendon ends were forced into apposition (Fig. 4-15). He abandoned this procedure because the tendon ends were frequently

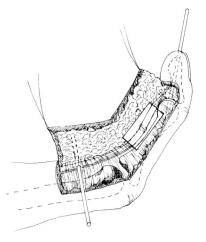

**Fig. 4-15.** Verdan displaced the lacerated tendons away from the sheath laceration and maintained this position with pins.

inadequately healed and spontaneously ruptured during the period of mobilization. The success of his technique depended on two factors: broad, firm contact of the tendon ends and minimal reaction by the undamaged parietal synovium. The technique failed because of its inability to *ensure* broad, firm contact of the tendon ends, particularly when the sublimis had been removed. Use of this technique in chickens frequently resulted in a slight gap between tendon ends, which allowed uninjured parietal synovium to become interposed between the tendon ends and to completely inhibit healing of the tendon ends (Fig. 4-16).

To ensure coaptation of the tendon ends and participation of the surrounding tissues in scar formation, he returned to the technique of resection of the sheath at the site of the tendon suture and approximation of the tendon ends with epitendinous sutures. Removal of a section of the fibro-osseous tunnel tendon sheath facilitates surgical repair and permits luxuriant ingrowth of fibroblasts from the peritendinous tissues to augment healing of the tendon ends.

The encirclement of a tendon by a for-

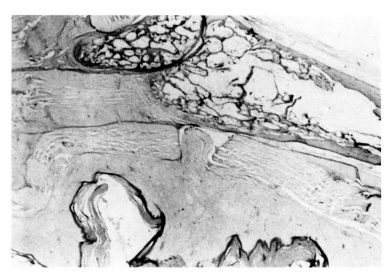

**Fig. 4-16.** Failure to maintain firm coaptation of the tendon ends results in herniation of the synovium between the tendon ends and no scar formation.

eign material that completely prevents adhesion formation noticeably delays tendon healing. Granulation tissue has been observed "creeping" under the device to reach the anastomosis. The observation that free tendon grafts completely encircled with a foreign material undergo necrosis has often been cited to support the need for peritendinous cells to participate in healing. This observation leads to the conclusion that any mechanical or technical procedure designed to prevent adhesion formation would impair tendon healing so severely as to render the method unfeasible. Actually, this conclusion is not valid, because it introduces many new variables not present in the healing of a simple tendon laceration. In the healing of a simple tendon laceration, the tendon ends are adequately perfused through the proximal and distal vasculature. In the tendon graft, no vascular anastomosis exists, so this must be established first.

The extratendinous origin of fibroblasts is based on observations following laceration of the sheath and tendon when healing occurs at that level. After direct tendon injury, which necessarily injures the fibrous portion of the fibro-osseous tunnel, cells within the parietal synovium proliferate and the distinct synovial cell layer disappears by the fourth day. Granulation tissue begins creeping into the digital sheath and between the tendon ends. Nascent collagen fibers are evident in the granulation tissue by the seventh day. The fibroblasts and collagen fibers that fill the defect between the tendon stumps are oriented perpendicular to the longitudinal axis of the tendon. Gradual reorganization and remodelling result in the fibroblasts and new collagen fibers becoming aligned along the long axis of the tendon, a phenomenon evident by the twenty-eighth day. By the ninetieth day there is evidence of collagen bundle formation. By this time, the nascent collagen in the adhesions, formed by the ingrowth of fibroblasts, remains delicate

and loose and does not interfere with the gliding function of the tendon. These observations pertain to the dog, an animal subsequently shown to react quite differently to tendon injury than humans do.

Surgeons agree that the formation of adhesions around a repaired tendon is a biological phenomenon that must be respected but that can be altered. Adhesion formation denotes extension of the normal healing process (which is occurring between the coapted tendon ends) to the surrounding tissues. These adhesions may be loose and filmy (favorable) or firm and nonyielding (unfavorable). This biological quality is determined by the associated structures injured and their individual healing characteristics that occur in the immediate vicinity of the tendon repair; for example, concomitant healing of either periosteum or dense fibrous structures induces unfavorable adhesion formation about a repaired tendon. Successful manipulation of tendon adhesions to aid functional recovery after tendon repair is facilitated by an adequate knowledge of the basic biology of wound healing.

The nature and degree of adhesions that form around tendon repairs determine the ultimate functional result. Scar formation is manifested primarily by new collagen production and organization into dense adhesions. The structural organization of collagen can be completely altered by changing its milieu without increasing the total collagen content. Examples of these structural changes associated with the accumulation of a glycosaminoglycan, hyaluronic acid, are frequent in humans. The presence of hyaluronic acid in synovial fluid may have more functional significance than just aiding lubrication and providing an osmotic gradient. When the cut end of a tendon retracts into the digital sheath, the tendon end rounds off and floats free within the sheath.

Coapted tendon ends heal within the sheath when the anastomosis is displaced

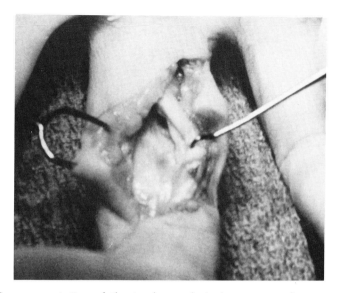

**Fig. 4-17.** Secure coaptation of the tendon ends in humans can be assured by direct suture. The synovial sheath has been excised 8 weeks after repair to demonstrate the lack of adhesions.

from the site of sheath laceration (Fig. 4-17). At 2 weeks filmy adhesions are present at the site of sheath laceration; however, the anastmosis displaced into the uninjured sheath is free of adhesions. At 3 weeks the adhesions at the site of sheath laceration become filmy. By 5 weeks the adhesions at the site of sheath laceration and tendon anastomosis are negligible.

## DEVELOPMENT OF GLIDING FUNCTION

As noted earlier, scar between tendon ends undergoes reorganization so that the nonpurposefully oriented fibrils and fibers disappear. If gliding function is to occur, scar along the longitudinal surface of the tendon must undergo a remodelling process quite different from that exhibited between the tendon ends (Fig. 4-18). For adhesions to permit satisfactory gliding function, a loose arrangement of the collagen bundles must exist to permit longitudinal gliding. Failure to glide appears to be related to the quantitative and qualitative characteristics of the adhesions surrounding the repair. Large quantities of scar, as occur

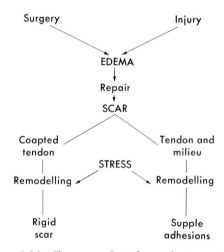

**Fig. 4-18.** The scar that forms between the tendon ends exhibits a different biological behavior than does the scar that forms between the tendon and its milieu.

after infection, can restrict motion. Scar induced by dense fibrous structures (that is, periosteum, bone, or palmar fascia) is slow to undergo satisfactory remodelling and may completely inhibit tendon gliding.

Repaired tendons fail to glide because adhesions undergo remodelling that produces unfavorable rather than favorable scar. Postoperative rehabilitative techniques are based on the concept of stressing scar tissue in an effort to accelerate or induce remodelling of the scar to form more favorable adhesions that will permit tendon gliding.

Many surgical techniques are based on the concept of preventing adhesions. Adhesion formation is a vital part of normal wound healing, and blood vessels that course through adhesions may be essential for nourishment of the tendon. Yet the clinical concept of minimizing adhesions is valid. After surgical repair of a lacerated tendon, gain of even an increment of motion is related to changes in the physical properties of the dense connective tissue around the tendon anastomosis. Why secondary remodelling of newly synthesized connective tissue in the healing tendon wound should produce different physical characteristics in portions of the same scar is unknown. The scar between the tendon ends becomes oriented along the long axis of the tendon and exhibits marked gain in tensile strength. The scar between the tendon and surrounding structures must become loose and filmy for gliding function to be regained. Possibly the newly synthesized connective tissue remodels in response to inductive influences of the tissue with which it is in intimate contact.

The surgeon has three avenues of treatment available to provide an optimum environment for the development of tendon gliding. These include: (1) biochemical methods for inducing favorable scar formation, (2) operative technique for inducing favorable scar formation, and (3) postoperative modification of scar tissue.

## CLINICAL CONTROL OF ADHESION FORMATION
### Biochemical methods for inducing favorable scar formation

Definition of the intracellular pathway of collagen biosynthesis and of the extracellular maturation of collagen has permitted investigation of the effects of agents that inhibit the orderly synthesis and maturation of collagen, the primary component of scar (Fig. 4-19). The ideal agent would be both specific for collagen and nontoxic at therapeutic levels. Biochemical agents have been identified that can modify collagen synthesis and organization, thereby quantitatively and qualitatively altering scar formation. Reduction in synthesis can be obtained by altering the synthesis of RNA or by disrupting the orderly incorporation of amino acids into polypeptide chains. The conversion of proline-rich protocollagen to tropocollagen may be interrupted by alteration of any of the five parameters necessary for proline hydroxylation. The chelating of iron, the absence of molecular oxygen, the blockage of alpha ketoglutarate, the absence of proline hydroxylase, and—most widely recognized—the lack of ascorbic acid—all interfere with the hydroxylation of proline and the normal production of mature collagen.

Only after the molecule contains a certain level of hydroxyproline, hydroxylysine, and glycosylated hydroxylysine can the molecule be extruded from the cell. The collagen molecule as first synthesized and secreted by cells is a precursor molecule (procollagen), which is larger than the collagen molecule that forms the fibers found extracellularly. This molecule contains a nonhelical amino acid sequence at the amino terminal, which may aid in its transport through the cell membrane and which precludes fiber formation. Soon after the molecule is secreted, the bulk of the nonhelical amino terminal is enzymatically cleaved, leaving the molecule tropocollagen.

Tropocollagen molecules form fibers by interaction with charged side groups of adjacent molecules. These fibers are indistinguishable by electron microscopy from more mature fibers, but they do not develop maximum tensile strength until the tropocollagen units undergo further cross-linking. These cross-links are formed from aldehydes that arise by enzymatic deamination of amino groups on the side chains of cer-

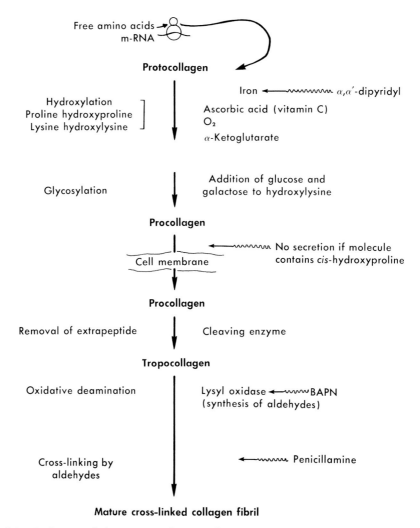

**Fig. 4-19.** Definition of the intra- and extracellular events in the biosynthesis of collagen has led to development of methods to interrupt collagen synthesis and organization.

tain lysyl and hydroxylysyl residues in the tropocollagen. These aldehydes form two types of cross-links: (1) two aldehydes can react with each other to form a stable aldol condensation product; and (2) an aldehyde can combine with an amino group from a nonaltered lysine or hydroxylysine to form a weaker, reversible bond known as a Schiff base. The number of aldol condensation products and Schiff bases in an intracellular collagen fiber gradually increases

with time so that tensile strength of the fiber continues to increase over weeks or months.

Study of the effects of four groups of compounds has been of particular interest and provides some early insight into possible ways of controlling or modifying scar formation and aggregation.

*Cis*-4-hydroxy-L-proline is a proline analogue that has been shown to be incorporated into the collagen molecule during the intracellular biosynthesis of collagen. The incorporation of the analogue indirectly produces an inhibition of collagen synthesis.

$\alpha,\alpha'$-Dipyridyl, a chelator of iron, has been used to inhibit the hydroxylation of proline and lysine in protocollagen by binding the iron used by proline hydroxylase.

Beta-aminopropionitrite-fumarate(BAPN) is a lathyrogen that irreversibly inhibits the extracellular enzymes that form aldehydes by the oxidative deamination of lysine and hydroxylysine in tropocollagen. The collagen, therefore, cannot cross-link and cannot be bound into fibers.

D-Penicillamine has been shown to inhibit cross-linking by binding to the aldehydes formed in tropocollagen and thereby preventing the formation of cross-links. It also disrupts previously formed Shiff bases.

Bora and associates studied the effects, in animals, of four compounds: *cis*-4-hydroxy-L-proline, $\alpha,\alpha'$-dipyridyl, beta-aminopropionitrite-fumarate and D-penicillamine. After inducing a tendon injury and allowing it to heal, they determined the extent of tendon gliding as a reflection of toe movement, thus providing an index of the degree of adhesion formation about the tendon repair. Daily treatment from the fourth to the twenty-first day after surgery revealed that D-penicillamine, *cis*-4-hydroxy-L-proline, $\alpha,\alpha'$-dipyridyl, and BAPN are effective. However, the latter two compounds were toxic at the level tested. No significant toxicity was observed in rats treated with *cis*-4-hydroxy-L-proline. The effects on collagen in the remaining tissues of the body were not determined. The most widely discussed agents that interfere with collagen organization are the lathyrogens. These agents—of which BAPN is the best known—interfere with the formation of aldehyde groups needed to form inter- and intramolecular cross-links as collagen matures. Since the ultimate functional result of a tendon repair graft is determined by the qualitative characteristics of the colla-

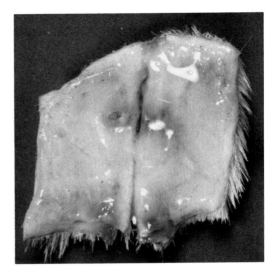

**Fig. 4-20.** The undersurface of a 10-day-old skin wound in an animal treated with a lathyrogen exhibits marked impairment of healing.

gen deposited in response to wounding, qualitative control of the scar could be beneficial. BAPN acts on newly synthesized collagen while having very little effect on mature collagen. Yet most mature collagen is subject to degradation by collagenase and remodelling by the deposition of nascent collagen. The most dramatic effects of a lathyrogen are on bone, vascular structures, and healing wounds. The effect on bone results in marked deformity of the animal. Collagen turnover in the major vessels of an animal treated with lathyrogens leads to the deposition of collagen of minimal tensile strength; thus aneurysm formation is frequent. The healing wound of the lathyritic animal contracts normally but does not gain significant tensile strength (Fig. 4-20).

Speer and associates report that alteration in the inter- and intramolecular bonds of nascent collagen around a tendon anastomosis can be produced without damage to other tissues. After a primary tendon repair in chickens had been performed, a secondary procedure—tenolysis—was performed, and the animals were given BAPN. The work required to produce longitudinal tendon motion was significantly less in the treated group. The difficulty of transferring these observations to humans is obvious. Above all, we do not know what the control values are for the development of tendon gliding in humans. Some patients produce favorable scar and develop gliding very rapidly, whereas others develop unfavorable scar and gliding is delayed or never develops adequately. And of course many patients' reactions are between these two extremes. Since the lathyrogens have a systemic effect, the results of administration could be disastrous. Biochemical control of scar formation has not been localized to the site in question, and certainly clinical use is not feasible at this time.

BAPN had one experimental trial in humans, with an early beneficial effect, but it had to be discontinued between 10 to 20 days because of fever, dermatitis, and hepatocellular toxicity, among other complications. Speer and associates attempted to overcome the systemic effects associated with administration of BAPN by synthesizing a large molecule that would remain localized and not produce systemic side effects. BAPN was linked with alternate salt and amide bonds to a copolymerisate of maleic acid anhydride, and methyl vinyl ether. The molecular weight of this compound is approximately $1 \times 10^2$. The resulting polymer is approximately 50% BAPN by weight. He has tested this polymer using the chicken toe model. Tendons were divided and repaired, and in one group of animals 0.05 ml of either the polymer alone or the BAPN-polymer was injected into the wound cavity. An additional group served as a control group. A fixed force was applied to the flexor tendon, and the degree of movement of the toe was recorded. No evidence of systemic reaction to either the BAPN-polymer or the polymer alone was observed. The results of these experiments suggest that potency of the BAPN-polymer was insufficient to produce sig-nificant biomechanical effects in scar tissue surrounding healing tendons. The failure to realize a significant effect may have been due to inadequate local concentration or local resorption of the BAPN-polymer.

### Operative techniques for inducing favorable scar formation

Failure to appreciate the significance of scar formation in the injured hand can result in impaired tendon gliding, joint motion, nerve regeneration, and skin compliance (Fig. 4-21). Tissues of the hand respond to injury and surgery (which is controlled injury) in virtually the same manner. Following injury or surgery, the wound healing processes outlined in Chapters 1 to 4 come into play and the reparative processes appear. The qualitative characteristics of the scar that forms determine the eventual functional result to be obtained. Functionally, the scar can be considered either unfavorable or favorable

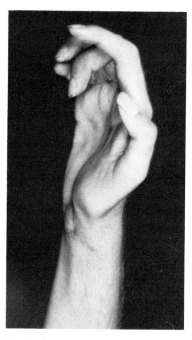

**Fig. 4-21.** Failure to appreciate the devastating results of scar can lead to total functional impairment of the hand from a simple laceration.

(Fig. 4-22). Scar formation and degradation occur simultaneously, providing a remodelling of both favorable and unfavorable scar and, ideally, functional reorganization. Through this remodelling and reorganizational activity, unfavorable scar can be converted to favorable scar. Yet in many instances this does not occur, and functionally the unfavorable scar persists to prevent functional recovery, that is, tendon gliding and joint motion.

Unfavorable scar interferes with all phases of restorative hand surgery—tendon gliding, joint motion, nerve regeneration, and skin compliance. Interference with tendon gliding results from the persistence of unfavorable scar adhesions. Scar may interfere with joint motion by interfering with the intracapsular and extracapsular movements associated with normal joint movement. Nerve regeneration is inhibited by interposition of new scar between the nerve ends, thereby inhibiting the return of nerve function in the hand. Finally, scar in the skin can interfere with joint motion and tendon gliding by producing severe contractures across flexion creases. Consequently, the "one wound" concept of scar formation after an injury or after surgery

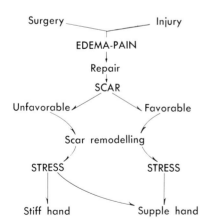

**Fig. 4-22.** Scar that results in injury can be biologically unfavorable or favorable; that is, its characteristics can determine the ultimate functional result.

has to be reevaluated. In the case of the repaired flexor tendon it is evident that the scar that forms between the coapted tendon ends undergoes remodelling to yield a rigid scar (certainly favorable for the transmission of the unmodified muscle action to the digits). Yet the same scar between the coapted tendon ends forms adhesions with the structures in juxtaposition to the tendon. This scar must undergo a totally different remodelling process to yield supple adhesions that will permit tendon gliding. Consequently there are many wounds produced by a single injury, for example, between the tendon ends, between the tendon and its milieu, between the bone ends, between bone and tendon, and between the nerve ends. Further consideration reveals that each injured structure induces the formation of scar that reflects its structural and physical characteristics.

Can we use this information to assist the natural healing processes in the induction of favorable scar? Development of operative methods for controlling or producing favorable scar formation requires recognition of the biological characteristics of the tissues that predispose to the development of unfavorable scar in a wound. A healing wound excites formation of tissues necessary for repair or for regeneration of the injured structures. For example, the fracture callus excites the production of extremely dense periosteal-like tissue. The presence of a repaired tendon within the immediate area of the fracture callus results in the formation of extremely dense scar between the fracture callus and the healing tendon. Similarly, lacerations or avulsions of the periosteum excite dense unfavorable scar formation between the healing periosteum and surrounding structures.

The dermis, palmar fascia, volar plates, and fibro-osseous tunnels (including the periosteum) are composed of dense interlacing bundles of collagen organized into a rigid nonyielding structure. Each of these structures excites the formation of scar

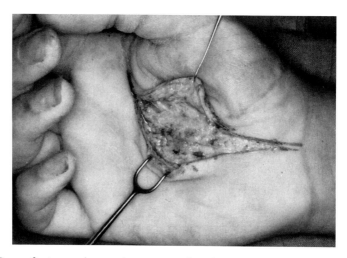

**Fig. 4-23.** Finger flexion and extension are significantly impaired by adhesions between the uninjured flexor tendons and the lacerated palmar fascia that was repaired.

that is unfavorable for tendon gliding. If tissue is deficient over exposed tendons (devoid of paratenon) coverage can be gained with free grafts or pedicle grafts. The base of the free graft is dense collagenous tissue in the form of dermis, which will heal directly to the recipient site. This fixes the nonyielding dermis of the free graft to the tendon and the surrounding structures, thus rendering free graft coverage undesirable in this circumstance. The dense fibrous tissue composing the palmar fascia is attached to the overlying palmar skin by multiple septa that extend into the dermis. In addition to the firm lateral attachments, fibrous attachments extend vertically to the metacarpals. This produces a rigid, nonyielding, immobile palmar fascia. Tendon injuries in the palm clearly injure the palmar fascia. If repaired or left unattended, the palmar fascia will develop dense adhesions between the repaired tendon and the palmar fascia. Since the palmar fascia is immobile, tendon gliding would be restricted. Let us consider the patient who sustained a palmar laceration that divided the palmar fascia without injuring the digital nerves or flexor tendons. The wound has been explored and the palmar fascia repaired (Fig.

4-23). Subsequently, the uninjured flexor tendons became adherent to the repaired palmar fascia and rendered tendon gliding inadequate. If the tendons had been lacerated, the restriction of movement would have been even more severe.

In the digit, the dense fibro-osseous sheath encircles the flexor tendons. The dense fibrous tissue forming the volar two thirds of the fibro-osseous tunnel is continuous posteriorly with the periosteum of the phalanx, which forms the posterior wall of the fibro-osseous tunnel (Fig. 4-24). These periosteal attachments—which encircle the phalanx—completely secure the fibro-osseous tunnel to bone. Consequently, these structures are rigid, nonyielding, and immobile. Repair of tendons in the palm and digits requires removal or avoidance of the structures that excite unfavorable scar formation. In the palm, the dense fascia is excised to expose the tendon anastomosis to the subcutaneous fat and muscle—structures that excite much less severe scar formation. In the digit the rigid fibro-osseous tunnel is excised when repairing tendons at the level of the sheath laceration. This is true only when repaired tendons are not mobilized early. If mobilization of the repaired tendon is begun in the

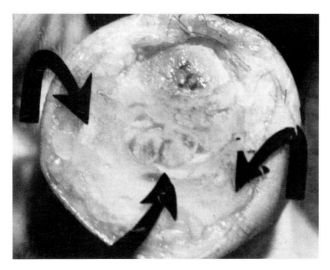

**Fig. 4-24.** A cross-section of the proximal phalanx in humans reveals the close approximation of the flexor tendons within the fibro-osseous tunnel.

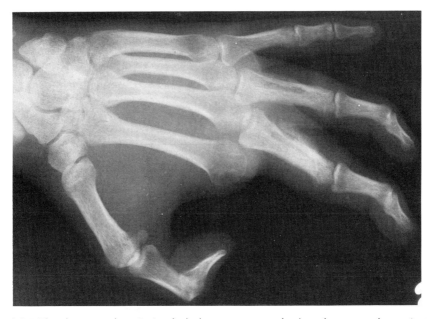

**Fig. 4-25.** The skin over the proximal phalanges was not broken; however, the periosteum was injured and resulted in callus formation that involved the extensor apparatus and prevented proximal interphalangeal joint flexion.

early postoperative period and if the sheath is cleanly injured, then the sheath is not excised; it is repaired. If the tendons are cut and the periosteum of the fibro-osseous tunnel is injured, repair may be delayed to avoid unfavorable scar formation as the peri-osteum heals. Preservation of the digital sheath in primary tendon repair was discussed earlier. Adhesion of the healing tendon to the injured periosteum results in an unfavorable scar.

Similarly, the healing fracture excites

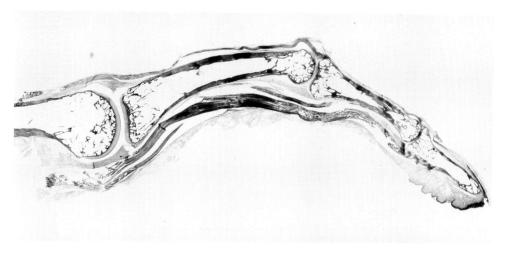

**Fig. 4-26.** Longitudinal section of human finger reveals the interrelationship of the flexor tendons to the posterior wall of the fibro-osseous tunnel.

bony callus formation resulting in dense adhesions between the bone and the adjacent structures. One should keep in mind that a phalangeal fracture that produces tears in the posterior wall of the fibro-osseous tunnel predisposes scar formation around the flexor tendons during the period of immobilization. Adhesions between the periosteum and flexor tendons can "check-rein" the interphalangeal joint and result in eventual fibrosis of the joint. Consequently, when one sees a phalangeal fracture, one concerns oneself with more than simply a fractured bone. The periosteum of the fibro-osseous tunnel may be violated; the fracture edge may have impinged or impaled the flexor tendons; and there may be associated tears of the anterior portion of the fibro-osseous tunnel. The extensor apparatus, the tendinous structures dorsal to the bony phalanges, is involved to a lesser degree because of the more rigid adherence of the fibro-osseous structures to the volar surface of the bony phalanx. Yet direct closed injury can excite intense periosteal reaction that incorporates the intact extensor apparatus into the resulting callus (Fig. 4-25). During immobilization, the joints become stiff in extension

by the check-reining effect of the scar on the extensor apparatus. A longitudinal section of the human finger reveals these interrelationships that should be immediately appreciated when encountering any fracture involving the phalanges (Fig. 4-26).

Let us consider further the avulsing injury over the dorsum of the hand, which eliminates all subcutaneous tissues and extensor tendons, and thereby exposes bare bone and joints (Fig. 4-27). The bony injury will excite new bone formation, and any dense fibrous tissue structure that is repaired in the vicinity will be bound to the callus by dense adhesion formation. The presence of dense dermis applied immediately to the bone will preclude subsequent tendon gliding through the area because of the nature of the adhesions formed (Fig. 4-28).

There are two basic tissues within the hand that predispose to favorable scar formation: subcutaneous tissue, and fat and synovial sheaths.

The application of loose subcutaneous tissue or fat onto an exposed tendon in the form of a flap minimizes dense scar tissue formation, thereby leaving the tendon in a bed of loose fatty tissue. Since fatty tissues do not excite a significant fibroblastic re-

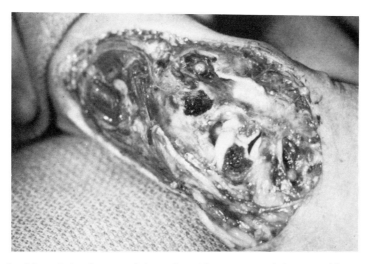

**Fig. 4-27.** Avulsion of the dorsum of the wrist with exposure of the carpal bones. Ultimate reactivation of the fingers will require bridging this defect with tendon transfers or grafts that must have an environment conducive to gliding.

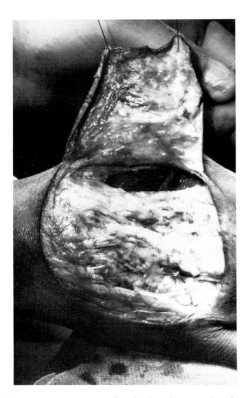

**Fig. 4-28.** Dense scar binds the dermis of a free skin graft and the underlying tendons that have sustained direct injury.

sponse, the pedicle flap results in minimal scarring between the recipient site and the graft. This is one of the major advantages of the pedicle flap. The pedicle flap does excite dense fibrous tissue formation around its periphery, that is, where the dermis of the flap abuts the dermis of the recipient site. As a result, use of a pedicle flap limits the area of unfavorable scar tissue formation to the periphery of the flap.

The deleterious effects of healing of the palmar fascia and the fibro-osseous tunnels can be minimized by surgical manipulation. For example, the dense palmar fascia can be excised in the area where tendon repair is to be performed. This exposes the remaining tissues, which are loose connective tissues and will form loose adhesions about the tendon to permit adequate tendon gliding (Fig. 4-29). Similarly, the volar portion of the fibro-osseous tunnel can be excised to expose the tendon anastomosis to the underlying subcutaneous fat that excites minimal tissue reaction (Fig. 4-30). Occasionally, tissue destruction predisposes to extensive scar tissue formation, necessitating elimination of the destroyed tissue

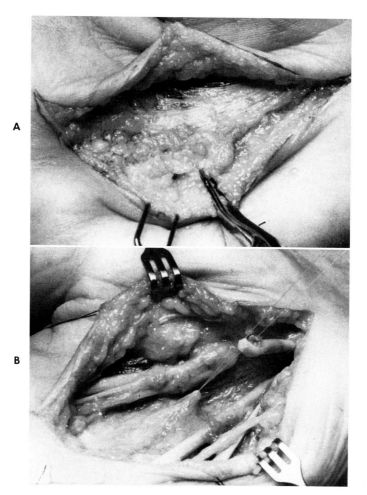

**Fig. 4-29. A,** The dense nonyielding palmar fascia is firmly attached in all planes. **B,** After excision of the palmar fascia, the more mobile underlying fatty tissues are exposed. Note the fatty tissues lining the reflected skin edges.

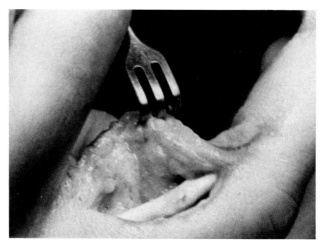

**Fig. 4-30.** The rigid fibro-osseous tunnel has been excised to expose the tendon anastomosis to the soft fatty tissues that facilitate gliding.

and replacement with tissues that induce favorable scar and provide an adequate bed for functional recovery. For example, an electrical burn through the volar surface of the wrist destroyed the flexor tendons and the median and ulnar nerves. The necrotic mass was excised and replaced with an abdominal pedicle flap that provided the loose fatty tissues that form an ideal bed for subsequent tendon grafts and nerve repairs (Fig. 4-31).

From these remarks we can develop a method for management of acute hand injuries based on operative control of scar formation. This method will be fully discussed in Chapters 6 through 10.

The synovial sheath can aid in the control of scar formation if properly utilized. Tendon laceration relative to digital sheath laceration is determined by the position of the digit at the time of injury. If the digit is cut in flexion, the site of tendon and sheath laceration will not coincide when the finger is extended. If the digit is cut in extension, the site of tendon and sheath laceration will coincide. If the tendon end retracts within the uninjured sheath and is not exposed to the area of the sheath lacer-

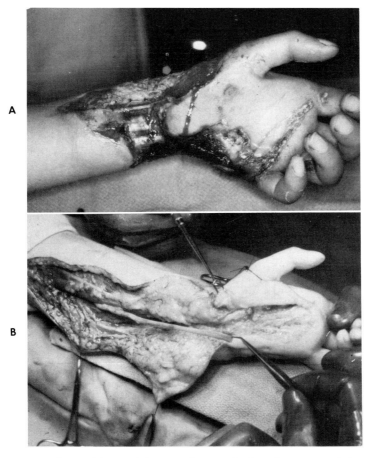

**Fig. 4-31. A,** An electrical burn of the wrist has resulted in destruction of the median and ulnar nerves and all the flexor tendons. **B,** All necrotic tissue has been removed and replaced with a pedicle flap that allows the transfer of fatty tissues to faciliate tendon gliding and nerve repair at subsequent procedures.

ation, there will be minimal reaction at the end of the tendon. The tendon end will round off and lie free within the uninjured synovial sheath (Fig. 4-32). If the tendon end remains in the area where the fibroosseous tunnel has been violated, the dense fibrous tissue of the fibro-osseous tunnel will stimulate extensive fibroplasia that results in dense adherence of the tendon ends to the fibrous sheath.

The salient points about healing of tendons within the synovial sheaths lining the fibro-osseous tunnels are: (1) a tendon cut and allowed to retract into the sheath does not swell and does not form adhesions; (2) laceration of a tendon in the distal palm may well preserve its gliding ability through-

out the length of the digital sheath (Fig. 4-33); (3) when coaptation of the tendon ends within the synovial sheath is not maintained, the parietal synovium herniates between the tendon ends and completely inhibits fibrogenesis; and (4) when coaptation of tendon ends is maintained, fibrogenesis occurs at the tendon anastomosis with minimal filmy adhesions at the site of sheath laceration (Fig. 4-34). Use of these principles can be most helpful in restoring function to the injured hand. Gradually opinion has shifted toward preservation of as much of the fibro-osseous tunnel as possible. Certainly in the patient with avulsion of the profundus tendon from its insertion and retraction of the tendon into the palm,

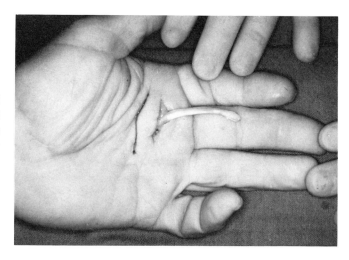

**Fig. 4-32.** The profundus tendon had been avulsed from its insertion and laid completely free of adhesions within the fibro-osseous tunnel for 6 weeks.

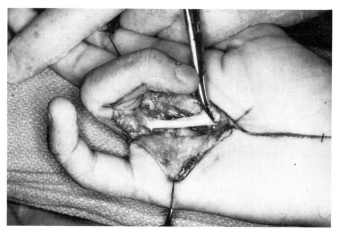

**Fig. 4-33.** Six weeks previously the profundus tendon had been lacerated at the level of the distal palmar crease. Note the unimpaired gliding of the distal segment of the tendon within the sheath.

excellent results are obtained by preserving the entire sheath and advancing the profundus for suture into the distal phalanx. Replacement of the digital sheath with prosthetic devices has been uniformly unsuccessful because the prosthetic devices completely inhibit adhesion formation, the key to free graft viability. More promising results have been demonstrated when the sheath is formed by normal biological processes. This sheath forms by reaction of the host's tissues to an implanted Silastic rod. After the sheath forms, the rod is removed and a free tendon graft is inserted in the autogenous sheath. The tendon graft adheres to the sheath wall in a spotty distribution, thus effectively reducing the number of adhesions between the tendon and its milieu.

*Effect of suture on tendon strength and gliding.* If a normal tendon is sutured using the technique of Bunnell, the tensile strength at 1, 3, and 4 weeks is 3,949, 2,045, 1,785, psi. Thus the sutured tendon does not gain tensile strength during the 4 weeks it is immobilized. If the above tendon is subjected to normal stress at 4 weeks, its tensile strength will be 6,177 and 6,656 psi, respectively, at 3 and 8 weeks after mobilization.

Similarly, if a tendon is completely divided, sutured, and immobilized for 4 weeks, its tensile strength will be 1,216, 904, and 816 psi at 1, 3, and 4 weeks, respectively. Thus no tensile strength gain is evident during the period of immobilization. If movement is allowed at 4 weeks, the tensile strength will be 4,842 and 7,128 gm at 3 and 8 weeks after mobilization is begun.

Thus suture markedly interferes with the tensile strength gain of a normal tendon and a partially severed tendon, and acts as a deterrent to wound healing in a completely severed tendon. This brings us to the problem of suture technique, which includes selecting the most effective suture for tensile strength gain and for producing minimal ischemia of the tendon ends.

*Selection of suture technique.* A study of the selection of suture material in vivo and in vitro demonstrated that steel is the strongest suture, but polyester is easier to handle. The tensile strength of any suture material is linear to the number of strands

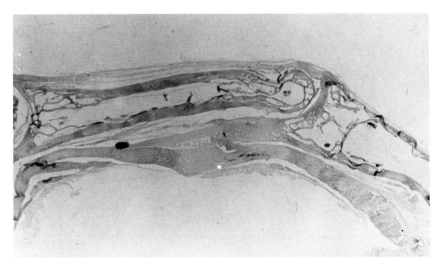

**Fig. 4-34.** The profundus tendon has been repaired within the sheath and displaced from the site of sheath laceration. Note the tendon has healed with minimal adhesions to the fibro-osseous tunnel.

and dependent on the technique of knotting. As is well known in nautical circles, a simple knot in a rope markedly depresses the tensile strength.

The strongest technique of tendon repair is the end weave or fish mouth repair, which is not adaptable for use in the digital sheath area. The Kessler, Bunnell, and Mason-Allen techniques provide essentially the same tensile strength.

*The effect of suture on gliding function.* The Kleinert, Kessler, Bunnell and Tsuge tendon suture techniques were utilized in the chicken toe model. The tensile strengths, movement of the joints when a standard load was applied to the tendon proximal to the repair site, and deformation of the scar were measured in each group at 28 days after repair. There were no statistically significant differences among the various repairs regarding tensile strength, tendon gliding, or scar deformation characteristics.

### Postoperative modification of scar tissue

Postoperative modification of favorable and unfavorable scar is required to allow function in the injured part. An ideal situation includes a team effort directed entirely toward the rehabilitation of the injured hand. Such a team would consist of a surgeon, a group of therapists whose interests are limited to the upper extremity, and a biomedical engineer. This group must concentrate all its efforts on the upper extremity to lessen distraction from other problems. This group, centered in a hand rehabilitation center, becomes an essential part of the surgical team, thereby permitting actual operating room observation and instruction.

*Effect of stress on tendon gliding.* The application of stress to a repaired tendon applies tension not only to the scar forming between the tendon ends but also to the adhesions forming around the tendon. To properly evaluate the effects of stress, we must define its effect on each site.

*Effect of stress on scar that forms be-tween the tendon ends.* Using the partial tendon laceration model, we completely immobilized one foot and mobilized the other from the time of surgery. Tensile strength determinations at 3, 7, 11, 16, 21, and 28 days after surgery revealed the following: (1) The tensile strength on the day of wounding (day 0) was always significantly greater than that of the immobilized tendons at 3, 7, 11, 16, 21, and 28 days after wounding; (2) tendon tensile strength significantly increased from the time of wounding until day 16 in the mobilized group; (3) by 11 days, the mobilized tendons were significantly stronger than the immobilized tendons; and (4) immobilized tendons did not gain tensile strength during the study.

We used the partial tendon laceration model to determine the ideal time to begin mobilization of partial tendon lacerations. After we partially severed the flexor tendon of the chicken, the long toe of one foot was maintained in acute flexion for 4 weeks while the opposite toe was mobilized on day 0, 3, 7, 11, or 16 after wounding. The results revealed that: (1) the tensile strength of mobilized tendons was greater than immobilized tendons regardless of the day of mobilization and (2) the tensile strengths of tendons mobilized at 0, 3, and 7 days were greater than those at days 11, 16, and 21. We concluded that mobilization of partial tendon lacerations should begin within 10 days after injury to ensure the greatest tensile strength gain.

Study of the effect of stress on completely severed tendons has revealed the following: (1) Mobilization results in significantly stronger repairs than immobilization; and (2) in tendons that were begun on mobilization at 3, 7, 11, 16, or 21 days after tendon repairs, testing of the tendon tensile strength at 28 days after repair revealed that the maximum tensile strength was noted in those tendons mobilized 11 days after repair.

*Effect of stress on adhesions that form*

*about a tendon repair.* Using the chicken model, we repaired lacerated profundus tendons. After 3 weeks of immobilization in acute flexion, a device was attached to the toe to apply constant stress to the site of tendon repair. Initial stresses of 50, 100, 150, 200, 300, and 400 gm were applied for a period of 48 hours in the respective groups. The tendon adhesions were tested to determine the amount of motion permitted in the toe when a load was applied to the tendon. There was no significant difference in any of the groups; the results in the control group were equal to those of the test animals.

In subsequent experiments, instead of killing the animals immediately after 48 hours of stress, we allowed them free mobility for 6 weeks. Testing at this time revealed no significant difference between those subjected to continuous stress and the control animals.

*When should a completely lacerated tendon be mobilized?* Under experimental conditions using the chicken model, we immobilized one tendon in acute flexion for 28 days while the tendon on the opposite foot was mobilized at 3, 7, 11, 16, or 21 days after tendon repair. An evaluation of tendon ruptures, tendon gliding, scar deformation, and bursting strength of the repair was made. The data reveal: (1) Mobilization results in significantly stronger repairs than immobilization; (2) maximum tensile strength at 28 days was observed in the tendons in which mobilization was begun at 11 days after tendon repair; and (3) mobilization had no effect on tendon gliding or deformation of the adhesions that form about the repaired tendon when tested at 28 days after repair.

Two camps of thought have developed regarding the time of mobilization after tendon repair. One camp recommends mobilization at 21 days. This appears to be based on the recommendations of Mason and Allen. However, review of their writings reveals that they actually recom-

mended 14 days of immobilization. Statistical analysis of Mason and Allen's data reveals no difference in the tensile strength between tendons mobilized at 10, 12, 14, 15, 16, 19, 28, 30, and 35 days and those mobilized at 21 days. Although Mason and Allen subjectively believed that unrestricted mobilization even after 21 days of immobilization "leads to bulbous proliferation at the site of union," they did not show that this interfered with tendon gliding. No randomized study has been reported that demonstrates increased tendon gliding following early mobilization. The data above reveal that tensile strength is increased and tendon gliding and rupture are unaffected, if tendons are mobilized at 11 days after injury.

Thus, the application of *continuous* stress to the adhesions that form about the repaired tendon have not been of significant benefit; however, the effects of *intermittent* stress have not been determined.

*Effective use of stress.* For stress to be most effective, it must be applied before significant adhesions form about the repaired tendon. Thus the recent clinical modes of treatment have evolved around this concept. Early motion of a primarily repaired tendon has many advocates who report excellent results. Passive motion of the repaired tendon is favored by all advocates of early movement of repaired tendons. The reason for this is that active motion is poorly controlled, and the aggressive patient may rupture the repair. Passive motion of flexion and extension of the finger has been advocated by Duran and Houser, who have reported excellent results.

*Technique of early mobilization after tendon repair.* The following method was adopted in its entirety from Duran. The essence of the method is as follows: At the operating table the wrist is flexed 20 degrees and the metacarpophalangeal joint of the finger is flexed 45 degrees. While observing the tendon repair, one moves the distal phalanx enough in extension to cause the flexor profundus to glide 3 to 5 mm (Fig. 4-35, *A* and *B*). Next the middle phalanx is moved into extension until both tendon repairs have moved 3 to 5 mm (Fig. 4-35, *C*). The amount of extension needed to produce this gliding at the distal interphalangeal and proximal interphalangeal joints is recorded.

A dorsal splint is applied to the level of the metacarpophalangeal joint while the wrist is flexed 20 degrees. A hole is placed in the nail, and a suture is placed through it and connected to an elastic. The elastic is attached to the volar aspect of the forearm dressing which thus holds the finger under slight tension. For the first 4½ weeks: (1) passive extension exercises are done to ensure 3 to 5 mm of flexor tendon excursion;

that is, approximately 30 degrees' extension at the proximal interphalangel joint and 40 degrees' extension at the distal interphalangeal joint; (2) patients are instructed to do these exercises 6 to 8 times at each joint twice daily; (3) uninvolved fingers are gently passively exercised at each session; and (4) between exercise sessions, all fingers are covered securely with stockinette. At 4½ to 5 weeks: (1) the dorsal splint is removed, (2) rubberband traction is attached to the wrist band, (3) passive motion is continued, and (4) gentle active extension exercises are initiated. At 5½ to 6 weeks, the nail suture and rubberband are removed and gentle active flexion is begun and increased with supervision. After 6 weeks, the repair is protected 2 additional weeks during active exercise; dy-

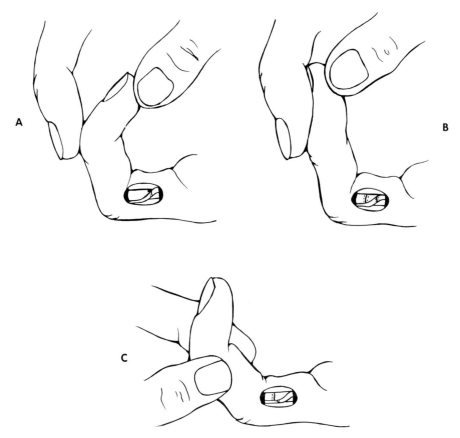

**Fig. 4-35.** Passive exercises (see text for details).

namic splinting may be initiated now, but with gentle tension only; and tension or force of dynamic splinting may be increased at 8 weeks.

The only difference in the use of active and passive motion is the increased ability to control the amount of stress produced through passive motion than through active motion. This immediate application of stress has two primary benefits: It reduces the amount of peritendinous participation in repair of the tendon (thus reducing restricting scar), and it accelerates the rate of tensile strength gain of the repaired tendon.

Between 5 and 21 days after repair (the intermediate time), the repaired tendon becomes embedded in peritendinous scar, and stress does not appear effective when weighed against the likelihood of repair rupture.

When one compares the number of ruptures during this period with the benefits of *active* motion, the ruptures exceed the benefits.

*Stress after the intermediate state.* The effects of stress beginning 3 weeks after tendon repair are well documented in clinical care. Typically, at 3 weeks the patient demonstrates minimal tendon gliding as reflected in joint movement. The continued application of *intermittent* stress is associated with a rather remarkable gain in tendon gliding. The rate of gain in movement after primary tendon repair has not been documented, but it has in flexor tendon grafts. At 6 and 12 weeks after surgery, the patient has regained 50% and 77% movement, respectively. The application of stress is useful as evidenced by this gain in motion. If the patient makes little effort to mobilize the tendon, that is, applies little or ineffective stress, there is minimal gain in tendon gliding.

Consider for a moment the stress applied by the patient after surgery. As he tries to flex the finger, stress of only 2 seconds' duration is applied, then reduced, then reapplied, until the discomfort or fatigue brings on a period of rest. This sequence is repeated many times per day according to our therapy program. We do not know how much stress is being applied to the tendon repair and peritendinous adhesions. However, Urbaniak and associates have measured the tension in a normal flexor tendon with the patient under local anesthesia both when the patient was at full relaxation and at maximal stress. In the index profundus tendon, the range of tension varied from 4,000 to 20,000 gm during maximum grip. Active flexion (defined as voluntary flexion of the digit until the fingertip touched the distal palmar crease against no resistance) recorded a tension of 500 to 2,600 gm. It is evident that active flexion of a digit after repair must be guarded to prevent rupture by the large loads applied to the repair.

*Effect of tendon tension on digital growth.* Occasionally a patient is seen who sustained a laceration of the flexor tendons as an infant or child and did not have it repaired. Gaisford and Fleegler reported two such cases. One was a 17-year-old boy who cut his ring profundus at 5 years of age. The right ring finger was 6 mm shorter than normal. The second patient, an 11-year-old, sustained a cut of the thumb flexor, the index profundus, and the median nerve distal to the motor branch in the palm. The nerve was repaired at age 8 years, but the tendon was not repaired until age 11 years. A roentgenogram at age 11 years revealed a normal thumb length but index shortening of 5 mm. They investigated the results of tendon laceration in young chicks. After reaching maturity, the chicks were killed, and the length of the toes was measured by roentgenogram. The toes in which functional tendons were not present exhibited significant shortening.

**BIBLIOGRAPHY**

Archer, R., and Weeks, J. M.: Intrasheath flexor tendon repair, presented at the meeting of the American Society of Surgeons of the Hand, 1967.

Birdsell, D. C., Tustanoff, E. R., and Lindsay, W.

K.: Collagen production in regenerating tendon, Plast. Reconstr. Surg. **37**:504, 1966.

Bojsen-Moller, F., and Schmidt, L.: The palmar aponeurosis and the central spaces of the hand, J. Anat. **177**:55, 1973.

Bora, F., Jr., Lane, J. M., and Prockop, J.: Inhibitors of collagen biosynthesis as a means of controlling scar formation in tendon injury, J. Bone Joint Surg. **54A**:1501, 1972.

Brockis, J. G.: The blood supply of the flexor and extensor tendons of the fingers in man, J. Bone Joint Surg. **35B**:131, 1953.

Caplan, H. S., Hunter, J. M., and Merklin, R. J.: Intrinsic vascularization of flexor tendons. In American Academy of Orthopaedic Surgeons: Symposium on tendon surgery in the hand, St. Louis, 1975, The C. V. Mosby Co.

Craver, J. M., Madden, J. W., and Peacock, E. E.: Biological control of physical properties of tendon adhesions, Ann. Surg. **167**:697, 1968.

Doyle, J. R., and Blythe, W.: Anatomy of the flexor tendon sheath and pulleys of the thumb, J. Hand Surg. **2**:149, 1977.

Duran, R. J., and Houser, R. G.: Controlled passive motion following flexor tendon repair in zones 2 and 3. In American Academy of Orthopaedic Surgeons: Symposium on tendon surgery in the hand, St. Louis, 1975, The C. V. Mosby Co.

Gaisford, J. C., and Fleegler, E. J.: Alterations in finger growth following flexor tendon injuries, Plast. Reconstr. Surg. **51**:164, 1973.

Greenlee, T. D., Beckham, C., and Pike, D.: A fine structural study of the development of the chick flexor digital tendon; a model for synovial sheathed tendon healing, Am. J. Anat. **143**:303, 1975.

Leffert, R. D., Weiss, C., and Athanasoulis, C. R.: The vincula with particular reference to their vessels and nerves, J. Bone Joint Surg. **56A**:1191, 1974.

Levine, M. D., Wray, R. C., Jr., Braitberg, R., and Weeks, P. M.: What suture technique should be used for primary tendon repairs? submitted to Hand, 1977.

Lindsay, W. K.: A synchronous study of collagen and mucopolysaccharide in healing flexor tendons of chickens, Plast. Recontr. Surg. **45**:493, 1970.

Lundborg, G., and Rank, F.: Experimental intrinsic healing of flexor tendons based upon synovial fluid nutrition, J. Hand Surg. **2**:417, 1977.

Mason, M., and Allen, H.: An experimental study of tensile strength, Ann. Surg. **113**:424, 1941.

Matthews, P.: The fate of isolated segments of flexor tendons within the digital sheath; a study in synovial nutrition, Br. J. Plast. Surg. **29**:216, 1976.

Ollinger, H., Wray, R. C., Jr., and Weeks, P. M.: Effects of suture on tensile strength gain of partially and completely severed tendons, Surg. Forum **26**:63, 1975.

Potenza, A. D.: Tendon healing within the flexor digital sheath in the dog, J. Bone Joint Surg. **44A**:49, 1962.

Resnick, D.: Roentgenographic anatomy of the tendon sheaths of the hand and wrist; tenography, Am. J. Roentgenol. Radium Ther. Nucl. Med. **124**:44, 1975.

Schedrup, E. W.: Tendon sheath patterns in the hand; an anatomical study based on 367 hand dissections, Surg. Gynecol. Obstet. **93**:16, 1951.

Speer, D. P., Peacock, E. E., and Chvapil, M.: The use of large molecular weight compounds to produce local lathyrism in healing wounds, J. Surg. Res. **19**:169, 1975.

Urbaniak, J. R., Cahill, J. D., and Mortensen, R. A.: Tendon suturing methods; analysis of tensile strength. In American Academy of Orthopaedic Surgeons: Symposium on tendon surgery in the hand, St. Louis, 1975, The C. V. Mosby Co.

Verdan, C. E.: Primary repair of flexor tendons, J. Bone Joint Surg. **42A**:647, 1960.

Wilner, H. I., Kay, R., and Eisenbrey, B. A.: Pharmacologic aids in angiography of the upper extremity, Am. J. of Roentgenol. Radium Ther. Nucl. Med. **121**:150, 1974.

Wray, R. C., Gangnes, R., Lowry, R., and Weeks, P. M.: Effect of stress on the mechanical properties of tendon adhesions, Surg. Forum **25**:342, 1974.

Wray, R. C., Jr., Levine, M., Moucharafieh, B., and others: When should a completely lacerated tendon be mobilized? submitted to J. Hand Surg., 1977.

Wray, R. C., Jr., Lowrey, R., and Gangnes, R. A.: A method for predicting the ultimate biological activity of scar about tendons and joints, J. Bone Joint Surg. **56**:1093, 1974.

Wray, R. C., Jr., Moucharafieh, B., Braitberg, R., and Weeks, P. M.: Effects of mobilization on partially lacerated tendons, Surg. Forum **32**:570, 1976.

Wray, R. C., Jr., Ollinger, H., and Lowrey, R.: Effect of continuous load on the mechanical properties of tendon adhesions, J. Bone Joint Surg. **57A**:727, 1975.

Wray, R. C., Jr., Ollinger, H., and Weeks, P. M.: Effects of mobilization on tensile strength of partial tendon lacerations, Surg. Forum **26**:557, 1975.

# CHAPTER 5
# Digital joint stability

For anatomical and clinical discussions, the structures composing or attaching to the joint capsule will be termed capsular, whereas those structures transversing the capsule without significant attachment to the joint capsular structures will be termed extracapsular. This discussion will be limited to the joints of the thumb, fingers, and skin.

## FINGERS
### Metacarpophalangeal joints

*Bony architecture.* The metacarpal heads are characterized by impressions that represent the site of ligamentous attachments. The rounded portion of the articular surface borders much of these sites of ligament attachment. As noted earlier, the collateral ligaments on the radial side of the index and middle fingers are expansive; consequently, the impressions on these bones are most distinct. These ligaments attach to the distal side of a tubercle on the metacarpal head. The position of these tubercles in relation to the metacarpal head varies from side to side and metacarpal to metacarpal.

The proximal aspect of the base of the first phalanx shows two volarly placed tubercles for reception of the metacarpophalangeal ligaments. The proximal phalanges of the index and long fingers exhibit a radiodorsal tubercle for the insertion of the phalangeal tendon of the first and second dorsal interosseous muscles, respectively. In the ring and little fingers dorsal tubercles are poorly defined. The radiovolar and ulnovolar tubercles are apparent on the proximal phalanges of all fingers.

The articular surface of the metacarpal head is contoured to provide mobility in extension yet stability in flexion. The articular surface of the metacarpal head describes a near-perfect circle (Fig. 5-1). Yet the cam effect of this joint is dictated by the origin of the collateral ligament dorsal to the axis of joint rotation. The cam effect at the metacarpophalangeal joint alters the function of the joint. If one plots the axis of rotation of the collateral ligament at its attachments to the metacarpal head, it becomes evident that the length of the ligament does not need to change as flexion proceeds from 60 degrees to 90 degrees (Fig. 5-2). That is, the radius of the circle from 60 degrees to 90 degrees does not change.

The topography of the metacarpal head contributes significantly to the stability of this joint in flexion. The articular surface of the index metacarpal presents a much

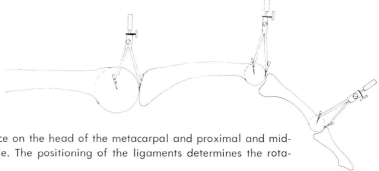

**Fig. 5-1.** The articular surface on the head of the metacarpal and proximal and middle phalanges forms a circle. The positioning of the ligaments determines the rotational effects.

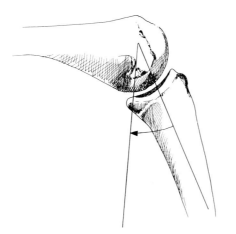

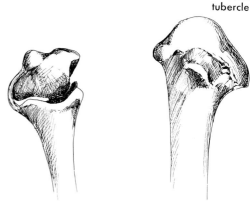

Radiovolar tubercle

**Fig. 5-2.** The articular surface of the metacarpal head forms a perfect circle. The length of the collateral ligament does not need to change from 60 to 90 degrees when only considered in two planes.

**Fig. 5-3.** The index metacarpal has a prominent radiovolar tubercle over which the radial collateral ligament must glide to allow full joint flexion. Note the prominent radiovolar tubercle on the index metacarpal head.

greater surface area to the proximal phalanx during full flexion than during full extension. This greater contact provides better stability. Of more significance is the bony prominence on the radial side of the volar portion of the metacarpal head. This prominence, covered with articular cartilage, appears to have been left over after the normal portion of the head was altered to receive the collateral ligament. As the joint goes into flexion, the radial collateral

ligament glides over the articular cartilage on this prominence. As flexion increases, tautness of the ligament is exaggerated by its being stretched over this bony prominence (Fig. 5-3).

Now let us consider the bony prominence on the radiovolar side of the metacarpal head. This ridge is most prominent proximally and less prominent distally (Fig. 5-4). Furthermore, on a lateral projection the ridge exhibits a 20-degree tilt,

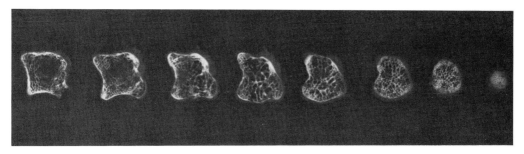

**Fig. 5-4.** Serial section of a metacarpal head reveals the prominent radiovolar tubercle and the thickening of bone for attachment of the collateral ligaments, especially the radial collateral ligament.

Dorsal

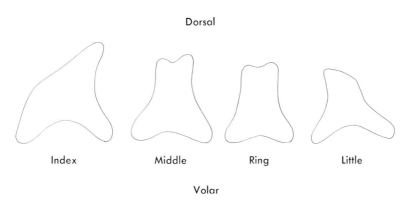

Index          Middle          Ring          Little

Volar

**Fig. 5-5.** Mapping the area of the articular cartilages of the metacarpal heads in two dimensions reveals the degree of contact between the articular surfaces in flexion and in extension.

and the proximal edge is more volar. It is evident that as flexion progresses from 60 degrees to 90 degrees, the collateral ligaments must be much longer at 90 degrees than at 60 degrees to allow accommodation of the ligament over the bony prominence. This radial prominence is much less evident as one progresses from the index to the little finger. Conversely, an ulnar bony prominence is most evident in the little finger and becomes less evident as one

proceeds to the index finger. This may explain the observation in our patients that the index and little fingers exhibit the greatest frequency of collateral ligament tautness that interferes with flexion. The articular surfaces of the long, ring, and little fingers similarly exhibit a greater area for contact in flexion than in extension. In fact, when the area of the articular surface is mapped in two dimensions, it resembles a frustum (Fig. 5-5).

In Fig. 5-6 radiopaque material was injected into the metacarpophalangeal joint to delineate the confines of the joint cavity in flexion and extension. In flexion, a very thin (less than 1 mm) rim of material covers the articular surface of the metacarpal (Fig. 5-6, *A*). The dorsal synovial pouch is very small, as is the volar pouch that is being compressed by the volar plate. Note the radiopaque material flowing over the radial prominence volarly placed on the metacarpal head. The attachments of the collateral ligaments are clearly defined. During extension of the metacarpo-phalangeal joint, the dorsal and volar recesses of the synovial capsule are readily outlined (Fig. 5-6, *B*). The volar pouch is no longer compressed by the volar plate; the dorsal pouch is no longer compressed by the extensor apparatus. These studies suggest that when the joint goes into full flexion, the volar plate is held snugly against the volar surface of the metacarpal by the taut metacarpoglenoidal component of the collateral ligament—a condition that resists volar dislocation of the proximal phalanx.

*Capsular support.* The ligaments around

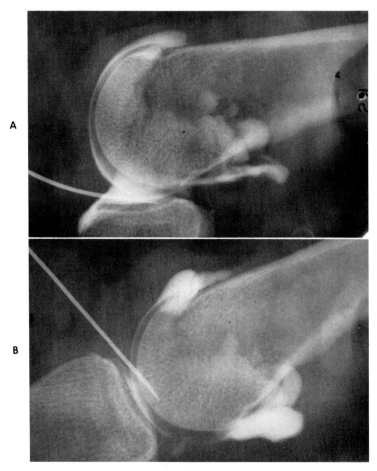

**Fig. 5-6. A,** Radiopaque studies of the metacarpophalangeal joint in flexion outline the volar and dorsal synovial sacs and the lateral extension of the joint capsule to the attachment of the collateral ligament. **B,** Radiopaque studies of the metacarpophalangeal joint in extension reveal the pooling of fluid in the volar sac.

the metacarpophalangeal joint include: the collateral ligaments (consisting of a metacarpophalangeal component and a metacarpoglenoidal component), the intermetacarpal ligaments, the volar plate, and the tendon-retaining ligaments.

The metacarpophalangeal contribution to the collateral ligaments can be readily separated from the metacarpoglenoidal component. The former is much thicker and more discrete than the latter and extends from the metacarpal head to the base of the proximal phalanx. The metacarpoglenoidal component is thinner and less discrete but extends perpendicularly from the metacarpal head to the volar plate of that joint. The metacarpophalangeal ligaments exhibit a conspicuous asymmetry within a single joint. There is a measurable variation in size, direction, and position. This variation is more marked in the index and becomes progressively less as one advances to the little finger. The metacarpophalangeal ligament on the radial side of the index is very large and strong. Its fibers attach to the dorsoradial aspect of the metacarpal head and run a lazy S course to insert on the volar tubercle at the base of the proximal phalanx. The size and position of this collateral ligament enable it to cover the radial aspect

of the metacarpal head. The ulnar collateral ligament of the index finger describes a direct course from the side of the metacarpal head—dorsal to the axis of rotation—to the volar lateral side of the proximal phalanx. The radial collateral ligaments of the long, ring, and little fingers describe a more direct course, each approaching the course of its companion ulnar collateral ligament. Yet all of the collateral ligaments of the metacarpophalangeal joints run an obviously oblique course—approaching 45 degrees in the little finger. Consequently, there is a considerable difference in the position, size, and orientation when the radial and ulnar collateral ligaments are compared. In general, it is assumed that the collateral ligaments of the metacarpophalangeal joint are in a slack position when the finger is extended. Landsmeer contends that the collateral ligaments are not, in fact, true collateral ligaments but are "oblique lateral ligaments." He further suggests that true collateral ligaments are taut in any position of the joint, provided that the joint surfaces maintain contact with each other.

One important function of the metacarpoglenoidal ligament is that it contributes to the stability of the metacarpophalangeal joint when the latter is in flexion. When the metacarpophalangeal joint is flexed and a force is applied to the base of the proximal phalanx in a volar direction, the metacarpoglenoidal ligaments become taut, thus resisting subluxation of the joint (Fig. 5-7). The metacarpoglenoidal liga-

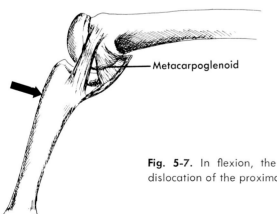

Metacarpoglenoid

**Fig. 5-7.** In flexion, the metacarpoglenoidal ligament resists volar dislocation of the proximal phalanx.

ment inserts into the volar plate of the joint, and this volar plate is rigidly attached to the volar lip of the proximal phalanx. Through this system of attachments the proximal phalanx is suspended in a sling that arises from the sides of the metacarpal head and passes under the metacarpal head, attaching to the base of the proximal phalanx.

The rectangular volar plate of the metacarpophalangeal joints is composed of dense fibrous tissue directed in a transverse plane. These fibers are more dense distally at their insertion into the base of the proximal phalanx. Laterally the volar plate is continuous with the metacarpoglenoidal ligament that suspends the proximal phalanx from the metacarpal head. Laterally the volar plate of the index receives the insertion of the transverse metacarpal ligament on its ulnar side and a slip of the first dorsal interosseous on its radial side (Fig. 5-8). The long and ring finger volar plates receive the insertion of the transverse metacarpal ligaments bilaterally. In the little finger, the abductor digiti quinti sends a slip into the ulnar side of the volar plate. The proximal attachment of the volar plate is membranous, blending with the deep palmar fascia. Thus, it lacks the firm skeletal fixation provided by the check

ligaments at the interphalangeal joints. The volar plate of this joint has a tensile strength of 5 to 8 kg as compared with 16 to 21 kg tensile strength of the volar plates in the interphalangeal joints. Of course these measurements reflect the weakest point of attachment of the volar plate. Since the metacarpophalangeal joint is capable of significant hyperextension, the volar plate attachments are assumed to be less rigid than in the interphalangeal joints where hyperextension is minimal. When the volar plate of the metacarpophalangeal joint is stressed to the point of rupture in hyperextension, the site of disruption is the proximal attachment of the plate.

Functionally, as metacarpophalangeal joint flexion approaches 60 degrees, the lateral oblique ligaments do become true collateral ligaments. From 60 to 90 degrees of flexion, the articular surface of the metacarpal head defines a semicircle with a fixed radius. Thus, one can surmise that if the collateral ligaments permit 60 degrees of flexion, they should be long enough to permit 90 degrees of flexion. Closer examination of the topography of the metacarpal head will reveal that this conclusion is inaccurate, as will be discussed later. In the fully flexed position, abduction is no longer possible and only slight rotation is allowed.

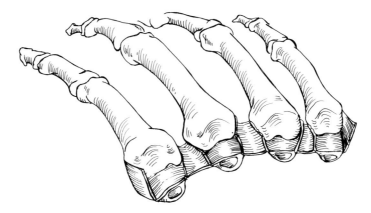

**Fig. 5-8.** The intermetacarpal ligaments attach to the volar plates, which in turn receive attachments laterally from the abductor digiti quinti and first dorsal interosseous muscles.

In this position of flexion these restraints to movement, other than flexion-extension, are provided by the collateral ligaments.

These observations support the concept that the metacarpophalangeal joint is tri-axial. Movement at this joint includes extension-flexion and abduction-adduction. Even though pure rotation is impossible, rotation can be accomplished through flexion and abduction of the joint. Adduction-abduction is possible only in the extended position because the collateral ligaments are slack in this position.

There are three intermetacarpal ligaments that interconnect the volar plates of the metacarpophalangeal joints in the fingers (Fig. 5-9). These broad flat ligaments, several millimeters wide, are placed transversely in the same plane as the volar plates into which they insert. It has been suggested that the ligaments are inappropriately named because the ligaments insert into the volar plates that are attached directly to the proximal phalanx. Yet the volar plate does attach to the metacarpal both through the metacarpoglenoid ligament and through less well-defined proximal attachments.

In the little finger the ulnar border of the volar plate receives an insertion of the abductor digiti quinti muscle. When the metacarpophalangeal joints have lost some of their inherent stability, as in rheumatoid arthritis, this structural arrangement predisposes to ulnar drift of all of the phalanges if the abductor digiti quinti muscle becomes spastic or shortened. The intermetacarpal ligament functions to limit lateral spread of the fingers and provide stability to the fingers. These ligaments provide a fulcrum for the lumbrical muscles as they course dorsally. The tendon-retaining ligaments will be discussed with the extracapsular tendon descriptions.

*Locking of the metacarpophalangeal joints.* Occasionally when doing a simple task, a finger will lock in flexion at the metacarpophalangeal joint. The locking phenomenon may disappear, only to reappear with increasing frequency. Examination reveals the metacarpophalangeal joint cannot be extended through the final 30 to 40 degrees to reach full extension, but flexion is normal. The proximal interphalangeal and the distal interphalangeal

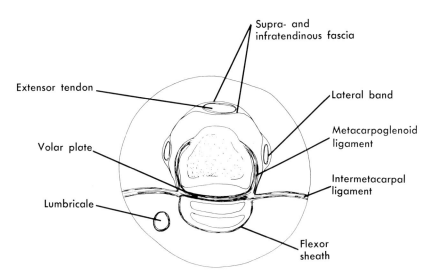

**Fig. 5-9.** A cross-section at the level of the metacarpophalangeal joint reveals the ligamentous attachments to the volar plate.

joints have a normal range of flexion and extension.

A ligamentous structure impaled or restricted from a normal range of motion by a bony prominence causes locking of a metacarpophalangeal joint in extension. The bony prominence may be either a normal but exaggerated volar-lateral tubercle on the metacarpal head or an osteophyte associated with degenerative disease. The normal but exaggerated volar-lateral prominence can result in locking if a portion of the accessory collateral ligament develops a band that will not glide over the metacarpal head during extension. At 30 to 40 degrees' loss of extension, the most proximal of the accessory collateral ligament fibers will abut the most prominent edge of the lateral-volar tubercle. Anatomically the lateral-volar tubercle describes a smooth, gradually enlarging arch when approached from its distal surface. The more prominent proximal edge is the site of ligamentous arrest. The index finger is always involved. Patients are young, ranging from 20 to 47 years.

Other causes of locking are as follows: (1) A sesamoid, present in the volar plate in 64% of hands, catches proximal to the volar ridge on the radial side of the index metacarpal head; (2) the index metacarpal head has a large bony prominence; or (3) the normal concavity of the palm exaggerates the prominence of the index metacarpal head.

A bony prominence produced by degenerative changes can be anywhere on the metacarpal head. If the bony prominence is on the volar surface on the metacarpal neck just proximal to the cartilage edge, the volar plate may be impaled and extension restricted. If the bony prominence is on the lateral surface, the collateral or accessory collateral ligament may be impaled. Actually it is the cuff formed by the accessory collateral ligaments that catches on osteophytes in this group. These osteophytes have been identified as etiologic agents in 11 of 24 cases reviewed with locking of the metacarpophalangeal joint. The 11 patients ranged in age from 47 to 83 years. The frequency of digit involvement for the index, long, ring, and little fingers was 0, 8, 2, and 1, respectively.

TREATMENT. Because spontaneous recovery has been reported (Aston, 1960), it is essential to observe the patient for 4 to 6 weeks depending on the patient's particular problem. Manipulation is usually ineffective and can result in fracture, for instance, of the head of the metacarpal.

Harvey reports two cases requiring surgery. In one, the capsule of the metacarpophalangeal joint was opened, and a prominent fold running proximally from the volar plate to the lateral side of the metacarpal head was noted. This fold was caught over the proximal side of the bony prominence on the anterolateral aspect of the metacarpal condyle. Division of the capsule (band) released the tension and permitted full extension. The bony prominence was removed. In the second patient a posterior incision was made; however, exposure was inadequate and the incision had to be continued into the palm to permit release of the joint capsule. When this occurs, a volar incision is recommended to facilitate division of the accessory collateral ligament from the volar plate on the radial side of the joint. If osteophytes are present, they may be removed. Surgery in this group is directed to the release of the taut band and/or excision of the bony prominence.

*Extracapsular support.* The intrinsic muscles of the hand can be classified into dorsal and volar interossei, lumbrical, and hypothenar and thenar muscles.

The dorsal interossei arise from the shafts of the metacarpals and are positioned dorsal to the axis of the hand. There are four. Each muscle arises from two muscle bellies attached to adjacent metacarpals. The first dorsal interosseous muscle is composed of a superficial and a deep muscle belly. The deep muscle belly arises from the radial side of the index metacarpal and terminates in a broad tendon that extends dorsally and obliquely to insert into the transverse lamina of the extensor apparatus. The superficial belly of the first dorsal interosseous muscle arises from adjacent sides of the thumb and index metacarpals and forms a single tendon. This tendon inserts into a tubercle at the base of the proximal phalanx. Thus, the tendon of the superficial belly is covered laterally by the tendon of the deep belly. The most volarward fibers of this lateral tendon and the fibers of the transverse lamina join the metacarpoglenoidal ligament to insert into the volar plate of the index metacarpophalangeal joint. As a consequence of these attachments, only a few fibers of the first dorsal interosseous muscle radiate into the radial wing of the extensor aponeurosis. This radial wing does receive fibers from the well-developed lumbrical of the index.

The second dorsal interosseous muscle, located on the radial side of the long finger, arises from two muscle bellies. The superficial belly arises from the adjacent sides of the long and index metacarpals. The tendon formed by these superficial bellies passes medial to the transverse lamina to insert into the tubercle at the base of the proximal phalanx. The deep belly arises from the radial side of the long finger metacarpal. Its tendon is positioned lateral to the transverse lamina and inserts into the wing of the extensor assembly. Certainly notable variations in these insertions are the rule rather than the exception.

The third dorsal interosseous muscle arises from a single muscle belly that usually forms a single tendon. Most frequently this single tendon passes lateral to the transverse lamina and inserts primarily into the wing of the extensor apparatus. Occasionally two tendons are evident, a deeper tendon lying medial to the transverse lamina and inserting into the wing of the extensor apparatus and a superficial tendon

forming the superficial layer of the wing. Consequently, when two tendons are present, the transverse lamina is encircled by both the superficial and deep tendons, and both tendons eventually insert into the wing of the extensor apparatus.

The fourth dorsal interosseous muscle is composed of superficial and deep bellies. The superficial belly arises from the adjacent sides of the ring and little finger metacarpals. The deep belly arises from the ulnar side of the ring metacarpal; its arrangement of insertion is similar to that described for the second dorsal interosseous muscle.

There are three volar interosseous muscles. The first volar interosseous muscle arises from adjacent sides of the index and long metacarpals and inserts into the base of the ulnar side of the proximal phalanx of the index finger. The second arises from the long and ring metacarpals and inserts into the radial side of the proximal phalanx of the ring finger. The third volar interosseous muscle arises from the ring and little finger metacarpals and inserts into the radial side of the proximal phalanx of the little finger. These tendons do not pass medial to the transverse lamina. They may participate to a variable degree in the transverse lamina or may contribute entirely to the wing portion of the extensor apparatus.

In summary, the insertions of the interossei onto the proximal phalanges are limited to the radial side of the index phalanx, the radial side of the long finger phalanx, the ulnar side of the ring phalanx, and the ulnar side of the little finger phalanx. In the little finger, the abductor digiti quinti inserts primarily into the base of the proximal phalanx. These dorsal and volar interosseous tendons are located dorsal to the deep transverse metacarpal ligament.

The range and power of lateral movement of the fingers was reported by Matheson and associates. The total range of lateral motion (obtained by adding maximum convergence and divergence of the proximal phalanx) at the metacarpophalangeal joint of the little, ring, long, and index fingers was 42, 17, 0.2, and 26 degrees, respectively. As suspected, the border digits showed the greatest range of motion, whereas the long digit had minimal lateral deviation at the metacarpophalangeal joint.

When the relative strengths of the fingers in lateral deviation were tested, the little, ring, long, and index fingers had an average thrust of 658, 357, 459 and 807 gm, respectively. Again, the border digits with the greater muscle masses showed the greatest strength.

The extensor communis tendon inserts on the proximal phalanx by a slip of tendon extending from the deep surface of the extensor tendon to the capsule of the metacarpophalangeal joint and the proximal part of the proximal phalanx. The deep layer of the tendon fuses with the distal part of the capsule to insert on the proximal phalanx through the capsular insertion. This insertion becomes taut by proximal displacement of the extensor aponeurosis when the interphalangeal joints are extended. Flexion of the interphalangeal joints results in relaxation of this attachment.

The sagittal bands arise from the transverse metacarpal ligament and terminate on the lateral border of the extensor tendon; some fibers pass over the dorsal surface and fuse with those of the other side. The proximal border of the bands is free, whereas the distal border is intimately associated with the aponeurotic expansion of the interossei with which it is often fused. In some cases, the aponeurotic expansion travels in the same tunnel as the phalangeal expansion. The sagittal bands stabilize the extensor communis tendon as it passes over the metacarpophalangeal joint, limit the excursion of the tendon, and form tunnels for passage of the interosseous expansions.

The interosseous aponeurotic expansions are formed on the radial side of the finger by the palmar interosseous and on the ulnar side by the volar part of the dorsal interosseous. On the radial side, this is reinforced by the lumbrical.

At the level of the midportion of the proximal phalanx, the extensor tendon divides into three bands—a medial extensor band and two lateral extensor bands (Fig. 5-10). The interosseous tendon from the interosseous muscles forms a fan in which three parts may be discerned. A lateral interosseous band is evident, which joins the lateral extensor tendon band. The lateral extensor bands cross the proximal interphalangeal joint and merge over the middle phalanx to form the terminal extensor tendon. On the radial side of the fingers, this interosseous lateral band is joined by the lumbrical tendon after it crosses the transverse metacarpal ligament. A medial interosseous band is discernible; this band joins the medial extensor band to form the medial extensor tendon. The medial extensor tendon inserts into the base of the middle phalanx. Finally, the terminal tendon is joined by the retinacular ligament that originates from the fibro-osseous tunnel at the level of the distal portion of the proximal phalanx. This ligament passes lateral to the proximal interphalangeal joint to insert into the lateral extensor tendon and then into the terminal extensor tendon. A transverse band covers the terminal tendon and attaches to the volar tendon sheath. The third contribution of the interosseous tendon is the interosseous hood that inserts into the extensor tendon at right angles over the metacarpophalangeal joint. Duchenne showed that the insertions of the interosseous muscle involve division of the whole muscle into two major independent actions, one as abductor of the finger, the other as extensor of the distal and middle phalanges and as flexor of the proximal phalanx.

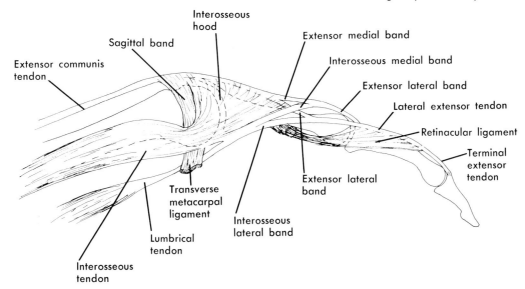

**Fig. 5-10.** The components of the extensor apparatus are represented schematically. (After Tubiana, R., and Valentin, P.: Surg. Clin. North Am. **44**:897, 1964.)

The extensor tendons are encircled by the infratendinous and supratendinous fascia. The infratendinous fascia extends across the metacarpophalangeal joint but can be separated from the joint capsule. This fascial layer inserts into the dorsal edge of the base of the proximal phalanx, where it fuses with the periosteum of the proximal phalanx. Distally, this layer is positioned beneath the transverse lamina of the extensor apparatus. Here it may fuse with the transverse lamina or may remain surrounded by loose connective tissue. The extensor tendon lies free over the infratendinous fascia with this loose connective tissue intervening.

The wing of the extensor apparatus is anchored to the deep transverse ligament by fibers either inserting into the deep part of the wing or forming a sling around the interosseous tendon. The interosseous tendon, which is positioned lateral to the transverse lamina, has to pierce it to gain access to the tubercle at the base of the phalanx. This perforation occurs either at the proximal border of the transverse lamina or within the lamina proper.

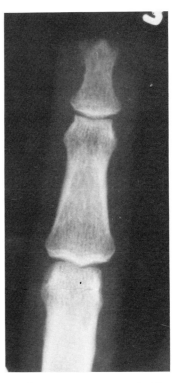

**Fig. 5-11.** The prominent central ridge of the base of the middle phalanx articulates with a central depression in the head of the proximal phalanx.

### Proximal interphalangeal joint

*Bony architecture.* The proximal interphalangeal joint is a hinge joint; that is, it permits movement—flexion and extension —in only one plane. Topographically, the head of the proximal phalanx presents two condyles separated by a deep cleft (Fig. 5-11). One condyle is slightly more prominent than its companion. The articular surface is broad and presents less change in surface area in extension and flexion than noted in the metacarpal. The base of the middle phalanx presents a mirror image of the head of the proximal phalanx; it presents two concave surfaces separated by a prominent central ridge. This ridge is concave in a lateral plane and convex in the anteroposterior plane. This architectural arrangement predisposes to lateral stability.

*Capsular support.* The ligaments around this joint include the collateral ligament, the volar plate, and the insertion of the medial extensor tendon into the dorsal lip of the base of the middle phalanx.

Each collateral ligament of this joint can be divided into three parts, a triangular ligamentous band immediately above and a fan-shaped ligament immediately below the true collateral ligament (Fig. 5-12). The true collateral ligament arises from a recess on the lateral surface of the head of the proximal phalanx and inserts into the lateral tubercle on the laterovolar surface of the base of the middle phalanx. In full extension the true collateral ligaments lie just dorsal to the apex of angulation of the head of the proximal phalanx. Kuczynski has described attachment of some of the lower fibers of the collateral ligaments to the palmar tubercle of the middle phalanx. Occasionally fibers from the flexor sheath were also noted to attach to this palmar tubercle. If the joint capsule is exposed and those fibers attaching to the palmar tubercle are divided, 20 to 25 degrees of hyperextension is demonstrable. At this point, further hyperextension is prevented by the volar plate.

The volar plate of the proximal interphalangeal joint is composed of dense fibrous tissue with extensive attachments along the entire volar lip of the base of the middle phalanx. Proximally, the volar plate presents two rigid lateral projections that are firmly attached to the laterovolar edges of the proximal phalanx (Fig. 5-13). Centrally, the proximal portion of the volar plate forms a free edge. More proximally, the periosteum of the proximal phalanx contributes to the formation of the fibro-osseous tunnel. An opening several millimeters in size separates the periosteum participating in the fibro-osseous tunnel from the proximal insertion

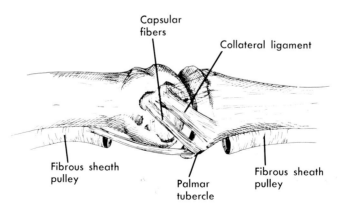

**Fig. 5-12.** The palmar tubercle of the middle phalanx receives fibers from the proper collateral ligament and from the proximal portion of the fibro-osseous tunnel.

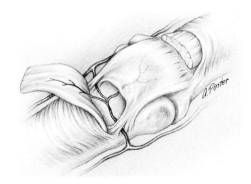

**Fig. 5-13.** The lateral edges of the proximal interphalangeal joint volar plate form two distinct bands that attach to the proximal phalanx and prevent hyperextension of the joint.

of the volar plate. Through this opening, the digital vessels send branches to the vinculum breve of the sublimis and the vinculum longum of the profundus tendons.

During flexion the volar synovial pouch located in the midaxial line of the finger can expand around the free proximal edge of the lax volar plate. Injection studies suggest that the vincula brevia are pulling the synovial pouch proximally to prevent their becoming trapped in the joint when extension is initiated (Fig. 5-14, *A*). It should be noted that in flexion the dorsal synovial pouch is compressed by the ex-

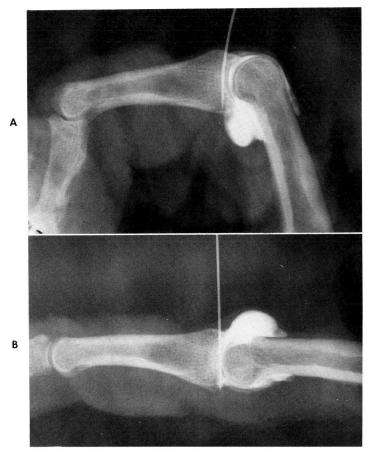

**Fig. 5-14. A,** A radiopaque study of the proximal interphalangeal joint in flexion reveals a large volar synovial sac. **B,** A radiopaque study of the proximal interphalangeal joint in extension reveals the extent and dimensions of the dorsal sac.

tensor apparatus. When the proximal interphalangeal joint is extended, the volar synovial pouch is compressed by the taut volar plate and flexor tendons, thus forcing the radiopaque material into the dorsal synovial pouch (Fig. 5-14, *B*).

The strength of this volar plate has been demonstrated in vitro. Moberg and Stener recorded a bursting strength of 19 kg in the volar plate of the proximal interphalangeal joint of the finger as compared with 6 kg in the volar plate of the metacarpophalangeal joint of the finger. The strength of this proximal attachment of the volar plate to the proximal interphalangeal joint is attested to by the fact that all ruptures of the volar plate occurred at the distal attachment to the base of the middle phalanx. When the volar plate is detached from the proximal or middle phalanx, hyperextension of the proximal interphalangeal joint is readily accomplished even with collateral ligaments intact.

***Extracapsular support.*** The sublimis and profundus tendons bridge the volar surface of the joint capsule but do not contribute fibers to the capsule. On the dorsal surface the interosseous medial band joins the extensor medial band. These two bands form the extensor medial tendon, which crosses the proximal interphalangeal joint before the tendon inserts into the dorsum of the base of the middle phalanx.

Laterally, the lumbrical tendon and interosseous tendon contribute to the interosseous lateral band, which unites with the extensor lateral band and crosses the proximal interphalangeal joint to receive fibers from the oblique retinacular ligament. The oblique retinacular ligament is composed of fibers extending from the flexor sheath (at the level of the distal third of the proximal phalanx) across the proximal interphalangeal joint to insert into the lateral extensor tendon.

Cleland's ligament arises from the edge of the osseous reflection of the flexor tendon sheath and extends laterally to the digital fascia (Fig. 5-15). During its distal migration the ligament is windowed to

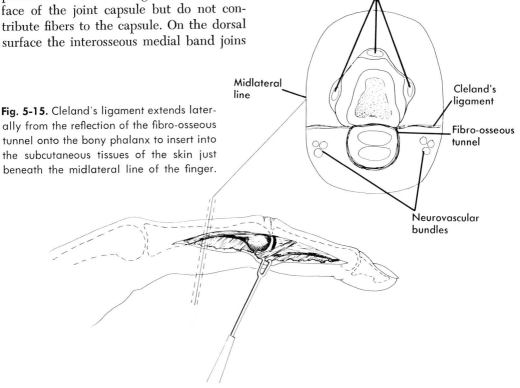

**Fig. 5-15.** Cleland's ligament extends laterally from the reflection of the fibro-osseous tunnel onto the bony phalanx to insert into the subcutaneous tissues of the skin just beneath the midlateral line of the finger.

permit the volar to dorsal course of the oblique retinacular ligament. The neurovascular bundles are volar to Cleland's ligament.

As a result of the tendinous and ligamentous structures bridging this hinge joint, its stability is further augmented.

### Distal interphalangeal joint

*Bony architecture.* The articular surface of the middle phalanx describes a perfect circle. The joint is a hinge joint, permitting only flexion and extension. The head of the middle phalanx presents two equally prominent condyles separated by a shallow cleft. The articular surface is broad, presenting the same surface area to the distal phalanx in extension and in flexion. The base of the distal phalanx presents an almost oval articular surface to the head of the middle phalanx. The central ridge between the two lateral recesses that receive the condyles is more apparent than real. This results from the volar and dorsal lipping of the distal phalanx, which is most prominent in the midaxial line.

*Capsular support.* This includes the collateral ligaments, the volar plate, an extensive dorsal and volar synovial pouch, and the terminal extensor tendon. The collateral ligaments are short and thick, extending obliquely across the axis of rotation of the joint. The ligament arises from a depression on the lateral side of the head

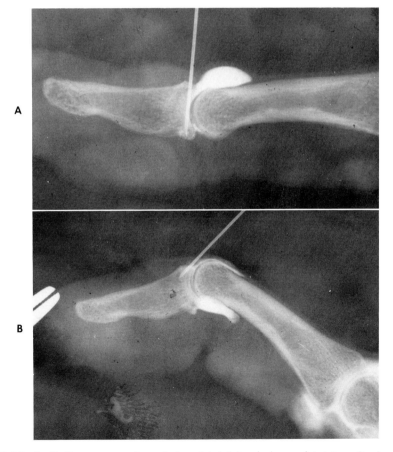

**Fig. 5-16. A,** Radiopaque studies of the distal interphalangeal joint cavity in extension reveal the proximal extension of the dorsal sac. **B,** Radiopaque studies of the distal interphalangeal joint in flexion reveal the proximal extent of the volar synovial sac.

of the middle phalanx and inserts into the prominent tubercle in the midlateral position of the distal phalanx. The more volar portion of this ligament extends obliquely to insert into the lateral edge of the volar plate. Distally, the volar plate attaches to the width of the volar edge of the base of the distal phalanx. Proximally, the volar plate inserts into the laterovolar ridge of the middle phalanx. The volar plate of the distal interphalangeal joint allows greater hyperextension than is possible at the proximal interphalangeal joint.

The terminal extensor tendon inserts into a ridge across the dorsum of the distal phalanx. One border of this ridge is the articular cartilage of the distal phalanx. Of necessity, a fracture of the dorsal ridge —for example, avulsion of the insertion of the terminal extensor tendon and a portion of its bony attachments—produces an intra-articular fracture.

Injection of radiopaque material into the distal interphalangeal joint reveals the large dorsal synovial sac when the joint is in extension (Fig. 5-16, *A*). When the joint is flexed, this radiopaque material is forced volarward to outline the large volar synovial sac, which extends 5 mm proximally (Fig. 5-16, *B*).

The compactness of the ligamentous structures and the major tendon insertion at or near the joint contributes to the notable stability of the distal interphalangeal joint.

*Extracapsular support.* The flexor profundus tendon inserts just distal to the insertion of the volar plate. A roughened triangular depression in the distal phalanx receives the insertion of the profundus fibers.

## THUMB
### Carpometacarpal joint

*Bony architecture.* Proximally, the thumb metacarpal articulates with the trapezium. The trapezium (from the Greek *trapezion*, small table) is firmly attached to the ad-

jacent scaphoid, trapezoid, and base of the index metacarpal by an extensive ligamentous system. When the trapezium is viewed from its volar side, a prominent ridge formed by a groove on the ulnar side of the bone is evident. This groove conveys the flexor carpi radialis tendon to its insertion in the base of the index metacarpal (Fig. 5-17).

The articular surface of the trapezium forms an angle of approximately 135 degrees with the index metacarpal in an anteroposterior plane. The articular surface of the trapezium is concave in the lateral direction and convex in the anteroposterior plane. The articular surface of the thumb metacarpal has the reverse arrangement to allow interlocking of the joint surfaces. This anatomical arrangement permits only

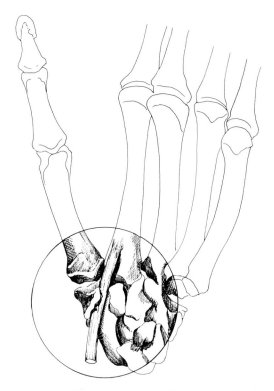

**Fig. 5-17.** The flexor carpi radialis tendon lies in a groove on the medial surface of the trapezium just proximal to its insertion into the base of the index metacarpal.

flexion and extension of this joint when the greater part of the surface areas of the two articular surfaces are contiguous.

Abduction and adduction occur along the ridge of the trapezium in a plane at 60 degrees to the plane of the dorsal surfaces of the index and long metacarpals. During abduction, the head of the thumb metacarpal moves in an anterolateral direction, whereas the base moves in a posteromedial direction. During adduction, the opposite directional changes occur. In flexion and extension of the abducted thumb metacarpal, the bone travels along the curved groove of the trapezium while the axis of movement changes continually. Kuczynski suggests that flexion is accompanied by medial rotation of the metacarpal, and extension by lateral rotation.

*Capsular support.* Haines described five discrete ligaments at the carpometacarpal joint of the thumb (Fig. 5-18). These include: the radial (lateral), the anterior oblique (ulnar), and the posterior oblique (dorsal). He further notes two intermetacarpal ligaments bridging the thumb and index metacarpals. These are the anterior and posterior intermetacarpal ligaments. The ulnar collateral ligament is a thick heavy ligament extending from the distal part of the ridge of the trapezium to insert in the volar beak of the thumb metacarpal base. This ligament is slack when the carpometacarpal joint is flexed but provides the entire restraining force to hyperextension.

The radial ligament attaches to the thumb metacarpal immediately proximal to the tendinous insertion of the abductor pollicis longus. This ligament bridges the carpometacarpal joint and inserts in the lateral side of the trapezium. In this position it is covered by the tendon of the abductor pollicis longus. The posterior oblique ligament attaches to the dorsal surfaces of the base of the thumb meta-

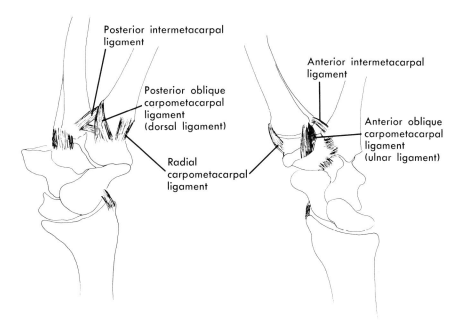

**Fig. 5-18.** Five major ligaments attach to the base of the thumb metacarpal; three of these ligaments insert into the trapezium and two into the base of the index metacarpal. (From Hollinshead, W. H.: Anatomy of surgeons; the back and limbs, ed. 2, New York, 1969, Harper & Row, Publishers, Inc.)

carpal and the trapezium. It is covered by the tendon of the extensor pollicis brevis. The anterior and posterior intermetacarpal ligaments extend between the radial edge of the index metacarpal base and the ulnar edge of the thumb metacarpal base. The joint capsule is lax; this is particularly important in that it permits greater mobility of the thumb. To accomplish abduction and extension, the beak of the thumb metacarpal base is elevated and pulled away from the trapezium. The ulnar collateral ligament checks the extent of retraction. If the volar beak of the thumb metacarpal is fractured (Bennett's fracture), the metacarpal proper is retracted posteriorly through the insertions of the abductor pollicis longus and extensor pollicis longus and brevis muscles.

*Extracapsular support.* The ulnar surface of this joint is bridged by the flexor pollicis longus within its sheath. Anteriorly the joint is covered by the musculotendinous origin of the abductor pollicis brevis and flexor pollicis brevis muscles. Radially, the abductor pollicis longus bridges the joint to insert into the base of the thumb metacarpal. More posteriorly, the extensor pollicis brevis spans the joint to which it is closely applied.

### Metacarpophalangeal joint

*Bony architecture.* The head of the thumb metacarpal is broad and thick. Its articular surface covers the single condyle to present almost as much surface area in extension as it does in flexion. The condylar head is usually rounded. There is a marked variation in range of motion at this joint within the general population. This may be caused by the shape of the joint surface, or by the supporting capsular structures, or both. In a significant segment of the population, this condylar head is flat. When the metacarpal head is flat, the joint acts as a hinge joint. The extent of movement is significantly limited and is achieved by prying the joint open. Consequently, in these individuals (10% of the population) the range of motion is achieved by the laxness of the joint capsule. The base of the proximal phalanx presents a large broad concave surface to accommodate the head of the metacarpal. A prominent volar ridge that receives the attachments from the volar plate is evident. A lateral tubercle provides insertion for the slip of the abductor pollicis brevis tendon.

*Capsular support.* The ligamentous structures about the joint include: the proper collateral ligaments, the accessory collateral ligaments, the volar plate, and the insertion of a slip of the extensor pollicis longus tendon into the proximal phalanx (Fig. 5-19). The proper collateral ligaments are broad and thick, extending from the sides of the metacarpal head in

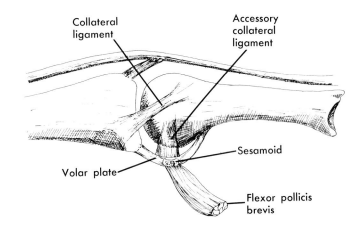

**Fig. 5-19.** The capsular structures of the metacarpophalangeal joint of the thumb include the collateral ligaments, the metacarpoglenoidal ligaments, and the volar plate with its special attachments.

Collateral ligament

Accessory collateral ligament

Sesamoid

Volar plate

Flexor pollicis brevis

an oblique direction to insert into the volarlateral side of the proximal phalanx. The tensile strength of these ligaments is 36 kg compared with 19 kg for the collateral ligaments of the interphalangeal joints of the fingers. In the thumb, rupture of a collateral ligament usually occurs from its insertion into the proximal phalanx. The accessory collateral ligament is a thin flat structure extending from the metacarpal head to insert into the volar plate.

The volar plate has a broad attachment to the volar edge of the proximal phalanx base. Stener suggests that the volar plate should be divided into a proximal and distal portion in relation to the location of the sesamoid bones within the plate. The distal volar plate is thick and rigid, whereas the proximal volar plate is thinner and more pliable. The tensile strength of the volar plate of the thumb metacarpophalangeal joint was found to be 16 kg compared with 6 kg for the volar plate of the metacarpophalangeal joint of the index finger. Rupture of the thumb metacarpophalangeal joint volar plate occurs at its proximal attachments to the metacarpals. The lateral sesamoid receives the inser-

tion of the flexor pollicis brevis, while the medial sesamoid receives the insertion of the adductor pollicis brevis muscle. Thus, through the volar plate, the sesamoids serve to transmit the actions of these two muscles directly to the proximal phalanx. In the midaxial plane the volar plate is thinned and supports the flexor pollicis longus tendon. Dorsally, a thin capsule is reinforced by the insertion of a slip of extensor pollicis longus tendon into the proximal phalanx.

***Extracapsular support.*** The intrinsic muscles of the thumb form a dorsal supporting sling somewhat akin to that seen in the fingers (Fig. 5-20). The abductor pollicis brevis arises from the radial half of the volar carpal ligament and extends toward the metacarpophalangeal joint of the thumb. Here its broad tendon that contributes fibers to the dorsal aponeurosis of the thumb appears. The remaining fibers insert into the lateral aspect of the joint capsule. The flexor pollicis brevis arises from the volar carpal ligament and from the crest of the trapezium. From these origins the muscle fibers converge into a tendon that lies on the radial side of the flexor pollicis longus tendon. The

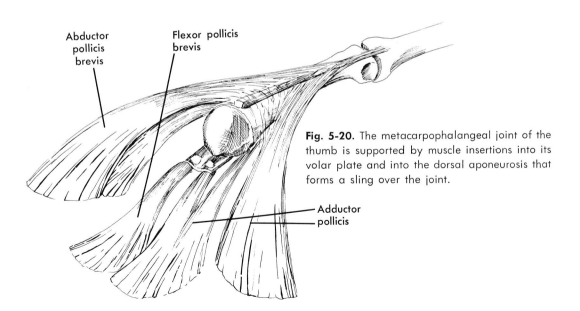

Abductor pollicis brevis

Flexor pollicis brevis

Adductor pollicis

**Fig. 5-20.** The metacarpophalangeal joint of the thumb is supported by muscle insertions into its volar plate and into the dorsal aponeurosis that forms a sling over the joint.

flexor pollicis brevis inserts into the radial sesamoid bone of the volar plate and by a second slip into the lateral tubercle at the base of the proximal phalanx. The opponens does not traverse the metacarpophalangeal joint but does insert along the lateral aspect of the thumb metacarpal.

The adductor pollicis arises from an oblique and a transverse head. The transverse head originates primarily from the long finger metacarpal, while the oblique head originates from the ligament covering the capitate and trapezoid bones and the tunnel of the flexor carpi radialis near its insertion. These two heads converge into a tendon whose major portion inserts into the ulnar sesamoid bone. A second small extension of the tendon inserts into the lateral tubercle of the proximal phalanx, while a third slip participates in formation of the dorsal aponeurosis of the thumb. Consequently, the dorsal aponeurosis of the thumb is formed by contributions of the extensor pollicis longus and brevis, the abductor pollicis brevis, and the adductor pollicis muscles. On the dorsal surface at the metacarpophalangeal joint, the extensor pollicis brevis provides a slip for attachment to the base of the proximal phalanx and a second slip that continues with the extensor pollicis longus to insert in the distal phalanx. Thus, the dorsal apparatus encloses the metacarpophalangeal joint and through the short muscles is anchored to the volar plate.

### Interphalangeal joint

The interphalangeal joint of the thumb is similar to those in the fingers except that the thumb joint is much bigger. The hinge joint structure is present with broad condyles providing added stability to the joint.

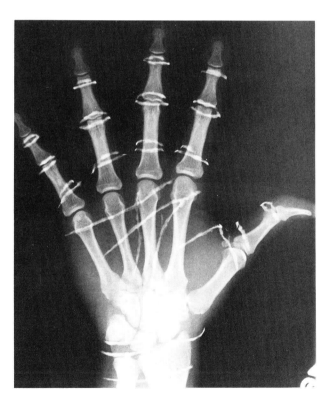

**Fig. 5-21.** The skin creases of the palmar surface are marked with radiopaque material.

The breaking strength of the collateral ligaments in the thumb interphalangeal joint has been measured at 10 kg as compared with 19 kg and 11 kg in the proximal and distal interphalangeal joints of the index finger respectively. No measurements are available concerning the tensile strength of the volar plate.

The extracapsular structures traversing this joint include the flexor pollicis longus tendon and the extensor pollicis longus tendon. The skin capsule is closely applied around this joint so that joint disruptions are frequently compound.

## SKIN JOINTS

On the volar surface of the hand, each joint has a corresponding flexure crease line (skin joint). Except for the proximal interphalangeal joint, these skin creases lie proximal to the respective joints (Fig. 5-21). The volar skin creases just proximal to the proximal interphalangeal joint do not overlie the metacarpophalangeal joint but actually are closer to the midpoint of the proximal phalanx. The distal palmar crease is just proximal to the metacarpophalangeal joints of the long, ring, and little fingers, whereas the proximal palmar crease curves to the carpal ligament area. The thumb carpometacarpal joint is represented by a long curving crease line extending from the midpalm to the first web space.

The thumb will be held in adduction if its carpometacarpal crease line is covered by a splint or a cast. Similarly, the distal palmar crease must not be covered if full flexion of the metacarpophalangeal joint is to be maintained.

The flexion crease of the thumb-index web space extends from the level of the index metacarpophalangeal joint in a proximal and curving line to join the flexion crease of the thumb carpometacarpal

crease in the midline of the proximal palm.

A roentgenogram showing these skin joints is particularly helpful when one is pinning fractures percutaneously.

## BIBLIOGRAPHY

Aston; J. N.: Locked middle finger, J. Bone Joint Surg. **42B**:75, 1960.

Duchenne, G. B.: Physiology of motion, translated and edited by E. B. Kaplan, Philadelphia, 1949, J. B. Lippincott Co.

Gad, P.: The anatomy of the volar part of the capsules of the finger joints, J. Bone Joint Surg. **49B**:362, 1967.

Haines, R. W.: The mechanism of rotation at the first carpo-metacarpal joint, J. Anat. 78:44, 1944.

Harvey, F. J.: Locking of the metacarpo-phalangeal joints, J. Bone Joint Surg. **56B**:156, 1974.

Joseph, J.: Further studies of the metacarpophalangeal and interphalangeal joints of the thumb, J. Anat. **85**:221, 1940.

Kaplan, E. B.: Functional and surgical anatomy of the hand, Philadelphia, 1953, J. B. Lippincott Co.

Kuczynski, K.: The proximal interphalangeal joint, J. Bone Joint Surg. **50B**:656, 1968.

Landsmeer, J. M.: Anatomical and functional investigation of the articulations of the fingers, Acta Anat. 25(Suppl. 24):1, 1955.

Landsmeer, J. M.: The anatomy of the dorsal aponeurosis of the human finger and its functional significance, Anat. Rec. **104**:35, 1949.

Matheson, A. B., Sinclair, D. C., and Skene, W. G.: The range and power of ulnar and radial deviation of the fingers, J. Anat. **107**:439, 1970.

Moberg, E., and Stener, B.: Injuries to the ligaments of the thumb and fingers; diagnosis, treatment and prognosis, Acta Chir. Scand. **106**:166, 1953.

Stener, B.: Displacement of the ruptured ulnar collateral ligament of the metacarpo-phalangeal joint of the thumb, J. Bone Joint Surg. **44B**:869, 1962.

Tubiana, R., and Valentin, P.: The anatomy of the extensor apparatus of the fingers, Surg. Clin. N. Am. **44**:897, 1964.

# SECTION TWO
# MANAGEMENT OF THE ACUTELY INJURED HAND

# CHAPTER 6

# A basic approach to the injured hand

## ESTABLISHING PRIORITIES

Injuries of the upper extremity are rarely life-threatening, yet the disability from residual deformity profoundly alters life. Care of the extensively damaged hand presents a special challenge. If the situation permits, the initial procedures should be discussed with the patient. However, the patient is usually so distraught that he does not comprehend an involved conversation.

Usually, it is impossible to preserve all of the components necessary to regain normal function in the hand. Yet preservation of as much functional tissue as possible is paramount to gaining at least a "basic hand." The basic hand is composed of a stable wrist and a radial digit with good sensation and mobility, separated by a deep cleft from at least one or two fingers or a "post" on the ulnar aspect of the hand (Fig. 6-1). A minimum of parts is required to provide this basic hand. If at least a basic hand can be preserved, it is much more functional and more acceptable to the patient than any prosthesis.

Primary treatment requires reestablishment or maintenance of adequate blood supply, realignment of the remaining skeletal elements, and obtaining adequate and complete skin coverage. Rarely are definitive reconstructive procedures performed during the initial treatment. Furthermore, the decision to salvage a part that is useless either in its original role or as a contributor to restoration of another part is unsound judgment. If one accepts this simple rule, it immediately places an added responsibility on the primary physician. To be able to discern whether a part is of value or not, one must be aware of the restorative techniques available for reconstruction or utilization of an injured part as a contributor to restoration of another part. Replantation, amputation, delay and observation, decompression, and reconstruction are all options the primary physician has available. The background required to select the proper technique and follow it through to its technical completion has created the specialty—surgery of the hand.

The loss of blood supply to a part was once considered an indication for amputation. However, the development of vascular surgery has modified this dictum. Presently, the only mandatory indication for amputation is irreversible loss of blood supply. An electrical burn at the wrist may completely devitalize the hand by direct destruction of the vasculature at the wrist, but a radial arteriogram will reveal a per-

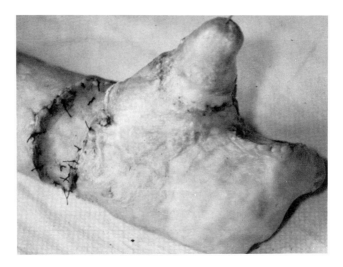

**Fig. 6-1.** A basic hand has been gained by transferring the index remnant to the thumb remnant, thereby providing a mobile thumb, a web space, and an ulnar post.

fectly normal-appearing vascular tree in the hand immediately after the injury. Restoration of vascular continuity at the wrist is successful for a short time. However, the vascular tree of the hand then becomes involved in an extensive vasculitis that precludes permanent reestablishment of circulation. When the vascular tree is not irreversibly destroyed, restoration of circulation in complete amputations at the arm, forearm, hand, and finger level is possible. Consequently, one must be prepared to make the decision to amputate or reimplant.

### REPLANTATION PRINCIPLES
#### At or proximal to wrist crease

Factors to consider in making the decision whether to close the stump or replant the part include: age of the patient, type of amputation, level of amputation, and general health of the patient. If all other factors are equal, the younger a patient is, the better the prognosis for functional recovery. The more peripheral the level of amputation is, the better the functional results. The functional prognosis in complete amputation above the elbow in an adult is such that, even if limb survival

is achieved, functional recovery is inadequate. In adults, the return of elbow function is expected; but the return of useful function in the hand and wrist is rare. Crushing injuries are associated with a poorer prognosis than clean sharp injuries. Consequently, the ideal setting for replantation is a clean, sharp amputation just proximal to the wrist in a young individual.

The principal factors necessary for successful limb replantation include: preservation of the severed limb, techniques of replantation, and postoperative management. The limb should be cooled as soon as possible to slow ischemic necrosis in the devascularized tissues. To do this, cover the amputated limb with a sterile gauze and place it within a plastic bag; then immerse the plastic bag in a mixture of ice and water. This will allow adequate cooling of the part but will prevent freezing and maceration. The vessel should not be cannulated in amputations distal to the wrist joint. In amputations proximal to the wrist, irrigation and flushing of the vessels may be beneficial. If irrigation is undertaken, the following technique is recommended. The vasculature of the hand should be flushed with a solution of 50 mg heparin in 500 ml 10% molecular weight dextran. Great care should be taken to cannulate the radial artery without causing trauma and to flush the vessels without creating excessive hydrostatic pressure. Inoue and associates recommend the use of decompressive incisions if the hand should begin swelling before replantation.

Operatively, the wounds should be debrided as conservatively as possible. The bones should be shortened to permit tendon, muscle, nerve, and vascular repair. After bony stabilization as many veins as possible should be repaired; autogenous vein grafts may be necessary. Then the arteries are repaired and circulation reestablished. Severed nerves should be repaired during the primary procedure unless they are so extensively damaged that it is impossible to determine the extent of nerve damage. A loss of a nerve segment precluding direct repair will require nerve grafts as a secondary procedure.

Postoperatively, uncontrollable edema may threaten survival of the extremity. Fasciotomies of the forearm and both dorsal and volar surfaces of the palm may be required either at the time of replantation or postoperatively. Fasciotomies are certainly easier and more expedient to accomplish during the primary procedure. Plaster splinting aids immobilization. Occasionally, shock not associated with blood loss develops after limb replantation. Treatment with bicarbonate may be required to correct the acidosis. After the wounds are healed, care must be taken to prevent the development of stiff joints.

### Digital replantation

The development of microsurgical techniques for replanting digits has been utilized to reestablish circulation in devascularized but incompletely severed digits. The techniques and results of digital revascularization and replantation will be presented in Chapter 7.

## TISSUE-ORIENTED EVALUATION AND TREATMENT

Injuries where the vascular supply to the parts is intact, but that extensively involve skin, bone, nerve and tendon, must be evaluated with regard to the potential available for functional restoration. In general, all innervated skin, isolated joints, and functional units (for example, the fingertips) should be preserved. At subsequent sittings these units may be restored either alone or in combination with other units to provide a single functional unit (Fig. 6-2).

Initial management of the injured hand, in which an adequate blood supply has been preserved, is directed toward restoring functional units, obtaining primary healing with minimal scar tissue formation, and providing an optimal environment for subsequent surgery as needed. A systematic evaluation of the tissues injured facilitates an accurate assessment of damage and aids in determining the extent and type of primary treatment necessary.

Our initial examination is tissue-oriented, beginning with skin and progressing through bone, joint, nerve, and tendon. Surgical reconstruction is similarly oriented, systematically progressing through each tissue complex until the restoration of motor unit function can be reestablished by repair, transfer, or grafting of tendons. The importance of continually reminding oneself of the digital joints and the need to keep them supple cannot be overemphasized.

As one evaluates the injury, obtaining information about each tissue requires answering the following questions. Is direct wound closure precluded by skin loss? If direct closure is not feasible, should a pedicle flap or a split graft be used to gain coverage? Which bones are fractured, what is the position of the fractured ends, what particular problems do the fractures present, and what type of fixation is re-

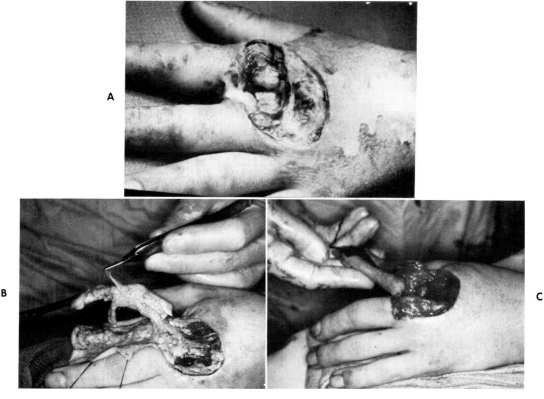

**Fig. 6-2. A,** An electrical burn has destroyed the extensor apparatus and the metacarpophalangeal joints of the index and long fingers. **B,** After the wound is healed, the proximal interphalangeal joint of the index finger is maintained on its ulnar neurovascular bundle for transfer to replace the destroyed metacarpophalangeal joint of the long finger. The filleted skin of the index finger maintains its nourishment through the radial neurovascular bundle and is used for coverage. **C,** The transfer in place.

quired? Are nerves severed, contused, or avulsed? Finally, if tendons are divided, one should consider where and under what circumstances the repair should be made, and what the timing of the repair should be.

Before one becomes irretrievably involved in operative manipulation of the injured hand, one must evaluate the general status of the wound (Fig. 6-3, *A*). Thorough cleansing of the wound is essential. In fact, wound irrigation and cleansing may require most of the initial operative time. This cleansing must be complete. The fine particles of grease, dirt, and emery dust associated with many industrial accidents evoke an intense, overwhelming inflammatory reaction and subsequent fibrosis that completely negates subsequent restorative procedures. Frequently, these foreign materials have been driven into the periosteum or into exposed cortical or cancellous bone. A steel bristle scrub brush may be used to remove these particles from bone (Fig. 6-3, *B*). In soft tissues, irrigation and excision are appropriate methods for removal of foreign material. Devices that produce pulsating jets of water are significantly more effective in removing foreign bodies and bacteria from traumatic wounds.

In cleanly lacerated wounds, trimming of the skin edges is usually unnecessary. The

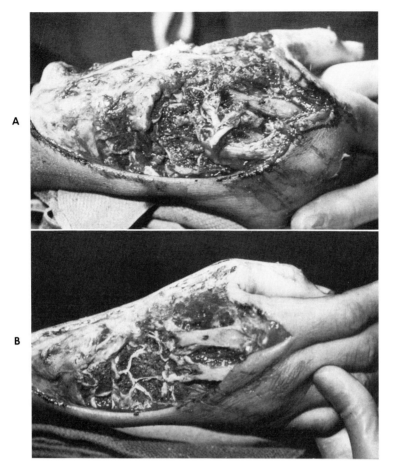

**Fig. 6-3. A,** This hand with a severe grinding avulsing injury of the dorsum had undergone surgery 4 hours prior to this picture. **B,** All devitalized tissues must be removed. When particles are ground into the bone, a scrub brush aids to removing the foreign particles.

skin of the hand possesses an excellent blood supply, and extensive débridement in the clean, sharp, lacerating injuries is not indicated. However, in crushing injuries the trauma associated with the blow can devitalize varying amounts of tissue adjacent to the area sustaining the brunt of the blow. The actual area of devitalized skin at the time of débridement can be difficult to determine accurately. Extension of thrombosis may result in the need for further débridement at a later sitting. The frequency of this spread of tissue damage requires that we reexamine the wound

within 48 hours of the initial trauma. Determining the status of crushed muscle, such as the interossei, is particularly difficult. Only by repeated examination of the wound can necrotic muscle be eliminated without eliminating viable muscle.

The question of wound closure evokes some controversy. Certainly when this question is raised, no definitive procedures should have been undertaken at the initial sitting. In grossly contaminated wounds every effect should be made to convert the injury to a clean surgical wound. If one feels he has accomplished this end, then loose closure is indicated. Obviously if the wound cannot be converted to a clean surgical wound, closure can be delayed. Delayed closure is indicated in certain crush injuries that will be discussed later. When there is any question concerning closure, one is obligated to inspect the wound within 48 hours. The use of antibiotics in the contaminated wound is routine, but the usefulness of antibiotics in such wounds has not been clearly shown. Although they are commonly employed in clinical practice, most retrospective and prospective reviews have not shown any benefit associated with the use of prophylactic antibiotics. Many have found instead that delayed primary closure is beneficial.

### Skin loss

When skin loss precludes wound closure, there are only two basic types of coverage available—free grafts and pedicle grafts (flaps). Free grafts may be either split-thickness or full-thickness. (Composite grafts will not be discussed, because there

are no indications for their use in acute hand injuries.) Free grafts differ from pedicle grafts in several respects. The free graft consists of epidermis and varying amounts of dermis. Since the free graft has no direct blood supply, it must obtain its nourishment from the recipient site. Thus, the dermis of the free graft must be in intimate contact with its recipient site. The dense collagen of the graft's dermis excites an intense reaction by the recipient area; consequently, the free graft becomes firmly adherent to the recipient site. Thus, free grafts are not utilized when the restoration of a gliding surface, such as a tendon stripped of its paratenon, is required. Split grafts are utilized when subcutaneous tissue or muscle is exposed in the depths of the wound and direct closure is not feasible (Fig. 6-4). If functional padding is desirable, increasing the thickness of the split grafts increases the amount of dermis transferred and provides more padding. The free full-thickness graft can be used in clean acute wounds in

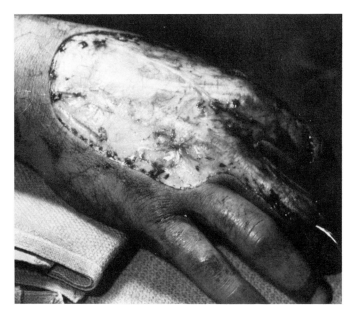

**Fig. 6-4.** When subcutaneous tissue or paratenon is exposed in the depths of a wound, a split-thickness skin graft provides an adequate functional coverage.

which function requires extra padding, that is, digital pulp and palmar areas.

Management of distally based flaps is difficult. We replace the flap if we feel certain that it is viable. Routinely we reexamine the wound within 48 hours. If the flap is viable, all is well. If the flap demonstrates areas of necrosis, it is trimmed until active bleeding is obtained. The defect is then covered with a free split graft. If we are uncertain of the viability of the flap or if closure places the flap under moderate tension, we allow the flap to remain retracted and place a skin graft in the defect.

Skin loss, as from thermal burns, presents an extraordinary challenge even though only one tissue—skin—may be damaged directly. Frequent development of stiff joints and inadequate tendon gliding makes the challenge more formidable. Usually the dorsum of the hand is more severely burned. Capillaries within the injured tissues become more permeable and a protein-rich fluid permeates the structures in the hand (Fig. 6-5). As a result of the relatively loose skin attachments, the dorsum of the hand exhibits the greatest amount of fluid collection. As edema fluid collects, the metacarpophalangeal joints assume a hyperextended position. The proximal interphalangeal joints become flexed. Fibrous tissue synthesis results around all of the structures involved in the edematous reaction (Fig. 6-6). This nascent collagen is deposited around the joint capsules, the extensor tendons, and to a lesser extent around the flexor tendons in dorsal injuries. As the dorsal wound responds with scar production and contraction, the malpositioning of the metacarpophalangeal and interphalangeal joints is exaggerated and becomes fixed. Thus, there are at least five major preventable changes associated with the production of deformity in the burned hand: persistent edema, improper positioning of the digital joints, prolonged immobilization, infection, and delayed (and frequently inadequate) skin coverage.

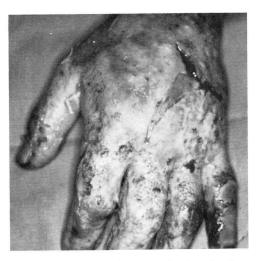

**Fig. 6-5.** Extensive edema of the hand reflects the severity of the injury and is an indication of the degree of the reparative processes that will be activated.

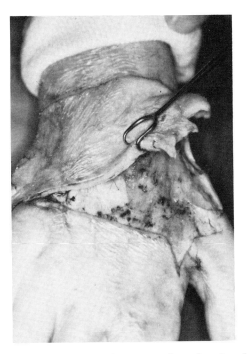

**Fig. 6-6.** Extensive fibrosis involves the dorsal skin and the dorsal fascia, obliterating the view of the underlying extensor tendons.

Edema has been treated by pressure dressings. Yet these dressings do not maintain constant pressure on the wound unless an elastic bandage is incorporated into the dressing. Even then, the dressing provides an ideal environment for bacterial proliferation. As bacterial colonization occurs, the wound is deepened and more tissue destroyed. When no dressings or light dressings are utilized, edema persists. Improper positioning of the digital joints can be overcome by an external apparatus that permits flexion of the metacarpophalangeal joints and extension of the interphalangeal joints. A gradual, gentle, passive range of motion should be accomplished in these joints daily, even when the grafts are in place.

When the burn is obviously third-degree or deep second-degree, early excision and grafting immediately reduce the edema formation and permit earlier motion in the joints (Fig. 6-7). When a second-degree burn is evident, strict attention to the joints during the repair and regenerative phase will aid in obtaining an optimal result.

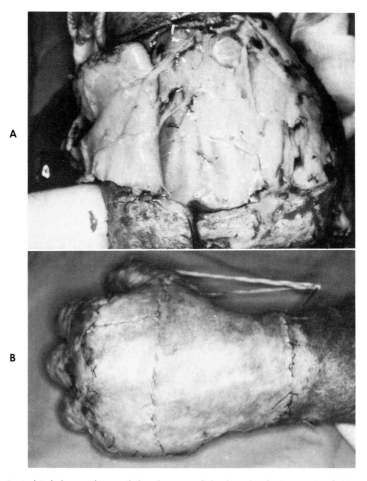

**Fig. 6-7. A,** A third-degree burn of the dorsum of the hand is being excised. Note the edema of the eschar and underlying subcutaneous tissues. The extensor tendons are faintly visible in a gelatinous milieu. **B,** Three days after excision and grafting, the edema has noticeably subsided. Note the positioning of the joints.

The pedicle flap consists of epidermis, dermis, and subcutaneous tissue that maintains its original blood supply during transfer. This blood supply, anatomically located in the subdermal plexus, may be carried by multiple fine branches in the pedicle or by a single artery and vein. The maintenance of blood supply permits the pedicle flap the luxury of the subdermal subcutaneous tissue and fat. This may be trimmed as needed.

Since the pedicle graft has its own blood supply, any combination of subcutaneous, neural, and bony tissue may be transferred with the flap. In fact, a spectrum of pedicle flaps is possible, extending from a simple broad flap of skin containing numerous fine capillaries to a pedicle flap containing all the digital components based on a single artery and vein.

The subcutaneous fat of the pedicle graft excites minimal scar formation by the recipient bed. Dense scarring is limited primarily to the periphery of the flap where the dermis of the flap and the recipient site abut. Pedicle flaps are utilized when local tissue loss precludes adequate coverage of tendons, bone, joints, and major neurovascular elements (Fig. 6-8). The premise for motor function is to allow gliding of tendons free from restrictive adhesions. Tendons are encircled by a specialized structure, paratenon, which aids gliding. Free skin grafts applied to paratenon do not interfere with tendon gliding, but when paratenon has been lost, flap

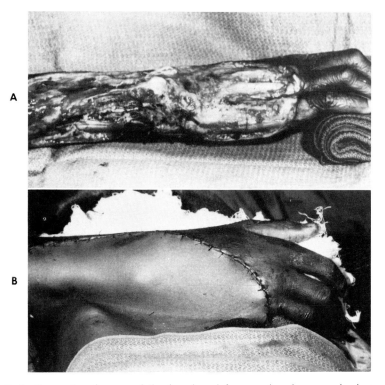

**Fig. 6-8. A,** The entire dorsum of the hand and forearm has been avulsed, exposing the metacarpals, carpals, and forearm. **B,** Coverage to preserve joint motion and allow later reconstructive procedures requires insertion of a pedicle flap. The metacarpophalangeal joints are improperly positioned in extension

coverage becomes necessary. Exposed tendon covered with a flap develops minimal scar tissue formation and adhesion between the tendon and underlying fat of the flap. Exposed bone that is or has been traversed by functional motor units requires pedicle flap coverage in anticipation of the restoration of motor units across the area. Certainly, periosteum readily accepts a split graft; but if tendon grafting, repair, or transfer is anticipated across that particular area, the split graft fails to provide an adequate gliding surface. An exposed joint in the hand, wrist, or elbow must be closed with a flap if joint mobility is to be preserved. When tissue is replaced over the dorsum of a joint, the joint is moderately flexed to ensure transfer of an adequate amount of pedicle tissue. Conversely, if the volar surface is covered, the pedicle graft is inserted with the wrist in moderate extension.

The variety of flaps available to provide optimal wound closure should be readily available to the surgeon for restoring function in an injured hand. The variety of techniques available are presented in Chapter 8.

**Fracture**

When treating any hand injury, and particularly fractures, one must be ever cognizant of edema formation. The notable edema formation associated with fractures probably is related to the severity of the force of injury required to produce the fracture. Edema is a manifestation of tissue damage with resultant alteration in capillary permeability. The protein-rich edema fluid attracts water into the interstitial spaces until normal capillary permeability is reestablished. This edematous fluid fills the interstices of the collateral ligaments and soft tissues surrounding joints and tendons. Edema is usually most noticeable on the dorsum of the hand because the palmar tissues are fixed and nonyielding, whereas the dorsal skin is freely moveable and lax. As edema collects on the dorsum

of the hand, the metacarpophalangeal joints are forced into hyperextension, and the proximal interphalangeal joints assume a flexed position. Collagen is then deposited about the collateral ligaments and the flexor and extensor tendons. The collateral ligaments, which are lax when the metacarpophalangeal joints are hyperextended, become fixed in their lax position. The flexor and extensor tendons are bound to the surrounding immobile structures. Consequently, optimal fracture treatment includes: (1) reduction and immobilization of the fracture, (2) maintenance of digital length and proper rotation, (3) preservation of joint motion, and (4) minimization of edema formation.

Immobilization can be accomplished with either external or internal splinting. External splinting, such as plaster casting, requires immobilizing more than just the two joints in juxtaposition to the fracture. If this external splinting is prolonged, stiff joint and tendon adhesions are more prone to develop. Dissatisfaction with external splinting has led to a greater interest in internal fixation, particularly with Kirschner wires. The advantages of internal fixation include: (1) firm approximation and immobilization of the accurately reduced fracture, (2) prevention of rotary movement, (3) maintenance of digital length, (4) minimal immobilization of juxtaposed joints, and (5) early tendon gliding and joint movement (Fig. 6-9). The disadvantages include infection, impingement of wires on tendinous structures, and edema formation secondary to surgery. Intra-articular fractures almost always require open reduction, accurate fixation, and early mobilization of the joints.

Successful fracture management is measured only by the ultimate functional result of the part and of the entire hand. The means by which this can best be accomplished is determined by the operator's experience and expertise. For final emphasis, the most common problem in the treatment of fractures is stiffness of the metacarpophalangeal joint in extension and of the interphalangeal joints in flexion.

## Nerve injury

There are three basic injury-regeneration patterns to consider: axonotmesis, neurapraxia, and neurotmesis.

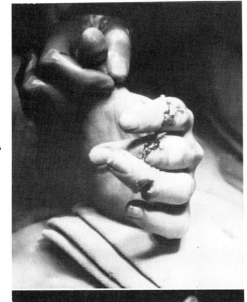

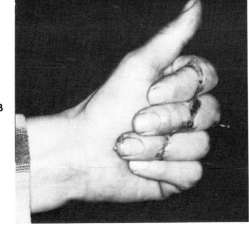

**Fig. 6-9. A,** Saw injury produced fractures of the middle phalanges of the long and ring fingers. **B,** The fractures have been reduced and immobilized with crossing Kirschner wires permitting a full range of motion at 5 days postoperatively. (From Remark, F. L., and Weeks, P. M.: Mo. Med. **68:**767, 1971.)

Axonotmesis is a phenomenon associated with a crushing injury that destroys the continuity of the axon but not the continuity of the supporting tissues of the nerve trunk. Since the nerve sheaths are intact, functional recovery is expected and occurs rapidly. Neurapraxia, in which the nerve is intact but conduction is impaired, can occur in the hand from dislocation of the lunate or from anterior fracture-dislocation of the wrist. The mechanism of action is increased pressure on the median nerve in the carpal tunnel. Saturday night palsy, that is, radial nerve compression, is another example of compressive injury interrupting conduction. In neurapraxia, recovery usually follows removal of the cause of the pressure. In neurotmesis, the connective tissues and axons of the nerve trunk are completely severed.

Sunderland has expanded the above classification, proposing five degrees of injury. Extending from least to most severe, these are: (1) loss of conduction in the axons, (2) loss of continuity of nerve fibers within the funiculi, (3) loss of continuity of the endoneurial tube and its contents, (4) loss of continuity of the perineurium and funiculi, and (5) loss of continuity of the nerve trunk.

The factors that determine the eventual functional result of a nerve injury and repair include: (1) age of patient, (2) type of injury, (3) composition of severed nerve trunk, (4) level of injury, (5) presence of associated injuries, and (6) skill of the surgeon. The disagreement concerning primary versus secondary nerve repair appears to have been resolved into the concept of delayed primary repair except in occasional circumstances. The factors championed by each group will be presented in order to understand the rationale of the delayed primary repair concept.

Factors favoring nerve repair at the time of acute injury are as follows: (1) Absence of scar tissue eliminates extensive dissection; (2) mobilization of the nerve ends is minimized because cut ends have not retracted and become embedded in scar; (3) one less operative procedure is required if the anastomosis is successful; (4) the earlier a nerve is repaired, the better the motor function recovery; (5) particularly good results are obtained in children with primary repairs; and (6) digital nerve lacerations almost always necessitate primary repair.

If primary nerve repair is elected, an advancing Tinel sign must be elicited after adequate time has elapsed for the regenerating axons to bridge the repair. The length of this latent period is determined by the time required for the cell's regenerative processes to become organized and for the regenerating fibers to traverse the repair. If the repair has been perfect, the latent period will be limited to the time required for the regenerative process to become organized, that is, 40 to 50 days. Yet a perfect repair is never obtained. Since regenerating nerve advances at approximately 1.0 mm per day, any delay beyond the latent period must stimulate one to question the adequacy of the anastomosis particularly in more distal nerve repairs. Thus, the position of an advancing Tinel sign must be examined carefully and recorded frequently. When advancement does not occur, the surgeon must recognize the need for secondary repair. This always seems easier when someone else performed the repair. If this decision is delayed, fibrosis and shrinkage of the distal nerve segment become extensive enough within a few months to interfere with regeneration.

Three indications for early repair after healing of injured tissues are: (1) nerve division by a blunt instrument that inflicts considerably more tissue damage than is readily apparent, (2) avulsion injuries that require primary attention to pedicle flap coverage, and (3) grossly contaminated injury. This form of repair also has the advantages that (1) if the damaged nerve is allowed to undergo degeneration and fibrosis over a period of 2 to 4 weeks, the level of viable nerve becomes strikingly obvious, and (2) fibrosis around the funiculi provides added purchase for the nerve suture. It is most helpful at the time of acute injury to overlap the nerve ends by 1 to 2 cm with a single suture (Fig. 6-10). This reduces the need for extensive mobilization of the nerve ends during the second procedure, thereby reducing tension at anastomosis, minimizing surgical

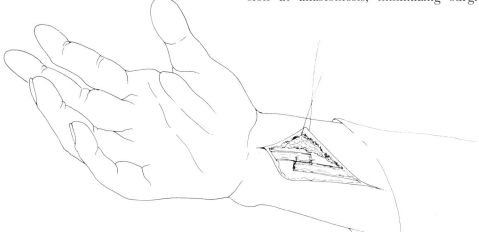

**Fig. 6-10.** Nerve repair as a secondary procedure is greatly facilitated if the nerve ends are overlapped as much as possible and held with sutures at the initial procedure.

interference with blood supply at the nerve ends, and permitting proper positioning of the joints to avoid stiffness.

### Tendon injury

Restoration of tendon function implies the restoration of tendon gliding, not simply surgical repair of the tendon ends. Surgical efforts are directed toward obtaining healing in a milieu that will produce a favorable scar, that is, that will undergo biological alteration to form adhesions that can be favorably modified by stress to permit tendon gliding. Ideally, a tendon repair is accomplished in a bed of loose areolar tissue or fat. These repairs must not be performed in the immediate vicinity of lacerations of the palmar fascia, fibro-osseous tunnels, periosteum, or near bony fractures (Fig. 6-11). As these structures composed of dense fibrous tissue heal, the tendon repair will become embedded in this dense nonyielding scar. In fact, it is for these reasons that the use of silastic rods has been greeted with such enthusiasm. Consequently, the concept of primary versus secondary tendon repair has developed.

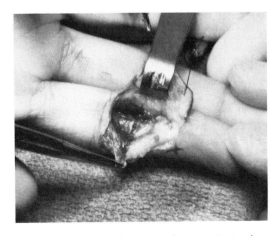

**Fig. 6-11.** Primary flexor tendon repair in the fibro-osseous tunnels, particularly where the sheath is thickened to form a pulley, can result in dense adhesions that restrict tendon gliding.

The flexor tendons are encircled by loose areolar tissue from the tendon origin to the distal palmar crease. From the distal palmar crease to the distal phalanx, the tendons are enclosed in the fibro-osseous tunnels. Primary repair of flexor tendons divided at the level of the forearm, wrist, palm, or over the distal phalanx may be indicated in clean wounds. Clean lacerations of the tendons within the fibro-osseous tunnels from the distal palmar crease to the midportion of the middle phalanx have evoked divided support for primary versus secondary repair. In this region, the main drawback to primary tendon repair is adherence of the tendon to the nonyielding fibro-osseous tunnel. If the unyielding fibro-osseous tunnels are completely excised, the tendons will bow-string from the palm to the distal phalanx. Thus, portions of the sheath must be retained to act as pulleys.

As a basic principle, if one has limited experience performing primary flexor tendon repairs, closure of the skin and referral of the patient are indicated. If transportation or referral is a problem, delayed primary repair can easily be accomplished within 2 weeks of the initial injury. The time limit of delayed primary repair has not been established; however, in our own experience, delayed primary repair has been successful even 40 days after the initial injury. In fact, the tendon ends at this time were very firm and provided excellent holding power for the sutures. The profundus and sublimis tendons had been severed, but there was no demonstrable shortening at 40 days after injury.

Extensor tendon lacerations can be treated more aggressively because of their short amplitude of motion and the absence of fibro-osseous tunnels—except at the wrist. The period of immobilization necessary after extensor tendon repair is longer than that following flexor tendon repair. This probably reflects the lack of scarring to fixed structures (which provides a splint for the repair) compared with the scarring that occurs on the volar surface.

### Joint mobility

The area most neglected when managing an injured extremity is the digital joint. It is of little value to obtain excellent skin coverage, bony union, and perfect nerve regeneration if the joints are allowed to become stiff. Tendon repairs or transfers in digits with stiff joints are futile. If a full range of passive motion is not obtained before tendon repair, then a full range of active motion cannot be expected after tendon repair. Constant awareness of joint mobility is essential. An understanding of the architecture of each joint, which pinpoints the structural arrangements permitting mobility, is essential for providing optimal management. The structural components of each joint are presented in Chapter 5. From a knowledge of these factors, it is evident that many anatomical factors can contribute to joint stiffness when coupled with alterations associated with the injury. The most common alteration, associated with every injury, is edema formation. Edema coupled with improper positioning is a potent deterrent to good function (Fig. 6-12). Edema must be minimized in the injured extremity. This should be accomplished by application of a snug dressing and constant elevation of the extremity. Adequate elevation does not mean simply raising the forearm for brief periods or carrying it in a sling. The hand, forearm, and arm must be elevated as high as feasible with the elbow extended. Elevation is maintained until the edema has completely subsided. Occasionally, edema recurs after elevation has been stopped, in which case it must be reinitiated. The pressure dressing is of particular importance. It provides immobilization of and exerts uniform pressure on the digits, wrist, and forearm. The nail beds should always remain exposed for use as an indicator of digital circulation. Reinforcement or replacement of the dressing assures maintaining its firmness. The necessity of preventing joint stiffness cannot be overemphasized.

### COMBINED INJURIES INVOLVING SKIN, BONE, NERVE, AND TENDON

When more than one tissue is involved, for example, skin loss, fractures, and nerve and tendon lacerations, one must adhere to the basic premise of obtaining primary healing with minimal scar formation and thereby provide an optimal environment for subsequent procedures as needed. Skin loss requiring replacement limits our initial definite surgical procedures to management of fractures and skin replacement. Definitive repair of injured tendons and nerves is best accomplished at subsequent sittings. When there is no skin loss, fractures and tendon lacerations (distant from the fracture site) may be repaired. Concomitant nerve and tendon repair can be performed; however, this can be most difficult to accomplish. If the nerve injury is repaired first, the manipulations incident to the tendon suture may endanger the deli-

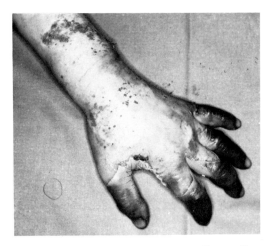

**Fig. 6-12.** Injury of the hand is usually manifest by severe edema on the dorsum of the hand. This forces the metacarpophalangeal joints into hyperextension and the thumb-index web space into adduction.

cate nerve repair. If the tendon injury is repaired first and the hand is flexed to protect the suture line, then the flexed position may obstruct repair of the nerve. As an alternative, repair of one structure is performed immediately, while repair of the other is deferred to a subsequent sitting. For example, some hand surgeons prefer primary repair of the tendon and delayed nerve suture. Certainly secondary tendon repair in the palm can be as successful a procedure as primary repair. The lumbrical muscle attachments to the long flexors help maintain forearm muscle tone. Comparison of the results of primary versus delayed digital nerve repair in the palm reveals equivalent results. If the procedures are performed at separate sittings, that is, primary tendon repair followed by secondary nerve repair, this requires prolonged immobilization of the hand at a time when the restoration of tendon gliding is critical. Primary digital nerve repair and later tendon repair permit mobilization of the tendons without superimposing a second period of immobilization. At the wrist level, flexor muscle tone is not maintained, and the muscles can develop significant myotatic contractures. At this level, primary tendon repair is favored. If segments of nerve are lost,

tendon repair is performed primarily because the need for nerve grafts is definitely a procedure for subsequent sittings.

## Volkmann's ischemia of the forearm or hand

Everyone involved in the management of upper extremity injuries should be thoroughly schooled in the natural history of Volkmann's ischemic contracture. Its general association with fractures of the humerus has lulled many into not considering the threat of ischemia when dealing with injuries other than fracture. Volkmann's ischemic contracture has developed after a variety of injuries, including closed crush injuries of the elbow, small caliber bullet injuries of the proximal forearm, burns, and many other conditions that evoke an intense reaction with edema formation (Fig. 6-13). The volar forearm muscles are enclosed by a dense forearm fasica anteriorly and laterally and by the radius and ulna with the intervening interosseous fascia posteriorly. As edema becomes more severe, the circulation in the volar forearm musculature is impaired. This impairment in circulation leads to further vascular injury that contributes to further edema. Much discussion has centered around whether the circulation is

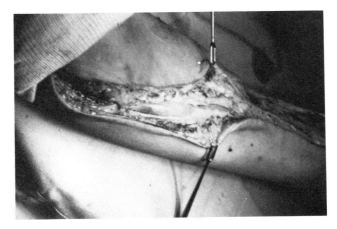

**Fig. 6-13.** As the thickened forearm fascia is opened, a transition from red muscle to white muscle to fatty replacement is observed in Volkmann's ischemic contracture.

interfered with primarily on the arterial or the venous side. Needless to say, there are data that are interpreted to support either viewpoint. Certainly a combination of arterial and venous insufficiency becomes prominent as the condition develops.

The cardinal signs of developing Volkmann's ischemia include pallor, pain, paresthesias, paralysis, and pulselessness. Presence of a radial pulse has been observed in patients developing Volkmann's ischemia. If the ischemic process is not recognized and treated immediately, a variable amount of muscle necrosis and nerve injury will ensue.

Seddon has suggested three main clinical types of Volkmann's ischemia in the forearm, depending on the severity of the necrosis. In the first, there is mild yet extensive flexor muscle involvement. In 3 to 6 months all involved muscles regain significant function even in the presence of contracture. Soon after the injury the median and ulnar nerves may be involved, but recovery is variable. In the second type, the deep flexors—flexor digitorum profundus and flexor pollicis longus—are severely involved. The sublimis flexors are minimally involved. Minimal or no recovery occurs in these muscles. The median and ulnar nerves recover but not completely. Finally, in the third type, there is extensive damage with destruction of all or most of the flexor muscles and some involvement of the extensor muscles. Nerve destruction may necessitate repair. Both nerves may be fibrotic for long segments. There are many shades between these three classifications. Each patient's condition has to be evaluated as a singular problem.

As soon as one suspects the development of Volkmann's ischemia, all dressings should be removed from the arm, forearm, and hand. If after complete removal of these dressings there is no improvement in the parameters heralding Volkmann's ischemia, the forearm musculature should be decompressed. This requires opening the forearm fascia from the lacertus fibrosus ligament to the distal forearm. If nerve compression is evident, the median nerve must be decompressed as it enters the forearm between the two heads of the pronator teres and the origin of the flexor digitorum sublimis. Further decompression in the carpal tunnel may be indicated. The ulnar nerve should be decompressed as it enters the forearm between the two heads of the flexor carpi ulnaris and more distally at the canal of Guyon. The degree of surgical decompression depends on the time since onset of ischemia and the extent of muscle and nerve involvement.

Volkmann's ischemia may involve the intrinsic muscles of the hand either in combination with forearm involvement or as a separate entity. The initial injury evokes an intense outpouring of fluid into the tissues of the hand and massive edema. Application of compressive dressings or casts aggrevates the increase in tissue pressure. The hand assumes a characteristic posture: the metacarpophalangeal joints in flexion, the interphalangeal joints in extension, and the thumb held in the palm. When Volkmann's ischemia is suspected in the hand, all dressings must be removed and the hand reevaluated. If there is no improvement, the hand must be decompressed; this requires dorsal and volar incisions to open the fascia of both sides. The thumb adductor seems to suffer most, so great care should be taken to decompress adequately the arterial and venous systems to this area. The fascia covering the interossei may require opening dorsally.

Finally, Volkmann's ischemia may develop in response to a variety of injuries. A high index of suspicion and prompt aggressive treatment are required to prevent or minimize the degree of contracture that develops as a result of the ischemia. Damage can occur during the first 6 to 48 hours of ischemia, and the contracture becomes progressively worse over the ensuing weeks.

### Injection injuries

Uncontrollable or massive edema can lead to circulatory embarrassment without necessarily producing a Volkmann's ischemic contracture response. With regard to pathophysiology and current concepts of management, two basic types of injuries will be discussed—the injection injury and the crush injury.

The airless paint gun injury is a typical injection injury. The airless paint gun delivers paint at pressures exceeding 3,000 psi through a nozzle with a bore of 0.031 inch. To enter the skin, the nozzle must be on or very close to the skin surface. The entry point appears rather insignificant (Fig. 6-14, *A*). Roentgenograms can reveal the extent of injection when radiopaque paints are involved (Fig. 6-14, *B*). Tissue destruction from injection of paint or products associated with painting is produced by the direct chemical action of the agent on the tissues and more significantly by the ischemia that develops secondary to edema formation. An intense and extensive inflammatory reaction is pro-

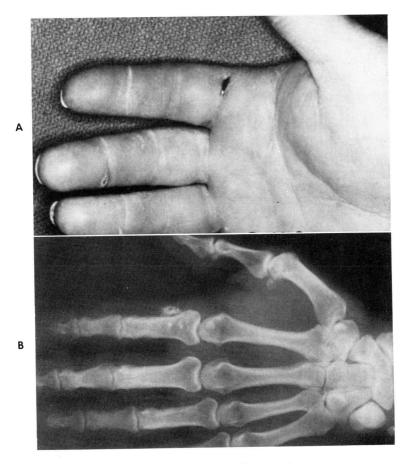

**Fig. 6-14. A,** The airless paint gun inflicts a small insignificant-appearing entry point at the base of the index finger. **B,** Roentgenogram reveals the extent of injection of radiopaque material. Commonly used paint thinners and cleaners are not radiopaque. (From Weeks, P. M.: J. Ky. Med. Assoc. **65:**1086, 1967.)

duced around vessels of the hand. Vascular thrombosis leading to necrosis of fat, muscle, and skin is observed. Treatment requires rapid and thorough removal of the offending agents and prevention of ischemia secondary to edema by thorough decompression of the hand. The palmar structures must be decompressed by opening the palmar fascia that forms rigid tunnels within the palm. The digit must be decompressed through a midlateral incision. Subcutaneously on the volar aspect of this incision, the thin band of fascia extending from the volar edge of the phalanges to the skin (Cleland's ligament) must be divided. This provides decompression of the volar compartment of the finger. Decompression of the dorsum of the hand requires only an incision in the skin and fascia; care must be taken to preserve the underlying veins. Before the need for extensive decompression and removal of the foreign material was appreciated, airless paint gun injection injuries uniformly resulted in at least ray amputation. With adequate decompression, amputation has become the exception rather than the rule. The intense inflammatory response subsides, and residual restrictive fibrosis is minimal.

A second type of injection injury is characterized by extravasation of intravenous fluids into the dorsum of the hand or forearm. Levarterenol extravasation, for example, produces noticeable local pallor, mottling of the skin, and a drop in skin temperature. These changes are ascribed to spasm of the venous, capillary, and arterial system, resulting from retrograde flow of the vasopressor into the capillaries and arterioles. Involvement of major vessels in the area of extravasation, as well as their vasa vasorum, leads to disruption of the vein wall integrity, increased vascular permeability, and massive brawny edema formation. Selection of the method of treatment is determined by the time elapsed between extravasation and its rec-

ognition. Within 18 hours after extravasation, the beneficial effects of multiple local injections of the antiadrenergic drug, phentolamine, are well established. If the phentolamine is injected locally within 12 hours after extravasation, tissue necrosis is prevented. From 12 to 18 hours after extravasation, the effectiveness of phentolamine injection is less predictable, and after 18 hours it is of no value. When the extravasation is detected after 18 hours, only supportive measures are of value.

Uncontrollable edema formation on the dorsum of the hand can lead to occlusion of the dorsal venous system, further edema formation, and ultimate occlusion of the volar venous system (Fig. 6-15). Digital necrosis ensues. Reestablishment of adequate digital venous drainage by surgical decompression of the palmar and digital

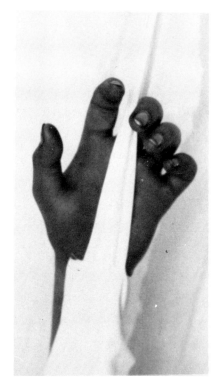

**Fig. 6-15.** Extravasation of levarterenol into the dorsum of the hand resulted in extensive edema and venous occlusion.

vasculature can prevent digital necrosis and minimizes necrosis in the immediate area of levarterenol infiltration. The role of mechanical tension in producing tissue hypoxia after levarterenol extravasation has been demonstrated experimentally. We have observed a similar chain of events when hypertonic dextrose is extravasated into the dorsum of the hand.

### Crushing injuries

A common industrial injury is the crushing injury usually produced by a press. If the face of the press is flat, the crushing force will be distributed over the flattened hand, producing a bursting of the skin along the lateral edges of the palm and more volarward in the digits. If the press

is beveled, then multiple fractures and bursting of the skin at the fracture level occurs (Fig. 6-16, *A*). These injuries produce extensive tissue damage resulting in marked edema formation. If these wounds are closed primarily, the resulting increased tissue tension may lead to more extensive vascular impairment. Because this resultant edema formation is inevitable, these injuries should be managed by gentle fracture reduction, stabilization of the wrist with a pin, meticulous wound débridement, and application of a snug but not tight dressing. Postoperatively, the hand should be maintained in an elevated position without any circumferential pressure being applied by the suspension apparatus. Circulation should be carefully

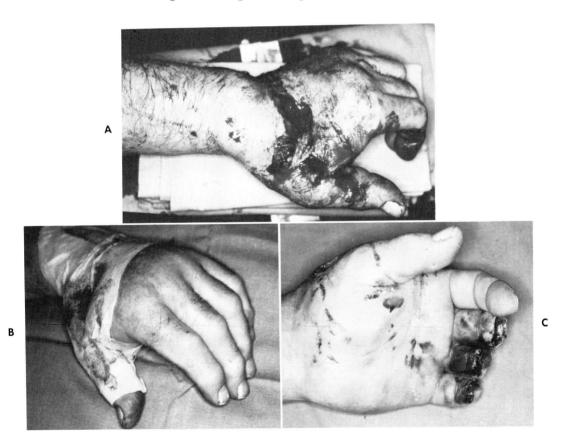

**Fig. 6-16. A,** The crush injury produces extensive damage to all the tissues of the hand. Edema that can lead to further tissue loss develops. **B,** The hand has been completely decompressed. **C,** Progressive necrosis of the fingers has occurred over a period of 3 weeks.

monitored, and if any evidence of vascular embarrassment is noted, the dressing must be removed. Forty-eight hours later the hand should be redressed under anesthesia. (Fig. 6-16, *B*). Débridement should be performed as indicated, and if the wounds appear clean, a split graft is then applied. In no instances have we used pedicle flaps in the initial management phase. As vascular thrombosis progresses, necrosis appears in one or more of the fingertips. These necrotic tips are amputated immediately (Fig. 6-16, *C*). Basically, no definitive procedures are carried out in these injuries during the initial management period. All efforts are directed toward preserving as much tissue as possible with as little manipulation as necessary. In many cases, if the tissues for reconstructing a basic hand can be preserved, our management has been successful. The crush injury, by its very nature, dampens our enthusiasm for early joint movement —at least until the extent of injury is manifest.

### The pneumatic tourniquet

The pneumatic tourniquet is used routinely in hand surgery to obtain a bloodless field. As such, it is frequently taken for granted—particularly since it is on the other side of the drape. Yet biochemical changes that occur must be appreciated by all who use the tourniquet in the ischemic forearm and hand during surgery.

Wilgis obtained venous blood samples preoperatively, intraoperatively, and after the tourniquet had been released. After inflation of the tourniquet, he observed a decrease in venous pH from 7.40 to 7.31 at 30 minutes of tourniquet ischemia. Thereafter a gradual decrease in pH to 7.19 at 60 minutes, 7.04 at 90 minutes, and 6.90 after 120 minutes was observed. A concomitant fall was reported in the partial pressure of oxygen from a normal level of 45 mm to 20, 10, and 4 mm of mercury pressure after 60, 90, and 120 minutes of

ischemia, respectively. After release of the tourniquet, return of these parameters to normal levels required up to 15 minutes when the arm had been ischemic for 90 minutes. Histologically, there is evidence of capillary and cell damage in striated muscle rendered ischemic for up to 2 hours. Severe acidosis (pH $< 7.2$) is associated with a hypocoagulability of blood. This might explain the profuse oozing that occurs after release of a tourniquet inflated for an extended period of time.

As a result of these observations, the following recommendations are made:

1. Keep tourniquet time to a minimum.
2. Two hours is the upper limit for a single application.
3. After removing the tourniquet, do not reapply it until the pH, $Pco_2$, and $Po_2$ have returned to normal.
4. Before attempting to stop the oozing, keep direct pressure on the wound and wait until the period of arteriovenous shunting has subsided.
5. Completely remove the tourniquet cuff and underlying padding after deflating to prevent constriction of the arm, which can lead to further venous congestion and oozing.
6. Between use, check pressure readings on the tourniquet to verify the actual pressure applied by the tourniquet at a particular sitting.

Care should be taken during the prepping of an arm to prevent the alcohol and iodine solution from impregnating the web roll beneath the tourniquet. This has been reported to cause skin burn at the distal end of the pneumatic cuff. Additional towels covering the tourniquet during prepping will prevent this complication.

### BIBLIOGRAPHY

Bruner, J. M.: Safety factors in the use of the pneumatic tourniquet in surgery of the hand, J. Bone Joint Surg. 33A:221, 1951.
Caldwell, P. C.: Studies on the internal pH of large muscle and nerve fibers, J. Physiol. **142:** 22, 1958.

Chase, R. A.: The severely injured upper limb, Arch. Surg. **100**:382, 1970.

Ellis, J. S.: The management of hand injuries, Practitioner **201**:730, 1968.

Entin, M. A.: Salvaging the basic hand, Surg. Clin. North Am. **48**:1063, 1968.

Flatt, A.: Tourniquet time in hand surgery, Arch. Surg. **14**:190, 1972.

Inoue, T., Toyoshima, Y., Fukusumi, H., and others: Factors necessary for successful replantation of upper extremities, Ann. Surg. **165**:225, 1967.

Klenerman, L.: The tourniquet in surgery, J. Bone Joint Surg. **44B**:937, 1962.

Moldaver, J.: Tourniquet paralysis syndrome, Arch. Surg. **68**:136, 1954.

Paletta, F. X., Willman, V., and Ship, A. G.: Prolonged tourniquet ischemia of extremities, J. Bone Joint Surg. **42A**:945, 1960.

Remark, F. L., and Weeks, P. M.: Management of the acutely injured hand, Mo. Med. **68**:767, 1971.

Seddon, H. J.: Surgical disorders of the peripheral nerves, Baltimore, 1972, The Williams and Wilkins Co.

Solonen, K. A., and Hjelt, L.: Morphological changes in striated muscle during ischaemia; a clinical and histological study in man, Acta Orthop. Scand. **39**:13, 1968.

Solonen, K. A., Tarkkanen, L., Närvänen, S., and others: Metabolic changes in the upper limb during tourniquet ischaemia: a clinical study, Acta Orthop. Scand. **39**:20, 1968.

Sunderland, S.: A classification of peripheral nerve injuries producing loss of function, Brain **74**:491, 1951.

Weeks, P. M.: Ischemia of the hand secondary to levarterenol bitartrate extravasation, J.A.M.A. **196**:288, 1966.

Weeks, P. M.: Airless paint gun injuries of the hand, J. Ky. Med. Assoc. **65**:1086, 1967.

Weeks, P. M.: Management of acute injuries of the upper extremity, J. Ky. Med. Assoc. **66**:705, 1968.

Wheeler, D. K., and Liscomb, P. R.: A safety device for a pneumatic tourniquet, J. Bone Joint Surg. **46A**:870, 1964.

Wilgis, E. F. S.: Observations on the effects of tourniquet ischemia, J. Bone Joint Surg. **53A**:1343, 1971.

Williams, G. R., and Frank, G. R.: Replantation of amputated extremities, Ann. Surg. **163**:788, 1966.

# CHAPTER 7
# The role of microsurgery in acute hand injuries

**DEVELOPMENT OF MICROSURGERY**

Microsurgery has assumed a major role in the field of hand surgery. Through use of the operating microscope, the hand surgeon has expanded his ability to preserve or reconstruct the fine structures of the hand. Recent advances in instrumentation and techniques in microsurgery have led to the development of the fields of free flap transfer, microneurorrhaphy, and replantation. These are rapidly becoming part of the armamentarium of the hand surgeon. The clinical applications of microsurgery are expanding and will be discussed, with emphasis on techniques that may provide improved functional results following hand surgery.

In 1960, Jacobson and Suarez demonstrated the value of the microscope in vascular surgery by markedly improving the results of arterial anastomosis in vessels less than 4 mm in diameter. As these pioneers predicted, the use of microsurgical techniques extended vascular surgery to many previously inaccessible areas.

Chase, Buncke, and Ackland, among others, provided the foundation for the development of microinstrumentation and microsutures. These instruments used in combination with proper magnification have allowed the transition of microsurgery from the experimental laboratory to the operative suite.

Transplantation of tissue by vascular anastomosis was introduced by Carrel in 1902 and Carrel and Guthrie in 1906. Experimental transplantation later incorporated the instrumentation of microsurgery, which lead to the development of clinical replantation. In 1964, human replantation became a reality when Malt successfully replanted the right arm of a 12-year-old boy. Later that same year, Kleinert successfully revascularized a crushed, devitalized thumb. Thus, the field of clinical replantation became a reality, and microvascular surgeons began reporting successful limb and finger replantations at an ever increasing rate.

Another aspect of microsurgery has been the development of immediate flap transplantation by microvascular anastomosis. In 1965 Krizek and later Strauch and Murray experimentally transplanted isolated composite grafts of skin and subcutaneous tissue. Using the pig for an experimental flap model, Daniel and Taylor demonstrated the feasibility of free transfer of axial pattern flaps. Soon thereafter, Daniel (1973) successfully performed on humans a free transfer of an island flap by microvascular anastomosis. In that same year,

Dr. Yang Don-Yoa of the Wasan Hospital in Shanghai and O'Brien in Australia performed free flap transfers that provided reconstruction of difficult defects in a single-stage procedure. The value of this aspect of microsurgery in hand surgery will be discussed in the section on the clinical applications of microsurgery.

These highlights of the development of the field of microsurgery include only a few of the many pioneers involved. Smith, Cobbett, and Buncke have provided excellent discussions of this field. Hakstian and Kleinert have outlined the role of microsurgery in hand surgery. Kleinert appropriately summarized this discussion with this statement: "The application of microsurgical techniques to the entire range of clinical hand surgery, from elective excision of soft tissue tumors to complicated digital reimplantation, will provide a higher standard of excellence with improved uniform results."

## INSTRUMENTATION

Proper instrumentation is the key to successful microsurgery. The early development of microsurgery largely consisted of advances in equipment that enable the surgeon to operate at magnifications ranging from 5× to 40×. At present, the equipment is readily available, allowing the novice to concentrate his efforts on perfection of manipulative techniques.

The operative instruments must be long enough to rest in the thumb-index web space. Spring control instruments without ratchets are required, because only pinch motion between the thumb and index finger will permit the control necessary to work under magnification. Essential to microsurgical procedures are the jeweler's forceps with finely polished tips for manipulation of vessels and nerves, suture handling, and knot tying. Small spring-loaded scissors enable the surgeon to prepare blood vessels and nerves for anastomosis or repair. Spring-loaded needle holders, either

curved or straight, should be capable of holding microneedles ranging in diameter from $140\mu$ to $50\mu$. These essential instruments must be used only under magnification to avoid misuse and must be cleaned carefully and stored in a separate instrument case to prevent damage.

A variety of clamps and microvascular clips are now available for blood vessel control. Ackland has designed a series of microclips that are light, gentle, and compact. His adjustable double approximating clamp is ideal for the actual vascular anastomosis (see Fig. 7-5, E and F).

The bipolar coagulator is an integral part of hand surgery and can be used in microsurgery. Because the current flow is limited to the contact points between the tips, there is no danger of injury to adjacent structures. Hemostasis is important during microsurgical procedures.

Ethicon, and Davis and Geck, each offer a variety of monofilament sutures that are suitable for nerve and vascular microsurgical procedures. Suture diameters in the range of $18\mu$ to $22\mu$ with needle diameters of $50\mu$ to $100\mu$ are suitable for vessels in the range of 0.6 to 1.5 mm in diameter. Thirty-five micron suture with $140\mu$ needles are appropriate for nerve repair and anastomosis of vessels ranging from 1.5 to 4 mm in diameter.

Although individual preferences will vary with experience, a general list of microvascular instruments and sources includes the following:

S & T microvascular instruments
S & T Chirurgische Nadeln
7893 Jestetten/BRD
Postfach 93, West Germany
  Jewelers forceps: straight #5, angulated #56
  Vessel stretcher
  Clamp-applying forceps
  Ackland pattern clamps: single 8, 11, and 14 mm
  Ackland pattern approximator with suture-holding frame
  ACC 1-8 mm
  ACC 2-11 mm
  ACC 3-14 mm

Sparta Instruments
305 Fairfield Avenue
Fairfield, N.J. 07006
 Razor blade holder 10-652
 Razor blades 10-655
 Scissors 12-380, 12-382
 Needle holder 13-311

Edward Weck & Co.
Weck Drive
PO Box 12600
Research Triangle Park, N. C. 27709
 Kleinert-Kutz microvessel clips
 10-mm blade (5 × 1 mm) 65105

Richards Manufacturing Co.
1450 Brooks Road
Memphis, Tenn. 38116
 McGee suction tube/20ga
  5¾-inch long angulated 13-0150

Codman
Randolph, Mass. 02368
 Bipolar microcoagulator

## CLINICAL APPLICATIONS

After the basics of microsurgery, including suture handling, knot tying, microdissection, and vessel anastomosis have been mastered, the applications for these techniques are vast. In the management of acute hand injuries, microsurgery may be needed for nerve repair, revascularization, replantation, and reconstruction. These areas will be discussed, including techniques pertinent to each procedure.

### Nerve repair

The importance of avoiding tension and connective tissue interposition during neurorrhaphy as advocated by Millesi is well appreciated when neurorrhaphy is accomplished using microtechniques. After the epineurium is excised at the proximal and

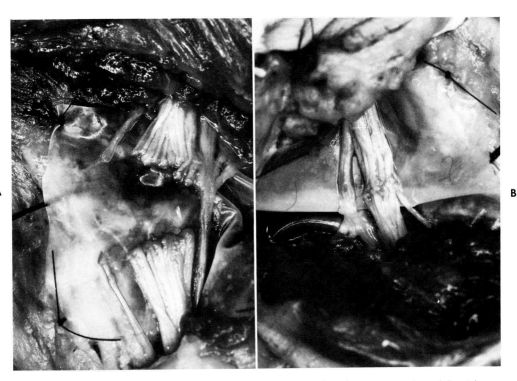

**Fig. 7-1.** Median nerve laceration at wrist. **A,** Epineurium has been resected, and fascicles are oriented for neurorrhaphy. (Note: two fascicles are intact.) **B,** Direct fascicular median neurorrhaphy is completed.

distal stumps under microscopic control, using microscissors or micro-razor blades in a holder (see instruments), the fascicles can be sutured with proper orientation (Fig. 7-1).

When the gap is greater than 2 cm, neurorrhaphy cannot be accomplished with microtechniques without graft interposition. In the digital nerves, the neurorrhaphy can be accomplished with interfascicular grafting, using the lateral antebrachial cutaneous nerve as a graft (Fig. 7-2). In the median, radial, and ulnar nerves, the sural nerve is ideal for interposition between groups of fascicles (Fig. 7-3). Microsurgical neurorrhaphy ensures accurate alignment of perineurial tubes at proximal and distal stumps without tension.

## Replantation

When a finger, a hand, or an entire extremity is either devascularized or completely amputated, revascularization and replantation must be considered. Although Douglas and recently Elsahy have demonstrated survival of completely avulsed portions of fingers reattached as composite grafts, this is clearly not feasible proximal to the level of the distal phalanx of the digit. The patient with any acute hand injury that results in amputation of digits or more proximal parts immediately requires untwisting of traumatic flaps, local wound cleansing, tetanus prophylaxis, antibiotics, and a general assessment for other critical injuries. The amputated portion should be cooled. This is best accom-

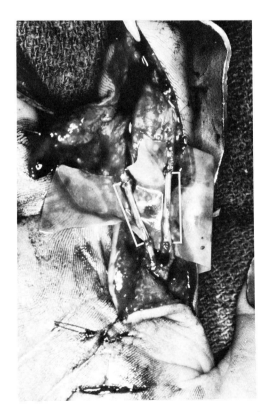

**Fig. 7-2.** Bilateral 3-cm interfascicular digital nerve grafts. (Donor nerve: lateral antebrachial nerve.)

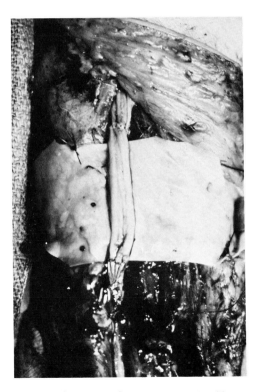

**Fig. 7-3.** Ulnar nerve laceration at wrist. Neurorrhaphy is accomplished with 3-cm interfascicular sural nerve grafts.

plished by placing the amputated part in a plastic bag and inserting the bag in a container of crushed ice and water. The ischemic digit or amputated part when cooled to 4° C can survive more than 21 hours. Only after fulfilling these steps should one seriously consider replantation or transfer of the patient and amputated part to a facility for replantation.

In this discussion of replantation, upper extremity amputations will be subdivided into three groups based strictly on importance of replantation for future hand function. The groups are as follows:

Group I
1. Entire hand or upper extremity
2. Thumb proximal to interphalangeal joint
3. Four digits proximal to interphalangeal joint

Group II
Three radial digits proximal to interphalangeal joint

Group III
1. Two or fewer digits
2. Portion of single or multiple digits distal to proximal phalanx

*Assessment of amputated part.* The mechanism of injury should be evaluated when a patient with an amputation is being assessed for replantation. In severe crush or avulsion injuries, only patients falling into Group I warrant further consideration for replantation. The amputated part should be radiographically evaluated; if fractures and soft tissue injuries are extensive, the value of replantation is seriously diminished. When the entire hand or upper extremity has multiple fractures, replantation of a Group II or III amputation may be detrimental to ultimate hand function. In the sharp amputations without crush or avulsion injury, replantation is generally advisable in Groups I and II.

*Patient assessment.* The patient who after initial assessment has multiple organ system injuries with either a Group I or II amputation may become a replantation candidate after stabilization of other injuries. In such a case, the digits should be maintained at 4° C over the next 6 hours. If the patient's condition is stable and if replantation does not impede other simultaneous surgical procedures, replantation may proceed.

*Concurrent disease.* In general, the risk of concurrent disease largely entails a consideration of anesthesia risk. Replantations are best performed while the patient is under general anesthesia where muscle activity is eliminated during the procedure. However, some microsurgical units advocate the use of regional anesthesia. Patients with diabetes or advanced atherosclerotic disease represent contraindications for replantations, especially in Group II and III amputations.

*Age and preinjury function.* Whereas a child is a likely candidate for replantation in all three groups, an adult appears to have less potential for eventual useful function in the replanted part. Patients with either a Group I or II injury whose occupation requires use of the injured hand should undergo replantation. Recommendation for replantation of Group III amputations is based solely on need of digits for specific hand function and cosmetic appearance and should not be undertaken without a discussion with the patient and family.

*Digital replantation technique.* Replantation is best performed by a team approach. Once either general anesthesia or regional anesthesia is established, one team begins treatment of associated injuries while the tourniquet is in place. This includes débridement of devitalized tissues. The hand in Fig. 7-4, *A* exemplifies a typical Group II amputation with a thumb injury and amputation of the radial three digits. The ring finger was severely traumatized and not a candidate for replantation. However, a portion of the tissues on the ulnar side of this digit was transferred to the thumb as an island flap (Fig. 7-4, *B*). These efforts

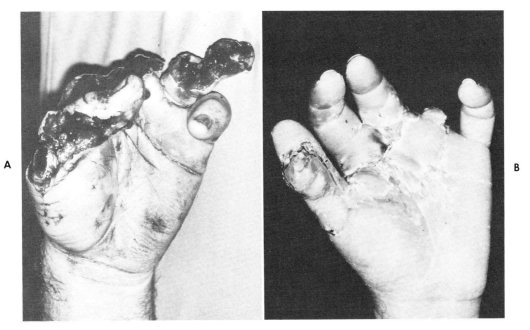

**Fig. 7-4.** Example of management of Group II amputation in hand. **A,** Traumatic amputation of radial three digits and partial amputation of radial aspect of thumb. **B,** The remaining portion of ulnar aspect of amputated ring finger is transposed as island flap to thumb defect. The index and middle fingers are replaced.

toward preservation of useful local tissue may aid reconstruction in conjunction with replantation.

A second team simultaneously prepares the amputated digits for replantation. The digital artery and nerves are best isolated through radial and ulnar midlateral incisions. An attempt is also made to locate dorsal veins on the amputated digit (Fig. 7-5, *A*). The vessels are marked with single vascular clips to facilitate later identification. The microsurgeon in charge should work on the second team to ensure his familiarity with vessel location and adequate vessel preparation. Both proximal and distal bone fragments are shortened approximately 0.5 cm to prevent tension on the vascular anastomosis (Fig. 7-5, *B*). If the amputation is through a joint, the joint surfaces are sacrificed and an arthrodesis is performed. The amputated part is secured to the proximal stump with Kirsch-

ner wires, either transmedullary or crossed, to obtain secure fixation (Fig. 7-5, *C*). The flexor and extensor tendons are repaired. If multiple replantations are planned, all digits are simultaneously prepared to this stage.

The tourniquet is now deflated and the digital vessels, nerves, and dorsal veins are isolated at the proximal amputation stump under the direction of the microsurgeon (Fig. 7-5, *D*). These vessels are also tagged with microclips. Next, the proximal artery stump is checked for pulsatile flow. If pulsatile flow is poor, the vessel must be dissected more proximally and again prepared for the anastomosis. The operating microscope is moved into place to aid neurorraphy and vascular anastomosis. A fascicular suture is accomplished with 9-0 monofilament nylon to each digital nerve. If dorsal veins have been isolated, the vein most accessible is anastomosed with 10-0

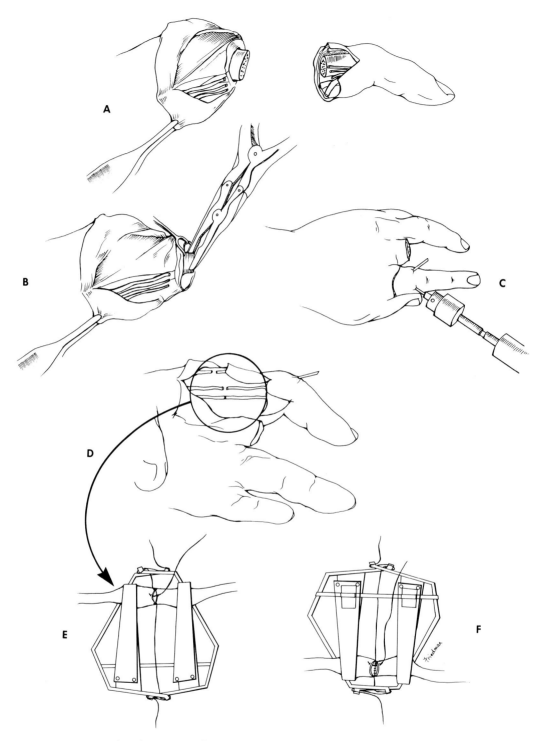

**Fig. 7-5.** Digital replantation technique. **A,** Isolation of digital vessels, nerves, and tendons at amputation sites. **B,** Bone stumps are shortened. **C,** Bone fixation. **D,** Extensor and profundus tendorrhaphy accomplished. Digital neurorrhaphy is performed with microscope. **E,** Anterior digital vessel anastomosis. **F,** Posterior digital vessel anastomosis.

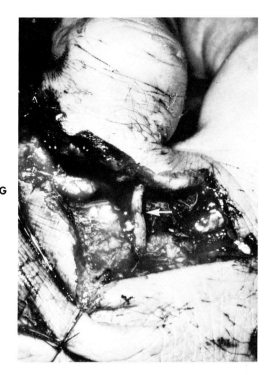

**Fig. 7-5, cont'd. G,** Completed vein anastomosis **(arrow)** on replanted digit.

are placed using absolute care to obtain correct apposition of the cut vessel edges. The clamp is rotated 180 degrees to facilitate the posterior anastomosis. Under maximum magnification, the lumen is flushed with the heparin-saline solution and the intimal side of the anterior anastomosis is examined. Any suture that is causing vessel overlap or penetrating the posterior wall is removed and reinserted (Fig. 7-5, *F*). The posterior row is completed with interrupted sutures. All microvascular clamps are released and exposed vessels are flooded with 1% lidocaine or 0.5% marcaine to minimize vasospasm. If a vein anastomosis has not been accomplished, the dorsal surface can again be examined for venous return, and after the distal veins are isolated, the first anastomosis can be accomplished (Fig. 7-5, *G*). A second vein should be isolated and repaired if possible because two venous repairs are preferable. If multiple digital replantations are planned, the second venous anastomosis should be delayed until the remaining digits have been vascularized. One digital arterial anastomosis per digit is adequate. Hemostasis should be carefully obtained. Split-thickness skin grafts meshed 1½ to 1 are advisable if skin tension prevents primary closure.

*Vein grafts.* When the vessel ends cannot be approximated without undue tension, a vein graft is required. A penrose tourniquet on the wrist will reveal several small veins on the volar surface. These can be easily harvested, and they function ideally as interposition grafts. When the mechanism of injury has an avulsion or crush force, or the intima appears injured, one should immediately proceed with vein grafts extending between uninjured portions of the proximal and distal vessel stumps. When arterial flow or venous return is inadequate in a technically satisfying anastomosis, an unrecognized intimal injury is likely. In this case, a vein graft spanning the area of possible injury should again be attempted.

*Adjuvant therapy.* Success or failure of

monofilament nylon. If veins are not readily isolated, one should immediately proceed with the arterial anastomosis. The vessel ends are placed in double approximating clamps (Fig. 7-5, *E* and *F*). Under 25× magnification, the adventitia is dissected from the vessel within the double approximating clamps. The end of the vessel is transected to remove traumatized intima; the lumen is flushed with heparin-saline solution (1,000 units/100 ml saline); and the intima is examined under maximum magnification. If the intima appears damaged, the vessel must be dissected proximally until uninjured intima is observed. The vessel lumen is then stretched by inserting a No. 2 forceps to double the internal diameter. The first two sutures are then placed at 120 degrees on the anterior wall of the vessel and attached to the hitches on the side of the frame (Fig. 7-5, *E* and *F*). Three to four more sutures replantation generally is related to the adequacy of the arterial and venous anastomoses. Many microvascular centers use central heparinization prior to the anastomosis and continue this anticoagulation treatment postoperatively. Others use low molecular weight dextran both intraoperatively and postoperatively. However, since platelet thrombus is the initial step in early thrombosis, the postoperative use of low molecular weight dextran along with aspirin orally may reduce platelet aggregation and is recommended for 7 to 10 days. Although infection has been an infrequent complication in successful revascularization, antibiotics should be continued in the postoperative period.

*Results.* Initial results are measured in simple terms of viability. O'Brien has reported an overall success rate of 61% for replantations. In the guillotine-complete amputations, a success rate in the 70% to 80% range can be expected. This obviously drops when attempts at revascularization of crush and avulsion injuries are included. In a recent review of 86 replantations in 71 patients at the Louisville Hand Service, Weiland noted a viability success rate of 53% of sharp amputations and of 28.5% of crush injuries. The majority of the failed replantations were the result of vascular thrombosis (68.4%) with most of these related to venous thrombosis (40.7%). In an addendum to this report, Weiland notes an increase in survival rate to 90% in their most recent 50 replantations. By proper case selection and careful attention to technique, replantation can be performed with a great potential for survival.

In the 32 patients with successful replantations, thirteen complications (40.6%) were noted. Tendon adherence represented the most common complication, occurring in six patients. Less common problems included delayed union of bone in three patients, postoperative infection in two patients, and atrophy of the replanted digit in one patient.

Long-term results depend largely on the success of the tendon and nerve repairs. Ideally, nerve and tendon results will be similar to those associated with acute hand injuries without vascular damage. In Weiland's report, the functional tendon results are reported on 17 of his 32 successful digital replantations. Complete primary flexor and extensor tendon repairs were performed on these 17 patients. Forty-seven percent of this group could flex a replanted digit within 1.5 cm of the distal crease with less than 15 degrees loss of extension. Thirty-five percent of these patients could not flex to within 3 cm of the distal palmar crease, or they demonstrated more than 15 degrees loss of extension, or both. O'Brien and associates do not report specific data, but they note that in 57 digital replantations, all patients have benefited from their final range of motion.

Weiland and associates include specific discussion on nerve repair results in the 32 successful replantations. In this group, 65.6% underwent primary nerve repair; 34.3% underwent secondary neurorraphy. In 18 successful digital replants that were specifically evaluated for two-point discrimination, 56% had two-point discrimination of 10 mm or less, and 44% had protective sensation. O'Brien and co-workers note that with primary digital nerve repairs, the two-point discrimination in their series ranges from 3 to 10 mm. The success of replantations has been satisfying to both patient and surgeon and warrants continuing efforts in this new area. As more complete long-term functional results become available, the exact role of replantation in acute hand injuries will be fully defined.

***Hand and arm replantation technique.*** The two team approach is again advisable in preparing both the proximal and distal stumps. The team handling the distal stump must carefully assess the distal extremity for associated injuries. If excessive muscle injury is present or if warm ischemic time has exceeded 6 hours, muscle ischemia will be excessive and success unlikely. Following simultaneous débridement, bone shortening is accomplished in the range of 5 cm, or greater if necessary. The bone is then internally fixed with Kirschner wires and intramedullary pins. If warm ischemic time approaches 6 hours, arterial anastomosis should first be accomplished, followed by venous anastomosis. However, if cooling has been adequate, wrist extensor and deep flexor tendonorrhaphy should precede the vascularization. The principles regarding the technique of anastomosis are the same as those discussed under digital replantation. Again, tension must be avoided. When tension is present or when vessels demonstrate intimal damage requiring resection of vessel ends; vein grafts should be incorporated in the revascularization procedure. The dorsal foot represents the best source for donor veins. Multiple dorsal venous anastomoses must be accomplished. Neurorrhaphy should be performed primarily using fascicular repair. When the gap is excessive, epineurial repair is indicated, which means delaying the use of nerve grafts for secondary elective procedures. If skin closure is difficult, split-thickness skin grafts meshed 1½ to 1 are indicated to prevent creating tension at the skin closure. Fasciotomy is advisable if edema is excessive, especially to decompress the intrinsic hand muscles. As we discussed in digital replantation, low molecular weight dextran, aspirin, and antibiotics should be used postoperatively for 7 to 10 days.

*Results.* Malt's initial hand replantations have been followed on a long-term basis and demonstrate remarkable functional recovery. Malt concludes that replantations are indicated in mentally alert, stable patients without central trauma whose amputated part of the upper extremity is well preserved. The injury should be isolated to the amputation site. Functional recovery is possible using these criteria in patients of all ages. His five successful replantations have demonstrated gross protective sensation, and in one case, a two-point discrimination of 1.5 to 2 cm in all fingers. All cases demonstrated motor function in the hand enabling a power grasp and finger motion.

O'Brien reports 13 successful replantations in 17 upper extremity amputations. Failures were due to infection and severe distal trauma. Five of the seven successful total hand replantations demonstrated good flexion and extension. Motor function results in replantations above the lower third of the forearm demonstrated considerable fibrosis in muscles with less digital movement. Sensory return in this series of replantations included a return of a two-point discrimination of 2 to 2.5 cm and protective sensation. These results and those observed in the Chinese experience support the value of total hand and extremity replantation.

### Reconstruction

Reconstruction following acute hand injuries is often hampered by the lack of adequate soft tissue and skin coverage. Skin grafting procedures provide inadequate coverage and may not even survive because of extensive fibrosis and poor vascularity. Distant flaps such as the McGregor groin flap, abdominal flaps, and others provide the needed full-thickness skin and subcutaneous tissue but necessitate multistaged procedures and immobilization of the hand in fixed positions. With the advent of microvascular surgery and identification of suitable donor flaps supplied by direct cutaneous arteries, it is now possible to provide this needed coverage in a single-stage reconstructive procedure.

The iliofemoral groin flap may be transferred directly as a free island flap based on the superficial circumflex iliac artery and vein. The flap may also include the superficial inferior epigastric artery and vein. The flap may be tailored to the exact size of the defect, a distinct advantage in free

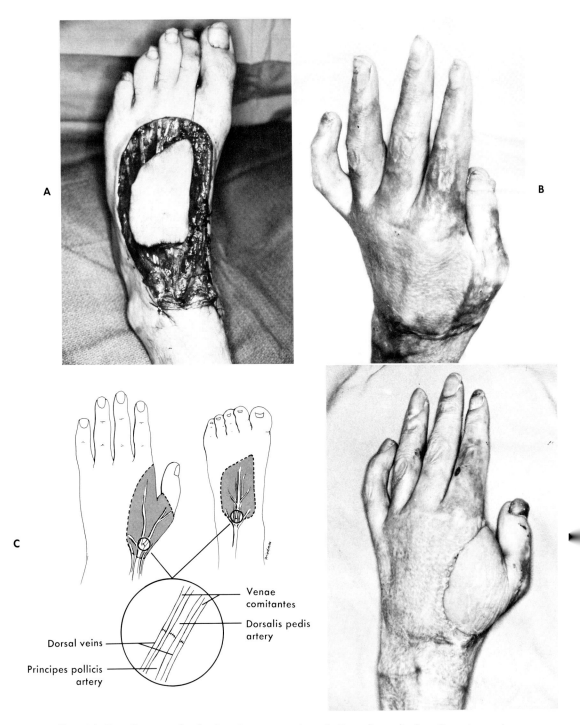

**Fig. 7-6.** Free flap transfer for hand reconstruction. **A,** Dorsalis pedis free flap elevated at donor site. **B,** Traumatic thumb-index web space contracture. **C,** Free transfer of dorsalis pedis flap to index-thumb web space. **D,** Six weeks following web space release and free flap transfer.

flap transfer, and the defect closed primarily. With this free flap, nerve, bone, and tendon grafting procedures may be performed primarily beneath a well-vascularized flap.

The dorsalis pedis flap as described by McCraw and Furlow is also suitable as a free flap donor region. This flap may be used as a neurovascular free flap incorporating the superficial peroneal nerve. The flap may also include underlying vascularized long extensor grafts and metacarpophalangeal joints. The flap extends from the level of the extensor retinaculum proximally to the toe web space distally and 5 cm medially and laterally to the dorsalis pedis artery (Fig. 7-6, *A*). The flap is drained by the long and short saphenous veins, and the venae comitantes of the dorsalis pedis artery. This flap is very thin and especially useful in the reconstruction of soft tissue defects in the hand. The donor area is skin grafted and generally does not provide future disabilities.

A patient who survived a burn of 50% of the body surface had a residual severe thumb-index web space contracture (Fig. 7-6, *B*). Following release of the web space contracture and the fibrosed short adductor muscle, local tissue was unavailable for reconstruction of the soft tissue defect; therefore, a dorsalis pedis flap was elevated for use in free flap transfer to this defect (Fig. 7-6, *A*). Microvascular anastomoses were accomplished between the princeps pollicis artery and the dorsalis pedis artery and between two dorsal veins and the venae comitantes of the dorsalis pedis artery (Fig. 7-6, *C*). A vascularized second long extensor was incorporated in the flap for later use in restorating the thumb extensor function. A single-stage reconstruction incorporating free transfer of an axial flap provided an improved hand function with no donor area disability (Fig. 7-6, *D*).

The ultimate goal of the hand surgeon is the restoration of the acutely injured hand to a functional normal status. Although the art of microsurgery, especially in the area of reconstruction, is still in its infancy, the microvascular free island flap, the free muscle flap, and vascularized bone and nerve grafts represent new reconstructive techniques that will greatly expand the ability of the surgeon to achieve this goal.

## BIBLIOGRAPHY

Ackland, R. D.: New instruments for microvascular surgery, Br. J. Surg. **59:**181, 1972.

Baxter, T. J., O'Brien, B. McC., Henderson, P. N., and Bennett, R. C.: The histopathology of small vessels following microvascular repair, Br. J. Surg. **59:**617, 1972.

Buncke, H. J.: The development of microsurgery. In Daniller, A. I., and Strauch, B., editors: Symposium on microsurgery, St. Louis, 1976, The C. V. Mosby Co.

Buncke, H. J., Buncke, C. M., and Schulz, W. P.: Experimental digital amputation and replantation, Plast. Reconstr. Surg. **36:**62, 1965.

Buncke, H. J., and Schulz, W. P.: Total ear reimplantation in the rabbit utilizing microminiature vascular anastomosis, Br. J. Plast. Surg. **19:**15, 1966.

Carrel, A.: The operative technique of vascular anastomosis and transplantation of organs, Lyon Méd. **98:**859, 1902.

Carrel, A., and Guthrie, C. C.: Complete amputation of the thigh with replantation, Am. J. Med. Sci. **131:**297, 1906.

Chase, M. D., and Schwartz, S. I.: Consistent potency of 1.5 mm arterial anastomosis, Surg. Forum **13:**220, 1962.

Chase, M. D., and Schwartz, S. I.: Suture anastomosis of small arteries, Surg. Gynecol. Obstet. **117:**44, 1963.

Chase, M. D., and Schwartz, S. I.: Technique of small artery anastomosis, Surg. Gynecol. Obstet. **116:**381, 1963.

Cobbett, J. R.: Microvascular surgery, Surg. Clin. North Am. **47:**521, 1967.

Daniel, R. K.: The free transfer of skin flaps by microvascular anastomosis, Plast. Reconstr. Surg. **52:**16, 1973.

Daniel, R. K., and Taylor, G. I.: Distant transfer of an island flap by microvascular anastomosis, Plast. Reconstr. Surg. **52:**111, 1973.

Daniel, R. K., Terzis, J., and Midgley, R. D.: Restoration of sensation to an anesthetic hand by a free neurovascular flap from the foot, Plast. Reconstr. Surg. **57:**275, 1976.

Douglas, B.: Successful replacement of completely avulsed portions of fingers as composite grafts, Plast. Reconstr. Surg. **23:**213, 1959.

Elsahy, N.: When to replant a fingertip after its complete amputation, Plast. Reconstr. Surg. **60:** 14, 1977.

Fisher, B., and Lee, S.: Microvascular surgical techniques in research surgery, Surgery **58:**904, 1965.

Grabb, W., BeMint, S., Koepke, G., and Green, R.: Comparison of methods of peripheral nerve suture in monkeys, Plast. Reconstr. Surg. **46:**31, 1970.

Hakstian, R. W.: Microsurgery; its role in surgery of the hand, Clin. Orthop. **104:**149, 1974.

Hurwitt, E. S., Altman, S., Borow, M., and Rosenblatt, M.: Intra-abdominal arterial anastomoses, Surgery **34:**1043, 1953.

Jacobson, J. H., and Suarez, E. L.: Microsurgery in anastomosis of small vessels, Surg. Forum **11:**243, 1960.

Kleinert, H. E., and Kasdan, M. L.: Anastomosis of digital vessels, J. Ky. Med. Assoc. **63:**106, 1965.

Kleinert, H. E., Kadsan, M. L., and Romero, J. L.: Small blood vessel anastomosis for salvage of severely injured upper extremities, J. Bone Joint Surg. **45A:**788, 1963.

Kleinert, H. E., and Neale, H. W.: Microsurgery in hand surgery, Clin. Orthop. **104:**158, 1974.

Komatsu, S., and Tamai, S.: Successful replantation of a completely cut-off thumb, Plast. Reconstr. Surg. **42:**374, 1968.

Krizek, T. J., Tani, T., Desprez, J. D., and others: Experimental transplantation of composite grafts by microsurgical vascular anastomoses, Plast. Reconstr. Surg. **36:**538, 1965.

Kutz, J. E., Hay, E. I., and Kleinert, H. E.: Fate of small blood vessel repair, J. Bone Joint Surg. **51A:**79, 1969.

Lapchinsky, A. C.: Recent results of experimental transplantation of preserved limbs and kidneys, Ann. N.Y. Acad. Sci. **87:**539, 1960.

Lendvay, P. G.: Anastomosis of digital vessels, Med. J. Aust. **2:**723, 1968.

Lendvay, P. G.: Replacement of the amputated digit, Br. J. Plast. Surg. **27:**398, 1973.

Malt, R. A., and McKhann, C. F.: Replantation of severed arms, J.A.M.A. **189:**114, 1964.

Malt, R. A., Remensnyder, J. P., and Harris, W. H.: Long-term utility of replanted arms, Ann. Surg. **176:**334, 1972.

Mathes, S., Vasconez, L., and Grau, G.: Direct fascicular repair and interfascicular nerve grafting of median and ulnar nerves in Rhesus monkeys, Surg. Forum **26:**545, 1975.

McCraw, J. B., and Furlow, L. T., Jr.: The dorsalis pedis arterialized flap; a clinical study, Plast. Reconstr. Surg. **55:**177, 1975.

McGregor, I. A., and Jackson, I. T.: The groin flap, Br. J. Plast. Surg. **25:**3, 1972.

Millesi, H.: Microsurgery of peripheral nerves, Hand **5:**157, 1973.

Millesi, H., Meissl, G., and Berger, A.: The interfascicular nerve grafting of the medial and ulnar nerves, J. Bone Joint Surg. **54A:**727, 1972.

Murray, J. E.: Current evaluation of human kidney transplantation, Plast. Reconstr. Surg. **34:** 93, 1964.

O'Brien, B. M., Henderson, P. N., Bennett, R. C., and Crock, G. W.: Microvascular surgical technique, Med. J. Aust. **1:**722, 1970.

O'Brien, B. M., MacLeod, A. M., Hayhurst, J. W., and Morrison, W.: Successful transfer of a large island flap from the groin to the foot by microvascular anastomosis, Plast. Reconstr. Surg. **52:** 271, 1973.

O'Brien, B. M., MacLeod, A. M., Hayhurst, W., and others: Major replantation surgery in the upper limb, Hand **6:**217, 1974.

O'Brien, B. M., MacLeod, A. M., Miller, G. D., and others: Clinical implantation of digits, Plast. Reconstr. Surg. **52:**490, 1973.

Phelan, J. T., Young, W. P., and Gale, G. W.: The effect of suture material on small artery anastomosis, Surg. Gynecol. Obstet. **107:**79, 1958.

Philipeaux, J. M., and Vulpian, A.: Note sur des essais de griffe d'un tronçon de nerf lingual entre les deux bouts de nerf hypoglosse, après excision d'un segment de ce denier nerf, Arch. Phys. Norm. Pathol. **3:**618, 1870.

Shambaugh, G. E., Jr.: Modified fenestration technic, Arch. Otolaryngol. **36:**23, 1942.

Sixth Peoples Hospital, Shanghai: Reattachment of traumatic amputations; the summing up of experience, Chin. Med. J. **5:**392, 1967.

Sixth Peoples Hospital, Shanghai: Replantation of severed limbs and fingers, Chin. Med. J. **1:**1, 1973.

Smith, J. W.: Microsurgery; review of the literature and discussion of microtechniques, Plast. Reconstr. Surg. **37:**227, 1966.

Smith, J. W.: Microsurgery and the vasa vasorum. In Donaghy, R. M., and Yasargil, M. G., editors: Micro-Vascular surgery, St. Louis, 1967, The C. V. Mosby Co.

Snyder, C. C., and Knowles, R. P.: Autotransplantation of extremities, Clin. Orthop. **29:**113, 1963.

Strauch, B., and Murray, D.: Transfer of composite graft with immediate suture anastomosis of its vascular pedicle, Plast. Reconstr. Surg. **40:**325, 1967.

Taylor, G. I., and Daniel, R. K.: The anatomy

of several free flap donor sites, Plast. Reconstr. Surg. **56:**243, 1975.

Terzis, J., Faibisoff, B., and Williams, B.: The nerve gap; suture under tension vs. graft, Plast. Reconstr. Surg. **56:**166, 1975.

Tose, L.: Autotransplantation of limbs, Master's thesis, Boston, 1961, Tufts University.

Ts'ui, C., and others: Microvascular anastomosis and transplantation, Chin. Med. J. **85:**610, 1965.

Weiland, A., Villarreal-Rios, A., Kleinert, H., and others: Replantation of digits and hands; analysis of surgical techniques and functional results in 71 patients with 86 replantations, J. Hand Surg. **2:**1, 1977.

# CHAPTER 8

# Skin and soft tissue replacement

When skin loss precludes direct wound closure, adequate coverage must be accomplished by using either free grafts or pedicle grafts. Free grafts include those which are split-thickness, full-thickness, or composite. The composite graft will not be discussed here because its use in acute injuries is very limited. Healing of split- and full-thickness free grafts necessitates adherence of the graft's dense, nonyielding dermis to the recipient site. Thus, free grafts are not utilized when the restoration of a gliding surface immediately beneath the graft is paramount.

The pedicle graft, which maintains its blood supply through the base of the flap, may incorporate any combination of subcutaneous, neural, and bony tissues into the flap. A spectrum of pedicle flaps is possible, extending from a simple broad flap of skin and subcutaneous tissue containing numerous fine capillaries to a pedicle flap containing all the digital components based on a single artery and vein.

## FREE GRAFTS

The free graft consists of epidermis and dermis. The graft is completely detached from the donor area and must derive its nourishment from the recipient site by osmosis. Consequently, the free graft must maintain intimate contact with the recipient site. Contact is aided through use of a stent (mechanic's waste pressed firmly against the graft by sutures attached to the wound margins and tied in a crossing fashion). Nourishment of the graft can be interrupted by anything that imposes itself between the recipient site and the free graft, such as a hematoma or seroma. The presence of bacteria that elaborate collagenase and thromboplastin activator results in vessel thrombosis and loss of the graft. The free graft derives its durability and functional qualities from the quantity of dermis included in the graft. Increasing the amount of dermis in the graft reduces shrinkage and adds functional padding over the grafted part. However, the thinner graft is more promptly revascularized, providing a higher success rate than the thick free grafts. Split grafts of 0.018 to 0.024 inch thickness provide sufficient dermis, unassisted healing of the donor site, and minimal risk of failure. The durability of the split-thickness and full-thickness skin grafts also depends on the characteristics of the recipient site. A bed of soft tissue that allows mobility and flexibility of the overlying graft is adequately covered by a split-thickness graft. The selection of the thickness of a free graft must take into consideration the location and size of the defect and the quality of the recipient bed.

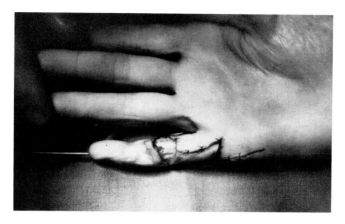

**Fig. 8-1.** A Kirschner wire immobilizes the interphalangeal joints to aid grafting and prevent contracture.

Contraction of split grafts is generally more severe on the palmar surface than the dorsal surface of the hand. This is probably because of the powerful flexor muscles that keep considerable tension on the graft over the dorsum of the hand. Thus, full-thickness grafts are used to cover flexion creases.

The steps in free grafting include: (1) preparing the recipient site, (2) immobilizing the part, (3) determining the size and thickness of graft required, (4) obtaining the graft, and (5) immobilizing the graft to provide firm contact with the recipient site.

The injury site is cleansed with copious irrigations. Minimal surgical débridement is usually required in the hand, except in the presence of foreign material. Immobilization of the recipient site is particularly important when a flexion crease is included in the area of tissue loss. Immobilization may be obtained by internal fixation, for example, Kirschner wires, or external fixation (strapping the injured part to a splint) (Fig. 8-1). After débridement and splinting have been accomplished, the tourniquet is released, and the hand is elevated for 5 to 10 minutes while gauze dressing is pressed against the wound. Ma-

jor bleeding is controlled with precision use of the cautery. If hemostasis was difficult to obtain during the operative procedure, inspection of the graft at 48 hours is justified. A major hematoma should be evacuated by removal of half the sutures and direct evacuation of the clot. Every effort should be made to obtain a dry bed before the graft is applied. Clear roentgenographic film is used to fashion a pattern of the skin defect. If a full-thickness graft is selected, it is cut according to the pattern. Fixation of the graft is accomplished with peripheral interrupted sutures that accurately align the dermal edges of the graft and recipient site. If the recipient site is loose fatty tissue, an occasional suture between the graft and bed reinforces fixation. The sutures are left long enough to allow further immobilization of the graft against the recipient site through the use of a cotton waste bolus. The donor sites for full-thickness grafts require direct closure. When closure of the donor site is precluded by the graft size, overgrafting with split-thickness grafts may be necessary. The split-thickness graft donor site heals by regeneration of the skin appendages remaining in the donor site.

We do not use the volar surface of the

forearm as a donor site for split-thickness grafts. Many of our patients have developed marked hypopigmentation of the donor area, which is unpleasing. Xavier and Lamb reported that of 67 patients with hand injuries who had had split-thickness grafts taken from the volar aspect of the forearm, none had hypertrophy or hyperpigmentation of the scar. However, 58 had mild to markedly hypopigmented scars. There were no other complications.

The split-thickness graft is fixed to the recipient site with the overlapping edge incorporated into the suture. If a depression is evident after graft fixation, a pattern of the graft is cut from gauze and made to overlap the graft to ensure uniform pressure by the next layer of dressing. Failure to gain hemostasis or immobilization is the primary cause for failure of graft survival. Movement between the graft and underlying bed may tear the nascent capillaries, predisposing the graft to hematoma formation and vascularization failure. Use of fine catgut suture is advisable in children because it avoids the traumatic removal of sutures in the apprehensive child.

Further immobilization and protection of the hand are gained through application of a large supportive dressing. Before this dressing is applied, one must determine exactly what he wants the dressing to accomplish and apply the dressing accordingly. A nonadherent single layer of gauze covers the wound. The bulk of the dressing consists of resilient mechanic's waste positioned to maintained the hand in the desired position. Wrist stabilization is gained through two abdominal pads placed across the volar and dorsal surfaces of the wrist. A final dressing with Kling gauze covered by tape maintains the consistency of the dressing. Reinforcement of the dressing may be required in the postoperative period. Occasionally, this dressing is termed a pressure dressing; this is misleading and inaccurate. The bulky hand dressing quickly loses its pressure effect and actually pro-

vides only immobilization—a task it must do well. The hand dressing can be converted to a pressure dressing by incorporating an elastic bandage into the dressing. These elastic bandages must be used with great care because improper use has led to disastrous results. During the postoperative phase, elevation and immobilization of the injured part are important. Elevation is continued until the dressing change at 10 to 14 days. Elevation through use of a sling is inadequate; one should simply keep the hand and forearm elevated above the level of the heart.

The dressing on an uncomplicated skin graft should not be disturbed for at least 7 days, since a second dressing application is never as effective as the initial dressing applied in the operating room. By the seventh day most grafts are well-vascularized, firmly adherent, and they can be inspected with care. Immobilization is continued for a total of 2 weeks; then guarded exercises are instituted.

Tissue coverage of finger pad losses presents problems peculiar to this area. The distal interphalangeal joint is immobilized with a transfixing Kirschner wire. A pattern of the tissue defect is prepared on clear roentgenographic film. This pattern is cut and traced on the recipient site. If the pattern is oval, the donor area is outlined as an ellipse to facilitate closure. The periphery of the graft is incised just to the depth of the dermis. A skin hook is used to elevate the point of the graft while countertraction is maintained on the surrounding skin. The graft is elevated by sharp dissection just superficial to the dermal attachments to the underlying subcutaneous tissues (Fig. 8-2). This provides a graft free of subcutaneous tissue. After the excess on each end has been excised, the graft is immediately transferred to the recipient site. The donor site is closed by direct suturing of the skin edges. A large donor site precluding direct closure must be covered with a split-thickness skin graft.

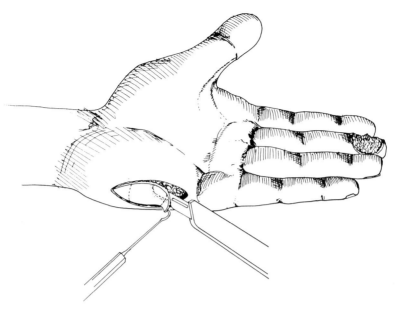

**Fig. 8-2.** A large full-thickness graft can be obtained from the ulnar border of the hand and the donor site closed directly.

Donor areas available for full-thickness grafts are determined by the size and functional requirements of the donor area. Small grafts can be obtained from the lateral side of the hypothenar eminence; the wrist, elbow, or groin flexion creases; and the inner aspect of the arm. Large full-thickness grafts are usually taken with the dermatome, and the donor site is over-grafted.

Use of the ulnar side of the hypothenar area as a donor area for obtaining coverage in the digits has the following advantages: (1) The morphology of the donor skin approaches that of the recipient site; (2) the donor site is readily available and inconspicuous; (3) primary closure of the donor site can be obtained and (4) excellent sensory function is eventually gained in the graft. Evaluation of the sensory function in the grafts as determined by light touch, pin-prick, and two-point discrimination revealed excellent function in 19 or 20 cases reported in one series.

Hyperpigmentation of free skin grafts on the flexor surface of the hand is particularly unsatisfactory to blacks. This can be avoided by using the plantar surface of the foot as the donor area. However, when overgrafting of the plantar defect is required, the period of immobilization of the entire patient is too prolonged.

## PEDICLE FLAPS

Pedicle flaps are used to provide coverage in areas where tendons or joints are exposed and in areas requiring sensory function. In addition, areas that must support tendon grafting or tendon transfer must be covered with a pedicle flap. A spectrum of pedicle flaps is possible. But first, one must consider the complications associated with pedicle flap utilization to minimize or avoid poor results.

Vascular insufficiency is the most frequent of flap complications. Vascular insufficiency implies either inadequate arterial supply or inadequate venous return. Inadequate arterial supply is characterized by the development of a "white" flap, whereas inadequate venous return presents a "blue" flap. Flap necrosis most often results from inadequate venous return. The factors that the surgeon can control in preventing flap necrosis include design, tension, edema, and inflammation of the flap. Proper design requires a knowledge of the vascular anatomy of the area, allowing incorporation of enough vascular canals into the pedicle to ensure adequate circulation. Flaps developed in areas that have no major vessels should maintain a 2:1 ratio, that is, the base is twice as wide as the length of the flap. However, special areas permit flap transfer on a single artery and vein. Undue tension embarrasses circulation, particularly venous return. Sutures tenting the flap can produce a white line across the flap resulting in ultimate necrosis of the flap distal to the line of tension. Acute angulation can lead to venous congestion and edema. As edema develops, it increases the intractable effects of tension and kinking. Finally, the presence of inflammation adds an additional metabolic burden on the flap.

Clinically, the flap that is progressing toward necrosis exhibits mottling, cyanosis, and edema. Digital pressure results in blanching of an area that rapidly refills when pressure is released. This blanching results when the stagnated blood has been expressed into the vessels of the surrounding area and returns to the emptied vessels when pressure is released. The appearance of a violet color signals inevitable necrosis. The process of necrosis extends much further proximally than is usually anticipated initially. If one waits until this time for surgical intervention, the flap must be returned to the donor site and trimmed until brisk bleeding is encountered.

The vascular supply of a flap can be enhanced by staged division of a portion of its vascular supply, thereby encouraging circulation through selected channels. This procedure is termed "delay." Flap delay permits the use of a greater length-breadth ratio than would be possible otherwise.

Anything that is interposed between the flap and the recipient bed inhibits healing and may predispose to infection and ultimate flap necrosis. Hematoma is the most frequent offender. Careful surgical technique is the best preventative. Edema is minimized if the flap can be positioned so that gravity aids venous drainage.

Local tissues may be developed into pedicle flaps, which are termed rotation, transposition, and advancement flaps. When adjacent tissue is rotated into a defect, the flap is termed a rotation flap. When tissue is displaced laterally into the defect, it is called a transposition flap. When the flap is elevated around its entire periphery (with circulation maintained through its subcutaneous attachments) and advanced distally, it is termed an advancement flap. Use of rectangular transposition or rotation flaps in the hand almost always requires free grafting of the donor site. Use of triangular flaps permits direct closure of the donor area and is termed a V-Y type advancement closure. These will be demonstrated in detail later in the chapter.

When the rotational-transposition flap has been sutured into the recipient site, a line of tension may result, which interferes with venous return and predisposes to necrosis. A cut-back at the base of the flap can eliminate this tension and permit free rotation of the flap into the defect. Great care must be taken so that the cut-back does not significantly reduce the circulation in the flap. One must remember that the limiting factor in transferring a local flap is the point of the pedicle farthest removed from the defect to be covered. This length of the flap must be measured directly and the flap designed to be long enough. Before any incisions are made, the pivotal point of the flap must be recognized and the flap designed to permit coverage without tension. Converting the tissue defect to a triangular shape facilitates local flap coverage.

## Classification of flaps according to blood supply

*Random pattern flaps.* The blood supply of these flaps is from perforating musculo-cutaneous vessels that are preserved at the base of the flap and communicate with the interconnecting dermal and subdermal plexus of the skin. The perforating vessels may arise from segmental, anastomotic, or axial arteries that lie deep within the muscles (Fig. 8-3).

*Axial pattern flaps.* The blood supply of these flaps arises from a segmental, anastomotic, or axial artery (often from a short perforator artery) that communicates with a direct cutaneous artery, which is positioned above the muscles and on the deep surface of the subcutaneous tissues. Thus the general outline of the flap is determined by the course of the direct cutaneous artery included in the flap. The size of the flap is determined by the anastomotic dermal and subdermal plexus communicating with the direct cutaneous artery.

In developing an axial pattern flap, one must carefully consider the anatomy of the arterial and venous supply even when a fairly constant anastomotic pattern has been noted. Axial flaps may be classified as either peninsular or island pattern flaps.

*Peninsular axial flaps.* The base of these flaps is maintained in continuity with the donor area, and the blood supply is provided by a direct cutaneous artery. The groin flap and the deltopectoral flap are examples (Fig. 8-4).

*Island axial flaps.* These differ from peninsular flaps in that the skin attachments to the donor area have been completely excised. The blood supply is provided through the pedicle of vessels; an example is Littler's island pedicle flap (Fig. 8-5). The refinement of microsurgical techniques has made it possible to completely divide this pedicle of vessels and transfer the flap to a distant place where circulation in the vessels is reestablished by vascular anastomosis.

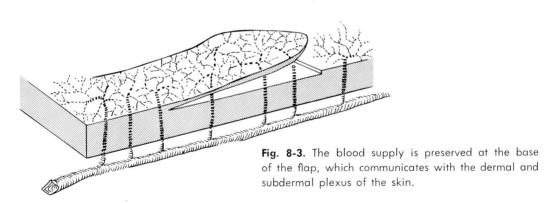

**Fig. 8-3.** The blood supply is preserved at the base of the flap, which communicates with the dermal and subdermal plexus of the skin.

**Fig. 8-4.** The base of the flap is maintained in continuity with the donor area.

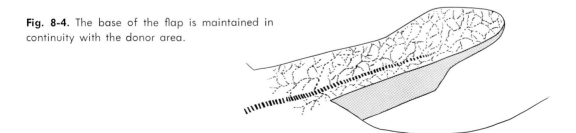

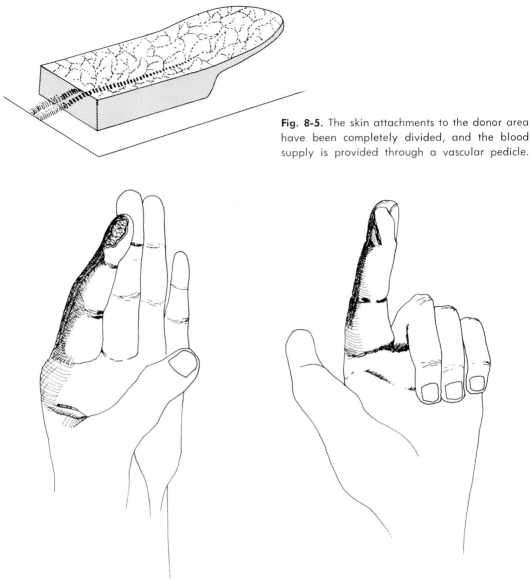

**Fig. 8-5.** The skin attachments to the donor area have been completely divided, and the blood supply is provided through a vascular pedicle.

**Fig. 8-6.** When the radiovolar pad of a finger is lost, its companion ulnovolar pad can be transferred with its neurovascular bundle.

### Classification of flaps according to function

Pedicle flaps, on a functional basis, can be divided into two groups—those that include major nerve branches in the pedicle (thus innervated) and those in which major nerve branches are not transferred in the pedicle (thus denervated). In the latter group, innervation must be accomplished by neural elements from the recipient site.

### Pedicle flaps that contain a major nerve branch

Innervated flaps are used primarily to provide coverage of the radiovolar surfaces of the finger pads and the ulnovolar

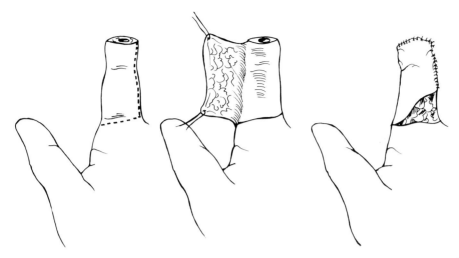

**Fig. 8-7.** A midlateral line incision is made from the amputation site proximal to the second flexion line it encounters. The incision is continued across the volar surface to the opposite midlateral line.

surface of the thumb pad. These can be developed locally as described by Kutler, Hueston, Kleinert, Littler, and Snow, or they can be developed at a distance from the injury site and transferred to the recipient site, as described by Littler and Horvitch.

### Local flaps that contain a major nerve branch

*Littler flap.* When a small defect exists on the radiovolar surface of a finger pad, coverage can be gained from the ulnar side of the pad with a flap into which are incorporated the digital neurovascular elements of the intact side. One edge of the flap is formed by the free edge of the injury wound. The flap is elevated adequately to allow transposition into the critical area of tissue loss (Fig. 8-6). Great care must be taken in planning the flap to permit complete coverage of the radiovolar pinch area without tension. Coverage gained with undue tension can result in a painful pulp. The donor area is closed with a free graft. This flap is of value only when the digital nerve on the radiovolar side of the finger has been damaged beyond repair and the ulnar digital nerve is intact.

*Hueston flap.* Hueston has devised a method of local flap repair that maintains one neurovascular bundle and provides excellent coverage of the fingertips with volar digital skin. The flap is outlined proximally from the site of injury along the midlateral line of the digit until it reaches the *second* flexion line along its course (Fig. 8-7). The incision then crosses the volar surface of the digit at this point. The flap is elevated superficial to the neurovascular bundle on the same side as the midlateral incision and deep to the neurovascular bundle on the opposite side. With distal transposition, a significant "dog ear" will appear which will require revision later. The donor area is closed with a full-thickness graft.

*Kutler lateral advancement flaps* (Fig. 8-8). Two triangular flaps are outlined, one on each side of the involved finger. The base of the triangle is formed by the edge of the tissue defect. The width of the flap is determined by the width needed to cover the end of the digit. Usually the apex of the triangle extends to the level of the distal joint. Mobilization of the triangles requires development of a subcutaneous pedicle containing the neurovascular elements. This is accomplished

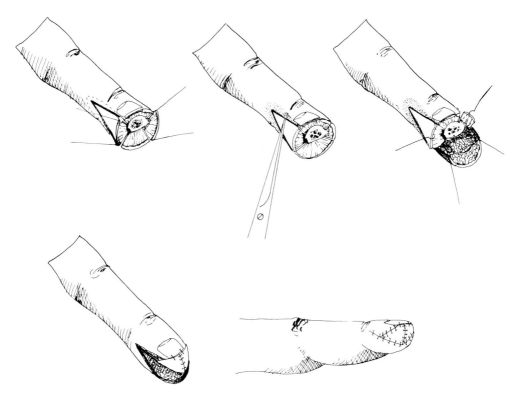

**Fig. 8-8.** Bilateral triangles are developed on subcutaneous pedicles and advanced distally for closure.

by detachment of the septa from the bony distal phalanx and the septa proximal to flap apex, which bind the subcutaneous pedicle to the skin proximally. During mobilization, a suture in the flap provides countertraction and minimizes tissue trauma. As mobilization of the flap proceeds, the bony phalanx is rounded to minimize tension during wound closure. If hemostasis is not complete, postoperative oozing can be a nuis..nce. The bases of the triangular flaps are approximated, and the united flaps are sutured to the nail to ensure coverage of the bony phalanx. The donor areas are closed directly, thus converting the V-shaped defect to a Y configuration. If obvious tension is encountered in closing the donor area, a single loosely tied suture is used. Closure of the volar part of the pad skin is facilitated by

trimming any excess pulp. Postoperatively, elevation and protection of the finger are most important. The dressing is left undisturbed for 10 to 14 days. Within 3 to 4 weeks, the finger pad is functional (Fig. 8-9).

*Kleinert volar advancement flap* (Fig. 8-10). A triangular flap is marked so that the base of the triangle is formed by the cut edge of skin at the amputation site. This base should be 2 to 3 mm wider than the edge of the nail matrix. The apex of the triangular flap reaches to the flexion crease of the distal interphalangeal joint. After the triangle is incised to the subcutaneous tissues, countertraction is applied to the triangular flap by a suture in the free end. The flap, including the entire thickness of subcutaneous tissue, is elevated by division of the septa at their at-

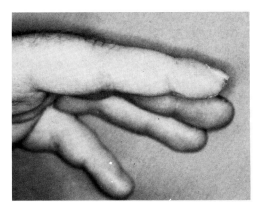

**Fig. 8-9.** The Kutler procedure can restore form and function to the fingertip.

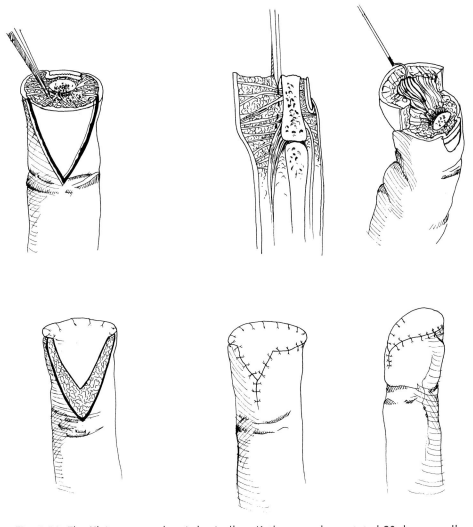

**Fig. 8-10.** The Kleinert procedure is basically a Kutler procedure rotated 90 degrees, allowing use of the volar pad for coverage.

tachment to the distal phalanx and the fibro-osseous tunnel. The septa attaching to the skin surrounding the triangle are detached from the subcutaneous pedicle. To gain adequate mobilization, division of the subcutaneous attachments at the apex of the triangle is necessary. Once this division is accomplished, the flap can be advanced more than a centimeter. If feasible, the bony phalanx and nail bed are cut straight across at the fingertip, and the flap is advanced for direct suture to the fingernail. The donor area is closed directly, yielding a V-Y closure pattern (Fig. 8-11). An external finger splint provides protection of the repair.

*Snow volar advancement flap* (Fig. 8-12). Midlateral incisions are made along the digit extending proximally from the amputation site to at least the level of the proximal interphalangeal joint and to the most proximal finger crease in large defects. After Cleland's ligaments are divided, the flap is sharply dissected from the fibro-osseous tunnel back to the level of the proximal finger crease. This allows advancement of the entire volar skin to gain coverage of the fingertip. Properly contoured coverage of the finger pad requires trimming the edges of the flap or taking a V-shaped wedge from the terminal end of the flap. The proximal and distal interphalangeal joints are flexed to allow construction of the finger pad with the volar flap. After the fingertip is completely covered, the midlateral line incisions are closed directly. If a large defect is covered, considerable tension may be encountered when closing the midlateral lines. This tension is alleviated by increasing the flexion of the distal and proximal interphalangeal joints. This degree of joint flexion can eventually be overcome by exercise and dynamic splinting.

*Littler volar advancement flap* (Fig. 8-13). Advancement of the entire volar pad as a visor flap based on both neurovascular bundles provides adequate coverage of small defects over the finger pads. Midlateral line incisions are made at both sides of the finger, beginning at the level of the amputation. Cleland's ligaments are detached, and the flap is elevated from the fibro-osseous tunnel as described above. However, a proximal transverse incision through skin and subcutaneous tissue (preserving continuity of neurovascular elements) permits distal advancement of the pedicle over the finger pad area. The neurovascular bundles can be stretched gently and will permit flap advancement of at least 1.5 cm. Advancement is facilitated by slight flexion of the finger joints. Free graft coverage of the donor area over the middle phalanx completes wound closure. The finger is immobilized in mild flexion at both interphalangeal joints for 10 days, after which exercises are begun gingerly.

*Distant island flap that contains a major nerve trunk.* The pedicle of this flap contains a major nerve branch in addition to the circulatory elements. Littler perfected the technique of island flap transfer incorporating a digital nerve branch from either the median or ulnar nerve. Many

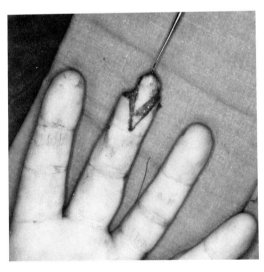

**Fig. 8-11.** The volar flap can be advanced to provide complete coverage of the amputated tip.

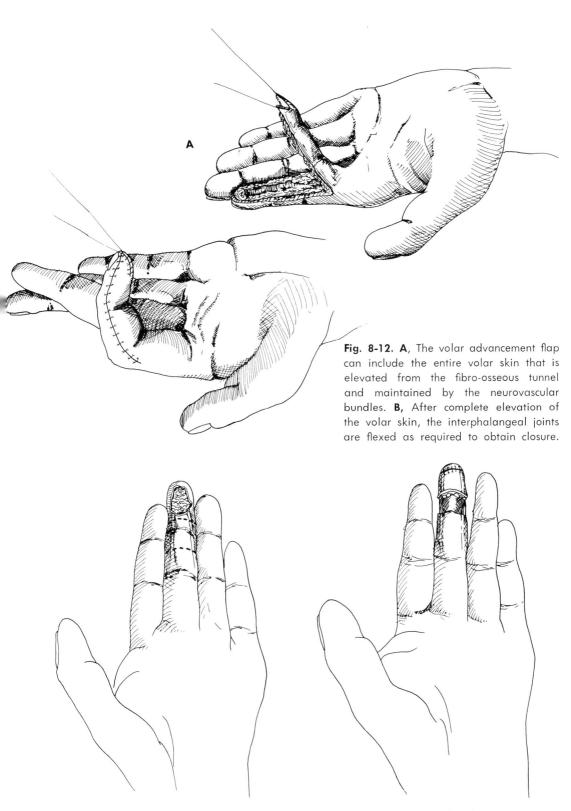

**Fig. 8-12. A,** The volar advancement flap can include the entire volar skin that is elevated from the fibro-osseous tunnel and maintained by the neurovascular bundles. **B,** After complete elevation of the volar skin, the interphalangeal joints are flexed as required to obtain closure.

**Fig. 8-13.** Loss of the finger pad may be repaired by advancement of volar skin on its intact neurovascular bundles.

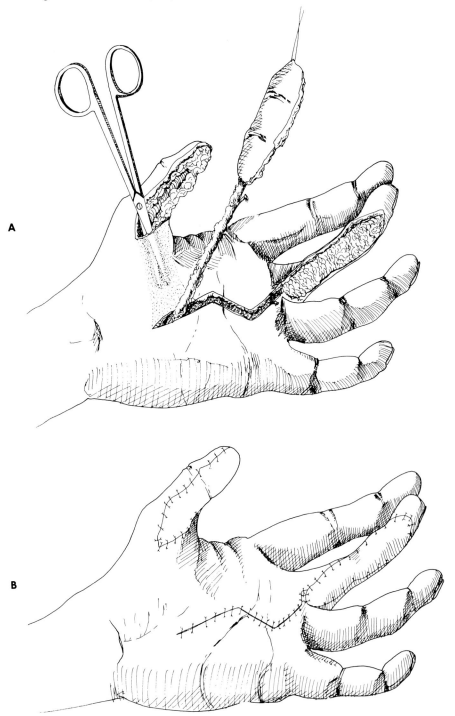

**Fig. 8-14. A,** An island of skin has been elevated with its neurovascular bundle intact and a subcutaneous tunnel prepared to provide access to the thumb defect. **B,** The island pedicle has been tunneled subcutaneously to the thumb defect and the donor area closed with a free graft.

modifications of the basic model have been presented, including islands in continuity from two adjacent fingers and islands innervated by a sensory branch of the radial nerve.

*Littler island pedicle transfer on a neurovascular bundle* (Fig. 8-14). A pattern of the recipient site is prepared and transferred to the ulnar side of a digit—usually the ring or long finger. The flap outline is modified to create a donor defect that conforms with favorable flexion lines (Fig. 8-15). After the skin incision, the neurovascular bundle is identified at the distal end of the island flap where it is divided and ligated. A skin hook provides countertraction allowing sharp dissection of the flap from the fibro-osseous sheath and the loose connective tissues over the extensor apparatus of the digit. The level of the superficial palmar arch is marked on the skin and a zigzag incision made from the origin of that digital artery to the proximal edge of the anticipated flap. After the palmar skin incision is made, the skin edges are freed by cutting the palmar fascia attachments to the skin. In the distal palm, the edge of the palmar fascia is identified and opened, exposing the underlying neuro-

vascular supply to the flap side of the digit. Because the opposing side of the adjacent finger derives its blood supply from a branch of the common digital artery, this branch is divided to preserve the continuity of the artery to the flap. The flap is elevated and the neurovascular bundle dissected proximally to the superficial vascular arch. To accomplish this degree of mobilization, the proper digital nerve contribution to the common digital nerve is sharply dissected back to the level of the vascular arch.

A subcutaneous or subfascial pocket is developed from the proximal palmar wound to the recipient site. The skin island and its long neurovascular pedicle are threaded through the pocket to the recipient site. Tension on the neurovascular pedicle is minimized by flexing the recipient digit. Acute angulation or constriction of the pedicle must be avoided. The pedicle flap is trimmed to fit the recipient site and sutured. The donor area is covered with a free skin graft immobilized with a stent. A dressing is carefully applied and left undisturbed for 7 to 10 days.

*Omer addition.* Utilizing the principles described above, the surgeon can develop

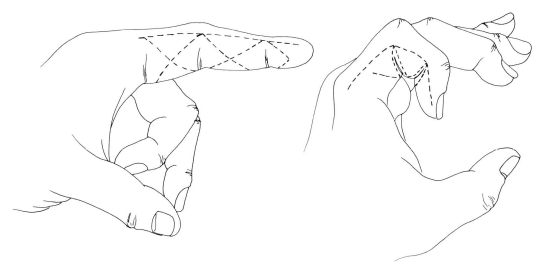

**Fig. 8-15.** The lines, as indicated in flexion and extension, do not participate in either of these movements.

a neurovascular pedicle in continuity from the radial and ulnar side of adjacent fingers. The cutaneous island is outlined along the ulnar aspect of the ring finger and the radial aspect of the little finger. The continuity of the adjacent flaps is maintained by including the skin forming the interdigital web. A pattern of the flap is transferred to the recipient site. The proximal radiovolar aspect of the index finger and the proximal volar aspect of the thumb are the preferred functional areas. The flap is transferred to the recipient site through a subcutaneous or subfascial tunnel and the donor site closed with a free graft. After all wounds have been sutured, a bulky dressing is applied and the hand is immobilized for 3 weeks.

*Holevich pedicle.* The principles of the volar-based island pedicle flap have been utilized to develop a flap innervated by the sensory branch of the radial nerve. Initially, the operative technique allowed for transfer of neurovascular elements as a subcutaneous implant into the thumb. Through a curved incision on the radial aspect of the index finger extending over the first metacarpal, the sensory branches of the radial nerve and the vessels are elevated with the subcutaneous tissues. The vessels within the area are preserved in a subcutaneous pedicle. The subcutaneous pedicle of neurovascular elements is transferred to the thumb through a volar tunnel in the thumb pad. No skin is transferred, and the technique is applicable only

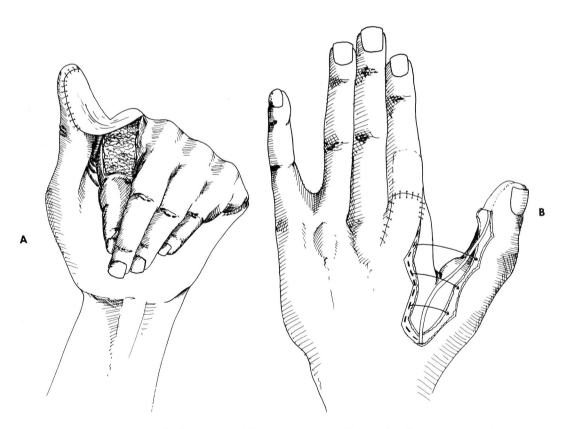

**Fig. 8-16. A,** A pedicle flap is raised from the dorsum of the index finger and contains a sensory branch of the radial nerve. **B,** At the time of division of the pedicle flap, the sensory branches of the radial nerve are tansposed intact to the thumb.

when coverage of the thumb is quantitatively adequate.

The technique has been modified to include a racquet-shaped skin flap from the dorsum of the proximal half of the index finger. This flap is several millimeters wide at the base to provide coverage from the thumb pad to the proximal edge of the thumb web space. The neurovascular elements are elevated with the skin flap, and the recipient site is prepared for transfer of the flap to the thumb. The proximal portion of the donor site is closed directly, while the more distal area requires free grafting for closure. The skin flap is sutured into the defect on the pulp of the thumb (Fig. 8-16, *A*). Three weeks later, the flap's cutaneous pedicle is divided, but the continuity of the branches of the radial nerve to the flap is preserved and transposed to the thumb. This is accomplished by making an incision proximally from the edge of the flap to the thumb web and then extending this incision distally to the base of the flap positioned on the thumb (Fig. 8-16, *B*).

### Pedicle flaps that do not include a major nerve

Denervated flaps are used primarily to gain coverage of the forearm (volar and dorsal surfaces) and the hand and fingers (volar and dorsal surfaces) except for the radiovolar area of the distal phalanges of the fingers and the ulnovolar area of the thumb pad. These flaps may be developed locally (from the dorsal or lateral surface of the involved digit) or from a distance (thenar eminence, palm, adjacent finger, chest, abdomen, or opposite arm).

*Local rotational flaps.* Flaps from the dorsal surface of the involved finger can be rotated into volar defects to provide coverage (Fig. 8-17). Careful planning is required to ensure complete coverage of the recipient site. The pedicle is based distally or proximally according to the need. Elevation of the flap is accomplished in the

loose areolar tissue plane overlying the extensor apparatus. A free graft is used to cover the donor area. These flaps are of particular value when volar coverage is needed—except for the finger pad. Use of volar skin to cover dorsal defects is rarely indicated.

*Local island flaps.* Occasionally the local rotational flap outlined in the previous paragraph cannot be mobilized adequately to cover a tissue defect. A local island flap that may be based either proximally or distally can be used. The extent of the tissue defect is obtained and positioned on the ulnar side of the proximal phalanx of the involved digit (Fig. 8-18, *A*). If the flap is to be positioned over the proximal inter-

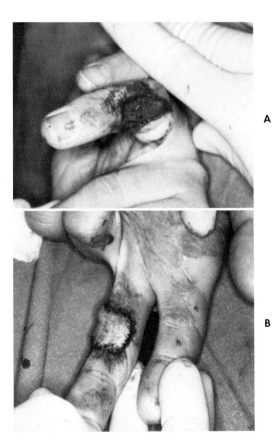

**Fig. 8-17. A,** A volar digital defect can be closed with a dorsal rotational flap. **B,** Note the limitations of volar coverage of the dorsal flap.

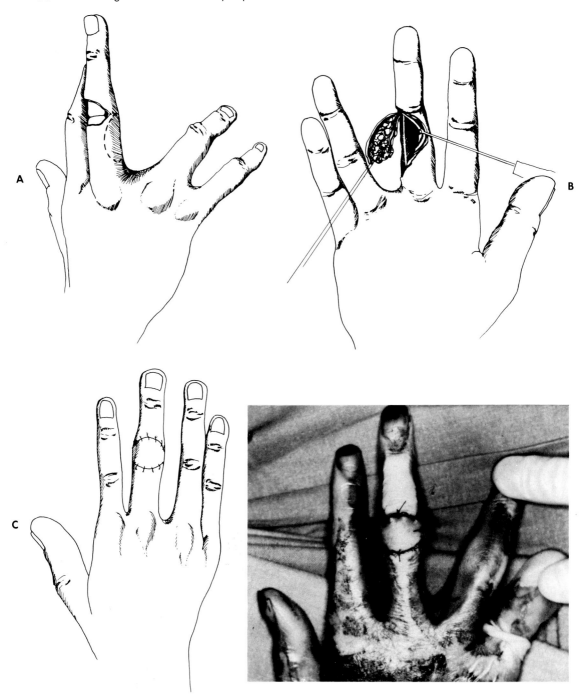

**Fig. 8-18. A,** When dorsal coverage of a proximal interphalangeal joint is required, the flap is outlined, as indicated. **B,** The flap may be based proximally or distally. Here it is based distally to facilitate coverage of the joint. **C,** The flap has been rotated into place over the dorsum of the joint and the donor defect closed with a free graft. **D,** The flap developed from the ulnar side of the long finger has been rotated to gain closure of the joint.

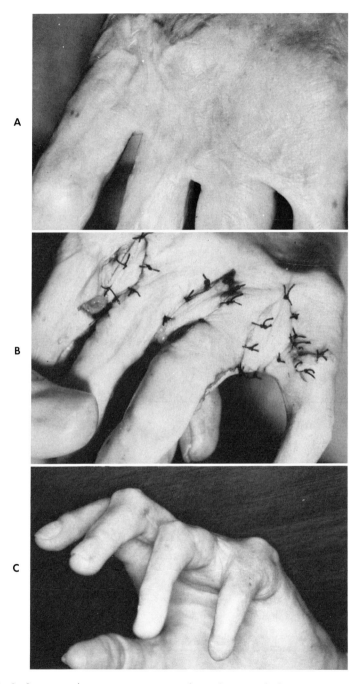

**Fig. 8-19. A,** Severe web contracture approaching the interphalangeal joint. **B,** Proximally based islands rotated into the digital webs. **C,** Postoperatively, marked improvement in web space freedom.

phalangeal joint area (volar or dorsal surface), the digital artery and vein are dissected free from the digital nerve to permit ligation of the vessels at the proximal extent of the flap (Fig. 8-18, *B*). The vessels with the attached subcutaneous tissue and skin flap are dissected from the digital nerve, leaving the nerve undisturbed in its bed. Frequently an arterial branch is encountered at the level of the midportion of the proximal phalanx, and this branch must be ligated and divided. As dissection of the digital vessels from the digital nerve proceeds, the skin flap is elevated and rotated into the defect (Fig. 8-18, *C* and *D*). If the defect to be covered is over the metacarpophalangeal joint or the interdigital web, the neurovascular bundle is identified distally and the vessels are divided at this point. The skin flap and attached vessels are dissected proximally from the digital nerve. The vessels may be freed from the nerve into the palm to provide a longer vascular pedicle, thus facilitating rotation of the flap either into the web space or over the metacarpophalangeal joint (Fig. 8-19). The flap donor site is closed with a full-thickness graft obtained from the midlateral surface on the ulnar side of the hypothenar area.

*Flag flaps.* The flag flap described by Iselin has a long, narrow, proximally based dorsal pedicle and a broad distal "flap" that includes the entire dorsal skin of the proximal or middle phalanx. The length of the pedicle allows transposition of the flap to any nearby location, such as the volar surface of the same digit, the dorsal surface of an adjacent digit, or the adjacent web space or palm.

Iselin has described a homodigital flag flap and a heterodigital flag flap. The homodigital flap is used to cover: (1) volar digital defects, even those located too far distally for reconstruction with a transverse standard cross-finger flap; (2) distal digital amputations when shortening is undesirable; and (3) dorsal defects. The heterodigital flag flap can be used: (1) to cover any proximal or distal dorsal defect of an adjacent finger; (2) to restore sensitivity to thumb stumps by using radial nerve–innervated tissues from the dorsal surface of the index finger, and (3) to lengthen a thumb stump as well as restore sensitivity.

The limitation of these flaps is their size. The flap cannot be longer than the dorsal surface of a phalanx; and the width of the pedicle should not exceed half the dorsal surface of the proximal phalanx.

The length of the flap is determined by the width of the defect. The pedicle is planned to be one-third the width of the dorsal surface of the proximal phalanx. The base of the pedicle may be located on either side of the finger (Fig. 8-20). The flap is elevated, preserving the peritendinous tissues over the extensor apparatus. All longitudinal vessels and nerves possible are included in the pedicle. The donor area is closed with a skin graft. After the flap has been inserted, the hand is immobilized in a dressing for 5 days. The dressings are removed, and passive and active motion in the joints possible is maintained.

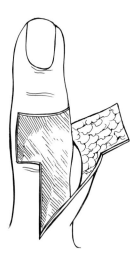

**Fig. 8-20.** The pedicle is one-third the width of the dorsal surface of the phalanx and is located on either side of the finger.

Iselin recommends resection of the pedicle 15 to 21 days later.

**Distant flaps.** For coverage of moderate size defects, the adjacent finger can provide an exceptionally good tissue match. The flap can be based laterally, distally, or proximally as needed.

*Laterally based cross-finger flap* (Fig. 8-21). This is the most common form of the cross-finger flap in use and provides the greatest amount of tissue for coverage. The defect on the injured finger is altered to conform to the favorable lines of flexion noted earlier. A pattern of the defect is prepared and transposed to the dorsum of the adjacent finger. The largest amount of tissue available for transfer can be obtained by a midlateral incision on the donor

finger and reflection of the flap toward the injured finger, much like turning the page of a book.

The flap is incised to the level of the loose areolar volar tissue over the extensor apparatus, and all tissue superficial to the deep fascia over the extensor apparatus is included in the flap. The flap is based on the side of the donor digit adjacent to the injured finger. As the flap is reflected, considerable relaxation and prevention of kinking are obtained by incising Cleland's ligament at the base of the pedicle. The fingers are positioned to maintain the joints in an optimal position, that is, metacarpophalangeal flexion and proximal interphalangeal joint extension. If the recipient area overlies the proximal or distal interphalangeal

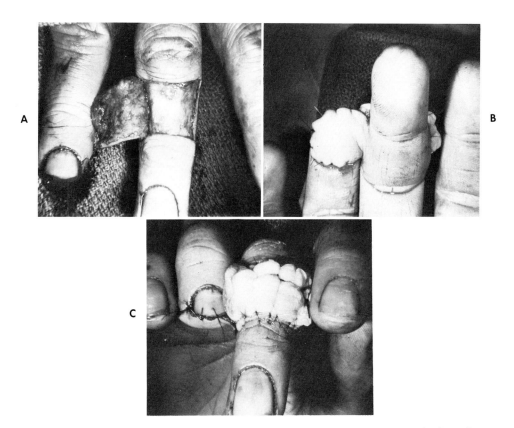

**Fig. 8-21. A,** Tip of ring finger has been amputated. The dorsal skin over the long finger is reflected. **B,** The skin flap has been set into the pulp defect of the ring finger. **C,** The donor area is closed with a full-thickness graft, and stent is applied.

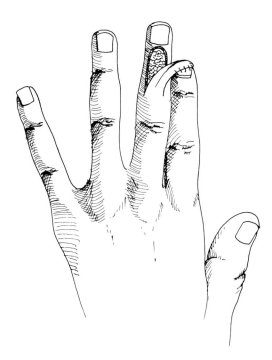

**Fig. 8-22.** The cross-finger flap may be based proximally or distally for coverage of defects in adjacent or distant fingers.

joints, a Kirschner wire may be used to aid in immobilization of the joint in extension. A full-thickness skin graft covers the donor area. After 14 to 16 days the flap is detached.

*Proximally or distally based cross-finger flap* (Fig. 8-22). A pattern of the defect is transferred to the dorsum of an adjacent finger or occasionally to a distant finger. The fingers are manipulated to determine the most comfortable and satisfactory position for joint immobilization. The flap is based to minimize tension. After the flap is elevated, the donor area is covered with a free graft before the flap is sutured to the recipient site. Kirschner wires impaling both digits provide excellent fixation but are not usually necessary. After 14 to 16 days the flap is divided.

*Thenar flaps* (Fig. 8-23). Tissue loss from the distal phalanges of the index or long finger can be replaced with a flap from the thenar area. A pattern of the tis-

sue defect is transferred to the thenar eminence immediately proximal to the metacarpophalangeal joint. The flap can be based either proximally or distally. The metacarpophalangeal and the distal interphalangeal joints of the injured finger are fully flexed to minimize flexion of the proximal interphalangeal joint. Some claim that in this position the proximal interphalangeal joint is only slightly flexed. It is virtually impossible to accomplish this position without at least 70 degrees of proximal interphalangeal joint flexion (Fig. 8-24). The donor area is closed, the flap attached, and immobilization gained with a strip of tape extending from the dorsum of the hand around the dorsum of the finger to the volar surface of the thenar eminence and palm. After 12 to 14 days the pedicle is severed. Mobilization of the joints by active and passive exercises is begun immediately.

Miller reviewed 39 patients with fingertip injuries treated by replacement with a thenar flap. He concluded that the main disadvantage of the thenar flap is the poor result obtained in the palmar donor site. Not only is the scar unsightly, but it is directly beneath the fingertip; and when the patient grasps an object, it may be tender.

This problem can be avoided if the flap is based laterally instead of proximally so that the skin comes from the central plateau of the thenar eminence. A square flap is designed to ensure adequate vascularity. A split-thickness graft is used to cover the donor area.

*Palmar flap.* The palmar flap can provide coverage only for small defects of the terminal phalanx of the thumb. A flap of the appropriate size is based on the radial side of the palm between the first digital crease of the index finger and the proximal transverse palmar crease. The donor site is closed with a free graft. The thumb is positioned in an adducted posture to allow placement of the flap into the recipient site without tension. After 12 to

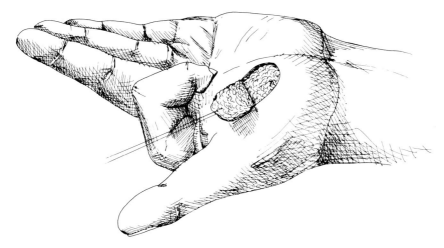

**Fig. 8-23.** The thenar flap can provide excellent tissue coverage for pad defect. Note the degree of joint flexion.

14 days the flap is divided. Discretion must be exercised in selecting this flap because it provides a minimum of tissue for coverage, and the positioning of the thumb is awkward.

*Anterior chest wall flaps.* White divides the anterior chest wall flaps into those from the anterolateral chest wall (either contralateral or ipsilateral), the epigastric region, and the infraclavicular region.

*Anterolateral chest wall flaps.* The advantages of flaps from this area compared with flaps from the lower abdomen are: (1) The skin is thinner; (2) the subcutaneous fat layer is thinner; (3) the skin is more pliable; (4) the donor area can be closed directly without the need for skin grafts; (5) the flaps can be raised in one stage without delay and applied directly to the recipient site; (6) hair growth is usually less in this area; and (7) the combination of the factors above allows more accurate outlining and cutting of the flap to fit the needs for coverage as accurately as possible.

*Contralateral chest wall flaps.* The blood supply to these flaps is from the intercostal

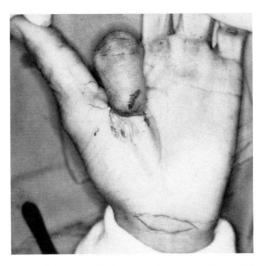

**Fig. 8-24.** Loss of fingertip tissue repaired with thenar flap. Note the degree of joint flexion required.

vessels and the thoracoepigastric system travelling in a transverse to oblique direction toward the midline. Circulation across the midline is inadequate to support a flap from the opposite side of the chest; thus these flaps are elevated in a transverse plane that does not cross the midline.

The donor area may be closed with a split-thickness skin graft or by direct suture. If it is determined that excessive tension will result from direct suture at the suture line, one should proceed immediately to skin grafting the defect. We have found it particularly helpful to place several sutures throughout the skin graft to fit it to the underlying bed. Movement of the extremity during convalescence does not cause movement of the skin graft.

The flap elevated in a transverse plane may be rotated either 90 degrees cephalad or 90 degrees caudad by a technique described by White (Fig. 8-25). Rotation is accomplished by extending either the upper or lower limb of the incision for a distance equal to the width of the flap. If the upper limb is extended, the flap

can be rotated 90 degrees cephalad. If the lower limb is extended, closure allows a rotation of 90 degrees caudad.

Use of the area above the umbilicus as a donor area allows the forearm to rest across the lower chest with the elbow flexed. This is not only comfortable, but permits free mobility of the patient in bending, stooping, walking, or sitting.

Great care must be taken in positioning the arm to avoid tension or kinking of the flap. If the arm is pushed too far toward the flap area, the flap can be kinked on its base. If the arm is not placed far enough across the chest, too much tension can occur in the flap. To ensure proper positioning, the relative position of the flexed elbow to the trunk is noted and maintained while the dressing is being applied. The

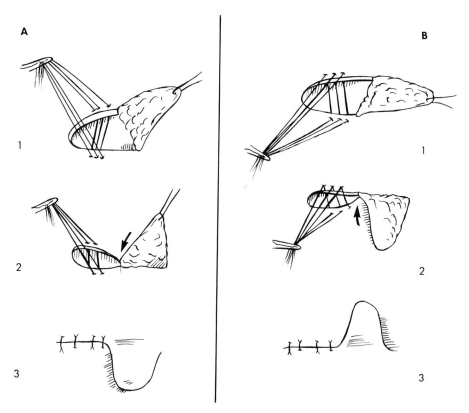

**Fig. 8-25. A,** The flap may be rotated cephalad by extending the upper limit of the incision. **B,** The flap is rotated caudad by extending the lower limb of the incision.

dressing consists of gauze and pads placed to conform to the surfaces. A skin protector is applied, and 4-inch strips of tape approximately 30 inches long are utilized. The tape is stuck to the back, then brought around the arm and over the dressing and hand and applied to the opposite posterolateral chest wall. After the dressing is completed, a window is cut over the flap. If the flap is under tension or is kinked, the tape is cut along the lateral edge of the arm and the extremity properly positioned and retaped.

The dressing is discarded after 7 days, the patient showers, and two strips of tape are reapplied to restrain the upper extremity. (The stent over the split-thickness skin graft is left in place.) Our patients shower daily and place a pad between the forearm and chest wall to reduce skin maceration.

The flaps are detached at 14 to 21 days, depending on the degree of inset accomplished, the healing of the flap edges, the configuration of the flap, and the size of the flap.

*Ipsilateral chest flaps.* The arm is difficult to immobilize when it is attached to an ipsilateral chest flap. Consequently, these flaps are used more often for coverage of the elbow, forearm, or wrist areas, that is, areas that lie across the ipsilateral side of the chest when the arm is rested on the chest or upper abdomen. These flaps may be based inferiorly, superiorly, or laterally. The donor site is closed with a split-thickness skin graft unless the flap is very small and the donor area can be closed without tension.

*Infraclavicular flaps.* The amount of tissue available from this area is so limited that coverage is limited usually to digital defects. Tubed flaps taken from the area immediately inferior to the clavicle are excellent for digital coverage. The skin is thin, yet it maintains an excellent blood supply. However, one must weigh the benefits from the use of flaps from this area against the scarring produced. Women particularly object to scarring in this area.

*Epigastric flaps.* Flaps from this area are particularly useful when coverage of a large defect is required in the distal forearm and/or hand (Fig. 8-26). The flap crosses the midline but maintains part of its base on each side of the midline. The dimensions potentially available for development of a flap are determined in one

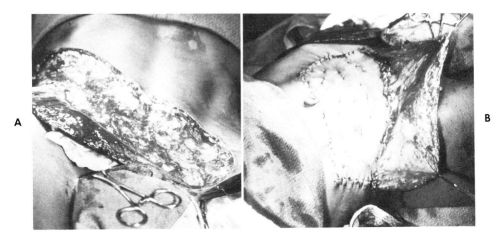

**Fig. 8-26. A,** An abdominal flap extending across the midline has been elevated with its base placed inferiorly. **B,** The donor area is covered with a skin graft that is fixed to the defect with sutures.

plane by the curvature of the trunk and in the other by the distance from the xiphoid to the umbilicus. Again, the arm is placed in a comfortable position across the lower chest and the flap planned as needed. Almost the entire circumference of the forearm can be covered by this flap. Again, the donor area is covered by a split-thickness skin graft.

*Abdominal wall skin flaps.* Flaps available from below the umbilicus are generally referred to as abdominal flaps. The skin in this area is the least desirable for flap coverage of the digits or hand. The abdominal flap has the following undesirable characteristics: (1) The texture and color do not match the recipient area; (2) the subcutaneous fat is usually abundant; (3) the skin is hairy; (4) weight gain is reflected in the flap; (5) the skin is thick and inelastic; (6) sensation that develops in the flap is poor; (7) the fatty layer of the flap prevents firm adhesion of the flap to bony areas or areas subjected to lateral stresses when fixation is desired; and (8) the flap dimensions are limited by the ratio of 1:1½, that is, if the base is 1, then the length of the flap is 1½ units. In spite of these difficulties, the abdominal flap is frequently used. The advantages are as follows: (1) Scarring of the donor area is in an area covered even by light summer clothes; (2) a large flap is available; (3) the need for bulk to replace a depression in a forearm is readily met by the abdominal flap; and (4) large tube pedicles can be developed and moved on a carrier with ease.

Coverage for the forearm or hand may be gained from the abdomen on the ipsilateral side. Use of skin from the opposite arm or pectoral region is satisfactory for coverage of small defects in particular locations, but the abdominal pedicle and chest flap remain the standbys for coverage of moderate to large defects. Since these flaps have no major vascular supply, attention must be paid to the length-to-width ratio and the anatomic positioning of the pedicle. Flap

length should be restricted to less than two times the width. Unless both quadrants of the abdomen are raised as a flap, the flap should not extend across the midline of the abdomen. Recently it has been demonstrated that the width of the distal end of the pedicle flap may exceed the width of the base by 20% to 30%. A pattern of the tissue defect is prepared and transferred to the donor area. Key points are tattooed on the recipient site and the flap to ensure accurate insertion of the flap into the defect. Darts are of particular value when covering the thumb-index web and the interdigital web spaces. As the flap is elevated, its subcutaneous tissues are trimmed until the transposed flap restores the normal contour of the recipient area.

A free skin graft is used to cover the donor site. Sutures are placed through the skin graft into the underlying bed for immobilization and protection of the graft from the friction of the overlying extremity. In addition, a stent may be used for added security. The flap is sutured into as much of the recipient site as possible—usually more than 90%. When a large defect is being covered, the flap and recipient bed are coapted by occasional mattress sutures tied over a bolus. After 2 to 3 days of limited activity, the patient is up and about without restriction. During the healing period, the dressing must be changed frequently to prevent accumulation of the discharge from the raw part of the flap. After 10 to 14 days, a very light dressing is adequate for support. At 21 days the flap is detached. Some favor immediate accurate insertion of the severed flap end; others postpone definitive insertion for 3 to 5 days after detaching the flap. Fastidious wound care before flap detachment can prepare the wound for definitive insertion at the time of flap division.

### Modifications of the abdominal pedicle flap

*Paired flaps.* Miura and associates reported the use of paired flaps to cover both the dorsal and volar surface of the hand.

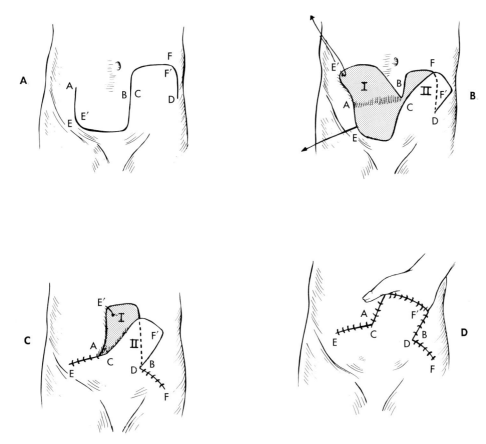

**Fig. 8-27. A,** The flaps are designed by the incision from *A* to *D*. **B,** Both flaps are reflected. Traction at points *E* and *F* allows rotation of the flaps into an opposing position. **C,** The flaps are in opposition. **D,** Both the volar and dorsal surfaces of the hand can be covered by the opposing flaps.

An S-shaped skin incision is marked on the abdominal wall (Fig. 8-27) to give adequate flap coverage of the defect. The flaps are raised and rotated to overlap. The edges are joined with raw surface facing raw surface. Thus a pocket is formed with a flap on both sides providing coverage for the volar and dorsal surfaces of the hand.

They have utilized this technique in 15 cases of circumferential avulsion of skin from the hand. This provides basically a mitten hand, which can subsequently be improved.

*Cone flaps.* Jeffs and Kemble describe a cone-shaped flap that they have found useful for covering any cone-shaped projection, such as a thumb, in which more soft tissue has been lost than bone. The dimensions of the flap are determined in the following manner: (1) The circumference of the quadrant is the same length as the circumference of the defect (Fig. 8-28); (2) the radii AB and AC equal 2BC; and (3) the flap may be based on either radius. To determine the radius, double the circumference and divide by $\pi$ ($\simeq 3$). The height of the cone is limited by the length of the circumference when the flap is sutured to the circumference of the defect.

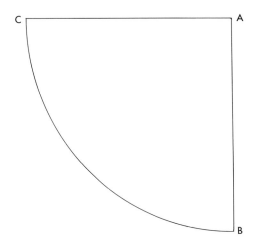

**Fig. 8-28.** Use of the cone flap is limited to coverage of avulsed or partially amputated digits.

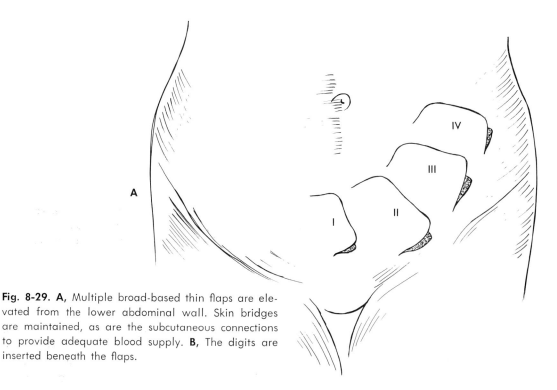

**Fig. 8-29. A,** Multiple broad-based thin flaps are elevated from the lower abdominal wall. Skin bridges are maintained, as are the subcutaneous connections to provide adequate blood supply. **B,** The digits are inserted beneath the flaps.

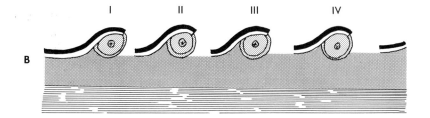

Use of the cone flap is limited to coverage of partially amputated and avulsed digits, particularly the thumb. It is unsuitable for resurfacing whole digits. The main advantages are its immediate availability, near total coverage of the defect, and minimal trimming needed to set in the flap.

*Louvre flaps.* Emmett has suggested the use of multiple broad, thin flaps based mainly on subcutaneous pedicles for resurfacing multiple, adjacent finger tissue defects. He suggests the use of the lower abdomen because of the natural skin looseness. Even though the flaps are nourished primarily from their subcutaneous connections, skin bridges are maintained to provide additional blood supply (Fig. 8-29). Each flap is raised of dermal

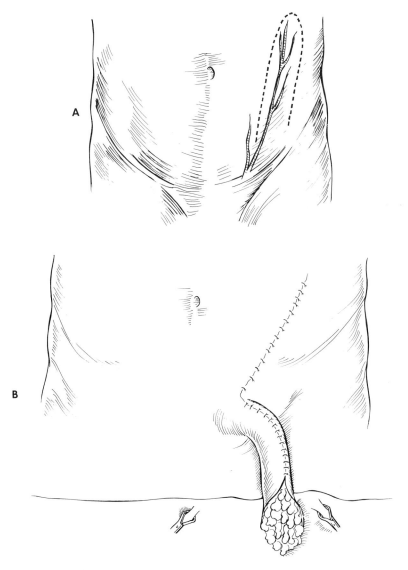

**Fig. 8-30. A,** Shaw developed a one-stage abdominal pedicle flap based on the superficial epigastric and circumflex iliac vessels. **B,** The flap may be tubed immediately and maintain an excellent blood supply.

thickness only in its distal half. Donor areas are covered with split grafts. The flaps are divided at approximately 3 weeks.

*Axial pattern flaps*

SHAW FLAPS. Shaw developed a one-stage abdominal pedicle flap that was based inferiorly on the superficial epigastric and superficial circumflex iliac arteries and veins (Fig. 8-30). He was able to tube the flap immediately, thus providing a one-stage tube flap with an excellent blood supply. The single pedicle tubes vary in length from 5 to 18 cm and in width from 2 to 7 cm. He noted that superficial veins can usually be seen through the skin and used as guides in outlining the flap. When the veins are not visible, their approximate location over the femoral triangle is used. The flap is elevated just superficial to Scarpa's fascia, or in some instances it includes this fascia. The attachment of the flap is undermined extensively to allow mobility in closing the angles when the base of the tube is formed. By staggering the inferior ends of the incisions, the base of the tube can be rotated through an arc of 180 degrees. If the medial incision is shorter than the lateral, the tube will rotate laterally. If the lateral incision is shorter than the medial incision, the tube can be rotated medially. If the recipient area is completely covered at the time of pedicle development, the tube can be divided in approximately 3 weeks. If, however, the tube itself is to be used to cover a portion of the defect, a delayed procedure is required. Shaw reports successful use of the flap in 31 cases, 25 of which covered defects of the hand and wrist.

Barfred reports use of the Shaw flap in 26 patients who required coverage of the hand or forearm. He notes that the length should not exceed three times the width of the flap. The flap is outlined parallel to the linea alba, but it overlies the inferior superficial epigastric artery and vein. The distal pedicle is thinned for application to the recipient site, and the proximal pedicle includes all tissues down to the level of the fascia. Direct closure of the donor area is usually possible. In 17 of 26 cases, the use of the flap was uneventful. In 6 cases the intended result was obtained in spite of minor marginal necroses that healed spontaneously. Major necrosis occurred in 4 cases. In 6 cases, thinning of the flap was the reason for reoperation. The color of the flap was darker than recipient site skin. In 2 cases, rupture of the sutured donor area occurred that required skin grafting.

Careful examination of the abdomen for previous surgical incisions must be undertaken before planning any flap.

GROIN FLAPS. The groin flap is an axial pattern flap popularized by McGregor. The flap is based on a single pedicle centered over the origin of the superficial circumflex iliac artery in the femoral triangle (Fig. 8-31). Since this is an axial pattern flap, one can raise without delay a flap whose ratio of length to width far exceeds that of the random pattern flaps. A firm grasp of

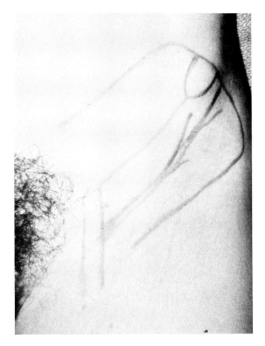

**Fig. 8-31.** The groin flap is centered over the origin of the superficial circumflex iliac artery.

the anatomy of the vascular supply of this flap is necessary.

The *superficial circumflex iliac artery* (Fig. 8-32) arises 2 to 3 cm below the midpoint of the inguinal ligament, usually from the femoral artery but, rarely, from the superficial epigastric artery at its origin. From this point it passes laterally, parallel to the inguinal ligament, as far as the medial border of the sartorius muscle. At the medial border of this muscle, it gives off a deep branch and at the same time becomes more superficial, passing into the tissue that is used as a groin flap. In this plane it continues its course laterally parallel to the inguinal ligament, dividing usually into an upper and lower branch just beyond the anterior superior iliac spine. Lateral to this point on the pelvis it is not really identifiable as a set vessel.

The *venous pattern* around the groin is more variable than the arterial pattern, although in general the veins resemble the arteries because they both have an overall system of "cartwheel" tributaries; in the case of the veins, these tributaries join the saphenous vein near its origin. This point is very close to the origin of the superficial circumflex iliac artery, and any flap incorporating it as an axial vessel could scarcely fail to include the corresponding venous system.

The anatomical points relevant to the raising of a groin flap are as follows: (1) The origin of the artery is 2 to 3 cm below the inguinal ligament with a course thereafter parallel to that ligament; and (2) the point of entry of the artery into the flap is at the medial border of the sartorius muscle.

By using the first of these facts we can design the flap with the vessel lying centrally along its axis; using the second, we know that if dissection is stopped short of the medial border of the sartorius muscle when the flap is being raised, the all-important axial artery will be quite safe.

The origin of the superficial circumflex iliac artery, which is the center of the base of this flap, is located in the following manner. Mark the anterior superior iliac spine and the pubic tubercle and draw a

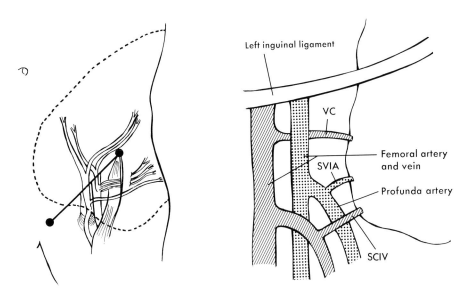

**Fig. 8-32.** The superficial circumflex iliac artery arises 2 to 3 cm below the midpoint of the inguinal ligament. *VC,* vena comitante; *SCIV,* superficial circumflex iliac vein; *SCIA,* superficial circumflex iliac artery.

line between the two; this marks the course of the inguinal ligament. Palpate and mark the femoral artery 2.5 cm below the ligament. This marks the point of origin of the superficial circumflex iliac artery. A line drawn laterally from this point and parallel with the inguinal ligament marks the course of the superficial circumflex iliac artery. Outline the flap with the vessels in the midportion. The actual width of flap that is supported by the vessel is unknown. In general, McGregor recommends a flap 10 cm wide to allow tubing the flap and to provide coverage. The length of the flap may be prolonged beyond the anterior superior iliac spine by a distance equal to the breadth of the flap.

Care must be taken to select the proper plane of elevation to prevent injury to the axial vasculature and to stop short of the vascular pedicle at the femoral artery. Dissection is begun laterally to facilitate finding the proper plane. The axial vessels are divided at this point; thus dissection deep to these vessels will protect the blood supply. As elevation proceeds medially, the fascia over the lateral border of the

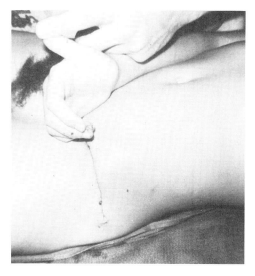

**Fig. 8-33.** Planning of the flap to allow transverse closure of the donor defect places the scar within the bikini area.

sartorius is incised and reflected with the flap. Thus the dissection continues between the sartorius muscle and the fascia. As the medial border of the sartorius is approached, elevation of the flap is considered complete.

When coverage of small to moderate defects is required, the flap can be designed to produce a donor defect within the bikini area. This allows direct closure of the donor area producing a straight line transverse scar well within the bikini area (Fig. 8-33). Limitation of the donor scar to this area is particularly appreciated by young people. Larger defects require closure with split-thickness skin grafts.

McGregor reports from his experience with 50 cases that the responses of the groin flap to elevation are quite different from those of random pattern flaps. Basically the differences are: (1) extreme pallor; (2) absence of transcient edema; and (3) longer time required for necrosis to develop.

Postoperative management is similar to that for pedicles from other areas. If the defect has been entirely covered by the flap, the pedicle is divided at 3 weeks, but not inserted until 7 days later. This is to prevent "rim necrosis." If all of the defect has not been covered, the flap is delayed by division of the axial artery 1 week prior to complete division of the pedicle.

## MANAGEMENT OF TISSUE LOSS FROM THE DISTAL PHALANGES
### Anatomical consideration

The requirement for functional sensibility in the radiovolar areas of the finger pads and the ulnovolar pad area of the thumb pad focuses particular attention on tissue replacement in these areas. Of the five types of nerve endings identifiable in the finger pad, Meissner's corpuscles have excited the most attention. Meissner's corpuscle is an ovoid organ with a thin lamellated capsule and a cellular inner core that is divided into three or four lobules. It is about $80\mu$ long by $30\mu$ wide, and its long axis lies perpendicular to the body surface, from which it may be less than $500\mu$ distant.

Before considering tissue replacement, let us digress for a moment to concern ourselves with the anatomy of a major component of the distal phalanx: the fingernail and its related structures. The fingernail consists of a plate and its supporting tissues. The nail plate is a keratinized structure that grows longitudinally from the nail groove, being replaced about every 5 months. The nail consists of a root embedded in the nail groove, a fixed middle portion, and a distal free edge. The growth center of the nail, the matrix, is a semilunar area of proliferating epithelial cells lining the volar surface of the nail groove. Externally, the matrix is identified by the lunula (the whitish area at the base of the nail). The nail is of particular value in splinting fractures of the bony phalanx or supporting soft tissue repairs. Failure to properly treat fragments of the nail bed can ultimately prove a nuisance.

Most fingertip injuries can be included in the following categories: (1) loss of skin and a minimum of subcutaneous tissue, (2) loss of skin and subcutaneous pulp, (3) loss of fingernail bed and bony phalanx with or without pulp loss, and (4) fractures of the distal phalanx associated with any of the other three types of injuries.

Before proceeding to selection of methods to manage these injuries, we must evaluate the various methods of coverage available in terms of function, sensory capabilities, and sensitivity. Previously, three types of skin coverage were identified: free grafts, pedicle grafts without a major nerve branch, and pedicle grafts with a major nerve branch incorporated into the pedicle. Each type of coverage will be evaluated for function, sensory reinnervation, and sensitivity.

### Sensory reinnervation of free grafts

Experimental studies in ducks revealed that if skin from the duck's bill and foot were interchanged, sensory corpuscles found only in the bill skin would not be formed in the transplanted foot skin. It was concluded that end-organ differentiation is controlled by the skin and not by the nerve fibers growing in from the recipient site. In humans, nonglabrous human skin grafts assume the sensory pattern of the skin adjacent to the recipient site, suggesting that the cutaneous nerve pattern in the graft is determined by the local sensory nerves and not the graft.

Meissner's corpuscle, a sensory end-organ present in large numbers in the glabrous skin on the volar aspect of the fingertip, is absent in the nonglabrous skin of other sites, such as the forearm. There is no evidence that these corpuscles undergo mitoses. Evaluation of forearm split-thickness grafts to the finger pads revealed that the two-point threshold was 4.5 mm, 2 mm, and 7.5 mm in three cases. Microscopic examination of these grafts revealed the failure of Meissner's corpuscles to develop in the forearm skin transplanted to the finger pad. The graft epidermis had thickened and assumed the morphologic characteristics of volar digital skin. Rete pegs in the grafts assumed the appearance of dermal papillae like that formed in normal volar pad skin. The dermal papillae of the grafts were completely devoid of Meissner's corpuscles. However, each graft did contain papillary and intraepidermal nerve fibers, and, on occasion, nerve endings resembling Merkel's discs were present. The failure of Meissner's corpuscles to develop in transplanted forearm skin implies that the development of cutaneous sensory endings, at least the complex encapsulated types, is controlled by the kind of skin in which the sensory nerve ends, rather than by the nerve cell. The proposal that Meissner's corpuscles are responsible for two-point discrimination requires reconsideration since one patient exhibited a two-point discrimination distance of 2 mm yet a biopsy revealed no Meissner's corpuscles.

Generally, the larger the graft, the poorer its sensation. This observation supports the theory of peripheral innervation of grafts and flaps. The available area for axon growth is proportional to the square of the periphery; that is, there are proportionally fewer axons per square millimeter available for a larger graft. Napier, in a detailed study of the sensory reinnervation of a small number of grafts, concluded that the grafts were innervated peripherally but that some deeper and larger nerves may link up with empty Schwann tubes within the graft.

### Clinical evaluation of tissue replacement methods

#### Free grafts

*Split-thickness grafts.* Evaluation of 51 patients who underwent coverage of finger pads (bone exposed in 18) with split grafts from the forearm area revealed the following:

1. Seventy percent of the patients could distinguish between points 3 mm apart, and over 90% could distinguish between points 4 mm apart.
2. Of 24 patients with injuries involving the thumb or index pad, 71% (17 patients) performed the pick-up test satisfactorily. The others substituted the middle finger for the index.
3. Sixty-two percent of the patients had no tenderness, whereas in 9% (5 patients) the tenderness interfered with the daily routine.

Residual tenderness was no more likely to develop in injuries that included bone injury than in injuries involving the skin and pulp alone.

In another series of 53 patients, in which free split grafts from the forearm were utilized, the following was reported:

1. Seventy percent complained of tenderness in the graft area, 41% reporting marked tenderness.
2. Forty-nine percent complained of cold sensitivity.

3. The average two-point discrimination test distance was 5 mm.
4. Thirteen of 27 patients having repair of the thumb or index pad avoided use of the repaired pad in the pick-up test.
5. The pain threshold on the injured finger was 4 gm compared with a control level of 20 gm.

*Full-thickness grafts.* In a series of 59 patients the following observations were recorded:

1. Sixty-eight percent complained of tenderness in the grafted pad.
2. Sixty-one percent complained of cold sensitivity (in 26% the sensitivity was severe).
3. Touch sensation was decreased in 51%, 37% exhibiting a decreased discrimination of size and texture.
4. An average two-point discrimination distance of 9 mm was achieved.
5. Eighty-one percent of the patients avoided use of their grafted fingertips in the finger-dexterity test.
6. The pain threshold averaged 9 gm on the repaired tips compared with a 20 gm control value.

#### Pedicle grafts

*Sensory evaluation of pedicle flaps that do not contain a major nerve branch.* Evaluation of one series of 20 patients with cross-finger flaps revealed the following: (1) Four complained of tenderness; (2) 3 complained of cold sensitivity, none severe; (3) all 15 patients with index finger or thumb repairs had good dexterity and function of pinch; (4) 25% of the flaps became obviously pigmented; (5) the average two-point discrimination distance was 6 mm; and (6) the average pain threshold was 6 gm compared with a control value of 20 gm. In a second series of 27 cases, an average two-point discrimination of 7.2 mm was noted.

In another series, two-point discrimination in 55 patients who underwent cross-finger flaps was analyzed according to the patient's age. The patients were divided into three groups: Group I, 1 to 12 years; Group II, 13 to 39 years; and Group III, 40 to 67 years (Table 8-1).

Other reports have not been so encouraging. In a review of 76 cross-finger pedicle flaps in Montreal, all 19 patients who had pedicle coverage of the index or thumb pad showed a loss of functional ability. Also, 66% demonstrated cold intolerance that was often associated with cyanosis of the graft, and 38% had hyperesthesia. Unfortunately, no two-point discrimination results are included in the report. Certainly the climate to which the patient is exposed must be considered when one attempts to compare results from different studies.

THENAR FLAPS. Miller was able to analyze 32 of 62 patients treated with thenar flaps. The average time off work was 8 weeks in those injured on the job and 3.7 weeks in those injured at home. The skin was assessed as normal in 25 patients, good in 5, and poor in 2 patients. The donor area was not satisfactory. In 20 patients, the palmar scar was either hypertrophic, dark, irregular, rough, or prominent. In 18 patients, two-point discrimination was tested. Eight were unable to discriminate, 3 were able to discriminate at 4 mm, 5 at 4 to 5 mm, and 2 at 5 to 6 mm. The range of motion of the finger was normal in 29, restricted in 3. In the 3 cases, the restriction in movement was at the distal interphalangeal joint.

PALMAR FLAPS. Evaluation of 21 patients

**Table 8-1.** Two-point discrimination in 55 patients who underwent cross-finger flaps

| Discrimination achieved | Number of patients in group | | |
|---|---|---|---|
| | I | II | III |
| 6 mm | 18 | 7 | 8 |
| 7- 8 mm | 1 | 2 | 2 |
| 9-10 mm | 1 | 4 | 4 |
| 10 mm | — | 2 | 6 |

has revealed the following: (1) Twenty-four percent complained of tenderness; (2) 67% complained of cold sensitivity; (3) of 10 patients in this group with index or thumb repair, one avoided use of this finger pad during the finger dexterity test; (4) the average two-point discrimination distance was 9 mm; and (5) the average pain threshold was 26 gm compared with a control value of 20 gm.

*Sensory evaluation of pedicle flaps that contain a major nerve branch*

ISLAND PEDICLE FLAPS THAT INCLUDE A MEDIAN NERVE BRANCH. Evaluation of 15 patients revealed the following:

1. In only one patient did two-point discrimination remain normal in the island pedicle flap. Two patients exhibited two-point discrimination distances of 20 and 16 mm. Two-point discrimination was absent in the other 12 patients.
2. Ninhydrin prints revealed return of sudomotor activity in all flaps.
3. There was no correlation between the return of sudomotor activity and sensation in the flap.
4. The ability to distinguish between sharp and dull was present in all flaps.
5. Cold sensitivity was present in 12 patients; in 5 this significantly interfered with hand function.
6. There was no decrease in cold intolerance in patients who exhibited this phenomenon preoperatively.
7. Hyperesthesia was reported in 7 patients.
8. Reorientation of sensation to the thumb occurred in 4 of 15 patients, requiring from 18 months to 8 years.
9. The island flap gave an excellent durable skin surface that possessed less than normal sensation.

Krag and Rasmussen reviewed six patients 1 to 11 years years after transfer of a neurovascular island flap to the thumb had been performed according to Littler's technique. All six patients referred pinprick in the flap to the donor finger. All had absent two-point discrimination in the flap even though it had been within normal limits a few months after surgery. All demonstrated functional improvement.

ISLAND PEDICLE FLAPS THAT INCLUDE A RADIAL SENSORY NERVE BRANCH. In a series of 14 patients, 9 exhibited a 2-point discrimination distance of less than 15 mm. Moberg has shown that this is the maximum distance at which tactile gnosis is functional. These 9 patients used the thumb in ordinary activities.

VOLAR OR LATERAL ADVANCEMENT FLAPS. No analysis of the parameters mentioned above are available in a group of significant size to be analyzed. Most reports state that normal sensation was maintained. Thus, the advantages of the local advancement flap include: (1) a relatively simple one-stage procedure, (2) early return to work with minimal joint complication, (3) normal or near normal sensation, and (4) a functional pad.

## MANAGEMENT OF SOFT TISSUE LOSS IN THE FINGER PADS
### Soft tissue loss

Loss of soft tissue without exposure of the bony phalanx is readily closed with a free graft. The advantages of the free graft are: (1) relatively simple, one-stage procedure, (2) excellent sensory return, (3) early return to work, and (4) minimal joint complications. Minimal skin losses of this type in small children can be adequately treated by simply allowing the wound to heal by contraction and epithelialization.

Conolly and others have advocated treating pulp injuries by allowing spontaneous healing by contraction and epithelialization of the wound. Eighteen distal pulp injuries in which a full-thickness skin loss of approximately 15% to 30% of the pulp surface area had been lost were treated in this manner. Spontaneous healing in all patients was accomplished within 3 to 4

weeks. In all but four patients, a satisfactory pain-free functioning fingertip resulted. The remaining four developed a tender scar. Avoiding the use of skin graft coverage in these cases allowed preservation of maximal tissue, finger length, and finger function through early movement.

Fox and associates report experience with 18 adult patients who sustained amputation injuries to 22 fingers without bone exposure. The area of full-thickness skin loss ranged from $0.4 \times 1$ cm to $1.8 \times 2.6$ cm. All wounds were covered directly with sterile aluminum foil and a dressing. Dressings were changed at 3, 5, and 7 days after injury and weekly thereafter. All patients returned to work within 10 days of injury. The range of motion in all joints of the injured fingers was normal. Complete wound healing was accomplished within 4 weeks. No breakdown of tissue occurred during the 6-month period of observation. Two-point sensory discrimination averaged 4 mm.

Illingwork reported excellent cosmetic and functional results in more than 300 children who had sustained fingertip tissue loss and who were treated with dressings only. In some patients the site of amputation extended through the base of the terminal phalanx below the nail. A long-term follow-up of a patient treated in such a manner is shown in Fig. 8-34.

### Soft tissue loss and bone exposure

If the loss is on the ulnovolar surface of the finger pad, a free graft is satisfactory. Available for coverage of an injury that results in loss of the pulp and a functional pad are the cross-finger and thenar flaps and the island flaps that include a major sensory branch of the median, ulnar, or radial nerves. Based on the reports evaluating the ultimate sensory function in each of these flaps, it is evident that if the thumb is involved, a flap that includes the sensory branch of the radial nerve should be used. If the finger pad of the index or long finger is involved, a thenar, a cross-finger, or an island flap (median or ulnar nerve innervated) is available. Since the majority of island flaps provide no better functional coverage than a cross-finger or thenar flap, there appears to be little reason to disrupt the normal function of an uninjured finger. The selection between a cross-finger flap and a thenar flap is simplified in patients over 40 because of the acute flexion of the proximal interphalangeal joint necessary for attachment of the thenar flap. In younger patients, either the thenar or cross-finger flap can be utilized for coverage of the index or long fingers.

### Soft tissue and bone loss

Coverage for these injuries may be obtained with local flaps, including the lateral advancement flaps of Kutler or the volar advancement flaps of Kleinert, Littler, or Snow. The selection of which flap to use is usually determined by the surgeon's past experience and familiarity with a technique. Apparently, all give excellent coverage and maintain normal sensation. When

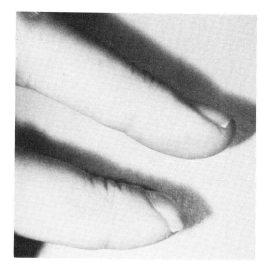

**Fig. 8-34.** Long-term follow-up of pulp injury treated by dressing changes only. Note volar curvature of nail and loss of pulp.

one is concerned with maintaining digital length and providing functional padding, the thenar or cross-finger flaps are prime candidates; the advantages of the cross-finger flap make it the usual choice. When one is confronted with soft tissue and bone loss resulting from a bevelling type amputation (more volar surface is lost than dorsal surface), the lateral and volar advancement flaps are inadequate to gain functional coverage of the fingertip and maintain length. Again the choice between thenar and cross-finger flaps must be made. When local advancement flaps or skin graft closure is not indicated, as discussed earlier, the cross-finger flap appears superior to the thenar flap—except in the thumb where the radial sensory nerve flap apparently maintains excellent sensory capabilities.

### Avulsion injuries

When the bony terminal phalanx is totally denuded, amputation is advised.

To summarize, the flaps transferred with a major nerve branch intact, that is, the lateral and volar local advancement flaps, maintain excellent sensory function. The radial sensory flap gives superior functional results when compared with the island flap containing a median or ulnar nerve branch. The flaps transferred without a major nerve branch in the pedicle (for example, thenar, cross-finger, palmar) provide needed bulk and functional surface but regain less discriminatory function than do free grafts. The poorest reinnervated flaps are those from the trunk.

In conclusion, each patient must be thoroughly evaluated and the operative procedure selected that fits his particular needs.

### BIBLIOGRAPHY

Alonso-Artieda, M.: Reimplantation of an avulsed ring finger using a sensory cross-finger flap, Br. J. Plast. Surg. 24:293, 1971.

Ashbell, T. S., Kleinert, H. E., Putch, S. M., and others: The deformed fingernail, a frequent result of failure to repair nail bed injuries, J. Trauma 7:177, 1967.

Atasoy, E., Ioakimidis, E., Kasdan, M. L., and others: Reconstruction of the amputated finger tip with a triangular volar flap; a new surgical procedure, J. Bone Joint Surg. 52A:921, 1970.

Barfred, T.: The Shaw abdominal flap, Scand. J. Plast. Reconstr. Surg. 10:56, 1976.

Baudet, J., and Lemaire, J. M.: The abdominal flap in the surgery of the hand; how does it stand? Ann. Chir. Plast. 20:215, 1975.

Beasley, R. W.: Principles and techniques of resurfacing operations for hand surgery, Surg. Clin. North Am. 47:389, 1967.

Beasley, R. W.: Reconstruction of amputated fingertips, Plast. Reconstr. Surg. 44:349, 1969.

Beasley, R. W.: Local flaps for surgery of the hand, Orthop. Clin. North Am. 1:219, 1970.

Bralliar, F., and Horner, R. L.: Sensory cross-finger pedicle graft, J. Bone Joint Surg. 51A:1264, 1969.

Brody, G. S., Cloutier, A. M., and Woolhouse, F. M.: The finger tip injury; an assessment of management, Plast. Reconstr. Surg. 26:80, 1960.

Brown, H. C., Williams, H. B., and Woolhouse, F. M.: Principles of salvage in mutilating hand injuries, J. Trauma 8:319, 1968.

Carroll, R. E.: Ring injuries in the hand, Clin. Orthop. 104:175, 1974.

Conolly, W. B.: The spontaneous healing of hand wounds, Aust. N.Z. J. Surg. 44:393, 1974.

Crawford, J., Horton, C. E., and Oakley, R. S.: Avulsion of ring finger skin, Plast. Reconstr. Surg. 10:46, 1952.

Cronin, T. D.: The cross finger flap; a new method of repair, Am. Surg. 17:419, 1951.

Cuperman, D. A.: The free flap, Rev. Lat. Am. Plast. Surg. 14:17, 1970.

Daniel, R. K., Terzia, J., and Schwarz, G.: Neurovascular free flaps, Plast. Reconstr. Surg. 56:13, 1975.

Daniel, R. K., and Williams, H. B.: The free transfer of skin flaps by microvascular anastomoses, Plast. Reconstr. Surg. 52:16, 1973.

Dobyns, J. H.: Rotation-transposition method for soft tissue replacement on the distal segment of the thumb, Plast. Reconstr. Surg. 54:366, 1974.

Emmett, A. J. J.: Finger resurfacing by the multiple subcutaneous pedicle or louvre flaps, Br. J. Plast. Surg. 27:370, 1974.

Fingertip injuries, Lancet 1:717, 1967.

Fisher, R. H.: The Kutler method of repair of finger-tip amputations, J. Bone Joint Surg. 49A:317, 1967.

Fox, J. W. IV, Golden, G. T., Rodeheaver, G., and others: Nonoperative management of fin-

gertip pulp amputation by occlusive dressings, Am. J. Surg. 133:255, 1977.

Gatewood, A.: Plastic repair of finger defects without hospitalization, J.A.M.A. 87:1479, 1951.

Gaul, J. S.: Radial-innervated cross-finger flap from index to provide sensory pulp to injured thumb, J. Bone Joint Surg. 51A:1257, 1969.

Gurdin, M., and Pangman, W. J.: The repair of surface defects of fingers by transdigital flaps, Plast. Reconstr. Surg. 5:368, 1950.

Haddad, R. J.: The Kutler repair of fingertip amputation, South. Med. J. 61:1264, 1968.

Harty, M.: The dermal papillae in the fingertip, Plast. Reconstr. Surg. 45:141, 1970.

Harvey, F. J., and Harvey, P. M.: A critical review of the results of primary finger and thumb amputations, Hand 6:157, 1974.

Holevich, J.: A new method of restoring sensibility to the thumb, J. Bone Joint Surg. 45A:496, 1963.

Holevich, J., and Paneva-Holevich, E.: Bipedicled island flaps, Acta Chir. Plast. 13:106, 1971.

Holm, A., and Zachariae, L.: Fingertip lesions; an evaluation of conservative treatment versus free skin grafting, Acta Orthop. Scand. 45:382, 1974.

Horn, J. S.: Full thickness hand skin flaps, Plast. Reconstr. Surg. 7:463, 1951.

Horner, R. L.: Finger tip trauma, Surg. Clin. North Am. 49:1373, 1969.

Hueston, J.: Local flap repair of fingertip injuries, Plast. Reconstr. Surg. 3:349, 1966.

Illingwork, C. M.: Trapped fingers and amputated fingertips in children, J. Pediatr. Surg. 9:853, 1974.

Iselin, F.: The flag flap, Plast. Reconstr. Surg. 52:374, 1973.

Jeffs, J. V., and Kemble, J. V.: The cone flap for resurfacing and reconstructing partial digits, Br. J. Plast. Surg. 26:163, 1973.

Johnson, R. K., and Iverson, R. E.: Cross-finger pedicle flaps in the hand, J. Bone Joint Surg. 53:913, 1971.

Joshi, B. B.: Dorsolateral flap from same finger to relieve flexion contracture, Plast. Reconstr. Surg. 49:186, 1972.

Joshi, B. B.: Sensory flaps for the degloved mutilated hand, Hand 6:247, 1974.

Kaplan, I.: The management of hand injuries, S. Afr. Med. J. 44:1011, 1970.

Keim, H. A., and Grantham, S. A.: Volar-flap advancement for thumb and finger-tip injuries, Clin. Orthop. 66:109, 1961.

Kelleher, J. C., Sullivan, J. G., Baibak, G. J., and others: The distant pedicle flap in surgery of the hand, Orthop. Clin. North Am. 1:227, 1970.

Kelleher, J. C., Sullivan, J. G., Baibak, G. J., and Dean, R. K.: Use of a tailored abdominal pedicle flap for surgical reconstruction of the hand, J. Bone Joint Surg. **52A:**1552, 1970.

Kislov, R., and Kelly, A. P.: Cross finger flaps in digital injuries with notes on Kirschner wire fixation, Plast. Reconstr. Surg. **25:**312, 1960.

Kleinert, H. E., McAlister, C. G., MacDonald, C. J., and Kutz, J. E.: A critical evaluation of cross finger flaps, J. Trauma **14:**756, 1974.

Krag, C., and Rasmussen, K. B.: The neurovascular island flap for defective sensibility of the thumb, J. Bone Joint Surg. **57B:**495, 1975.

Kutz, J. E., and Kleinert, H. E.: A critical evaluation of cross finger flaps, J. Trauma **14:**756, 1974.

Li, C. S., Nahigian, S. H., Richey, D. G., and Shaw, T.: Primary application of the one-stage abdominal tubed pedicle, Hand **1:**184, 1972.

Lie, K. K., Magargle, R. K., and Posch, J. L.: Free full-thickness skin grafts from the palm to cover defects of the fingers, J. Bone Joint Surg. **52A:**559, 1970.

Lie, K. K., and Posch, J. L.: Island flap innervated by radial nerve for restoration of sensation in an index stump, Plast. Reconstr. Surg. **47:**386, 1971.

Lister, G. D., McGregor, I. A., and Jackson, I. T.: The groin flap in hand injuries, Injury **4:**229, 1973.

Littler, J. W.: Principles of reconstructive surgery of the hand. In Converse, J. W., editor: Reconstructive plastic surgery, vol. 4, Philadelphia, 1964, W. B. Saunders Co.

McCash, C. R.: Cross-arm bridge flaps in the repair of flexion contractures of the fingers, Br. J. Plast. Surg. **9:**25, 1956.

McCraw, J. B., and Furlow, L. T.: The dorsalis pedis arterialized flap, Plast. Reconstr. Surg. **55:**177, 1975.

McGregor, I. A., and Jackson, I. T.: The groin flap, Br. J. Plast. Surg. **25:**3, 1972.

Micks, J. E., and Wilson, J. N.: Full-thickness sole-skin grafts for resurfacing the hand, J. Bone Joint Surg. **49A:**1128, 1967.

Miller, A. J.: Single finger tip injuries treated by thenar flap, Hand **6:**311, 1974.

Miura, T., and Nakamura, R.: Use of paired flaps to simultaneously cover the dorsal and volar surfaces of a raw hand, Plast. Reconstr. Surg. **54:**286, 1974.

Moberg, E.: Methods for examining sensibility in the hand. In Flynn, J., editor: Hand surgery, Baltimore, 1966, The Williams & Wilkins Co.

Moller, J. T.: Lesions of the volar fibrocartilage in finger joints, Acta Orthop. Scand. **45:**673, 1974.

Murray, J. F., Ord, J. V., and Gavelin, G. E.: The neurovascular island pedicle flap, J. Bone Joint Surg. **49A:**1285, 1967.

Napier, J. R.: The return of pain sensibility in full thickness skin grafts, Brain **75:**147, 1952.

O'Brien, B.: Neurovascular island pedicle flaps for terminal amputation and digital scars, Br. J. Plast. Surg. **21:**258, 1968.

O'Brien, B. McC., Morrison, W. A., Ishida, H., and others: Free flap transfers with microvascular anastomoses, Br. J. Plast. Surg. **27:**220, 1974.

O'Brien, B. McC., and Shanmugan, N.: Experimental transfer of composite free flaps with microvascular anastomoses, Aust. N.Z. J. Surg. **43:**285, 1973.

Omer, G. E., Jr.: Evaluation and reconstruction of forearm and hand after acute traumatic peripheral nerve injuries, J. Bone Joint Surg. **50A:**1454, 1968.

Omer, G. E., Jr., Day, D. J., Ratliff, H., and others: Neurovascular cutaneous island pedicles for deficient median-nerve sensibility, J. Bone Joint Surg. **52A:**1181, 1970.

Onizuka, T., and Ichinose, M.: Lengthening of the amputated fingertip, J. Trauma **14:**419, 1974.

Patton, H. S.: Split-skin grafts from hypothenar area for fingertip avulsions, Plast. Reconstr. Surg. **43:**426, 1969.

Porter, R. W.: Functional assessment of transplanted skin in volar defects of the digits, J. Bone Joint Surg. **50A:**955, 1968.

Quilliam, T. A., and Ridley, A.: The receptor community in the finger tip, J. Physiol. **216:**15, 1971.

Ridley, A.: A biopsy study of the innervation of forearm skin grafted to the finger tip, Brain **93:**547, 1970.

Robinson, D. W., and Masters, F. W.: Severe avulsion injuries of the extremities including the degloving type, Surg. Clin. North Am. **47:**379, 1967.

Salomon, J. R.: Partial-thickness skin grafting of fingertip injuries, Lancet **1:**705, 1967.

Shaw, D. T., and Payne, R. L.: One stage tubed abdominal flaps, Surg. Gynecol. Obstet. **83:**205, 1946.

Shaw, D. T., Li, C. S., Richey, D. G., and others: Interdigital butterfly flap in the hand (the double-opposing Z-plasty), J. Bone Joint Surg. **55A:**1677, 1973.

Shaw, M. H.: Neurovascular island pedicle flaps for terminal digital scars; a hazard, Br. J. Surg. **55:**161, 1968.

Smith, J. R., and Boon, A. F.: An evaluation of finger-tip reconstruction by cross-finger and palmar pedicle flap, Plast. Reconstr. Surg. **35:**409, 1965.

Snow, J.: The use of volar flap for repair of finger-tip amputation; a preliminary report, Plast. Reconstr. Surg. **40:**163, 1967.

Strickland, J. W., and Dingman, D. L.: Avulsions of the tactile finger pad; an evaluation of treatment, Am. Surg. **35**:756, 1969.

Sturman, M. J., and Duran, R. J.: Late results of finger-tip injuries, J. Bone Joint Surg. **45A**:289, 1963.

Tajima, T.: Treatment of open crushing type of industrial injuries of the hand and forearm; degloving, open circumferential, heat-press, and nail-bed injuries, J. Trauma **14**:995, 1974.

Taylor, G. I., and Daniel, R. K.: The anatomy of several free flap donor sites, Plast. Reconstr. Surg. **56**:243, 1975.

Tempest, M. N.: Cross-finger flaps in the treatment of injuries to the finger tip, Plast. Reconstr. Surg. **9**:204, 1952.

Thomson, H. G., and Sorokolit, W. T.: The cross-finger flap in children; a follow-up study, Plast. Reconstr. Surg. **39**:482, 1967.

Thompson, R. V.: Essential details in technic of finger amputations, Med. J. Aust. **2**:14, 1963.

Weiner, D. L., Silver, L., and Aiache, A.: Preservation of traumatically amputated fingertips, Plast. Reconstr. Surg. **49**:609, 1972.

White, W. L.: Flap grafts to the upper extremity, Surg. Clin. North Am. **40**:389, 1960.

Woolf, R. M., and Broadbent, T. R.: The four-flap Z-plasty, Plast. Reconstr. Surg. **49**:48, 1972.

Wood, R. W.: Multiple cross-finger flaps, "piggy back" technique, Plast. Reconstr. Surg. **41**:54, 1968.

Xavier, T. S., and Lamb, D. W.: The forearm as donor site for split skin grafts, Hand **6**:243, 1974.

# CHAPTER 9

# Management of bone, joint, and ligament injuries

Before one undertakes the management of bone, joint, and ligament injuries, a thorough review of digital joint stability and movement (Chapter 5) is essential. In any case, a cursory anatomical review of each injured joint discussed will be provided. A joint is stabilized by capsular and extracapsular structures. The capsular structures are primarily ligamentous, whereas the extracapsular structures are musculo-tendinous.

## HYPEREXTENSION INJURIES
### Thumb

*Metacarpophalangeal joint.* The capsular structures stabilizing this joint are the volar plate and the proper and accessory collateral ligaments. The extracapsular structures include: the adductor pollicis insertion into the ulnar sesamoid bone, the flexor pollicis brevis insertion into the radial sesamoid bone, and the tendinous hood mechanism formed by the adductor pollicis and abductor pollicis brevis coalescing into the long extensor.

It has been suggested that the volar plate of the metacarpophalangeal joint be designated as the proximal and distal volar plate with respect to the location of the sesamoid bones within the plate. Thus, the distal volar plate inserts into the proximal pha-

lanx, whereas the proximal volar plate inserts into the metacarpal neck.

Resistance to hyperextension of the metacarpophalangeal joint is encountered as the volar plate becomes taut. Severing the proximal portion of the volar plate permits an average of 20 degrees further hyperextension, at which point the accessory collateral ligaments become taut, impairing further hyperextension (Fig. 9-1). Division of these accessory collateral ligaments allows 80 degrees of hyperextension (Fig. 9-2). Division of the volar part of the proper collateral ligaments is necessary for hyperextension to exceed 90 degrees (Fig. 9-3). Consequently, hyperextension injuries require rupture of the volar plate, the accessory collateral ligaments, and at least part of the proper collateral ligament as determined by the degree of hyperextension injury.

Careful questioning of the patient concerning the range of motion at the metacarpophalangeal joint before the injury is particularly important. Evaluation of metacarpophalangeal extension in normal subjects reveals a wide variation (Fig. 9-4). Anyone with a "normal" exaggerated degree of hyperextension is aware of this hypermobility. Comparison with the uninvolved hand is useful but must not be

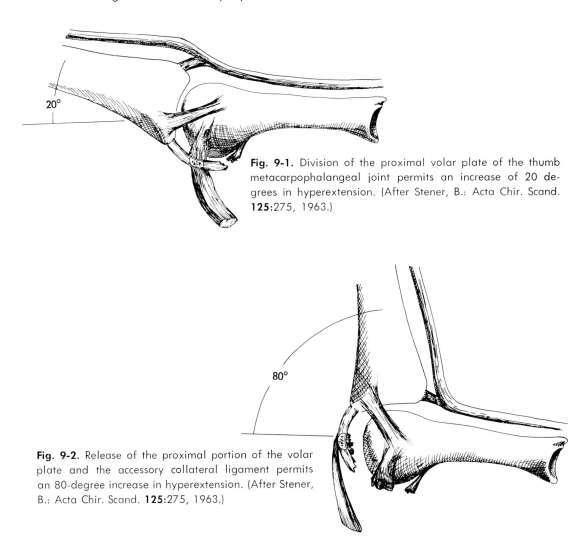

**Fig. 9-1.** Division of the proximal volar plate of the thumb metacarpophalangeal joint permits an increase of 20 degrees in hyperextension. (After Stener, B.: Acta Chir. Scand. **125**:275, 1963.)

**Fig. 9-2.** Release of the proximal portion of the volar plate and the accessory collateral ligament permits an 80-degree increase in hyperextension. (After Stener, B.: Acta Chir. Scand. **125**:275, 1963.)

overinterpreted. An exact diagnosis of the extent of injury demands a thorough clinical examination: inspection for hematoma or abnormal positioning, localization of a tender area, and testing of active and passive function. A patient's inability to oppose hyperextension of the joint actively should lead one to suspect injury to the muscles that prevent hyperextension, that is, the flexor pollicis brevis and the transverse head of the adductor pollicis. The functional state of the flexor pollicis brevis can be checked by palpation as the patient pinches the thumb pulp against the pads of the long and index fingers. Normally, the muscle is clearly palpable. When injured, it cannot be palpated as a firm mass. When the injury is limited to the ligaments checking hyperextension, muscle contraction may be eliminated by regional anesthesia before joint instability can be demonstrated. Flexion of the interphalangeal joint of the thumb relaxes the flexor pollicis longus while passive motion in the metacarpophalangeal joint is evaluated.

Ligament rupture usually results in tenderness and swelling over the site of rupture. When stress is applied to the liga-

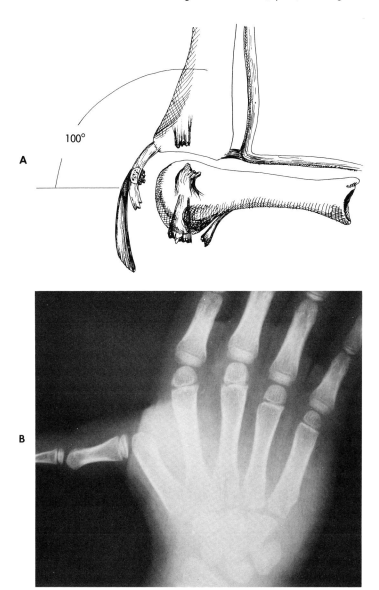

**Fig. 9-3. A,** Division of the volar plate and the proper and accessory collateral ligaments allows a marked increase in hyperextension. **B,** Patient sustained a laceration of the flexor pollicis brevis without injury to any capsular structures. Note marked hyperextension present only after injury. (**A** from Stener, B.: Acta Chir. Scand. **125**:275, 1963.)

ment, pain is localized to the torn ligament. The physical signs of swelling, tenderness over the ligament, pain on stressing the ligament, and positive stress roentgenograms obtained while the joint is anesthetized indicate ligament tear.

Roentgenographic examination is of particular value in making the correct diagnosis. The relationship of the sesamoid bones to the proximal phalanx on a scout film and during passive motion is most important. An increased distance between the joint surfaces indicates the interposition of tissue to the joint. Scout films should be

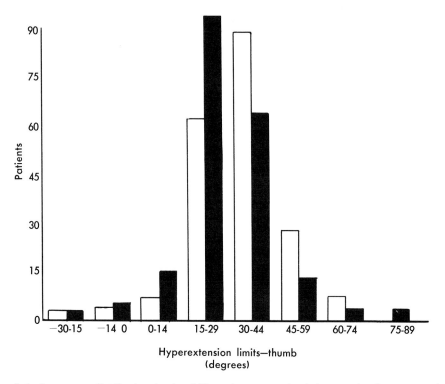

**Fig. 9-4.** Frequency distribution in the 200 patients examined for passive hyperextension of the metacarpophalangeal joint of the thumb. The black columns represent right, and the white, left.

scrutinized for evidence of bone chips at the sites of ligament attachment. Stress films made without anesthesia of the involved part are of no value unless they are positive. Negative films with the hand anesthetized must be obtained before ligamentous rupture can be excluded.

Examination after regional anesthesia is informative. The metacarpophalangeal joint is hyperextended until resistance is encountered, and a lateral roentgenogram is obtained. The degree of hyperextension and the position of the sesamoid bones provide the clues necessary for accurate assessment of the extent of injury.

If hyperextension is possible and the sesamoid bones do not follow the proximal phalanx as it rotates around the metacarpal head, the distal volar plate has been disrupted (Fig. 9-5). In this event the flexor pollicis brevis and adductor pollicis, which

insert into the volar plate, retract proximally.

If hyperextension is possible and the sesamoid bones are fractured, injury is limited to the accessory collateral ligaments and the volar plate through the level of the sesamoid bones. However, if the sesamoid bones remain in a normal relationship with the proximal phalanx during exaggerated hyperextension, the ligamentous disruption will be in the proximal volar plate. Abnormal hyperextension to +80 degrees with the sesamoid bone accompanying the phalanx and joint instability permitting dorsal displacement indicates rupture of the proximal volar ligament and tear in the muscle units attaching to the sesamoid (Fig. 9-6).

Coonrad reports that the metacarpophalangeal joint of the thumb in 1,000 normal subjects exhibits a range of hyper-

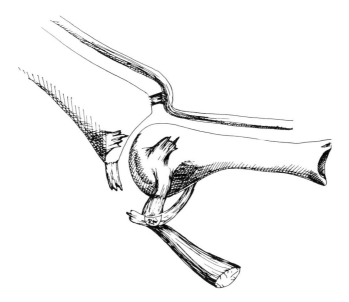

**Fig. 9-5.** When the volar plate is disrupted distal to the sesamoid bones, these bones do not follow the proximal phalanx into extension.

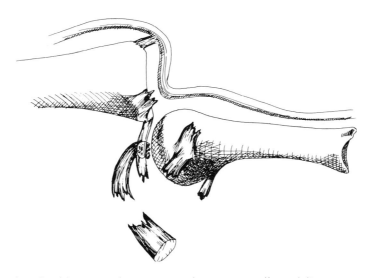

**Fig. 9-6.** In dorsal subluxation, the proper and accessory collateral ligaments and volar plate are disrupted; on occasion muscle units are also disrupted.

extension from 0 to 90 degrees, averaging 20 degrees in motion. Demonstration of this wide variation in range of motion has made interpretation of hyperextension injuries more difficult.

Operative treatment is indicated when there is reason to suspect disruption of the adductor pollicis or flexor pollicis brevis muscles. These muscles are particularly vulnerable, as shown in Stener's cases. Because these muscles contribute significantly to grip and pinch strength, it is important that they be repaired. If the proper collateral ligaments are intact and the accessory collateral ligaments ruptured, direct repair of the accessory ligaments is not required.

Exposure of the volar plate is obtained through an incision along the thumb's most proximal skin crease. The incision is curved proximally along the thumb metacarpal. The insertions of the adductor pollicis and short flexor into the sesamoid bones are identified. If disrupted, they are reattached to the distal portion of the volar plate. Avulsion of the volar plate is repaired by using the pullout wire technique. Fracture through the sesamoids with marked distraction can be reduced and held with suture in the surrounding ligament. Immobilization for 4 weeks is adequate.

### Fingers

*Metacarpophalangeal joint.* Hyperextension without dislocation implies that the collateral ligaments are at least partially intact. The locked position in hyperextension should be carefully discerned from dislocation at this joint (Fig. 9-7). Once dislocation has been excluded, the hyperextended metacarpophalangeal joint can be reduced by traction on the proximal phalanx and gentle flexion. Once the joint is reduced, the condition of the collateral ligaments should be determined. If reduction required anesthesia, stress films may be made immediately; otherwise, the region should be anesthetized and the collateral ligaments tested. If the ligaments of the index or little finger are ruptured, the metacarpophalangeal joint should be immobilized in 50 to 70 degrees flexion for 10 to 14 days before motion is begun. A night splint that holds the metacarpophalangeal joints in 50 to 70 degrees flexion is recommended.

*Proximal interphalangeal joint.* Normally the proximal interphalangeal joint cannot exceed 10 degrees of hyperextension. Hyperextension is prevented by the volar plate that bridges the volar surface of the joint attaching to the base of the middle phalanx and the neck of the proximal phalanx. This volar plate is extremely durable. The sublimis tendon contributes to the checkreining effect because division of the tendon may result in gradual increase in hyperextensibility of the joint. Usually a hyperextension injury at this level results from a direct force on the fingertip. This force is transmitted to the proximal interphalangeal joint.

When the continuity of the volar plate is disrupted, it usually occurs at the base of the middle phalanx (Fig. 9-8). However, on occasion the plate is avulsed from its proximal attachment. Operative reattachment of the volar plate is required to prevent persistence of the hyperextension and snapping at the joint when flexion is initiated. At surgery, if the volar plate is within the joint, it is extracted and reposi-

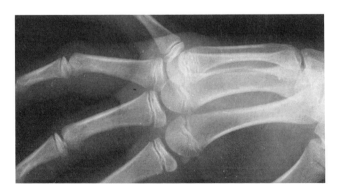

**Fig. 9-7.** The metacarpophalangeal joint of the little finger is locked in hyperextension.

tioned. If the avulsion is distal, the plate is reapproximated with a pullout suture tied over a dorsal button. When the tear is proximal, drill holes in the proximal phalanx allow direct suture of the volar plate to the phalanx. This produces a 10 to 15 degree flexion contracture at the proximal interphalangeal joint. A fine pin traverses the proximal interphalangeal joint and stabilizes it in 10 to 15 degrees flexion for 4 weeks, when active and passive exercises are instituted.

Hyperextension of the proximal interphalangeal joint may be accompanied by herniation of the head of the proximal phalanx through an aperture in the palmar aspect of the capsule, which is bounded distally by the base of the middle phalanx and proximally by the edge of the avulsed capsule. If hypertension of the proximal interphalangeal joint is maintained, it is the result of bowstringing of the lateral bands over the phalangeal head. In some instances, the head of the proximal phalanx may be trapped between the decussations of the sublimis tendon.

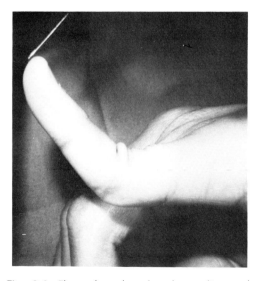

**Fig. 9-8.** The volar plate has been disrupted, permitting hyperextension of the proximal interphalangeal joint.

## DISLOCATIONS

The dislocated joint must be thoroughly examined to rule out fracture, ligament rupture, and partial ligament rupture, in that order. Sprain has been defined as an injury of a joint ligament or capsule resulting in stretching of the ligaments. Of course, ligaments stretch so little as to be insignificant, so the injury is actually one of tearing of the ligamentous fibers. Tears involving a few fibers should be classified as sprains. This is a diagnosis of exclusion.

From roentgenograms one determines the absence of a fracture. Particular attention must be paid to the position of the sesamoid bones when a fracture is present.

Stress roentgenograms may be obtained to demonstrate ligament rupture. These roentgenograms cannot be interpreted as normal until the injured part has been anesthetized.

Often the ligament avulses a fragment of bone at its attachment rather than rupturing through its substance, and this displaced fragment can be detected on a roentgenogram. For a complete dislocation to occur, joint ligaments must be disrupted. It is our purpose to review joint dislocations and to provide the anatomical derangements associated with the injuries and methods for management.

### Thumb

*Carpometacarpal joint.* The base of the thumb metacarpal articulates with the saddle-shaped trapezium bone. It is maintained in this saddle by an ulnar ligament, which bridges the joint attaching to the volar beak of the thumb metacarpal and the tuberosity of the trapezium. A thinner dorsal ligament is reinforced by the broad insertion of the abductor pollicis longus into the base of the metacarpal. Frequently, a second slip of abductor tendon overlying the joint anteriorly is present.

Dislocation at this joint is almost always dorsal; that is, the metacarpal overrides the trapezium dorsally (Fig. 9-9). For this displacement to occur, the ulnar ligament must rupture. More often the ulnar ligament avulses a portion of the volar beak of the metacarpal base—a condition discussed later.

Even though anatomic reduction is readily accomplished and maintained by proper

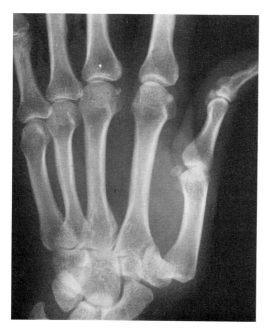

**Fig. 9-9.** The thumb metacarpal has been dislocated from its seat in the trapezium.

casting, subsequent instability in the joint is frequent. Apparently the healing process reconstitutes a ligament that is not adequate to stabilize the joint. Littler suggests open reduction and reconstruction of the disrupted ligament, because direct suture repair is difficult to obtain. He partially transects the flexi carpi radialis above the wrist and longitudinally splits the tendon distally toward its insertion, which is preserved (Fig. 9-10). The strip of tendon is threaded through a drill hole in the base of the thumb metacarpal, which enters at the site of the ligament avulsion and exits radial to the abductor pollicis longus insertion. The tendon is looped around the long abductor insertion, to which it is sutured, and threaded into flexor carpi radialis tendon, to which it is sutured. This provides an excellent prognosis for a stable joint.

*Metacarpophalangeal joint.* Dislocations of the metacarpophalangeal joint may be dorsal, volar, lateral, or any combination. Each will be discussed.

*Dorsal dislocations.* Hyperextension injury of the metacarpophalangeal joint is the penultimate occurrence before dorsal dislocation. The hyperextension injury ruptures the volar plate attachments, the ac-

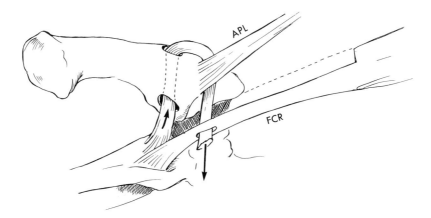

**Fig. 9-10.** The flexor carpi radialis has been partially transected above the wrist and split longitudinally distally, where it is threaded through a drill hole at the base of the thumb metacarpal.

cessory collateral ligaments, and at least the volar part of the proper collateral ligaments.

Physical examination can reveal much concerning the degree of injury, even if the joint has been reduced before examination. Observation of both localized swelling and point tenderness and functional assessment are mandatory. Unopposed passive hyperextension of the joint not present before injury is indicative of interruption of the adductor pollicis or flexor pollicis brevis. Palpation of the flexor pollicis brevis during thumb-to-index pinch can reveal the functional state of this muscle. If the examination is normal, regional anesthesia is necessary to determine the extent of capsular damage. Stener notes that if the accessory collateral ligaments are injured but the proper collateral ligaments are intact, the proximal phalanx can be incompletely dislocated; that is, the volar surface of the proximal phalanx lies in a plane with the dorsal surface of the metacarpal. Complete dislocation indicates injury of the proper collateral ligaments (Fig. 9-11). Asymmetrical injury of the proper collateral ligaments produces rotation of the proximal

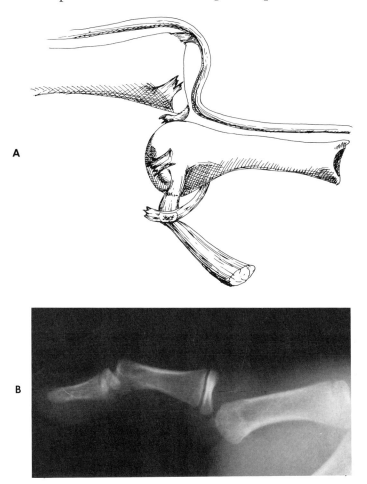

Fig. 9-11. **A**, Dorsal dislocation of the thumb metacarpal associated with disruption of the joint capsular structures, as indicated. Position of the sesamoid on roentgenogram determines the level of involvement of the volar plate. **B**, Dorsal dislocation of the thumb metacarpophalangeal joint. Note the sesamoid bone following the base of the proximal phalanx. Thus, any injury to the volar plate is proximal to the sesamoid bone.

phalanx as it is dislocated. If the volar plate is avulsed proximal to the insertions of the adductor pollicis and flexor pollicis brevis muscles, the sesamoids are noted on roentgenogram to follow the proximal phalanx into extension. If a fracture through the sesamoids is demonstrated on roentgenogram, the sesamoids are sewn together with sutures through the volar plate proximal and distal to the fracture. If the volar plate tear passes distal to the sesamoids, the sesamoids do not follow the displacement of the proximal phalanx.

In complete dislocations, the proximal phalanx base overrides the metacarpal. To allow such positioning, at least the major part of one collateral ligament and probably both ligaments are disrupted. Roentgenograms are of prime importance in determining the level of injury to the capsular structures. If the sesamoids follow the proximal phalanx dorsally, the volar plate may be lying atop the metacarpal, interposed between the joint surfaces, or trailing along the contour of the joint.

The most common site of volar plate rupture is proximal to the sesamoids; thus, in dorsal displacement of the proximal phalanx, the tendons of the flexor pollicis brevis and the oblique head of the adductor pollicis straddle the metacarpal head. The flexor pollicis longus tendon is displaced laterally. Reduction is facilitated if the insertions of the intrinsic muscles to the sesamoids are intact; that is, the muscles guide the volar plate back into proper positioning. If the metacarpal is flexed into the palm, the tension on the intrinsic muscles is lessened, thereby permitting gradual traction and flexion to complete reduction. After reduction, adequate stress films are obtained to detect any lateral instability in the collateral ligaments. Furthermore, dorsal stability must be verified. If one can readily dislocate the proximal phalanx dorsally, the intrinsic muscles are torn and should be repaired. Instability following pure dorsal dislocations is un-

common. Postreduction roentgenogram verifies proper positioning of the joint surfaces, width of the joint space, and positioning of the sesamoids. In pure dislocations of the proximal phalanx (in the absence of collateral ligament disruption or intrinsic muscle disruption), excellent results can be expected by splinting the properly reduced joint in slight flexion for 3 weeks.

Operative treatment is indicated when there is a reason to suspect disruption of the adductor pollicis or flexor pollicis brevis muscles or the collateral ligaments. When both proper collateral ligaments have been ruptured, both are repaired. Isolated tears of the accessory collateral ligaments in the absence of injury to the proper collateral ligament require immobilization only until the pain and swelling have subsided.

Surgical exposure is gained through a dorsal incision over the metacarpophalangeal joint. Any structures trapped within the joint space are extracted and repositioned, and the tension on the dislocated proximal phalanx is reduced by flexing the carpometacarpal joint, applying traction on the proximal phalanx, and gently flexing the proximal phalanx.

Dorsal and lateral stability of the joint must be inspected. If the joint is dorsally unstable, the adductor pollicis and flexor pollicis brevis muscles are exposed to determine the extent of injury so that they can be repaired. If the volar plate has been avulsed from the proximal phalanx, it is reattached, using the pullout wire technique. Disruption of the tendons at their insertion into the sesamoids is repaired. When lateral instability is present, the disrupted collateral ligament is repaired. Immobilization in slight flexion for 6 weeks is sufficient.

In a retrospective study of 26 complete dorsal dislocations, treatment was as follows: "Some were immobilized for 2 weeks, others for 4 weeks and a few had no immobilization." One patient required open reduction after closed manipulation failed. Follow-up revealed that two patients developed an unstable joint. All other patients had stable thumbs and a normal range of motion. One can conclude from this study that brief immobilization of pure dorsal dislocations provides an excellent prognosis.

Though Stener reports excellent results following surgical repair of dorsal dislocation of the thumb, excellent results can also be expected through splinting the anatomically reduced joint in slight flexion for 3 weeks. Hyperextensibility to stress test in itself does not justify open reduction, because many individuals can voluntarily and painlessly hyperextend their thumb metacarpophalangeal joints to 45 or even 60 degrees yet have no clinical weakness or subsequent degenerative changes.

Operative intervention in dorsal dislocations is indicated in the following situations: (1) when the dislocation is irreducible or after reduction the joint space is abnormally wide, (2) when the joint is unstable in the flexion-extension plane (careful attention must be paid to the positioning of the

sesamoid bones on roentgenogram), and (3) dislocations that after reduction exhibit lateral instability of greater than 40 degrees with radial or ulnar stress.

*Volar dislocation.* When the proximal phalanx is displaced volar to the metacarpal head and telescoped into the palm (Fig. 9-12), the collateral ligaments have been disrupted and the posterior joint capsule has been torn. Membranous attachments of the volar plate may be torn or intact. Closed reduction can be readily accomplished. Stress roentgenograms are obtained to determine the integrity of the collateral ligaments. If the ulnar collateral ligament is disrupted, operative intervention is indicated. Otherwise, the joint must be held in flexion to ensure proper length of the collateral ligaments as they heal by scar formation. Active motion is begun early.

*Lateral dislocation.* The factors contributing to lateral stability of the metacarpophalangeal joint include: (1) the broad head of the metacarpal, (2) the radial and ulnar collateral ligaments, (3) the accessory collateral ligament and volar plate, and

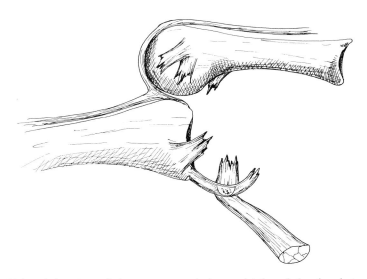

**Fig. 9-12.** Volar dislocation of the metacarpophalangeal joint of the thumb is associated with disruption of the capsular structures, as noted. Usually the patient reduces the dislocation at the time of injury.

(4) the intrinsic muscles inserting into the sesamoids, proximal phalanx, and extensor apparatus. These provide great stability to the joint, yet dislocation is more frequent at this joint than in the metacarpophalangeal joints of all the fingers.

After dislocation the patient usually has pain and swelling of the joint but normal joint alignment. Flexion and extension are normal; however, when lateral stress is applied to the radial or ulnar collateral ligaments, instability may be demonstrated (Fig. 9-13). To state conclusively that the collateral ligaments have not been ruptured, one must anesthetize the thumb and again stress the collateral ligaments. If significant lateral deviation is noted, stress roentgenograms must be obtained. Complete rupture of a collateral ligament must occur before significant lateral displacement is evident. The joint angulates more than 40 degrees when total disruption of a collateral ligament has occurred.

Complete tear of the ulnar collateral ligament without accompanying bony fracture usually occurs at its attachment to the proximal phalanx. Careful review of the roentgenograms may reveal fragments of bone (usually at the collateral ligament's distal insertion), indicating ligament detachment (Fig. 9-14). The radially directed stress draws the aponeuroses of the adductor pollicis taut across the joint capsule, squeezing the collateral ligament proximally. This doubles the ligament on itself with the free end pointing proximally—a situation that hardly promotes adequate healing of the ligament ends (Fig. 9-15). Stener reported this malposition in 25 of 39 patients operated upon for ulnar collateral ligament tears. Consequently, all metacarpophalangeal joints ex-

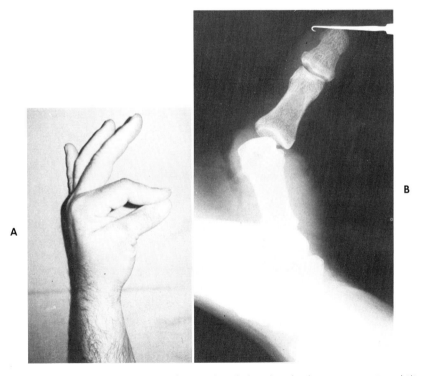

**Fig. 9-13. A,** Stress applied to the ulnar side of the thumb demonstrates instability at the metacarpophalangeal joint. **B,** Roentgenograms reveal instability at the metacarpophalangeal joint and absence of fracture.

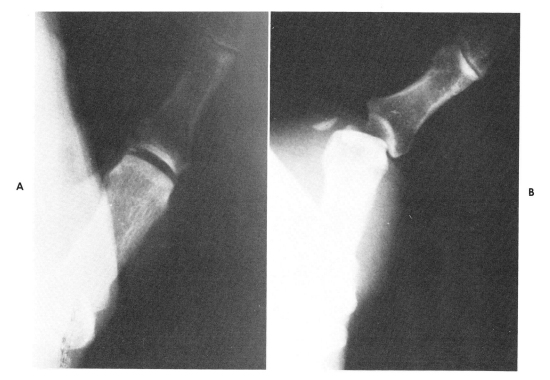

Fig. 9-14. A, A slightly displaced chip fracture is evident at the base of the proximal phalanx. B, As lateral stress is applied to the thumb metacarpophalangeal joint, the aponeurosis of the adductor pollicis is drawn taut across the joint capsule, and the bony fragment and ulnar collateral ligaments are dislocated proximally.

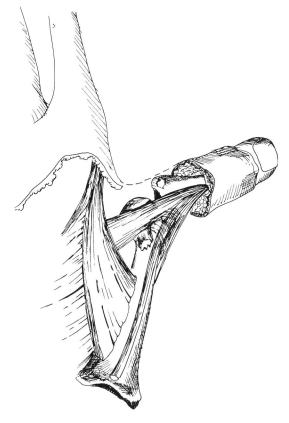

Fig. 9-15. The ulnar collateral ligament is avulsed from the proximal phalanx and reflected proximally, where it is held by the fibers of the adductor pollicis muscle.

hibiting a major disruption of the ulnar collateral ligament, that is, greater than 40 degrees of lateral motion on stress roentgenograms, should undergo operative repair. Surgical exposure is gained through a curved dorsoulnar incision over the metacarpophalangeal joint. The folded collateral ligament is identified at the proximal end of the adductor aponeurosis. This aponeurosis is divided parallel to the fibers of the extensor pollicis longus tendon. As the adductor aponeurosis is reflected, the frayed ends of the ligament and its detachment site from the proximal phalanx are exposed. The collateral ligament is reattached to the proximal phalanx, using the pullout wire technique (Fig. 9-16). A 5-0 double arm wire suture is passed in a crisscross fashion through the collateral ligament. When a significant bone fragment is attached to the ligament, a single small hole is drilled in the center of the fragment. The wire suture is passed through the drill hole; if this is not done, the bony fragment attached to the ligament will be diverted

either medially into the joint or laterally. A second drill hole is made by introducing a Kirschner wire through the site of fracture at the base of the proximal phalanx and directing it out the radial side of the proximal phalanx. We use a Kirschner wire with a hole drilled in its point. The wire sutures are threaded through the hole in the Kirschner wire, and the Kirschner wire with the attached suture is pulled (not drilled) out the radial side of the proximal phalanx. The suture is passed through a pad and a button. Before the suture is tied, the metacarpophalangeal joint is positioned in 15 degrees flexion and pinned with a transfixing Kirschner wire. The ligament is advanced up to the side of the base of the proximal phalanx and its wire suture tied over the button. The adductor aponeurosis is repaired. In Stener's series of 39

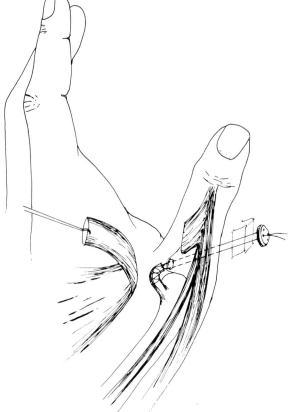

**Fig. 9-16.** The adductor pollicis insertion into the dorsal hood has been reflected and the ulnar collateral ligament reattached to the base of the proximal phalanx.

cases, all obtained excellent results for stability and pinch strength, and all were painless.

*Interphalangeal joint.* Contributing to the stability of the interphalangeal joint are: (1) the broad insertions of the flexor and extensor tendons spanning the joint; (2) the short thick collateral ligaments, (3) the volar plate, (4) snug fixation of the skin envelope, and (5) single plane of joint mobility.

Dislocation requires major ligament rupture, yet the flexor and extensor tendon insertions almost always remain intact (Fig. 9-17). Closed reduction is readily accomplished. However, most of these dislocations are associated with skin wounds. Postreduction roentgenograms must be obtained for verification of the reestablishment of joint congruity. The joint is immobilized in 10 to 15 degrees flexion for 3 weeks.

### Fingers

*Carpometacarpal joint.* Dislocation of the metacarpal base is not uncommon. Most frequently the dislocation is in a dorsal direction in response to a volar force (Fig. 9-18). Roentgenographic examination in the true lateral position is essential in making the diagnosis. Usually closed reduction is possible. Yet a significant incidence of instability and recurrent subluxation necessitates internal fixation by inserting a Kirschner wire transversely into the adjacent stable metacarpal. Three weeks of immobilization are adequate. Failure to obtain complete reduction often leaves the

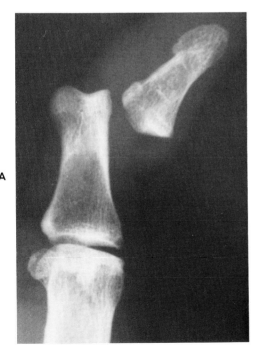

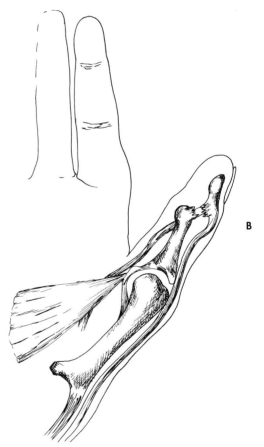

**Fig. 9-17. A,** The distal phalanx of the thumb has been dislocated dorsally. The head of the proximal phalanx appeared in the skin wound. **B,** Dorsal dislocation of the distal phalanx is usually associated with disruption of the capsular structures, but the continuity of the extensor and flexor apparatus is maintained.

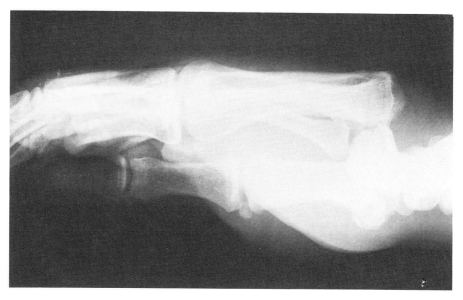

**Fig. 9-18.** Dorsal dislocation of the metacarpals has occurred at the carpometacarpal joints.

patient with a weak grip, a tender bony prominence, and a persistent aching in the fracture site.

Generally, carpometacarpal dislocations of the ulnar side of the hand are reduced with ease, but if closed reduction is incomplete, open reduction and Kirschner wire fixation is necessary. If open reduction is not required, then closed reduction and percutaneous insertion of a Kirschner wire through the metacarpal into the normal adjacent metacarpal base ensures maintenance of reduction. Three to 4 weeks of immobilization are required for stability.

*Metacarpophalangeal joint.* Dislocations of this joint may be either volar or dorsal, the latter being much more frequent.

*Dorsal dislocation.* Dorsal dislocation of the base of the proximal phalanx at the metacarpophalangeal joint in the fingers occurs most frequently in the index finger. The proximal phalanx is usually positioned atop the metacarpal head (Fig. 9-19, *A*). The volar plate of the joint is disrupted most frequently from its loose filmy attachments to the metacarpal, thus remaining attached to the proximal phalanx through its dense fibers. As the proximal phalanx is displaced dorsally, the volar plate follows and usually is found dorsal to the metacarpal head. The collateral ligaments are slackened during this displacement and may not be ruptured. Occasionally, however, the radial collateral ligament tears, resulting in ulnar deviation of the finger. The flexor tendons are taut as a result of the dislocation and slip over the ulnar side of the smooth metacarpal head. This ulnar displacement occurs because the intermetacarpal ligament that inserts into the proximal fibro-osseous tunnel is present on the ulnar side of the index but absent from the radial side. The lumbrical muscle encircles the metacarpal head on its radial side, and the palmar fascia completes the encirclement of the metacarpal head proximally (Fig. 9-19, *B*). Generally, closed reduction is impossible and should not be pursued.

OPERATIVE REDUCTION. A volar incision is made exposing the prominence of the metacarpal head. After the skin is reflected proximal to the metacarpal neck, the palmar fascia is split longitudinally to ex-

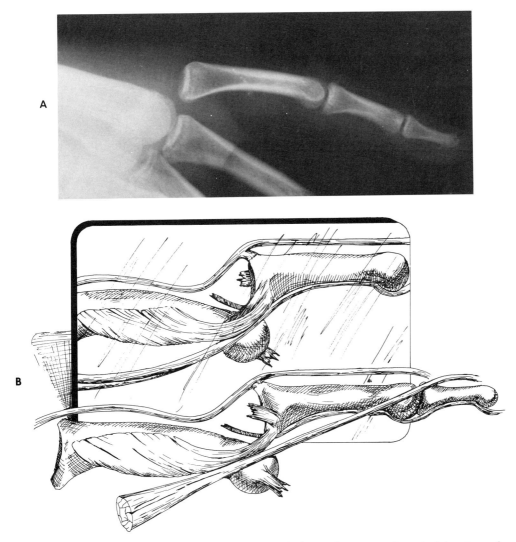

**Fig. 9-19. A,** Dorsal dislocation of metacarpophalangeal joint. **B,** Dorsal dislocation of metacarpophalangeal joint of the index finger reflected in a mirror. The collateral ligaments are disrupted as is the volar plate that is displaced dorsal to the metacarpal head. The long flexor tendons are displaced to the ulnar side of the metacarpal head.

pose the lumbrical muscle and flexor tendon sheath. The tension in the long flexor tendons on the ulnar side of the metacarpal head is released by incising the flexor tendon sheath along its attachments to the volar plate of the metacarpophalangeal joint. As the flexor tendon tension is released, the displaced volar plate can be extracted from its dorsal location and re-positioned. Distal traction permits reduction of the proximal phalanx. Fixation of the volar plate to the metacarpal or the deep fascia discourages dorsal instability. Immobilization in 60 degrees flexion prevents significant shortening of the torn collateral ligaments as they heal.

Dorsal dislocation of the proximal phalanx in the little finger is much less

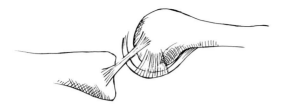

**Fig. 9-20.** The volar plate has been ruptured from its attachment to the proximal phalanx and is displaced into the joint space.

frequent than in the index finger. The anatomical disarrangement is similar to that seen with the index finger except that the flexor tendons of the little finger are displaced to the radial side of the metacarpal head, and the abductor digiti quinti tendons complete the encirclement of the metacarpal head on the ulnar side. Open reduction is required. Dislocation at the long and ring metacarpophalangeal joints is rare. This is probably because of the presence of the transverse metacarpal ligament on both sides of these joints.

*Volar dislocation.* Volar dislocation of the proximal phalanx in any finger is rare. McLaughlin has reported one case that involved the long finger. The dorsal joint capsule had been interposed between the joint surfaces and required open reduction. Renshaw and Louis reported a case in which the volar plate was ruptured from its insertion into the proximal phalanx and displaced over the head of the metacarpal (Fig. 9-20). If the collateral ligaments are intact, closed reduction through manipulation is impossible.

OPERATIVE REDUCTION. Louis utilized a transverse volar incision made in the distal palmar crease over the metacarpophalangeal joint of the involved finger. Extension of the incision was necessary over the ulnar border of the hand both proximally and distally. The displaced base of the proximal phalanx was encountered immediately beneath the skin. Exposure was improved by transection of the tendon of the abductor digiti quinti allowing access to the medial

aspect of the joint. The volar plate was lifted from between the joint surfaces and reduction accomplished.

***Proximal interphalangeal joints.*** Dislocations of this joint may be in a lateral, dorsal, or volar direction. The anatomical changes with each will be discussed.

*Lateral dislocation.* Collateral ligament injuries of the proximal interphalangeal joints of the fingers are not uncommon. Frequently they are the result of athletic encounters. Collateral ligament injuries are caused by abduction or adduction force applied to the extended finger and are characterized clinically by unilateral pain, swelling, and sharply localized tenderness.

Stress roentgenograms of the injured joint should be obtained and, if abnormal, compared with the corresponding finger joint of the uninjured hand. Extreme tenderness requires anesthesia to overcome muscle spasm. The median nerve may be anesthetized at the wrist by inserting a long spinal needle along the proper digital nerve in the web space and passing the needle proximal to the level of the wrist. The ulnar nerve is blocked by following the common digital nerve to the little finger subcutaneously to the level of the hook of the hamate (see Fig. 14-6). Partial tears of the ligament are differentiated from complete tears by the degree of lateral mobility in the joint. Partial tears of the ligament usually cause pain, swelling, and localized tenderness with minimal lateral mobility on stress roentgenograms. Adequate treatment of partial tears requires immobilization in the slightly flexed position; the period of immobilization depends on the apparent severity of the injury. Incomplete ligamentous ruptures respond satisfactorily to immobilization. However, complete ligament tears, inadequately treated, result in disability of the finger by continued swelling, stiffness, and sensitivity to minor trauma (Fig. 9-21). Complete ligament tear requires operative repair.

Redler and Williams reported operative

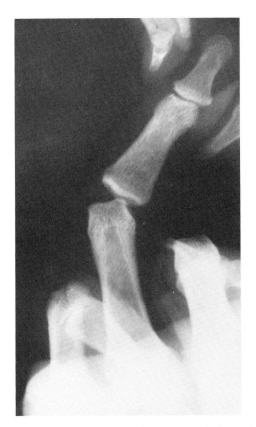

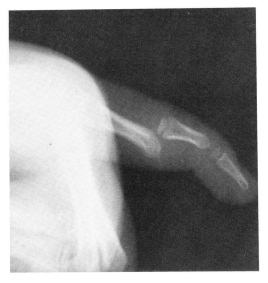

**Fig. 9-22.** Dorsal dislocation of the proximal interphalangeal joint. For this dislocation to occur, the volar plate must be ruptured.

**Fig. 9-21.** Stress roentgenogram reveals lateral instability of proximal interphalangeal joint.

repair of ruptured collateral ligaments in 14 of 18 patients. Rupture of the radial collateral ligament was present in 15 patients, whereas the ulnar collateral ligament was ruptured in 3. In every case the ligament had disrupted at its attachment to the proximal phalanx. The ligament was dislocated into the proximal interphalangeal joint in 7 cases. Operative repair was accomplished with the pullout wire technique, and immobilization of the proximal interphalangeal joint in full extension was maintained for 3 or 4 weeks with a plaster cast. Within 12 to 16 weeks motion was regained, and no patient had lost more than 10 degrees of flexion or extension.

*Dorsal dislocation.* For dorsal dislocation to occur at the proximal interphalangeal joint, the volar plate must be detached,

either from the base of the middle phalanx or from the neck of the proximal phalanx (Fig. 9-22). Most frequently, the disruption occurs at its insertion into the middle phalanx. The joint is exposed through a midlateral incision. The filmy portion of the fibrous digital sheath is excised. As the tendons are retracted, the volar plate is exposed, usually having ruptured from its insertion in the middle phalanx (Fig. 9-23). To gain access to the volar plate, the lateral attachments of the volar plate to the accessory collateral ligaments are divided. A crisscross suture is inserted into the volar plate and passed through two drill holes in the base of the middle phalanx. The suture is tied over a padded button on the dorsum of the middle phalanx.

The volar plate tear may extend posteriorly, dividing the collateral ligament into segments parallel to the direction of its fibers. Thus, the volar plate maintains its attachment to the proximal phalanx and its lateral attachments to the accessory collateral ligament. A segment of the proper collateral ligaments may maintain its attachments to the proximal phalanx while

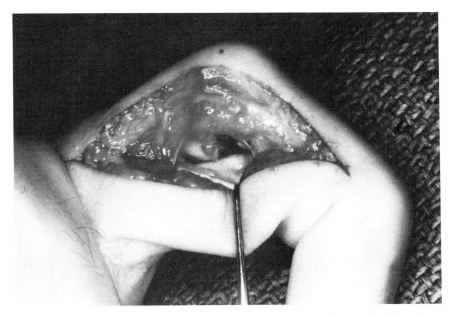

**Fig. 9-23.** The long flexor tendons are retracted, exposing the free end of the disrupted volar plate.

the remaining segment is attached to the anterolateral surface of the dorsally displaced middle phalanx. When the middle phalanx is dorsally dislocated, the collateral ligaments are slack. Traction and gentle flexion facilitate reduction of the dislocation. If the collateral ligament attachments between the proximal phalanx head and the middle phalanx base are intact, the reduction will be stable. Immobilization with splinting is adequate to allow healing of the ligamentous tear and volar plate tear. If the collateral ligament is torn from its insertion, open reduction and direct suture are required; the volar plate should be repaired at the same sitting.

*Volar dislocation.* Spinner and Choi reported that rupture of the central slip of the extensor hood, identified at surgical exploration or by clinical examination, occurred in five consecutive cases of volar dislocation at the proximal interphalangeal joint (Fig. 9-24, A). All cases were treated by closed reduction and immobilization; the fingers exhibited some malfunction of

the extensor apparatus, such as a boutonnière deformity. They reported on experimental studies undertaken to determine the position and direction of forces required to produce a volar dislocation of the middle phalanx at the proximal interphalangeal joint. From these studies it was concluded that traumatic anterior dislocation of the proximal interphalangeal joint, with or without fracture, is produced by a combination of forces. Initially a lateral force ruptures one collateral ligament and the volar plate; this leads to a second anteriorly directed force that displaces the base of the middle phalanx anteriorly and ruptures the central slip of the extensor mechanism. Rupture of the central slip and triangular ligament predisposes to development of a boutonnière deformity unless operative repair is accomplished.

Consequently, an anterior dislocation of the proximal interphalangeal joint should be viewed as a disruption of the central tendinous slip, an avulsion of the collateral ligament (which may be displaced be-

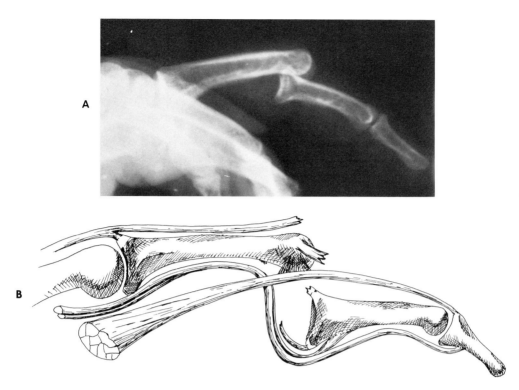

**Fig. 9-24. A,** Volar dislocation of the proximal interphalangeal joint. **B,** Volar dislocation of the proximal interphalangeal joint requires rupture of the collateral ligaments, the volar plate, and the extensor tendon insertion, which ultimately produces a boutonnière deformity if untreated.

tween the lateral band and the oblique retinacular ligament), and a tear of the volar plate in addition to the bony dislocation (Fig. 9-24, *B*). Prompt reduction and repair of these structures (middle slip, collateral ligament, and volar plate) combined with stabilization of the proximal interphalangeal joint in extension with a fine Kirschner wire for 3 weeks are mandatory. Mobilization is begun gradually, protecting the joint with splinting for several subsequent weeks.

Stress roentgenograms of the proximal interphalangeal joint after reduction will verify the degree of ligament injury.

Eaton reported five cases of volar dislocation of the proximal interphalangeal joint and developed a method of approach to treatment somewhat different from that

of Spinner as recorded above. Eaton suggests that if the collateral ligaments and volar plate are disrupted, volar dislocation is possible, yet the extensor tendon may remain intact. If the dislocation is reducible, the articular surfaces congruent on roentgenogram, and the extension lag less than 30 degrees, then surgery is not indicated. Surgery is indicated if the dislocation cannot be reduced, if the articular surfaces are not congruent, or if the extension lag is greater than 30 degrees. The degree of collateral ligament tear also influences the decision regarding surgery.

IRREDUCIBLE DISLOCATION. Occasionally an injury will rupture the radial collateral ligament of a proximal interphalangeal joint and force the middle phalanx into volar rotation and lateral deviation. This ad-

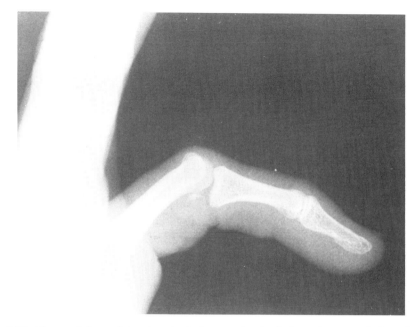

**Fig. 9-25.** The radial condylar head of the proximal phalanx is rotated dorsally and markedly distracted from the middle phalanx.

vances the extensor hood on the condyle of the proximal phalanx. With continued lateral deviation of the middle phalanx, the condyle of the proximal phalanx produces a rent in the extensor hood. When the deviating force is removed, the distal edge of the rent in the extensor hood becomes entrapped within the intercondylar groove. Roentgenograms reveal a classical picture (Fig. 9-25). The proximal phalanx is slightly rotated in relation to the middle phalanx. The joint surfaces are distracted on the side of rotation while they are still in contact, although imperfectly, on the opposite side. Occasionally a bony chip is evident that has been avulsed from the proximal phalanx with the collateral ligament. Repeated attempts at closed reduction may be unsuccessful. A serpentine dorsal incision provides excellent exposure (Fig. 9-26). Entrapment of the herniated condyle between the lateral band and the central portion of the extensor tendon becomes evident. The distal edge of the rent

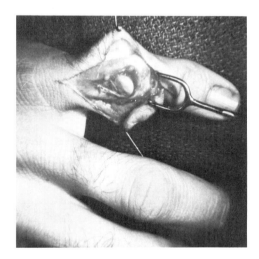

**Fig. 9-26.** Through a dorsal skin incision, herniation of a single condyle through the extensor hood is evident.

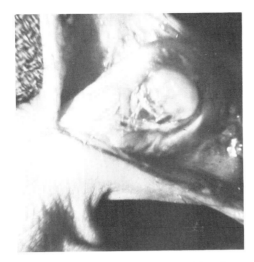

**Fig. 9-27.** The condyle is entrapped by the extensor hood.

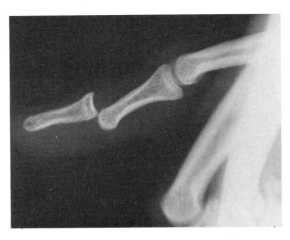

**Fig. 9-28.** Dorsal dislocation of distal interphalangeal joint. The volar plate and collateral ligaments are disrupted.

is held firmly in the recess between the condylar heads (Fig. 9-27). When this portion of the extensor tendon is lifted out of the intercondylar head recess, the subluxation is immediately corrected. The collateral ligament is reattached proximally with a wire suture. Because of the collateral ligament injury, the proximal interphalangeal joint is immobilized for 3 weeks with a Kirschner wire across the joint.

***Distal interphalangeal joint.*** Stability in this joint is contributed by the flexor and extensor tendons bridging the joint, the short stout collateral ligaments, and the dense volar plate and the firm skin-ligament capsule.

Dislocations are frequently associated with open skin wounds because of the firm skin-ligament capsule. Dorsal dislocations are associated with rupture of the collateral ligaments and the volar plate (Fig. 9-28). Disruption of the extensor and flexor tendons is uncommon. Usually the long flexor is displaced laterally. In twisting injuries the extensor tendon insertion may be avulsed. Careful attention to the roentgenograms may reveal bone chips associated with the extensor tendon avulsion. If a

significant sized chip is associated with avulsion of the extensor tendon, then direct suture repair is indicated. Rarely is the profundus tendon avulsed from the distal phalanx, but if it is, it should be repaired immediately using the pullout wire technique (see Fig. 11-12).

Usually reduction of the dislocation is readily accomplished after local anesthesia has been administered. Dislocations that cannot be reduced by simple traction are rare. However, buttonhole tears in the volar plate with the middle phalanx head that protrudes through the rent may not be reducible by simple traction and may require operative intervention. Pohl reported a dorsal dislocation at the distal interphalangeal joint in which closed reduction attempts were unsuccessful. During surgery the head of the middle phalanx was found lying subcutaneously, and the profundus tendon was displaced behind the ulnar condyle of the middle phalanx. The volar plate and collateral ligaments were disrupted at their proximal attachment. Traction on the distal phalanx forced the middle phalangeal head more volarward, precluding reduction. Flexing the digit provided

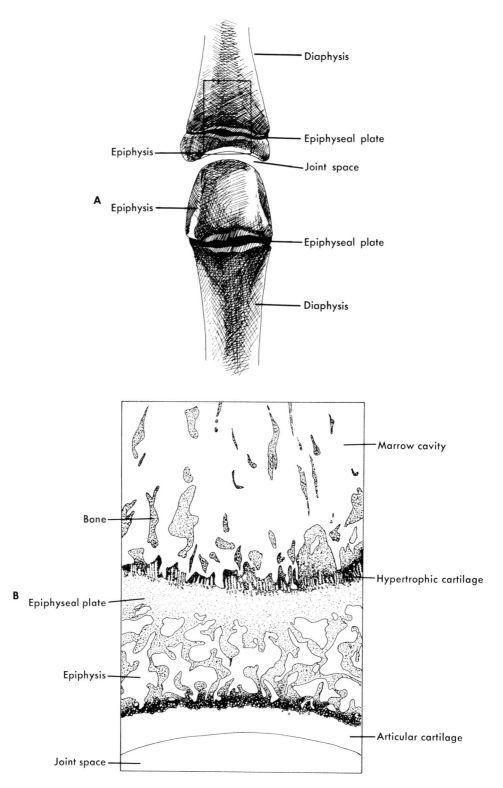

**Fig. 9-29. A,** The relative positions of the epiphyseal plates of the metacarpophalangeal joint as seen on roentgenogram. **B,** An enlargement through the articular surface of one joint reveals the relative position of the epiphyseal plate.

adequate relaxation of the profundus tendon to permit lifting it over the condylar head and reducing the joint dislocation.

Immobilization in 5 to 10 degrees flexion with a transfixing Kirschner wire minimizes the need for dressings and ensures immobilization. In the absence of extensor tendon injury, active and passive motion is begun after 3 to 4 weeks of immobilization. A stable functional joint can be expected.

## EPIPHYSEAL INJURIES

Since the epiphyseal plate is weaker than bone, ligament, or tendon, traumatic separations of the epiphyseal plate are more frequently seen in children, than tendon and ligament injuries. The epiphyseal plate can be divided into four distinct zones of cells: the resting cell zone, the proliferating cell zone, the hypertrophying cell zone, and the endochondral ossification zone (Fig. 9-29). The latter zone is structurally the strongest, whereas the resting cell and the proliferating cell zone are weaker. The hypertrophying cell zone is the weakest; most epiphyseal fractures occur through this zone.

The vascular supply of the epiphyseal plate is derived from vessels on both the epiphyseal and metaphyseal sides that are located in the layer of endochondral ossification. When an epiphysis is completely covered with cartilage, its blood vessels penetrate the rim of the epiphyseal plate to enter the epiphysis, and the vessels are very vulnerable to injury.

The most common epiphyseal fractures involve the phalanges, especially the base of the proximal phalanx. Frequently the fracture results from a twisting injury that rotates and angulates the distal fragment. These fractures are difficult to reduce because the small proximal fragment cannot be grasped. Closed reduction should be attempted, but often the displacement cannot be fully corrected, resulting in some persistent angulation. In this event, the involved finger is strapped to the adjoining finger, and both are splinted in a position of slight flexion for a period of 4 weeks. Any persistent angulation disappears with active use, and the normal excursion of the fingers in flexion and extension becomes restored.

Growth disturbances because of fractures of the epiphyses are most unusual, and shortening is rarely seen. Open reduction is rarely indicated.

### Classification of injuries to the epiphyseal plate

Injuries to the epiphyseal plate have been divided by Salter into five types.

*Type I.* Separation of the epiphysis occurs through the hypertrophying layer of cartilage cells (Fig. 9-30, *A*). Since the proliferating cells are intact, the epiphysis will survive unless the nutrient vessels are disrupted. If the vascular system remains intact, healing is rapid and complete within 3 weeks, and the prognosis is good.

An example of Type I epiphyseal fracture is separation of the epiphysis of the distal phalanx (Fig. 9-30, *B*). Usually the phalanx is flexed and displaced laterally. The epiphysis remains extended relative to the phalanx. Closed reduction by traction and application of lateral and vertical pressure on the joint and phalanx corrects lateral and volar displacement. If external splinting is inadequate, the finger can be immobilized with a smooth Kirschner wire threaded through the distal phalanx, its epiphysis, and the distal interphalangeal joint. After 3 weeks, the pin is removed and motion begun. Occasionally the fibers of the extensor tendon become interposed in the fracture line, necessitating open reduction. A single pin is inserted through the tip of the terminal phalanx into the base of the epiphysis.

*Type II.* In this group the epiphysis is separated, together with a triangular seg-

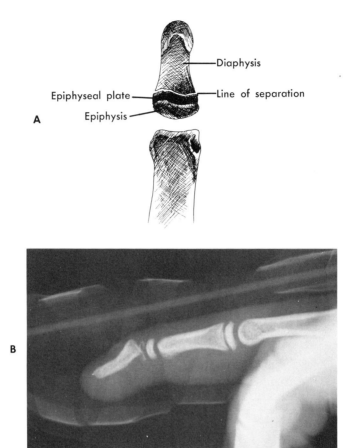

**Fig. 9-30. A,** In a type I epiphyseal fracture, the epiphysis is separated throughout its extent from the diaphysis. **B,** The epiphysis has been separated, although a ring of calcified bone is still intact.

ment of the metaphysis (Fig. 9-31). The periosteum is preserved on one side and helps to stabilize the epiphysis following reduction. Generally, the blood supply to the epiphysis is not damaged, so the prognosis is good. The small triangular portion of the metaphysis is displaced with the epiphysis, allowing the proximal phalanx to rotate on the epiphysis. Closed reduction can be readily accomplished. While steady traction is applied to the finger, the finger is rotated in the opposite direction of the deformity. A roentgenogram confirms reduction. The finger is immobilized by extension of a posterior plaster shell from the midforearm to the tip of the fin-

ger with the metacarpophalangeal and interphalangeal joints in slight flexion. The plaster is removed in 3 weeks, and motion is encouraged.

*Type III.* In this group the fracture line extends from the articular surface of the epiphysis to the hypertrophying layer of cartilage cells of the plate, then laterally through this zone to the periphery (Fig. 9-32). As in other joint injuries, it is essential to restore the congruity of the articular fragments. The prognosis is good because the vascular supply is intact.

*Type IV.* In this group the fracture line extends vertically across the full thickness of the epiphysis, the epiphyseal plate, and

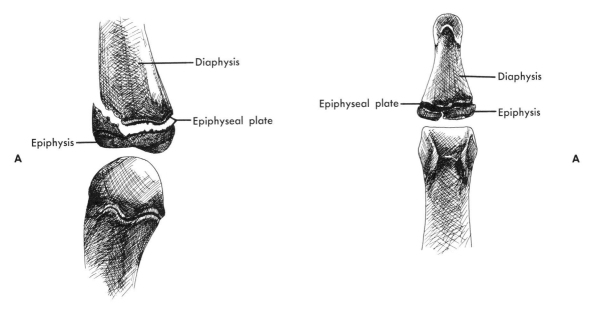

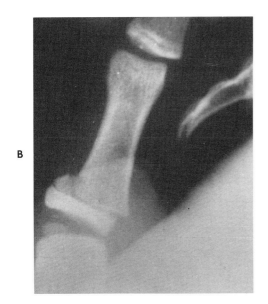

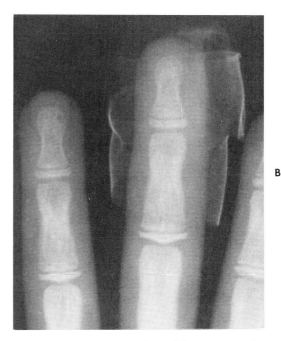

**Fig. 9-31. A,** Type II epiphyseal injuries involve fracture of a portion of the epiphyseal plate and of the metaphyseal bone. **B,** The fracture through the base of the proximal phalanx of the thumb crosses the epiphysis and laterally involves the metaphysis.

**Fig. 9-32. A,** Type III epiphyseal fracture extends from the articular surface through the epiphysis and into the epiphyseal plate. **B,** Fracture of the distal phalanx, extending from its articular surface through the epiphysis and into the epiphyseal plate.

a triangular-shaped wedge of metaphysis (Fig. 9-33). The incongruity of the articular surface should be noted. Complete anatomic reduction in this lesion is essential in order to realign the plate and to restore a smooth articular surface. Some form of internal fixation may be necessary to maintain reduction. The extent of epiphyseal plate damage is unknown—it may be severely damaged—so the prognosis is guarded.

*Type V.* In this group, a portion of the epiphyseal plate is crushed by compression. This is most often encountered in joints moving in only one plane. Displacement of the epiphysis is unusual. Usually roentgenograms give no indication of the extent of injury. Premature closure of the plate with loss of growth and angular deformity is the rule. The prognosis is poor (Fig. 9-34).

**Factors governing prognosis of injuries to the epiphyseal plates**

Lesions of types I, II, and III have a good prognosis, provided the blood supply to the epiphysis is not disrupted. In type III, anatomic realignment of the plate must be achieved. Type IV lesions are accompanied by a less favorable prognosis, but the sequelae can be minimized by restoring alignment of the plate. Severe crushing injuries of part or all of the epiphyseal plate, as seen in Type V lesions, carry a poor prognosis. Forceful manipu-

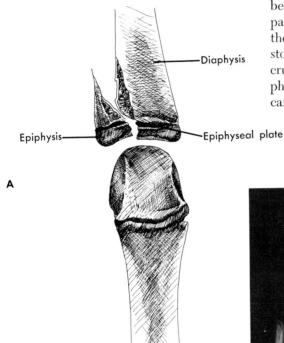

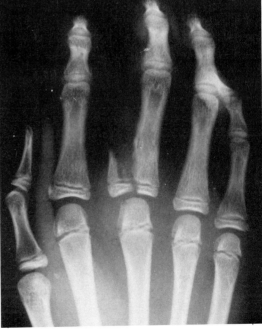

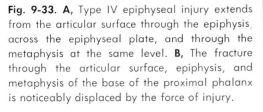

**Fig. 9-33. A,** Type IV epiphyseal injury extends from the articular surface through the epiphysis, across the epiphyseal plate, and through the metaphysis at the same level. **B,** The fracture through the articular surface, epiphysis, and metaphysis of the base of the proximal phalanx is noticeably displaced by the force of injury.

lation during closed reduction or instrumentation during open reduction may further traumatize the epiphyseal plate and influence the final result. Parents should be informed of the possibility of growth disturbances which may not be apparent for 6 to 12 months.

If the epiphyseal plate is not severely disrupted and its alignment is intact, as in types I and II lesions, considerable displacement of the epiphysis can be tolerated. Remodeling will restore the anatomic position of the epiphysis. If the plate is out of alignment and articular incongruity is present, as in types III and IV, it is essential that anatomic alignment be restored even if open reduction must be employed.

## ARTICULAR FRACTURE DISLOCATION

Articular fractures may or may not be associated with dislocations of the injured bone. Fractures extending into an articular

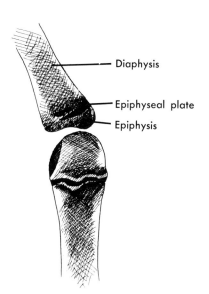

**Fig. 9-34.** Type V epiphyseal injury involves compression and destruction of a portion of the epiphyseal plate, with premature closure on one side. This type of injury can result in deviation of the finger to the injured side.

surface present problems not encountered in diaphyseal fractures. These problems are created by: (1) the reactions evoked in healing of fractures extending through articular cartilages, (2) the need to maintain a smooth gliding surface for proper joint function, and (3) edema formation after injury. Healing of joint injuries was discussed in Chapter 2 and should be reviewed before proceeding. Disruption of the smooth cartilaginous articular surfaces can lead to the development of a traumatic arthritis. Recognition of the hazards of edema formation is mandatory. If the collateral ligaments and soft tissues surrounding the joints are allowed to participate in the healing phenomenon in a shortened position, the joint becomes stiff. Similarly, edema around tendons leads to new collagen deposition that binds the tendon to the fixed underlying structures limiting gliding function.

### Thumb

*Carpometacarpal joint.* Because the thumb plays such a major role in hand function, any injury involving the thumb is significant. As noted earlier, the base of the thumb metacarpal articulates with the saddle-shaped trapezium. The metacarpal base presents the reciprocal of the saddle joint to aid in stability. The radial lateral ligament, which is covered by the abductor pollicis longus tendon, inserts into the thumb metacarpal. The volar edge of the metacarpal base (called the volar beak) receives the insertion of the ulnar ligament. This ligament inserts proximally into the ridge on the tubercle of the trapezium and the intercarpal ligaments. The dorsal capsular area consists of a ligamentous structure covered by the tendons of the extensor pollicis brevis and longus. The entire capsule is redundant.

The ulnar ligament functions to limit the range of abduction and extension of the thumb. If this ligament is not functioning, the unopposed pull of the abductor pollicis longus and extensor pollicis longus and brevis dislocates the metacarpal shaft radially and proximally (Fig. 9-35). Fracture dislocations involving this joint require accurate reduction and maintenance of this reduction to minimize the chances of traumatic arthritis, pain, and instability developing in the joint. Fractures involving the articular surface of the base of the thumb metacarpal are generally classified as either a Bennett or a Rolando fracture.

*Bennett's fracture.* When the volar beak at the base of the thumb metacarpal is fractured, the ulnar ligament no longer stabilizes the base of the thumb metacarpal. As noted above, the pull of the ab-

ductor pollicis longus and extensor pollicis longus and brevis dislocate the thumb metacarpal dorsally and proximally.

TREATMENT. There is much discussion concerning the best method of treatment of a Bennett fracture. Two opposing groups have developed with regard to the issue of how to best maintain reduction. Those favoring closed reduction and simple plaster immobilization have reported that even though the late anatomical results, as judged radiographically, are poor, the functional results are often excellent, despite poor reduction. Gradually the opposing fraction began stressing the fact that closed reduction of the fracture dislocation was not difficult to obtain but was extremely

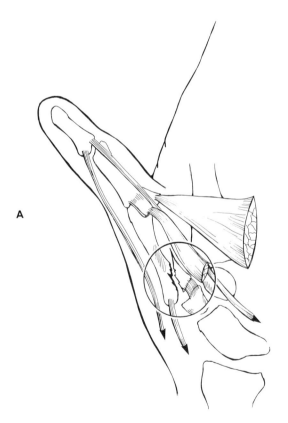
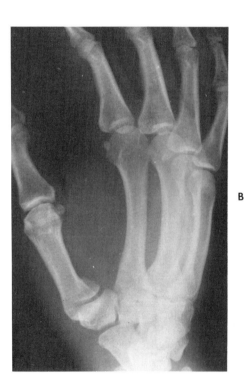

**Fig. 9-35. A,** Fracture of the volar lip at the base of the thumb metacarpal subjects the thumb to the unopposed pull of tendons and muscles bridging the fracture site. **B,** Fracture of the volar lip at the base of the thumb metacarpal has allowed proximal displacement of the thumb.

difficult to maintain during the healing phase. Traction was introduced to counteract the unopposed pull of the abductor pollicis longus and the short and long extensors. Skin traction proved inadequate, even dangerous. Skeletal traction was more satisfactory, and with time, recommendations for placement of the pins for traction moved closer to the fracture site (Fig. 9-36).

Since the primary difficulty in treating a Bennett fracture is maintaining accurate reduction of the fracture, the methods of treatment have revolved around techniques for maintaining this reduction. Closed reduction and casting exponents contend that if great care is taken to ensure adequate

lateral pressure against the dorsum of the metacarpal base, reduction will be maintained. Others contend that traction is required, in addition to casting, to counteract the pull of the long abductor and extensors of the thumb. Advocates of internal fixation to maintain reduction have suggested the following techniques: (1) percutaneous pinning across the reduced fracture site (Fig. 9-37), (2) percutaneous pinning of the thumb metacarpal to the index metacarpal after the fracture has been reduced (Fig. 9-38), (3) percutaneous pinning across the fracture site and into the trapezium, and (4) open reduction and direct fixation with pins or screws. Study of the results obtained by the meth-

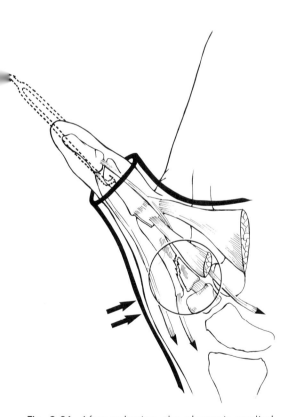

**Fig. 9-36.** After reduction, the plaster is applied to maintain pressure on the base of the thumb metacarpal. Concurrent use of traction has been recommended.

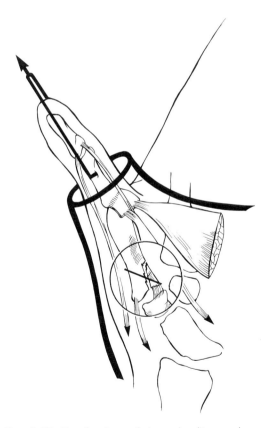

**Fig. 9-37.** The fracture of the volar lip can be pinned directly, and a cast that permits incorporation of a traction device can be applied.

ods mentioned above does not allow a clear-cut selection of the procedure of choice. This is precipitated by the fact that Bennett's fracture covers a spectrum extending from those with small chips off the volar beak to those fractures involving the majority of the articular surface. Furthermore, the degree of proximal displacement of the metacarpal shaft may vary from no dislocation to complete dorsal dislocation.

CLOSED REDUCTION AND PLASTER IMMOBILIZATION. Usually closed reduction can be accomplished without difficulty. Maintaining this reduction requires constant pressure on the base of the metacarpal fracture until union has occurred, usually 4 to 6 weeks. This requires a snugly fitting cast that must be adequately padded to prevent

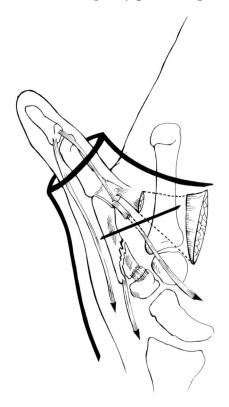

**Fig. 9-38.** Reduction of the fracture and direct pinning of the thumb metacarpal to the index metacarpal has been advocated. Notice the additional use of the plaster.

skin necrosis at the points of pressure. It has been suggested that a preliminary reduction be undertaken without anesthesia to recognize the feel of reducing the fracture. Frequently a palpable click can be detected as the bone is reduced. Adhesive felt is used to pad the pressure points, such as the base of the thumb metacarpal and the bony prominences of the wrist. Plaster is applied, a strip at a time, to allow molding to the contour of the hand, wrist, and forearm. While the plaster is still soft, traction is applied to the thumb and the fracture reduced by direct pressure over the base of the thumb metacarpal. This position is maintained until the plaster has hardened enough to permit further reinforcement with plaster. Radiographs are taken and repeated at 1 and 2 weeks after reduction to confirm that reduction has been maintained. At 4 to 6 weeks the plaster is discarded and gradual motion begun.

If the surgeon elects to use traction, skeletal traction is the safest and most efficient. A Kirschner wire is inserted across the metacarpal shaft near the condylar neck, and an outrigger is incorporated into the cast. The cast must extend from the upper part of the forearm across the wrist and to the thumb. It is carefully molded around the base of the thumb, the palmar aspect of the head of the metacarpal, and the radial side of the thenar eminence.

OPEN REDUCTION AND INTERNAL FIXATION. A transverse incision at the base of the thenar eminence is curved to proceed distally along the metacarpal projection. The skin flap is reflected, and the thenar muscles are retracted after dividing their fine aponeurotic origin. This exposes the carpometacarpal joint. The joint capsule is entered laterally, preserving the dorsal and volar ligamentous attachments. The bony fragment is identified and impaled with a fine Kirschner wire. The fracture is reduced, aided by traction on the thumb and pressure on the dorsum of the metacarpal base, and the wire is drilled into the base of the thumb metacarpal. Care must be taken to ensure accurate anatomical reduction of the fragments. The wire is cut, the thenar muscles are reattached, and the skin edges are sutured. Plaster cast immobilization is used for 6 to 8 weeks; then the plaster is discarded and the Kirschner wire removed. This method, as reported by Moberg, has subsequently been adopted by Gedda—an earlier advocate of closed reduction and plaster cast immobilization.

*Rolando's fracture.* Rolando described an intra-articular fracture involving the thumb metacarpal base that produced two fragments, one volar and one dorsal. This eponym has come to include the more se-vere comminuted fractures involving the metacarpal base. In fact, as a result of modern machinery we see more comminuted fractures than pure Rolando fractures (Fig. 9-39, *A*). Green has recommended open reduction and internal fixation only if the volar and dorsal fracture components are single large fragments. Certainly restoration of the articular surface is difficult if not impossible. However, a much closer restoration of the articular surface and more precise placement of Kirschner wires for fixation are possible by open reduction. An incision is made along the radial border of the extensor pollicis brevis tendon from the metacarpophalangeal joint level to the proximal wrist crease. The sensory nerve branches are carefully retracted. The abductor pollicis brevis is reflected to expose the area of the fracture. The periosteal attachments of each fragment are preserved. While gentle traction is maintained

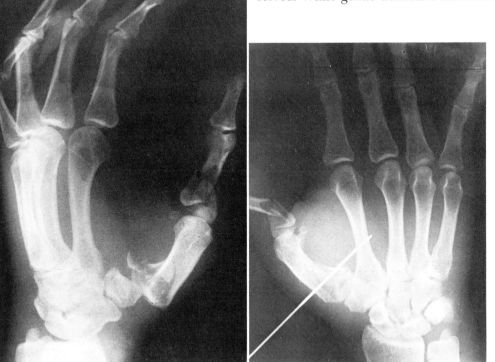

**Fig. 9-39. A,** Crush injury resulted in comminuted fracture involving the articular surface at the base of the thumb and the proximal phalanx. **B,** Open reduction of the base of the thumb metacarpal is obtained as described in the text and maintained with Kirschner wire.

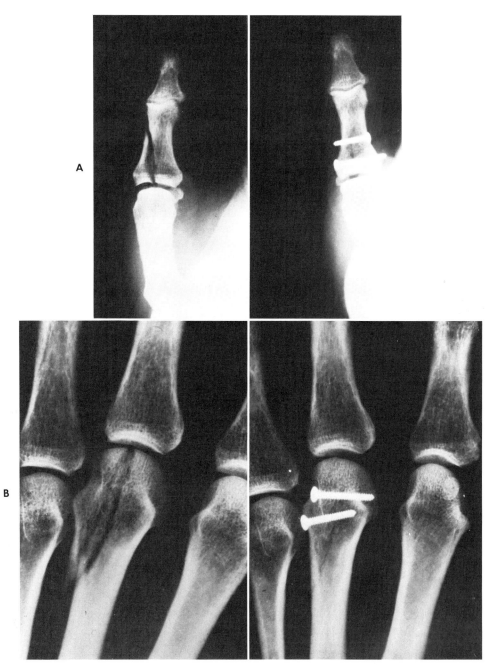

**Fig. 9-40. A,** Displaced fracture through base of proximal phalanx is reduced and fixed with compression screws. **B,** Restoration of joint surface is possible by open reduction. Fixation is maintained with compression screws.

on the thumb, the fragments are manipulated as closely as possible into proper alignment. While traction is maintained and the fragments are compressed into reduction, a Kirschner wire is passed through the thumb metacarpal into the index metacarpal. Roentgenograms must be obtained to verify satisfactory reduction (Fig. 9-39, *B*). The wire is left in place 4 to 6 weeks; then gentle passive and active motion is begun.

## FINGERS

*Metacarpophalangeal joint.* Obviously fractures involving the metacarpophalangeal joint may be of the proximal phalanx base or the metacarpal head, or both. If there is significant separation of the fragments, open reduction with anatomical restoration of the articular surface and use of a compression screw to maintain reduction and allow early motion is recommended (Fig. 9-40, *A*).

Fracture of the articular head of the metacarpal is an infrequent variant of the "boxer's fracture." The blow is received directly on the metacarpal head, producing a fracture through the joint surface (Fig. 9-40, *B*). Displacement of the fragment is frequent. Open reduction with anatomical restoration of the articular surface and the use of a compression screw to maintain

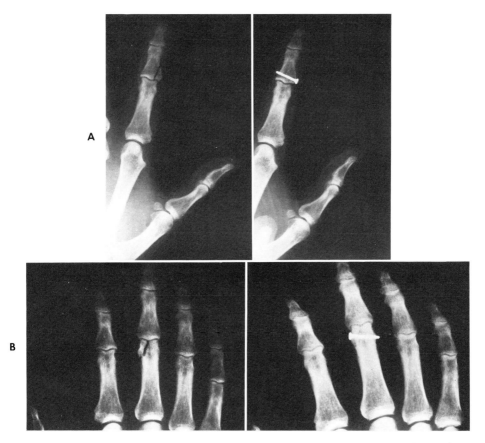

**Fig. 9-41. A,** Fracture involving condyle of proximal phalanx is secured after reduction with a compression screw. **B,** Early painless motion is possible after reduction and fixation with a compression screw.

reduction and permit early motion is recommended (Fig. 9-40, *B*).

***Proximal interphalangeal joint.*** Fractures involving the proximal interphalangeal joint can involve the head of the proximal phalanx or the base of the middle phalanx (Fig. 9-41). If a large fragment is present, open reduction and internal fixation with a compression screw is recommended (Fig. 9-41). Usually fractures of the head of the proximal phalanx result from a direct blow, such as a punch press, which produces varying degrees of crushing of the bony head. Fractures of the base of the middle phalanx principally involve either the volar lip, the dorsal lip, or the entire base.

*Volar lip fractures.* A fracture subluxation at the proximal interphalangeal joint level is usually a fracture of the ventral rim of the base of the middle phalanx (Fig. 9-42, *A*). The size of the fragments may involve more than 50% of the articular surface; however, the usual fragments involve 20% to 40%. Since the volar plate of this joint is attached to this fragment, the accessory collateral ligaments, volar plate, and bony fragment maintain their normal relationships (Fig. 9-42, *B*). Subluxation occurs because the joint surfaces have lost their structural congruity, and the central slip of the extensor apparatus pulls the middle phalanx dorsally and proximally. The larger the fragment, the greater the chance of dislocation. The proper collateral ligaments may remain attached to the middle phalanx and become slack as the middle phalanx is dorsally displaced. In some cases the collateral ligaments (at least one) are torn. The subluxation may be easily reduced; however, repositioning of the volar fragments is more difficult.

A variety of methods of management

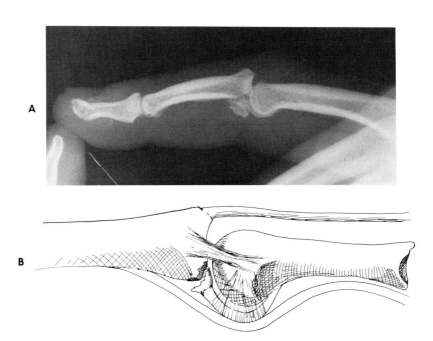

**Fig. 9-42. A,** Fracture of the volar lip of the middle phalanx negating the restrictive effects of the volar plate and allowing dorsal subluxation of the middle phalanx. **B,** Fracture of the volar lip of the base of the middle phalanx frees the middle phalanx from the restrictive effects of the volar plate.

have been suggested, ranging from closed reduction alone, to closed reduction with skeletal traction, to open reduction and internal fixation. Treatment by acutely flexing the proximal interphalangeal joint and maintaining this position is mentioned only in condemnation.

CLOSED REDUCTION AND EXTENSION-BLOCK SPLINTING. McElfresh and associates have suggested the use of a dorsal splint that is incorporated into a forearm plaster gauntlet so that the more proximal joints are maintained in the position of function and the proximal interphalangeal joint cannot extend to more than 10 to 15 degrees short of the demonstrated position of instability (Fig. 9-43). Free flexion is permitted from the onset. To reduce the hazard of a flexion contracture developing in the proximal interphalangeal joint, the angle of extension blocking is reduced about 25% each week. They reported that 70 to 90 degrees of flexion was regained in 3 weeks, whereas full extension was not permitted for 6 to 12 weeks. Twelve of seventeen patients regained full extension, whereas three lacked 10, 5, and 15 degrees at 3 months. Sixteen of seventeen patients regained 90 to 105 degrees flexion at the proximal interphalangeal joint. However, the fragment size (percent of articular surface) was in the 10% range in thirteen

of seventeen patients. None had fractured greater than 50% of the articular surface even by estimate. They recommend this method of treatment in patients with less than 30% of the total articular surface involved in fracture.

CLOSED REDUCTION AND SKELETAL TRACTION. The object of this method is to reduce the subluxation of the middle phalanx and provide countertraction in three directions to prevent recurrent subluxation and maintain the fracture site in close proximity to the fragment. Pins to be used for traction are inserted into the proximal phalanx, the base of the middle phalanx, and the neck of the middle phalanx (Fig. 9-44). A cast that extends from the proximal forearm to the proximal palmar crease is applied. A wire splint is incorporated into the cast to form a circle about the finger in the flexion-extension plane. The involved joint is flexed about 20 degrees and traction applied to each direction to secure reduction. This reduction must be confirmed by roentgenogram after a few hours and after the first week. Robertson and associates report good results with this method. In seven cases, all patients regained 65 to 85 degrees active painless motion at the proximal interphalangeal joint. Careful attention must be paid to the traction rig, which is large and cumber-

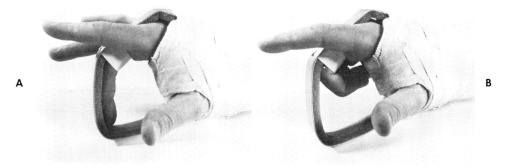

**A**  **B**

**Fig. 9-43. A,** A dorsal finger splint is incorporated into a short arm cast, which maintains the position of the metacarpophalangeal joint and proximal phalanx. Extension of the proximal interphalangeal joint is limited to 10 to 15 degrees short of the angle at which subluxation occurs. **B,** Full flexion of the proximal and distal interphalangeal joints is permitted immediately.

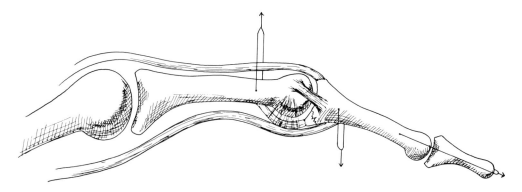

**Fig. 9-44.** Traction in three planes corrects the subluxation and allows reattachment of the volar plate through its bony fragments.

some. This is an excellent method to use when the volar lip fracture involves a large portion of the articular surface and is severely comminuted. When the fragment is very small and joint stability is not impaired, closed reduction and splinting are adequate.

OPEN REDUCTION AND INTERNAL REPAIR. A midlateral incision is made on the radial side of the finger and extended from the distal interphalangeal joint to the proximal crease of the proximal phalanx. Reflection of the skin edges exposes Cleland's ligament, which is divided. The neurovascular bundle is identified beneath Cleland's ligament and is maintained in the volar tissue flap, which is freed from the flexor tendon sheath. The dorsal skin flap is elevated to expose the extensor apparatus and underlying joint. The filmy portion of the flexor tendon sheath overlying the proximal interphalangeal joint is excised. This exposes the sublimis and profundus tendons as well as the volar surface of the volar plate. A longitudinal incision is made through the center of the collateral ligament. The dorsal half of the collateral ligament is elevated in continuity with the periosteum of the proximal and middle phalanges (maintaining its attachment to both). The volar half is detached from the volar plate, exposing the articular surface. The fracture

site is identified, and the volar rim fragment is brought into the center of the wound (Fig. 9-45).

To allow free mobility of the volar plate and facilitate suturing, the accessory collateral ligament on the opposite side is detached from the volar plate. This can be done without a separate incision on the ulnar side of the finger unless the injury is longstanding, in which case contracture of the collateral ligaments may make a second incision necessary.

When a single, large volar rim fragment is present, the continuity of the articular surface of the joint can be restored by reducing the fracture dislocation under direct visualization. With the proximal interphalangeal joint held in slight flexion, the reduction is maintained by inserting a Kirschner wire through the volar rim fragment and into the middle phalanx. When a small or shattered fragment is present, a smooth articular surface is more difficult to achieve. If articular continuity cannot be readily restored, resection of the bony fragment from its attachment to the volar plate is indicated.

In either case (retention or resection of the bony fragment) a Bunnell stitch is placed through the volar plate using a 5-0 stainless steel wire suture. If a bony fragment has been retained, it is important

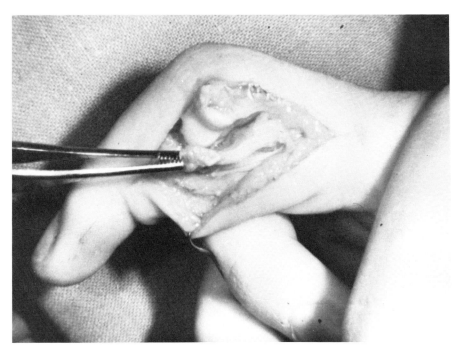

**Fig. 9-45.** The volar plate with the attached bony fragment has been freed from the accessory collateral ligaments to facilitate suturing.

to make a fine drill hole through the center of the fragment. A corresponding drill hole is placed in the fracture site to exit laterally through the middle phalanx. This allows the fracture segment to be accurately repositioned. If the hole is not made in the center of the fragment, the fragment will be deflected either into the joint or volarward when the suture in the volar plate is tied. Both suture wires are passed through a single hole in the middle phalanx and out through the skin and through a padded button. Passage of the suture wires through the middle phalanx is much simpler if the hole has been drilled with a Kirschner wire that has a hole in its tip to receive the wires.

After placement of the wire but before it is tied, the proximal interphalangeal joint is completely reduced, flexed 10 to 15 degrees, and fixed in this position by a Kirschner wire transfixing the proximal

interphalangeal joint. A roentgenogram is necessary at this point to be sure that proper reduction of the middle phalanx has been obtained. Even slight subluxation should not be tolerated. The wire ends are tightened over the button to adjust the tension on the volar plate (Fig. 9-46). If the bony fragment has been resected, tension must be adjusted so that the distal end of the volar plate fits snugly into the fracture site of the middle phalanx. The collateral ligament is repaired with fine absorbable suture, and the skin is closed.

The finger is immobilized for 5 to 6 weeks postoperatively; then the Kirschner wire transfixing the proximal interphalangeal joint is removed and gentle active and passive motion is begun. The wire suture used to reattach the volar plate is removed 2 weeks later by cutting the suture over the button and pulling on the knot.

RESULTS. The best results in treatment

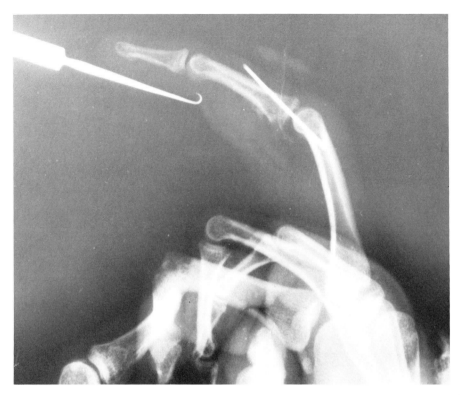

**Fig. 9-46.** Congruity of the articular surface has been reestablished and is maintained with transfixing Kirschner wire. A wire suture has been placed in the volar plate and through the base of the middle phalanx to be tied over a button.

of fracture dislocation of the proximal interphalangeal joint are obtained if treatment is carried out promptly after the injury has occurred. This necessitates early, accurate diagnosis and selection of proper treatment.

A spectrum of deformities results from injuries involving the volar plate of the proximal interphalangeal joint. These range from simple disruption of the volar plate from its insertion into the base of the middle phalanx to extensive comminution of the base of the middle phalanx. In the latter case, the volar plate remains attached to the fracture fragment, which retains its normal anatomical position. Varying degrees of dorsal subluxation of the middle phalanx may be present, including dislocation. Failure to recognize the spectrum

of deformities has led to some confusion in selecting the proper treatment.

Either immobilization alone or direct surgical repair is an acceptable mode of treatment in the following instances: (1) simple disruption of the volar plate without associated subluxation of the middle phalanx, and (2) avulsion of a small volar rim fragment in continuity with the volar plate without associated subluxation of the middle phalanx.

In those instances in which the injury to the proximal interphalangeal joint involves dorsal subluxation of the middle phalanx, we believe treatment must be directed toward reduction of the subluxation and restoration of the articular surface continuity. In our experience it is impossible to maintain anatomical reduction

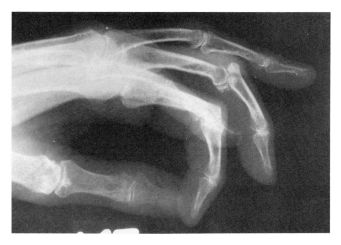

**Fig. 9-47.** Failure to completely reduce and restore the articular surfaces results in the development of a traumatic arthritis.

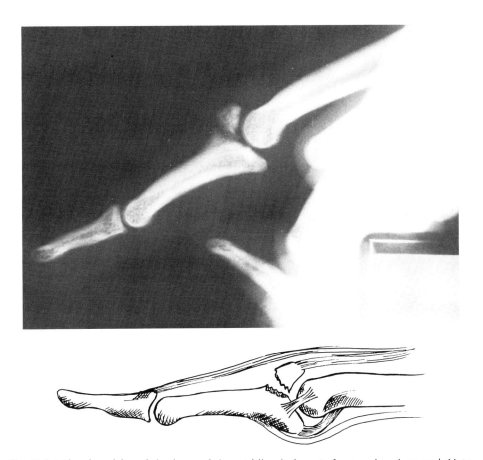

**Fig. 9-48.** The dorsal lip of the base of the middle phalanx is fractured and rotated. Note volar subluxation of the middle phalanx.

and restore articular surface continuity without open reduction and internal fixation.

Following immediate treatment of a fracture dislocation of the proximal interphalangeal joint by open reduction and internal fixation, the average total range of motion that can be expected is 78 degrees. These results are consistent with good function.

Wilson and Rowland's analysis of their cases was "difficult to evaluate" because the range of painless motion after operative treatment varied greatly with age and reaction of the patient's joints to surgery. McCue reported excellent results with this technique in a large series.

The consequences of delay of treatment or improper diagnosis and treatment include traumatic arthritis with ultimate destruction of the articular surface, pain on motion, or ankylosis (Fig. 9-47). Treatment of late traumatic arthritis is limited to fusion of the painful joint, replacement of the joint with a prosthesis, or amputation of the finger.

*Dorsal lip fractures.* Isolated fractures of the dorsal lip occur much less frequently than other fractures involving the middle phalanx base. A spectrum of deformities exists according to the extent of articular surface disrupted. Subluxation associated with the fracture is common (Fig. 9-48). Usually the collateral ligaments, volar plate, and flexor tendons are intact. The dorsal fragment remains attached to the central slip of the extensor tendon. Treatment is directed toward reduction of the subluxation or dislocation and reattachment of the bony fragment with its concomitant central slip.

OPEN REDUCTION AND INTERNAL FIXATION. Through a dorsal skin incision, the edge of the lateral band is identified and carefully elevated. This exposes the fracture site and fragment. The subluxation is corrected and the proximal interphalangeal joint pinned in full extension with a transfixing Kirschner wire. If the fragment is large enough, a fine Kirschner wire is used to transfix it to the middle phalanx (Fig. 9-49). If the

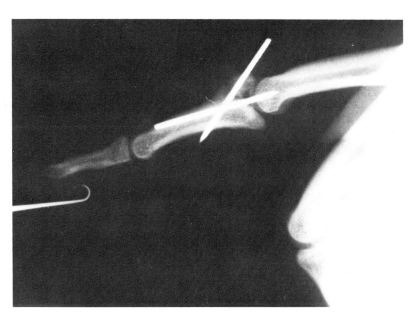

**Fig. 9-49.** The volar subluxation has been corrected and the fragment reduced and fixed with a single Kirschner wire.

fragment is too small for pin fixation, simply reducing the fracture and allowing the tension in the dorsal hood to hold it in place are adequate. In either case, the subluxation is reduced and proper alignment maintained for 4 to 6 weeks with

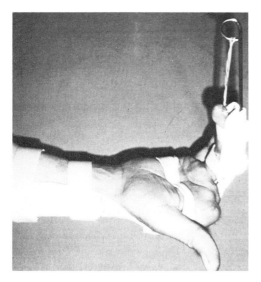

**Fig. 9-50.** The splint maintains the metacarpophalangeal joint in 70 to 90 degrees flexion and the interphalangeal joints in full extension. Traction is applied through a hook attached in the nail.

a Kirschner wire, which transfixes the proximal interphalangeal joint.

*Comminuted fractures.* This injury is most often seen in heavy equipment operators, for instance, punch press operators. The finger is usually crushed in a posteroanterior plane. The tendons bridging the joint are usually intact; however, the central slip and the volar plate may be detached because of fragmentation of their insertion. It is impossible to accurately reconstruct the articular surfaces by open reduction and hold this reduction by any fixation device. To make the best of a bad situation, we recommend fabrication of a polyform splint that positions the metacarpophalangeal joint in 70 to 90 degrees flexion and the proximal interphalangeal joint in full extension (Fig. 9-50). A wire loop is incorporated into the outrigger and positioned 2 to 3 inches beyond the fingertip. A bra hook is glued to the finger nail. The finger is anesthetized, and with gentle traction, the fragments are manipulated into the best alignment possible. Traction is maintained with a rubberband attached to the bra hook and the loop on the splint. The finger is supported dorsally in a trough formed by the splint.

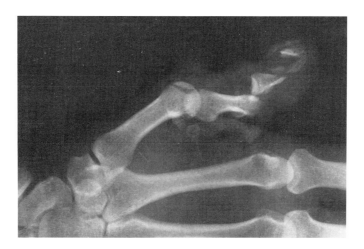

**Fig. 9-51.** Crush injury of the thumb results in displacement of the distal phalangeal fragments.

At 2 and 3 weeks after reduction, the rubberband is disconnected, and the joints are gently extended and flexed, actively and passively. The apparatus is discarded at 4 weeks and therapy begun in earnest to regain as much function as possible.

*Distal interphalangeal joint.* Fractures involving the distal interphalangeal joint usually result from crush injuries and may be compounded. These fractures require splinting for 3 to 4 weeks followed by gradual increase in intensity of mobilization efforts. Occasionally longitudinal fractures of the middle phalanx extend between the condylar heads. Again, these are usually crush fractures; the crushing force dislocates the fragments laterally. If a large fragment is present, open reduction and internal fixation with a compression screw is recommended (Fig. 9-51). This allows early movement and minimizes adhesion formation between the bony fragments and the adjacent extensor and flexor tendons. If fixation and early mobilization are not instituted, significant adhesion formation may result.

## DIAPHYSEAL FRACTURES

Optimal treatment of diaphyseal fractures includes: (1) reducing and immobilizing the fracture, (2) maintaining digital length and proper rotation, (3) preserving joint motion, (4) minimizing adhesion formation to gliding structures, that is, tendons, and (5) minimizing edema formation.

Usually closed reduction can be accomplished, but occasionally open reduction is required. Immobilization can be accomplished with either external or internal splinting. External splinting, that is, plaster cast, requires immobilization of more than just the two joints in juxtaposition to the fracture. If external splinting is prolonged, stiff joints and tendon adhesions are more prone to develop. Dissatisfaction with external splinting has led to a greater interest in internal fixation. The advantages of inter-

nal fixation include: (1) firm approximation and immobilization of the fracture, (2) prevention of rotatory movement, (3) maintenance of digital length, and (4) minimal immobilization of juxtaposed joints. The disadvantages include infection and impingement of wires on tendinous structures and the reparative process evoked by surgery.

## Metacarpal fractures

Certain metacarpal fractures may directly affect the metacarpophalangeal joint. These include transverse fractures just proximal to the origin of the collateral ligaments, and longitudinal fractures extending into the articular surface.

*Transverse fractures just proximal to the origin of the collateral ligaments.* In the fingers, a fracture at this level completely frees the metacarpal head from any proximal stabilizing influence. The only attachments to the metacarpal head, the collateral ligaments, remain attached to the proximal phalanx. If the metacarpal head tilts volarward and the proximal phalanx is in a neutral position, the joint is actually hyperextended and the collateral ligaments become slack. If this is not corrected, the resultant repair processes will fix the collateral ligaments in a shortened position, thus blocking flexion—as seen so often in the claw-hand. Inadequate reduction leaves a prominent metacarpal head in the palm, which may produce discomfort when grasping objects. This fracture can be reduced by gaining control of the metacarpal head through the collateral ligaments. Grasping the proximal phalanx and flexing the metacarpophalangeal joint to at least 90 degrees produce tightening of the collateral ligaments about the metacarpal head (Fig. 9-52). While this control is maintained, pressure is directed dorsally onto the metacarpal head while the metacarpal shaft proximal to the fracture is forced volarward. After the fracture is reduced, the proximal phalanx is maintained in 70 to 80

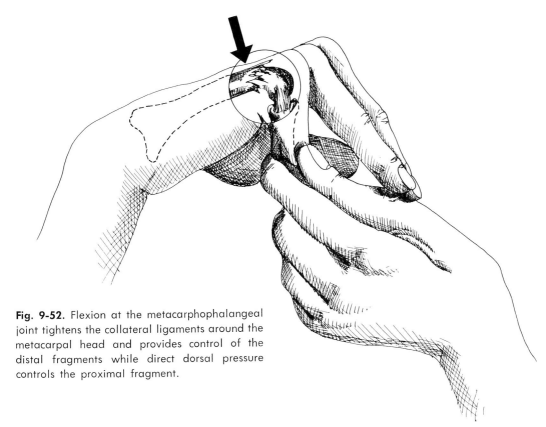

**Fig. 9-52.** Flexion at the metacarpophalangeal joint tightens the collateral ligaments around the metacarpal head and provides control of the distal fragments while direct dorsal pressure controls the proximal fragment.

degrees flexion during the 3 weeks of immobilization. Malrotation can be prevented by including the adjacent fingers in the splint. After 3 weeks exercises are begun gingerly.

The following metacarpal fractures are more prone to be unstable and require open reduction and internal fixation: (1) oblique fractures crossing more than one metacarpal shaft, (2) fractures through either the second or fifth metacarpal, (3) comminuted fractures, and (4) fractures in which segments of the bone are lost. When there is comminution of the fracture at the condylar neck, external fixation is difficult to maintain. Digital length can be maintained by a transverse Kirschner wire impaling the metacarpal head and penetrating the adjacent stable metacarpal. Yet a single wire does not prevent rotation of the metacarpal head on the wire. A second wire is required to provide complete immobilization. Exposure of the metacarpal may be necessary for accurate placement of these wires. Internal fixation is particularly helpful in the individual in whom the risk of developing a stiff joint is high. Movement is begun early, that is, 2 to 3 days after surgery, to minimize the opportunity to develop stiff joints.

### Fracture of metacarpal shaft

*Fingers.* Fractures of the metacarpal shaft may be transverse, oblique, or comminuted. The transverse fracture angulates dorsally, producing volar displacement of the metacarpal head. Dorsal angulation results from the pull of the intrinsic and long flexor muscles, all of which are volar to the fracture plane. Treatment of these fractures in the index and little fingers is more difficult than in the long and ring fingers because of the mobility of the index and little fingers.

Usually transverse fractures are stable

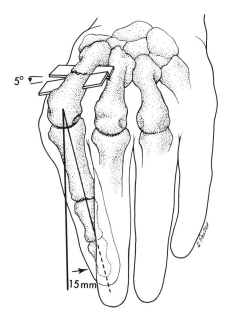

**Fig. 9-53.** Five degrees malrotation in the shaft of the metacarpal can result in 15 mm of lateral displacement when the finger is fully flexed.

after reduction. Oblique fractures have a marked tendency toward telescoping because of the proximal pull of the intrinsic muscles. Rotational deformity is common in oblique fractures. The effect of slight malrotation at the metacarpal shaft on the distal phalanx is deceptively great. If 5 degrees of malrotation is accepted at the shaft of the metacarpal, the distal phalanx will exhibit 15 mm of overriding (Fig. 9-53). The importance of preventing malrotation cannot be overemphasized. Malrotation is minimized by passive or active flexion of all fingers into the palm while the fractures are pinned and again after internal fixation.

When there is a tendency toward shortening, length may be maintained by gentle closed reduction of the fracture and cross-pinning to the adjacent metacarpal. Skeletal traction to prevent shortening of the metacarpal is used infrequently, since the pin for traction must be in the proximal phalanx, and positioning for adequate trac-

tion predisposes to the development of a stiff metacarpophalangeal joint. Pulp or skin traction is difficult to maintain and can lead to circulatory embarrassment of the skin or entire digit.

Fractures in the midshaft or the neck of the metacarpal usually result in volar angulation of the distal fragment, displacing the metacarpal head into the palm. The metacarpal shaft fracture is reduced by flexing the metacarpophalangeal joint to gain control of the distal fragment of metacarpal and forcing the metacarpal head dorsally while maintaining pressure in a palmar direction on the proximal fragment of the metacarpal to complete reduction. If the reduction is not stable because telescoping or shortening cannot be corrected and maintained, then internal fixation with a Kirschner wire driven transversely through the fractured metacarpal head and into the stable adjacent metacarpal is the treatment of choice. One should remember that a second wire is needed to ensure stability. Fractures of the shaft of the long and ring fingers, which are stable after reduction, can be reinforced by a dorsal splint, thereby permitting active motion of the fingers.

When a fracture site is adequately reduced and immobilized, pain around the site subsides rapidly. If pain persists, one should be alerted to further investigate its cause. Disastrous results have been associated with fracture management when pain persists in a well-reduced, well-immobilized fracture.

Open reduction and internal fixation of metacarpal fractures are necessary in the following circumstances: (1) when a displaced fracture involves a joint, (2) when the fracture is markedly displaced so that the interposition of soft tissue prevents reduction, (3) when the fracture is unstable in a reduced position, and (4) when multiple fractures preclude proper reduction and immobilization.

TRANSVERSE FRACTURES. Closed reduction

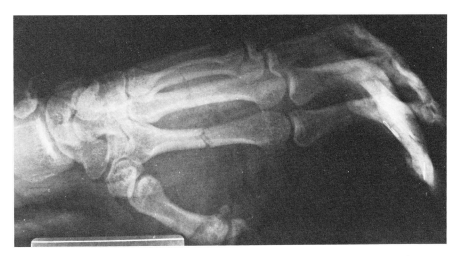

**Fig. 9-54.** Transverse fracture of the ring, long, and index finger metacarpals are non-displaced and stable. Casting is adequate.

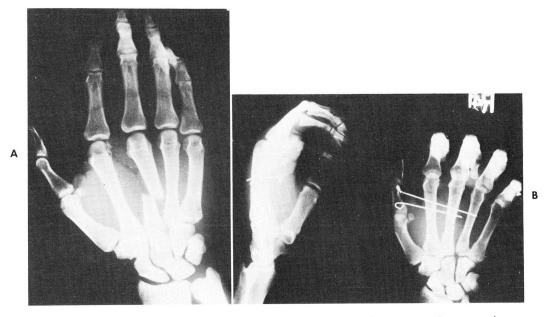

**Fig. 9-55.** A crush injury of the hand with fracture of a single metacarpal, **A,** may be treated to advantage by internal fixation, **B.**

and external fixation (cast) are adequate in most transverse fractures (Fig. 9-54). The cast must be checked often during the first 10 days to be sure it fits snugly and has not become ineffective as the edema subsides. Occasionally circumstances may dictate internal fixation of a transverse fracture. The patient in Fig. 9-55 sustained a crushing injury that burst the palmar skin in addition to fracturing the long finger metacarpal. Prolonged swelling of the hand was anticipated. Early motion was particularly desirable in this patient. The transverse pins allowed digital motion with

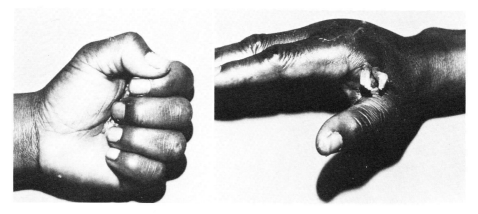

**Fig. 9-56.** Early motion in the edematous hand helps maintain joint motion and tendon gliding and encourage reduction of edema.

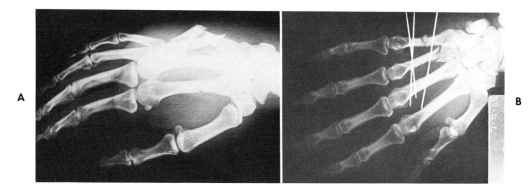

**Fig. 9-57. A,** Comminuted fractures are present in the midshaft of the fifth metacarpal and base of the fourth metacarpal. **B,** Fractures have been reduced and immobilized with transfixing Kirschner wires.

minimal discomfort within 24 hours of surgery (Fig. 9-56). The volar wound was closed as the edema subsided.

OBLIQUE FRACTURES. Because of the tendency in oblique fractures toward telescoping and rotational deformity, we frequently utilize internal fixation. The Kirschner wires are introduced percutaneously while closed reduction is being maintained. If we are unable to obtain adequate closed reduction and fixation after two attempts at percutaneous pinning, we perform an open reduction.

COMMINUTED FRACTURES. Press injuries and low velocity missile injuries are associated most often with comminuted fractures.

The degree of shortening is eventually checked by the intermetacarpal ligaments. These ligaments interconnect the metacarpals (through the collateral ligaments), and shortening of a fractured metacarpal is limited by the stable adjacent metacarpal. Fractures of the metacarpals of the index and little fingers are more difficult to treat than are those of the long and ring finger metacarpals because the latter are splinted by intact metacarpals on either side. When there is a comminuted fracture of the long or ring finger and the adjacent border finger metacarpal is fractured, open reduction and internal fixation are necessary (Fig. 9-57). Closed reduction

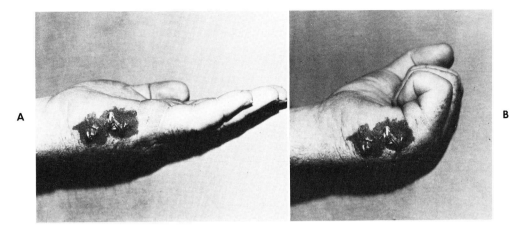

**Fig. 9-58.** When the fracture sites are completely reduced and immobilized, **A,** full range of early painless motion is possible, **B.** (Same patient as in Fig. 9-57.)

and percutaneous pinning are attempted initially. This should not be pursued further if after two attempts proper reduction and fixation have not been accomplished. Exposure is limited to one of the fractures so that adequate reduction and fixation may be obtained. The adjacent fracture is manipulated and the Kirschner wires continue into and through the adjacent fracture. To maintain adequate stabilization of adjacent metacarpal fractures, the Kirschner wires must be continued into an adjacent normal metacarpal. Furthermore, two pins must be used distal to the shaft fracture. If this is not done, when early mobilization is begun, motion will occur at the fracture site producing pain, which limits the patient's range of motion, thus defeating the benefits of early mobilization. When proper reduction and fixation are obtained, the patient can begin early painless motion without restriction (Fig. 9-58).

*Thumb.* The principles of treatment presented previously are applicable to fractures of the thumb metacarpal. Yet the thumb is so important in hand function that particular care must be exercised to ensure proper reduction, alignment, and immobilization. The plane of metacarpal rotation across the palm must be fully ap-

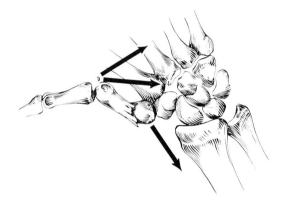

**Fig. 9-59.** Tendinous structures that traverse the fracture site result in characteristic displacement shown above.

preciated when the thumb is positioned after fracture reduction. Fractures through the base or shaft are displaced by the tendinous structures inserting into each fragment (Fig. 9-59). The distal metacarpal fragment is flexed into the palm by the pull of the thenar muscles described earlier. The proximal fragment serves as an insertion for the abductor pollicis longus and produces extension-abduction of this fragment. Since extension of the proximal fragment is limited by the ulnar ligament, the distal fragment should be manipulated to effect and maintain reduction.

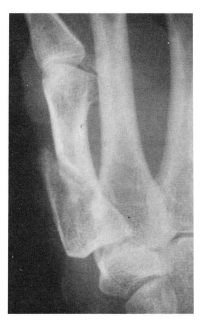

**Fig. 9-60.** Proximal muscle pull telescopes the oblique metacarpal fracture proximally.

Oblique and comminuted fractures predispose to shortening and malrotation (Fig. 9-60). If the reduction is unstable, skeletal traction applied by a transverse Kirschner wire through the metacarpal is satisfactory. An outrigger is incorporated into the cast to permit traction.

### Proximal phalanx

Transverse fractures of the phalanges, particularly midshaft, heal slowly. The surface area of the midshaft is small and composed primarily of cortical bone. Five to 6 weeks of immobilization may be needed before adequate callus forms. The time of immobilization is determined by the type of fracture (transverse, oblique, or comminuted), the adequacy of reduction, the method of fixation (internal or external), and clinical assessment of the healing process. Roentgenograms are helpful in confirming fracture reduction, but the decision to begin mobilization is made through clinical assessment of the fracture.

Generally, fractures of the proximal and middle phalanges are unstable. These phalanges are supported by the snug skin capsule and are subjected to the pull of tendons and tendinous aponeuroses transversing or inserting into the phalanges. Fractures of the proximal phalanx are usually held in a displaced position by the pull of the extensor mechanism and the interosseous muscles. The interosseous muscles tend to flex the metacarpophalangeal joint, pulling the proximal fragment of the proximal phalanx into flexion. Displacement of the flexor tendons within the fibro-osseous tunnel into flexion pulls the distal fragment of the proximal phalanx volarward. The extensor mechanism accentuates this volar displacement. Slight to considerable flexion of the proximal interphalangeal joint may occur. The fractures may be transverse, oblique, or comminuted, and the principles earlier established are applicable here. Yet two additional factors must be appreciated. One is that the periosteum of the proximal and middle phalanges forms the dorsal wall of the fibro-osseous tunnel wherein the flexor tendons glide. Consequently, any fracture of these phalanges necessarily interrupts the continuity of the gliding surfaces of the flexor tendon sheath. Furthermore, impingement of the fracture site on the flexor tendons can produce direct damage to the tendons (Fig. 9-61). If the digit is immobilized for an extended period of time (beyond 3 weeks), the flexor tendons can become scarred to the unfavorable scar associated with the healing periosteum. Thus, in this type of injury it is paramount to maintain gliding of the flexor tendons while the phalangeal fracture is healing. To accomplish these goals, open reduction and internal fixation are required. Placement of Kirschner wires in the proximal phalanx is facilitated by acutely flexing the metacarpophalangeal joint so that the shoulders of the base of the proximal phalanx are palpable (Fig. 9-62).

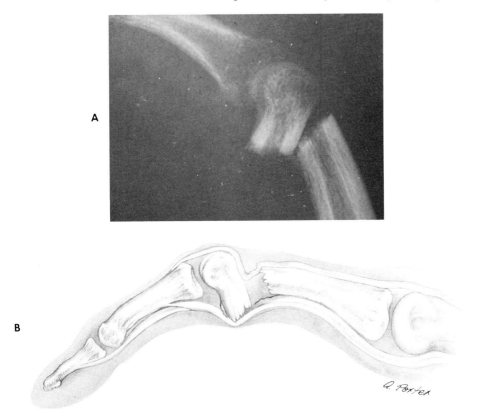

**Fig. 9-61. A,** Volar displacement of the distal segment of the proximal phalanx fracture. **B,** Fracture violates the posterior wall of the fibro-osseous tunnel, and the bony fragments impinge on the trapped flexor tendons.

Use of a high speed drill is necessary for the proper placement of the Kirschner wires. The Kirschner wire pierces the skin and penetrates the shoulder at the base of the proximal phalanx. When the wire enters the medullary cavity, it encounters the opposite wall of the phalanx and is deflected within the cavity across the fracture site and into the head of the proximal phalanx. Drilling is continued until the proximal interphalangeal joint cannot be flexed. This means the wire has crossed the joint and entered the middle phalanx. The wire is backed out until the proximal interphalangeal joint can be moved freely. Placement of the second wire is accomplished in this same manner. An intraoperative roentgenogram in two planes is always obtained. Placement of the wires in

this manner almost ensures proper placement of the wires and fixation of the fracture. Furthermore, the metacarpophalangeal joint can be fully flexed and extended to –10 degrees without impingement of the wires on the skin.

A second factor in the management of diaphyseal fractures of the phalanges is an appreciation that the joints are not directly injured. The subsequent stiffness that develops in the joints is a result of the tissues' reaction to injury. If one accepts the concept that the joints are not injured directly, then active and passive motion of the joints can begin very early after open reduction and internal fixation of the fracture. The case of J. H., who sustained a compound crushing fracture of the proximal phalanx and dislocation of the distal interphalangeal joint, illustrates this point (Fig. 9-63, *A*). The proximal phalangeal fracture was reduced and pinned directly. Three days after surgery the patient exhibited 70 degrees of active proximal interphalangeal joint flexion and 70 degrees of active metacarpophalangeal joint flexion (Fig. 9-63, *B*). Shortly thereafter he accomplished a normal range of active motion at the metacarpophalangeal and proximal interphalangeal joints. Less aggressive treatment may have resulted in loss of control of the proximal fragment, adhesion of the flexor tendons to the site of fracture callus, and checkreining of the proximal interphalangeal and the metacarpophalangeal joints. Of course each fracture must be evaluated and treatment provided to acquire the best possible result according to the needs of that particular case.

Any method that advocates immobilization of the proximal interphalangeal joint in acute flexion must be suspect, as has been mentioned earlier.

### Middle phalanx

Fractures across the shaft of the middle phalanx involve a maximum amount of cortical bone and a minimum of cancellous bone. Such fractures will heal slowly. Conversely, fractures at the base or neck of the phalanx heal rapidly because of the greater exposure of cancellous bone.

Occasionally a fracture is impacted in proper alignment. This is treated by immobilization with a padded metal splint

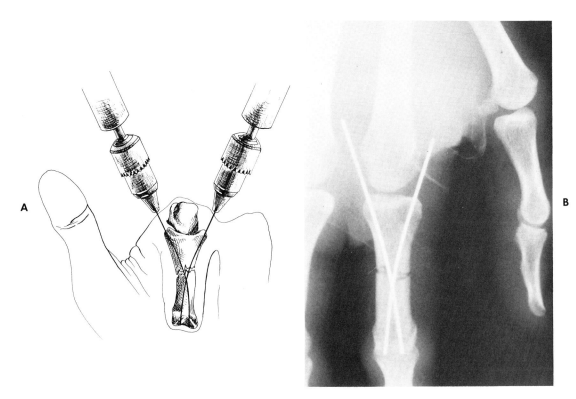

**A**

**B**

**Fig. 9-62. A,** Pinning of a proximal phalanx shaft fracture is facilitated by inserting the wire into the shoulders of the proximal segment. **B,** The fracture site has been stabilized by crossing Kirschner wires introduced through the base of the proximal phalanx.

bent to hold the metacarpophalangeal joint in at least 60 degrees flexion and the interphalangeal joint in 10 to 20 degrees flexion.

When the fracture is displaced, correction of the angulation is essential. Displaced fractures that are unstable when reduced are best treated by reduction and internal fixation or external traction fixation. Fine, smooth Kirschner wires are selected. Introduction of the wire through an articular surface does not give the cortical bone fixation desired and, if the wire is left projecting, interferes with joint motion. More suitable fixation is obtained by passing the wire obliquely through the cortex of the proximal fragment, across the fracture site, and obliquely out the cortex of the distal fragment (Fig. 9-64). If needed (and it usually is for transverse fractures), a second wire is placed to cross the first in the frac-

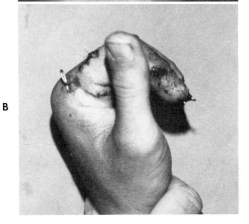

**Fig. 9-63. A,** Metaphyseal fracture involving the base of the proximal phalanx has been reduced and is held with a single wire. (See Fig. 2-17, A for preoperative picture.) **B,** Note active range of motion 3 days postoperatively.

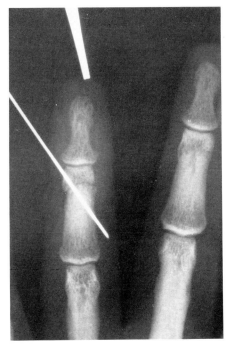

**Fig. 9-64.** Transverse fracture of the middle phalanx after open reduction, removal of interposed soft tissue, and insertion of the initial Kirschner wire.

ture site, again penetrating the thick cortex of the diaphysis. Care must be taken to prevent the second wire from wedging open the fracture site; this occurs when the wire passes across the fracture site and enters the cortical bone with the fracture site not held in firm, accurate reduction.

Comminuted phalangeal fractures require external traction to maintain proper reduction and immobilization. Skeletal traction is utilized by placing a transverse pin through the distal end of the fractured phalanx. This leaves the distal joints free for movement.

Maintenance of reduction can be troublesome. If one becomes too concerned about getting the nail bed to point toward the tubercle of the scaphoid, the result may not be as satisfactory as when one concentrates more on the relationship of the fractured finger to the other fingers. Proper alignment is determined by fully flexing and extending the fingers. If the normal relationships are not maintained in both positions, then reduction is not adequate. Occasionally normal relationships may be maintained in flexion but not in extension or vice versa. Both positions must be satisfactory.

Traction combined with direct pressure over the fracture site is sufficient to reduce most fractures of the middle phalanx. If external fixation is selected, the finger must be splinted with the metacarpophalangeal joint in at least 60 to 70 degrees flexion and the proximal interphalangeal joint from –10 to 0 degrees extension for 3 weeks.

### Distal phalanx

Fractures of the distal phalanx usually result from crushing injuries that produce significant soft tissue injury. In such cases our primary concern is to obtain soft tissue repair. When the fracture is comminuted, the fragments are molded into position and splinted. These fractures frequently fail to unite; however, firm fibrous union occurs, which is adequate. Chip fractures must be evaluated carefully to rule out an avulsion of the extensor tendon insertion into the base of the distal phalanx. Less common is the chip fracture on the volar surface that results in detachment of the long flexor tendon from the distal phalanx.

## MANAGEMENT AFTER FRACTURE REDUCTION AND FIXATION (INTERNAL OR EXTERNAL)

We use the management scheme presented below in the Milliken Hand Rehabilitation Center; the results will be discussed later in this chapter. The first step in planning a treatment program is evaluation of the patient's hand. This establishes a baseline for determining progress and indicates treatment priorities. Surgical management of fractures influences therapy and can be divided into two main categories: closed reduction with external fixation, and open reduction with internal fixation. Treatment during the initial phase depends on the method of reduction and type of fixation utilized. In the first category, fractures are immobilized by a plaster cast or a splint. Therapy is directed at increasing and maintaining range of motion of uninvolved joints and digits. In the case of a patient with a metacarpal or wrist fracture immobilized by a cast, the aim of early treatment is to increase and maintain mobility of the metacarpophalangeal, proximal interphalangeal, and distal interphalangeal joints. When the cast is removed, exercises and splints that further increase the range of motion of the digits and the wrist are initiated. Specific treatment methods will be discussed later.

When open reduction and internal fixation are indicated, therapy involves nearly all the joints of the hand, as it may not be necessary for the transfixing pins to cross any joints in order to stabilize the fracture. For example, good active and passive range of motion can be achieved in both the metacarpophalangeal and proximal interphalangeal joints of a digit with a proximal phalanx fracture. However, even when the pins do cross a joint, it is possible to work with all the other joints in that finger, as well as the rest of the hand, to prevent associated stiffness and to promote maximum hand function as early as possible.

As stated earlier, evaluation is the first step in treatment. The following methods of management are applied to all joints not immobilized by a cast, splint, or Kirschner wire.

In the initial phase of treatment, whirlpool or hand soaks may be used to assist in débridement of wounds and to relax the hand. Patients are given sponges to squeeze, which provide gentle exercise while their hands are soaking. Then gentle active range of motion exercises are performed at each joint to increase and maintain joint mobility and to increase tendon gliding. It is especially important to focus on extensor tendon gliding, as these tendons frequently become adhered to the fracture site. The therapist stabilizes the part proximal to the joint, and the patient is instructed to move through as complete a range of motion as he can accomplish. In general, proximal joints are exercised before distal joints. When the patient has performed isolated motion at each joint of a digit, he is asked to flex the finger toward the palm. When all fingers and the thumb have been exercised in this manner, the patient actively works on making a fist and touching his thumb to each finger. Passive range of motion exercises are similarly performed at each joint as the therapist firmly stabilizes the part proximal to the joint before applying force. This is done by flexing and extending a few degrees beyond the patient's own arc of movement. Traction may also be applied as the part is moved into more degrees of motion. Contract-relax, rhythmic stabilization, and joint mobilization are additional methods used

to passively increase joint range of motion. The patient then performs active exercises in order to maintain gains made by passive stretching. This is facilitated by the use of various pieces of exercise equipment that provide goal orientation for the patient. Fig. 9-65 illustrates the use of an exercise board. Vinyl straps enable the patient to stabilize his finger proximal to a joint and work independently on increasing active range of motion.

In most cases, patients are provided with a dynamic splint to further increase and maintain joint mobility. Dynamic splints provide an ongoing effect of treatment as patients are instructed to wear their splints several times daily and wear them often at night. If all joints in a finger are stiff, the proximal joints should be splinted first (see Fig. 12-21). When 60 to 80 degrees of metacarpophalangeal flexion has been achieved, the patient is fitted with a dynamic proximal interphalangeal flexion splint (see Fig. 12-22). If proximal interphalangeal joint contractures begin to develop, a static finger extension splint is fitted. This is used as a preventive measure, and the patient generally wears one at night only. However, if a patient displays

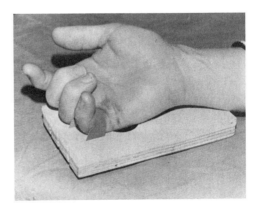

**Fig. 9-65.** The slotted board allows adjustment of the vinyl straps to support either the proximal or middle phalanx.

marked limitation in both proximal inter-phalangeal joint extension and flexion, he may be fitted with a Wynn-Parry dynamic extension splint (see Fig. 12-28). He is instructed to alternate use of the dynamic splints during the day and to wear the static extension splint at night. Distal inter-phalangeal joint flexion assumes more attention when the patient displays good metacarpophalangeal and proximal inter-phalangeal joint motion. A dynamic distal interphalangeal flexion splint is shown in Fig. 12-23. Common splints have been illustrated, but it is important to note that each splint is individually designed and constructed for each patient. The therapist must be creative in fabricating a splint in order to meet each patient's specific needs. When a splint is no longer effective, it must be adjusted or another splint made in order to meet new objectives.

Edema is often present during the initial treatment phase. The primary method of reducing edema is elevation. The patient must be well informed of the importance of keeping his hand elevated at the level of his head. During therapy sessions, the patient rests his arm on an elevated board, which is adjustable, as shown in Fig. 9-66. An arm sling that maintains elevation of the hand and forearm in bed may be provided; however, many patients are successful in using pillows to keep their hands and arms elevated at night. If swelling is noted in a single digit, the patient is fitted with an elastic finger stocking made from an ace bandage. This provides constant pressure to reduce swelling and is an easy method for a patient to apply independently several times daily. An infant blood pressure cuff is used around a single digit to apply intermittent pressure. If edema is present in the entire hand, the Jobst compression unit may be used before and after the exercise program to decrease swelling. A temporary measure involves the use of T-Foam or Temper Stick on the dorsum of the hand and then wrapping the hand firmly with an ace bandage. A Jobst pressure garment can be ordered if edema in the hand persists.

It is essential for the patient to resume use of his injured hand for light everyday activities. If the fracture occurred in the dominant hand, the patient is instructed to begin using the hand in activities such as eating and writing. When the nondominant hand is injured, various light activities that can be performed unilaterally or bilaterally are suggested. Ongoing activity helps to prevent stiffness, and patients can often see their own progress more clearly as they are able to accomplish increasingly difficult tasks.

As further healing occurs and the patient's hand is less tender, massage is done with firm pressure to soften the scar. Deep friction massage is done in a distal direction as the patient actively extends his joint in order to stress adhesions around the extensor tendon. Modalities such as hot packs or paraffin may be used to temporarily decrease discomfort. More resistive exercises

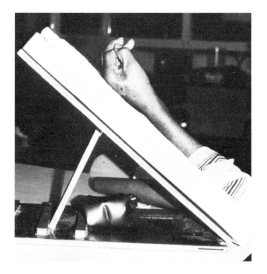

**Fig. 9-66.** During exercises, the upper extremity is maintained in an elevated position by the apparatus above.

are added to the patient's treatment program, and he is encouraged to perform more repetitions to increase endurance and hand strength. Often a patient will benefit from performing a task that requires a sustained grasp. Activities such as hand printing, woodworking, and leatherwork can be graded in order to provide the patient with a challenging and goal-directed activity. Handles can be built up and weights added in order to meet each patient's needs. Further treatment often includes strenuous heavy work activities in order to prepare the patient for his return to work.

The success of this treatment scheme depends on the patient's ability to understand his specific treatment goals and his reliability in following his home program. Written instructions are provided, and the patient is often asked to repeat verbal directions to avoid misconceptions in the use of splints and exercise equipment. It is important to realize that improvement is the result of a wide range of treatment techniques that are administered in a manner most beneficial to each patient's specific needs.

## FACTORS AFFECTING FUNCTIONAL RECOVERY
### Immobilization

Careful evaluation of function after immobilization reveals that patients with comminuted injuries of the metacarpals and phalanges have the poorest results. Furthermore, there is a direct relation between the period of immobilization and the final result. Wright observes that uniformly poor results are obtained in fractures immobilized for more than 3 weeks. In patients whose fractures of metacarpals and phalanges were immobilized for longer than 3 weeks, over 60% demonstrated significant loss of hand function. This loss of hand function was seen when the initial fracture was relatively minor. He suggests that this length of immobilization is not justified.

Early mobilization decreases edema and reduces the severity of adhesions around tendons and joints. Concern for the elbow and shoulder must be maintained.

### Traction

Moberg observes that poor results from the use of traction are common because no effective method of traction is available. He classifies the methods available for the application of traction according to their manner of attachment. These include skin, skeletal, and pulp traction.

Skin traction, most often used for closed fractures of the metacarpals and phalanges, is difficult to apply and to maintain effectively. The danger of constriction is always present. Skeletal traction with a transverse wire piercing the phalanges has been used extensively. This provides firm attachment for adequate traction. Yet the phalanges are basically covered by tendons on the volar, lateral, and dorsal surfaces, severely limiting the uncovered areas for purchase on the phalanges. Consequently, any transverse wire impaling the proximal or middle phalanges may result in impalement of the extensor apparatus. The third method of traction is the use of pulp traction with a wire through the pulp of the finger. This is used extensively and has been found to be very effective. Criticism has included the risk of infection, injury to nerves and vessels of the pulp, and the development of pressure necrosis. The risk of these complications has made this a less than totally satisfactory method of applying traction.

Moberg has modified nail traction and suggested vertical placement of a wire through the fingertip, the periosteum of the distal phalanx, and the nail (Fig. 9-67). This method is easy to perform and entails minimal risk of infection. Necrosis from pressure is prevented by using a wire spreader. This spreading device prevents

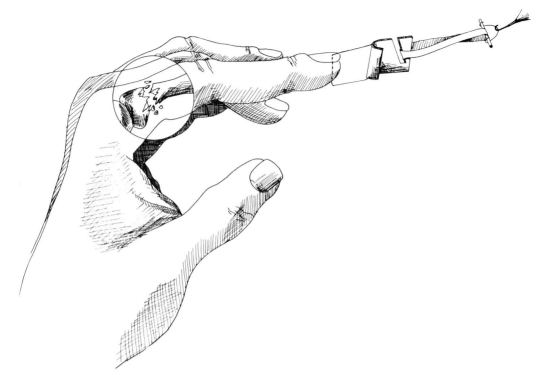

**Fig. 9-67.** Traction on a proximal phalangeal fracture can be maintained with a suture in the terminal phalanx and the use of a spreader device. (After Moberg E.: Emergency surgery of the hand, London, 1967, E. & S. Livingstone, Ltd.)

the wires from pressing on the intervening fingertip.

**FUNCTIONAL RESULTS**

During the five-year period 1971 to 1976, we have been involved in the management of 566 cases with fractures of the meta-carpals and phalanges. To make analysis of these cases meaningful, we have grouped them as follows:

Group I: Single fractures involving either a metacarpal or phalanx
Group II: Single fractures involving a meta-carpal
Group III: Single fractures involving the proximal phalanx
Group IV: Single fractures involving the middle phalanx
Group V: Single fractures involving the distal phalanx
Group VI: More than one fracture per hand
Group VII: More than one fracture per finger
Group VIII: Crush injuries with multiple fractures
Group IX: All fractures combined

The total active motion and total passive range of motion of each joint of the injured finger were determined. The values for active motion were added, as were those for passive motion for each finger. These were obtained by recording the amount of active motion and subtracting from this figure the loss in active motion. Similarly, the passive range of motion was determined. A study of Table 9-1 reveals the following:

1. Patients obtaining the best results were those in Group II (single meta-carpal fracture), Group IV (single middle phalanx fracture), and Group

**Table 9-1.** Functional recovery of patients with metacarpal and/or phalangeal fractures

| | No. of fractures | Average total active motion | Average total passive motion |
|---|---|---|---|
| Group I | 75 | 196 ± 53 | 221 ± 43 |
| Group II | 25 | 201 ± 72 | 227 ± 60 |
| Group III | 29 | 174 ± 60 | 207 ± 40 |
| Group IV | 11 | 199 ± 34 | 217 ± 29 |
| Group V | — | — | — |
| Group VI | 58 | 174 ± 30 | 210 ± 24 |
| Group VII | 15 | 131 ± 52 | 183 ± 56 |
| Group VIII | 27 | 128 ± 69 | 177 ± 57 |
| Group IX | 155 | 182 ± 62 | 214 ± 48 |

I (single metacarpal or phalangeal fracture). The results obtained in these three groups were not significantly different.

2. Patients in Group VI (more than one fracture per hand), and Group III (single proximal phalangeal fracture), obtained results that were not as good as those in the three categories mentioned first.

3. The least successful recoveries were obtained in patients sustaining either a crush injury with multiple fractures (Group VIII) or those who had more than one fracture per finger (Group VII).

4. A significant difference between the active range of motion and the passive range of motion is noted in all cases. This indicates that therapy has provided an active range of motion that the patient is never able to fully realize as active motion because of scarring along the musculotendinous unit.

**BIBLIOGRAPHY**

Ahern, G. S.: Hand injuries; what to do, what not to do, Tex. Med. **66:**72, 1970.

Althorp, C. F.: A case of irreducible dorsal dislocation of the proximal phalanx of the index finger, Lancet **1:**701, 1901.

Aufranc, O. E.: Fracture dislocation of the proximal interphalangeal joint of the finger, J.A.M.A. **204:**815, 1968.

Barnard, H. L.: Dorsal dislocation of the first phalanx of the little finger; reduction by Farabouef's dorsal incision, Lancet **1:**88, 1901.

Bate, J. T.: An operation for the correction of locking of the proximal interphalangeal joint of finger in hyperextension, J. Bone Joint Surg. **27:**142, 1945.

Becton, J. L., Christian, J. D., Jr., and Jackson, J. G. III: A simplified technique for treating the complex dislocation of the index metacarpophalangeal joint, J. Bone Joint Surg. **57A:**698, 1975.

Belpomme, C.: External osteosynthesis of distal fractures of the phalanges by reposition-fixation of the fingernail, Int. Surg. **60:**219, 1975.

Bennett, E. H.: On fracture of the metacarpal bone of the thumb, Br. Med. J. **2:**12, 1886.

Bora, W., Jr., and Didizian, N. H.: The treatment of injuries to the carpometacarpal joint of the little finger, J. Bone Joint Surg. **56A:**1459, 1974.

Brown, P. W.: The management of phalangeal and metacarpal fractures, Surg. Clin. North Am. **53:**1393, 1973.

Bunnell, S., editor: Surgery of the hand, Philadelphia, 1970, J. B. Lippincott Co.

Clawson, D. K., Souter, W. A., Carthum, C. J., and others: Functional assessment of the rheumatoid hand, Clin. Orthop. **77:**203, 1971.

Clinkscales, G. S.: Complications in the management of fractures in hand injuries, South Med. J. **63:**704, 1970.

Coonrad, R. W., and Goldner, J. L.: A study of the pathological findings and treatment in soft-tissue injury of the thumb metacarpophalangeal joint, J. Bone Joint Surg. **50A:**439, 1968.

Coonrad, R. W., and Pohlman, M. G.: Impacted fractures in the proximal portion of the proximal phalanx of the finger, J. Bone Joint Surg. **51A:**1291, 1969.

Curtis, R. M.: Joints of the hand. In Flynn, J. W., editor: Hand surgery, Baltimore, 1966, Williams & Wilkins Co.

Dennyson, W. G., and Stother, I. G.: Carpometacarpal dislocation of the little finger, Hand **8:**161, 1976.

Eaton, R. G.: Joint injuries of the hand, Springfield, Ill., 1971, Charles C Thomas, Publisher.

Eaton, R. G., and Littler, J. W.: Dislocations and ligamentous injuries of the hand. Sound slide presentation at American Academy Orthopaedic Surgeons, New York City, 1969.

Gedda, K. O., and Moberg, E.: Open reduction and osteosynthesis of the so-called Bennett's fracture in the carpo-metacarpal joint of the thumb, Acta Orthop. Scand. **22**:249, 1953.

Green, D. P.: Pins and plaster treatment of comminuted fractures of the distal end of the radius, J. Bone Joint Surg. **57A**:304, 1975.

Green, D. P., and Anderson, J. R.: Closed reduction and percutaneous pin fixation of fractured phalanges, J. Bone Joint Surg. **55A**:1651, 1973.

Green, D. P., and O'Brien, E. T.: Fractures of the thumb metacarpal, South. Med. J. **65**:807, 1972.

Green, D. P., and Terry, G. C.: Complex dislocation of the metacarpophalangeal joint, J. Bone Surg. **55A**:1480, 1973.

Hazlett, J. W.: Carpometacarpal dislocations other than the thumb; a report of 11 cases, Can. J. Surg. **11**:315, 1968.

Hsu, J. D., and Curtis, R. M.: Carpometacarpal dislocations on the ulnar side of the hand, J. Bone Joint Surg. **52A**:927, 1970.

Hunt, J. C., Watts, H. B., and Glasgow, J. D.: Dorsal dislocation of the metacarpophalangeal joint of the index finger with particular reference to open dislocation, J. Bone Joint Surg. **49A**:1572, 1967.

Johnson, F. G., and Greene, M. H.: Another case of irreducible dislocation of the proximal interphalangeal joint of a finger, J. Bone Joint Surg. **48A**:542, 1966.

Kaplan, E. B.: Extension deformities of the proximal interphalangeal joints of the fingers; an anatomical study, J. Bone Joint Surg. **18**:781, 1936.

Kaplan, E. B.: Dorsal dislocation of the metacarpophalangeal joint of the index finger, J. Bone Joint Surg. **39A**:1081, 1957.

Kettlekamp, D. B.: Experimental and clinical autogenous distal metacarpal reconstruction, Clin. Orthop. **74**:129, 1971.

Kuczynski, K.: The proximal interphalangeal joint; anatomy and causes of stiffness in the fingers, J. Bone Joint Surg. **50B**:656, 1968.

Linscheid, R. L., and others: Fracture conference; fractures of the phalanges, Minn. Med. **51**:1599, 1968.

Lipscomb, P. R., Southall, R. C., and Johnson, E. W.: Fracture conference; posttraumatic affections of the metacarpal joints of the thumb, Minn. Med. **52**:285, 1969.

McCue, F. C., Honner, R., Johnson, M. C., and others: Athletic injuries of the proximal interphalangeal joint requiring surgical treatment, J. Bone Joint Surg. **52A**:937, 1970.

McElfresh, E. C., Dobyns, J. H., and O'Brien, E. T.: Management of fracture-dislocation of the proximal interphalangeal joints by extension-

block splinting, J. Bone Joint Surg. **54A**:1705, 1972.

McLaughlin, H. L.: Complex "locked" dislocations of the metacarpophalangeal joints, J. Trauma **5**:632, 1965.

Meyers, M. H.: Dislocations; diagnosis, management and complications, Surg. Clin. North Am. **48**:1391, 1968.

Moberg, E.: The use of traction treatment for fractures of phalanges and metacarpals, Acta Chir. Scand. **99**:341, 1949.

Moberg, E.: Fractures and ligamentous injuries of the thumb and fingers, Surg. Clin. North Am. **40**:297, 1960.

Moller, J. T.: Lesions of the volar fibrocartilage in finger joints, Acta Orthop. Scand. **45**:673, 1974.

Murakami, Y.: Irreducible volar dislocation of the proximal interphalangeal joint of the finger, Hand **6**:87, 1974.

Petrie, P. W., and Lamb, D. W.: Fracture-subluxation of base of fifth metacarpal, Hand **6**:82, 1974.

Pohl, A. L.: Irreducible dislocation of a distal interphalangeal joint, Br. J. Plast. Surg. **29**:227, 1976.

Redler, I., and Williams, J. T.: Rupture of a collateral ligament of the proximal interphalangeal joint of the finger; analysis of 18 cases, J. Bone Joint Surg. **49A**:322, 1967.

Renshaw, T. S., and Louis, D. S.: Complex volar dislocation of the metacarpophalangeal joint; a case report, J. Trauma **13**:1086, 1973.

Riordan, D. C.: Hand fractures, Industr. Med. Surg. **37**:103, 1968.

Robertson, R. C., Cawley, J. J., Jr., and Faris, A. M.: Treatment of fracture-dislocations of interphalangeal joints of hand, J. Bone Joint Surg. **28**:68, 1946.

Rolando, S.: Fracture de la base du premier metacarpien; et principalement sur une variété non encore décrite, Presse Med. **33**:303, 1910.

Rüedi, T. P., Burri, C., and Pfeiffer, K. M.: Stable internal fixation of fractures of the hand, J. Trauma **11**:381, 1971.

Salter, R. B., and Harris, R. W.: Injuries involving the epiphyseal plate, J. Bone Joint Surg. **45A**: 587, 1963.

Schulze, H. A.: Treatment of fracture-dislocations of proximal interphalangeal joints of fingers, Mil. Surg. **99**:190, 1946.

Smith, R. J., and Sturchio, E. A.: The locked metacarpo-phalangeal joint, Bull. Hosp. Joint Dis. **29**:205, 1968.

Specht, E. E.: Epiphyseal injuries in childhood, Am. Fam. Physician **10**:101, 1974.

Spinner, M., and Choi, B. Y.: Anterior dislocation

of the proximal interphalangeal joint, J. Bone Joint Surg. **52A**:1329, 1970.

Stener, B.: Hyperextension injuries to the metacarpophalangeal joint of the thumb-rupture of ligaments, fracture of sesamoid bones, rupture of flexor pollicis brevis; an anatomical and clinical study, Acta Chir. Scand. **125**:275, 1963.

Tsuge, K., and Shoichi, W.: Locking metacarpophalangeal joint of the thumb, Hand **6**:255, 1974.

Wiley, A. M.: Chronic dislocations of the proximal interphalangeal joint; a method of surgical repair, Can. J. Surg. **8**:435, 1965.

Wilson, J. N., and Rowland, S. A.: Fracture-dislocation of the proximal interphalangeal joint of the finger, J. Bone Joint Surg. **48A**:493, 1966.

Wright, T. A.: Early mobilization in fractures of the metacarpals and phalanges, Can. J. Surg. **11**:491, 1968.

# CHAPTER 10
# Repair of severed nerves

The spectrum of functional return in extremities sustaining similar nerve injuries varies from near-normal restoration of function to virtual uselessness of the hand. Why the marked discrepancy? The following is a discussion of how near-normal function can frequently be obtained after nerve injury and of methods one might utilize to increase the percentage of patients who obtain a gratifying result.

## EXAMINATION FOR NERVE INJURY

The general historical data concerning the how, why, when, and where of the injury are obtained. The sensory tests for nerve function are subjective. In young children and uncooperative adults, such tests are of questionable value. With these patients one must maintain a high index of suspicion. If the location or depth of the wound leads one to suspect nerve injury, the wound may be explored in the operating room under optimal conditions; that is, the limb is anesthetized, and a tourniquet renders the operative field bloodless. Conversely, even in the cooperative adult the lack of demonstrable nerve function does not necessarily mean that the anatomical continuity of the nerve is disrupted. Knowledge of the history of injury and of the extent and location of the wound assists the surgeon in arriving at the correct diagnosis.

Examination to determine the level and extent of nerve transection includes evaluation of sensory function and evaluation of motor function. One must recall the variability of innervation, particularly between the ulnar and median nerves. On occasion all the thenar muscles may be innervated by the ulnar nerve. Sensory function is examined by testing for sensation to light touch and pin prick in the selected area. Specific tests for motor function are restricted to particular muscle groups. Nonfunctional muscle groups are correlated with the area of sensory loss and with the nerve that normally innervates these structures. Electromyography and nerve conduction studies can provide objective evidence of nerve injury but are not practical in evaluating an acute injury. The anatomical relationships of the major nerve trunks within the arm and forearm will be described along with the evaluation of motor and sensory function of the hand.

### Radial nerve

*Anatomy.* The radial nerve arises from the posterior cord of the brachial plexus. The radial nerve in the upper part of the arm lies posterior to the brachial artery and anterior to the long head of the triceps muscle. It then turns laterally and posteriorly with the deep brachial artery

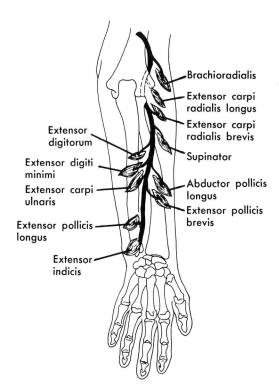

Brachioradialis

Extensor carpi
radialis longus

Extensor carpi
radialis brevis

Supinator

Abductor pollicis
longus

Extensor pollicis
brevis

Extensor
digitorum

Extensor digiti
minimi

Extensor carpi
ulnaris

Extensor pollicis
longus

Extensor
indicis

**Fig. 10-1.** The usual sequential motor distribution
of the radial nerve.

beneath the long head of the triceps muscle
to contact the posterior aspect of the humerus. As it continues its spiral course
along the posterior surface of the humerus,
it maintains contact medially with the
medial aspect of the triceps and laterally
with the lateral head of the triceps. At the
lateral border of the medial head of the
triceps, the radial nerve pierces the lateral
intramuscular septum and continues its
spiral course closely applied to the lateral
side of the brachialis muscle. Subsequently, it lies between the brachialis and
the extensor carpi radialis longus and
passes in front of the lateral epicondyle
to enter the forearm. In the arm the radial
nerve gives off muscular branches to the
triceps, anconeus, and extensor forearm
muscles arising from the lateral epicondyle
(Fig. 10-1).

As the radial nerve spirals forward

around the brachialis muscle, it lies between
the brachialis and the origins of the brachioradialis from the humerus. Branches supply
the brachioradialis, and as the nerve continues distally beneath the extensor carpi
radialis longus and the extensor carpi
radialis brevis, branches to these muscles
are evident. It is at this level that the radial
divides into a deep branch and a superficial branch. The deep branch penetrates
the supinator muscle, whereas the sensory
branch continues superficial to the supinator and beneath the brachioradialis muscle.
This division of the superficial and deep
branches occurs about the level of the
lateral epicondyle of the humerus. The
motor branches up to this point include the
brachialis, the brachioradialis, extensor
carpi radialis longus, and extensor carpi
radialis brevis. The superficial radial nerve
may occasionally supply the extensor carpi
radialis muscle; otherwise, it has no muscular branches. It reverses in the forearm
under the cover of the brachioradialis to
emerge on the ulnar side of the brachioradialis tendon at the junction of the middle
and distal two thirds of the forearm. The
deep branch or posterior interosseous nerve
may supply the extensor carpi radialis
brevis. In turn it penetrates and supplies
the supinator muscle. As it emerges from
the distal edge of the supinator, it is positioned deep to the superficial group of
muscles. It supplies branches to the extensor tendon and terminates at the wrist
with branches to the wrist joint. It supplies
in turn the extensor carpi radialis brevis,
supinator, extensor digitorum communis,
extensor digiti minimi, extensor carpi
ulnaris, abductor pollicis longus, extensor
pollicis longus, extensor pollicis brevis, and
extensor indicis. Thus, in compressive injuries, such as a Saturday night palsy, one
would expect to see motor return in the
order presented. Variation of innervation
occurs, but it is not common.

*Evaluation of motor function.* The most
common motor distribution of the radial

nerve is given in Fig. 10-1. Radial nerve injury is most frequently associated with a fracture of the shaft of the humerus. Injury to the nerve may result from direct laceration in the arm or forearm area. Lacerations of the radial nerve in the arm divide the muscle bellies overlying the nerve but do not directly injure the wrist and digital extensors, all of which are located in the forearm. Thus, the test for radial nerve function in the hand indicates only nerve injury. If, however, the laceration is over the dorsal forearm, then radially innervated muscles are directly injured, and demonstration of their malfunction can be construed as evidence of direct nerve injury while, in fact, the nerve might be intact. At the elbow the radial nerve divides into a motor branch—the posterior interosseous nerve—and a sensory branch. The most distal muscle belly innervated by the posterior interosseous branch of the radial nerve is the extensor pollicis brevis; thus when a laceration of the mid or proximal forearm without direct division of the muscle belly of the extensor pollicis brevis is observed, the continuity of the posterior interosseous nerve can be determined by evaluating the motor function of the extensor pollicis brevis. When the extensor pollicis brevis is directly lacerated, this positions the laceration far distal to the more proximal muscle branches of the posterior interosseous nerve. One knows then that the posterior interosseous nerve is intact even though all the tendons of the wrist and digital extensors have been divided by the injury.

Lacerations in the arm allow evaluation of distal muscles to determine the continuity of the radial nerve.

An intact nerve supply to the brachioradialis is demonstrated by palpation of its tendon along the radial border of the volar surface of the forearm as the patient flexes the elbow against resistance. The brachioradialis inserts into the distal radius. The extensor carpi radialis longus can occasion-

ally be distinguished from the extensor carpi radialis brevis because the long muscle inserts on the radial side of the index metacarpal and is primarily a radial deviator of the wrist. The extensor carpi radialis brevis inserts on the dorsal surface of the long finger metacarpal and is primarily a wrist extensor. When the longus is functional and the brevis nonfunctional, the radial nerve has usually been divided at the bifurcation of the posterior interosseous nerve and the superficial sensory branch. Furthermore, the more distally innervated muscles (that is, common extensor, independent extensors of index and little fingers, extensor pollicis longus and brevis, and abductor pollicis) will be nonfunctional. The extensor carpi radialis longus is palpated by having the patient radially deviate the wrist against resistance. The tendon is palpable at the base of the index metacarpal just medial to the extensor pollicis longus tendon. As the wrist is extended against resistance, the extensor carpi radialis brevis is palpable just proximal to the base of the index and long metacarpals.

Activity of the supinator is demonstrated if the patient can supinate the forearm with the elbow fully extended. The presence of an intact extensor digitorum communis is demonstrated by the ability of the patient to extend the fingers and the metacarpophalangeal joints with the wrist held in extension. Care must be taken to keep the wrist extended, because flexion of the wrist advances the extensor hood proximally and allows extension of the fingers through the intrinsic muscles of the hand. The extensor carpi ulnaris tendon can be palpated in the area of the radial styloid process by having the patient dorsiflex and ulnarly deviate the wrist.

Contraction of the abductor pollicis longus can be demonstrated by palpation of the tendon along the radial aspect of the "anatomical snuff box" as the patient abducts the thumb while the thumb metacarpophalangeal and interphalangeal joints are held in extension (Fig. 10-2). The extensor pollicis brevis tendon can usually be felt just dorsal to the abductor pollicis longus tendon as the thumb is abducted with its metacarpophalangeal joint and interphalangeal joint held in 15 degrees of flexion. Although extension of the interphalangeal joint of the thumb can be produced by a slip from the abductor pollicis brevis muscle, function of the extensor pollicis longus muscle can usually be demonstrated by having the patient extend the metacarpophalangeal and interphalangeal joints while abducting the thumb. During this maneuver the tendon stands out clearly on the radial aspect of the anatomical snuff box. If the long and ring fingers are held in the fully flexed position, the action of the independent extensors of the index and little fingers can be demonstrated.

*Evaluation of sensory function.* The superficial branch of the radial nerve at the elbow continues distally beneath the brachioradialis muscle until it surfaces in the distal forearm. Generally this sensory branch forms three divisions at the wrist. One supplies the dorsum of the thumb; the other branches supply the web

space (the anatomical snuff box) and possibly the dorsal surface of the index finger. There is great variability in sensory innervation, and the definite overlap makes sensory examination difficult. Lacerations in the distal forearm, base of the thumb, and web space should be inspected for radial nerve division because painful neuromas are common. However, lack of sensory function of the radial nerve does not prevent essentially normal use of the hand (Fig. 10-3).

**Ulnar nerve**

*Anatomy.* The ulnar nerve does not supply any muscles of the arm. The ulnar nerve arises from the anterior medial cord of the brachial plexus. In the axilla it is positioned between the axillary vein and artery. As it descends in the arm, it lies medial to the brachial artery and at the midarm pierces the intermuscular septum to lie on the anterior surface of the medial head of the triceps muscle. It continues on the distal course and passes posterior to the medial epicondyle of the humerus. It enters the forearm by passing behind the epicondyle and between the humeral and ulnar heads of the flexor carpi ulnaris

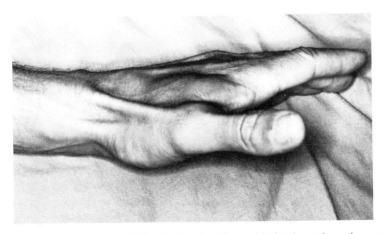

**Fig. 10-2.** The "anatomical snuff box" showing the medial (ulnar) boundary tendon of the extensor pollicis longus and the lateral (radial) boundary tendons of the abductor pollicis longus and extensor pollicis brevis.

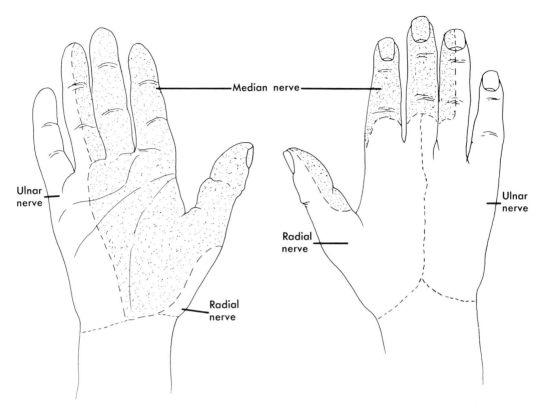

**Fig. 10-3.** Common sensory distribution of median, radial, and ulnar nerves in the hand.

muscle (Fig. 10-4). Occasionally muscle branches to the flexor carpi ulnaris arise above the level of the epicondyle. After entering the forearm, the ulnar nerve lies between the deep surface of the flexor carpi ulnaris muscle and the superficial surface of the flexor digitorum profundus muscle. Its course is virtually a straight line to the tunnel of Guyon. The muscle branches in the forearm include the first branch, which arises just below the level of the medial epicondyle and supplies the flexor carpi ulnaris (Fig. 10-4). There may be more than one branch to the flexor carpi ulnaris. The remaining motor branch in the forearm extends to the ulnaris side of the flexor digitorum profundus muscle. The sensory branches of the ulnar nerve include the dorsal sensory branch, which arises at the

junction of the distal fourth and proximal three fourths of the forearm. This nerve becomes subcutaneous by migrating dorsally and medially under the flexor carpi ulnaris and over the ulna. A second sensory branch is a small palmar branch that supplies an area of skin over the hypothenar eminence. At the wrist the ulnar nerve passes lateral to the pisiform bone and medial to the hook of the hamate within the tunnel of Guyon. Within this tunnel, the ulnar nerve divides into a deep and a superficial branch. The deep branch migrates dorsally between the heads of the abductor digiti minimi and the flexor digiti minimi brevis muscles. The superficial branch continues its distal course in the palm superficial to the muscles. The superficial branch divides into two terminal branches; a proper digital

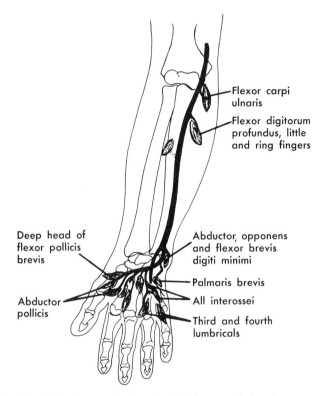

Flexor carpi
ulnaris

Flexor digitorum
profundus, little
and ring fingers

Deep head of
flexor pollicis
brevis

Abductor, opponens
and flexor brevis
digiti minimi

Palmaris brevis

Abductor
pollicis

All interossei

Third and fourth
lumbricals

**Fig. 10-4.** Usual segmental motor distribution of the ulnar nerve.

branch supplies sensation for the ulnar side of the little finger, and a common digital branch supplies sensation for the adjacent sides of the little and ring fingers. After penetrating the hypothenar muscles, the deep branch of the ulnar nerve extends transversely across the palm toward the thumb. In its course the ulnar nerve supplies one or more branches to each of the three hypothenar muscles. After penetrating the hypothenar muscles, the deep branch turns to run almost perpendicular to the arm. The interosseous muscles are innervated in turn as are the lumbricales to the little and ring fingers. As the motor branch progresses across the palm, the final innervations are the adductor pollicis, the deep head of the flexor pollicis brevis, and finally the first dorsal interosseous muscle. Consequently, a test of the first dorsal interosseous activity serves as a test of the final

innervation of the motor branch of the ulnar nerve.

The usual distribution of the ulnar nerve is shown in Fig. 10-4. All motor and sensory function in the hand and forearm is nonfunctional when the ulnar nerve is lacerated in the arm. As noted earlier, the ulnar nerve enters the forearm by passing around the medial epicondyle of the humerus and between the two heads of the flexor carpi ulnaris muscle. Several centimeters proximal to this entering point the ulnar nerve displays several muscle branches that supply the flexor carpi ulnaris and possibly the flexor digitorum profundus to the little and ring fingers. The nerve progresses through the forearm beneath the flexor carpi ulnaris muscle. Near the junction of the proximal three fourths and distal fourth of the forearm, the dorsal sensory branch of the ulnar nerve surfaces dorsally from beneath the flexor carpi ulnaris to supply the dorsum of the hand and the ring and little fingers. A laceration of the nerve proximal to this sensory branch exhibits loss of sensitivity in the aforementioned area in addition to the motor loss in the hand. Laceration of the nerve distal to the sensory branch deployment allows normal sensation over the dorsum of the hand and little and ring fingers. Associated tendon or muscle injuries are evaluated and will be discussed in Chapter 11.

*Evaluation of motor function.* The ulnar nerve is severed most frequently by a sharp laceration at the wrist. Thus, thorough examination of the motor and sensory deficits in the hand is of great clinical importance. Function of the palmaris brevis can occasionally be demonstrated by electromyography; it is the only muscle supplied by the superficial branch of the ulnar nerve. To demonstrate function of the abductor digiti minimi, the muscle is palpated for developed tension while the patient forcibly abducts the little finger. The hand should be placed on a flat surface during this examination to prevent trick movements. Abduction and adduction of the long finger can be examined for by testing the strength of these two motions and comparing it with the uninjured hand. It is impossible to directly palpate the muscles responsible for this motion of the long finger. The first dorsal interosseous can be palpated directly for developed tension during forced abduction of the index finger. Function of the adductor pollicis flexion of the interphalangeal joint (Froment's sign) (see Fig. 11-3). In about 1% of persons, the median nerve may supply both the first dorsal interosseous and the adductor pollicis; testing for function of the abductor digiti minimi then becomes vital.

Lacerations of the ulnar nerve just below the elbow usually lead to denervation of the flexor digitorum profundus of the little and ring fingers (and, very rarely, the long finger) and the flexor carpi ulnaris.

Function of the flexor carpi ulnaris is demonstrated by palpation of the tendon over the ulnar border of the volar surface of the wrist as the patient flexes and ulnarly deviates the hand. Normal function of the flexor digitorum profundus can be demonstrated directly by having the patient flex the distal interphalangeal joints of the appropriate fingers. To distinguish direct muscle laceration from nerve laceration, one has only to evaluate the motor function of the hypothenar muscles, that is, the abductor digiti minimi, the opponens digiti minimi, and the flexor digiti minimi brevis. The abductor digiti minimi can be evaluated by direct palpation as the little finger is abducted against resistance.

Lacerations in the palm can involve the motor branch without involving the sensory branches. Thus, if only the sensory examination for ulnar nerve function is utilized in evaluating a laceration of the palm, division of the motor branch may be overlooked. Similarly a palmar laceration that divides the sensory branches of the median nerve may divide the motor branch of the ulnar nerve. Since the last muscle innervated by the ulnar nerve is the first dorsal interosseous, testing its function should be mandatory in all palmar lacerations.

*Evaluation of sensory function.* The ulnar nerve has two sensory branches in the hand and forearm. The dorsal cutaneous branch supplies a variable area of the ulnar and dorsal aspect of the hand (to approximately the level between the third and fourth metacarpals) and the dorsal surface of the little finger. The palmar cutaneous branch supplies the palm to approximately the level of the fourth metacarpal and the skin of the volar surface of the little finger and ulnar side of the ring finger. The most constant areas supplied by the ulnar nerve are the dorsal and volar surfaces of the little finger. On a rare occasion the median nerve may supply sensation to the entire palmar surface of the hand (Fig. 10-3).

## Median nerve

*Anatomy.* The median nerve arises from the medial cord of the brachial plexus. The median nerve traverses the arm lateral to the brachial artery to the midarm where the nerve assumes a position anterior and medial to the artery. In the lower arm the lacertus fibrosus covers the median nerve and brachial artery. During its passage through the arm, the median nerve does not have any motor branches. As the median nerve enters the forearm (Fig. 10-5), it is positioned medial to the brachial artery and lies on the anterior surface of the brachialis muscle. Near the origin of the pronator teres, the median nerve passes between the two heads of this muscle and emerges on the deep surface of the pronator teres muscle. As it emerges from beneath the pronator teres, the nerve is positioned on the deep surface of the flexor digitorum superficialis; it maintains this position to the level of the musculotendinous junction, then the nerve appears on the radial side of the flexor digitorum superficialis muscle. The branches in the forearm extend to the pronator teres, flexor carpi radialis, palmaris longus, flexor digitorum superficialis, flexor digitorum profundus (index and long finger portions), flexor pollicis longus, and pronator quadratus. In the forearm, the anterior interosseous nerve arises about 5 cm below the level of the medial epicondyle of the humerus and is positioned on the surface of the flexor digitorum profundus. It then passes between this muscle and the flexor pollicis longus to rest on the interosseous membrane. It progresses distally, lying on the interosseous membrane to innervate the

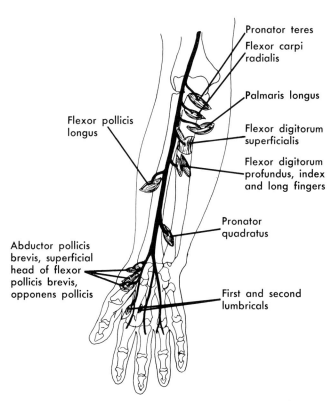

**Fig. 10-5.** Usual segmental motor distribution of the median nerve.

pronator quadratus muscle (the last major muscle in the forearm innervated by the median nerve). At the wrist the median nerve appears on the radial side of the flexor digitorum superficialis tendons. A small palmar branch pierces the forearm fascia and supplies the skin at the base of the palm. As the median nerve progresses through the carpal tunnel, it lies anterior to the flexor tendons and immediately beneath the flexor retinaculum. Near the distal border of the flexor retinaculum, the median nerve divides into the following: (1) a motor branch for the thenar muscles; (2) proper digital nerves for the thumb and radial side of the index finger; and (3) common digital nerves for the adjacent sides of the index, long, and ring fingers. The motor branch of the median nerve runs a short course to enter the muscles of the thenar eminence, that is, the abductor pollicis brevis, the flexor pollicis brevis, and the opponens pollicis. The lumbricales are innervated by motor branches accompanying the proper digital nerve to the index finger and the common digital nerves to the adjacent sides of the index and long fingers. The terminal sensory innervations of the median nerve are on the volar surface of the hand and include the thumb, index finger, long finger, and the radial side of the ring finger (Fig. 10-3).

*Evaluation of motor function.* The common distribution of the median nerve is shown in Fig. 10-5. The level of the laceration of the median nerve in the forearm can be detected by the functional muscle groups remaining. Of course, direct laceration of muscle bellies and tendons may temporarily confuse the diagnosis. Evaluation of the median innervated muscles in the hand confirms the diagnosis of nerve injury. The extent of direct muscle injury can be defined at the time of surgery. The median nerve is most frequently injured at the wrist. Thus, tests for the function of the thenar muscles assume the greatest clinical importance. However, part or all

of the thenar muscles may occasionally be supplied by the ulnar nerve. The abductor pollicis brevis produces palmar abduction of the thumb and is examined by having the patient move his thumb to a position approximating a right angle to the plane of the palm. Function of the opponens pollicis can be demonstrated by having the patient move the plane of his thumb nail through an arc of 90 degrees. The thumb nail is placed in the midpalm perpendicular to the palm; then the thumb is palmarly abducted and simultaneously opposed to a vertical rod placed in the palm (Fig. 10-6). The plane of the thumb nail comes to lie virtually parallel to the plane of the palm. Function of the flexor pollicis brevis may be demonstrated in the presence of an intact flexor pollicis longus only by palpa-

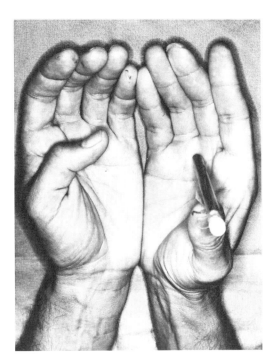

**Fig. 10-6.** Opponens pollicis muscle function is tested by placing the thumb in the midpalm so that the plane of the nail is perpendicular to the plane of the palm *(left)*. The thumb is then palmarly abducted and simultaneously opposed to a vertical rod placed in the palm *(right)*.

tion of the tendon of the flexor pollicis brevis as it inserts into the radial sesamoid bone of the thumb. One can demonstrate function of the lumbricales of the index and middle finger only by electromyography.

In the forearm a functioning pronator teres can be palpated directly as the patient attempts pronation of the forearm. The flexor carpi radialis tendon can be palpated overlying the ulnar border of the radius as the patient flexes and radially deviates the wrist. The palmaris longus is demonstrated by palpation of the tendon at the wrist as the patient opposes the thumb and little finger lightly while simultaneously trying to move them out of opposition (see Fig. 11-4). Function of the flexor digitorum superficialis is demonstrated by having the patient flex the proximal interphalangeal joint of the long, ring, or little finger while the other fingers are held in full extension by the examiner. Function of the flexor pollicis longus is demonstrated by flexion of the interphalangeal joint of the thumb. Examination for function of the flexor digitorum profundus of the index and long fingers is accomplished by having the patient produce independent flexion of the distal interphalangeal joint of the appropriate finger. Occasionally the ulnar nerve will supply the flexor digitorum profundus to the long finger. An intact nerve supply to the pronator quadratus is very difficult to demonstrate.

*Evaluation of sensory function.* The usual sensory distribution is shown in Fig. 10-3. The most constant area supplied by the median nerve is the skin over the distal phalanx of the index finger.

### Digital nerve

The digital nerves are the terminal branches of the median and ulnar nerves. Each proper palmar digital nerve supplies sensation to at least the volar aspect of one half of the finger. Functional continu-ity of the digital nerve is demonstrated by testing for perception of light touch just volar to the midlateral line of the distal phalanx.

### INDICATIONS AND CONTRAINDICATIONS TO PRIMARY NERVE REPAIR

Although some authors favor primary repair, others are equally strong advocates of secondary nerve repair. None of these authors has presented a controlled series to demonstrate the advantage of his proposed technique. Primary and secondary repair of sharply lacerated nerves were compared in a well-controlled experimental study; the interval between primary repair and evaluation was the same as the interval between secondary repair and evaluation. Early after repair nerve action potentials, electromyographs, and tetanic contraction strength were studied. These results supported primary repair, but by 52 weeks after repair there seemed to be little difference between the two repairs. However, an insufficient number of animals were used to allow statistical comparison of primary and secondary repairs. Even retrospective studies have failed to demonstrate whether primary or secondary nerve repair will give better functional results. No controlled prospective clinical study comparing primary and secondary nerve suture has been reported.

For the reasons discussed under the heading "Results of Repair" (p. 284) many authors have proposed primary suture for pure motor or pure sensory nerves. In practice this would limit primary repair to the digital nerves, the motor branch of the median nerve in the palm, the terminal motor branches of the ulnar nerve, the posterior cutaneous nerve of the forearm, and the terminal superficial radial nerve.

All would agree that primary repair is indicated only in a tidy wound, for example, one in which there is limited damage to the nerve or surrounding tissues (see Fig. 11-1). We feel that an untidy, contaminated, or infected wound should be a definite contraindication to primary repair.

## TECHNIQUE OF NERVE REPAIR
### Without loss of a major portion of nerve length

*Primary treatment other than neurorrhaphy.* Many authors have suggested simply "tacking" the nerve ends together with one or two stitches at the time of the acute injury. Other authors have recommended suturing the nerves in the overlapped position. These techniques are designed to prevent retraction of the nerve ends and to reduce the gap created by resection of the neuroma at the time of secondary neurorrhaphy. No improvement in return of nerve function has been shown to follow tacking or overlapping nerve ends, but these techniques do facilitate secondary neurorrhaphy.

*Epineurial repair.* The classic technique for repair of nerve lacerations is epineurial suture. If the nerve has been divided by a very sharp instrument, little or no resection of the nerve ends is required. If the nerve ends are contused, the contused portion should be removed. A miter box has been developed to aid in cleanly resecting the damaged nerve ends (Fig. 10-7); however, most surgeons believe that simply dividing the nerve with a portion of a razor blade is sufficiently accurate. The two nerve ends are joined with simple interrupted sutures of 6-0 or 7-0 silk placed in the epineurium around the periphery of the nerve (Fig. 10-8).

If secondary epineurial nerve repair is elected, the inevitable neuroma and glioma must be resected. The proximal and distal nerve stumps are resected until their funiculi protrude from the surface of the cut nerve end (Fig. 10-9). The nerve ends are oriented by the vessels on their surface or by the pattern of funiculi and are approximated with epineurial sutures as described previously for the primary repair.

*Funicular (fascicular) repair.* Langley

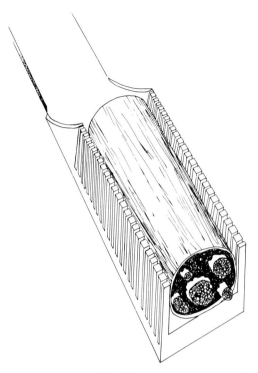

**Fig. 10-7.** A miter box for trimming nerve ends.

and Hashimoto were the first to mention the potential advantages of funicular suture. The technique did not gain popularity, however, until 1964 when Smith introduced the technical refinement of the operating microscope in peripheral nerve surgery. Goto states that many of the axons pass into connective tissue following epineurial suture. He found microscopic evidence of better distal passage of nerve fibers following funicular suture. Goto, Bora, Hakstian, and Grabb have all reported favorable results following funicular suture in both animals and humans. In further investigations since then at least one of these authors, as well as others, has contradicted the work, suggesting improved results with funicular repair.

Bora conducted a controlled study in cats. He found return of muscle function in 3 out of 10 cats whose nerves were sutured by the epineurial technique and in 8 out of

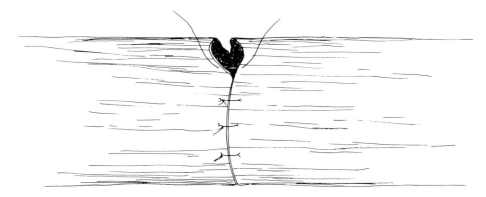

**Fig. 10-8.** The classic epineurial repair.

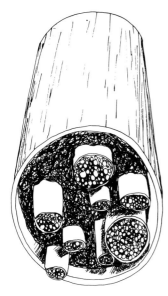

**Fig. 10-9.** Trimmed nerve end showing protruding funiculi and the "foreskin" effect of the epineurium.

10 cats whose nerves were sutured by the funicular technique. Sensation return appeared to be the same in both groups. From these data, he recommended use of funicular suture in nerve repair. When the fourfold contingency tables are used, however, these results are not significantly different at the 5% confidence level.

More recently Bora and co-workers studied the effectiveness of epineurial and perineurial suture techniques, as well as a combined epiperineurial suture technique in severed sciatic nerves in rabbits. They measured the myelin content of the posterior tibial nerve and found relatively more myelin in the epineurial repair group (60% of normal) versus the perineurial repair group (28.3% of normal); thus they concluded that other criteria for measuring nerve regeneration were worthy of investigation.

Grabb repaired the median and ulnar nerves of monkeys after resecting a 5-mm segment. The nerves were repaired by the following techniques: (1) epineurial suture, (2) funicular suture choosing the corresponding funiculi on the basis of their size and position, or (3) funicular suture following identification and pairing of predominantly motor or sensory funiculi by electrical stimulation. His evaluation was based on integrated electromyographic recordings of muscle activity in the opponens pollicis and the abductor digiti minimi. There was no difference in the rate of return following the two methods of funicular suture. Results after funicular repair were better than results after epineurial repair only at the 7% confidence level.

Orgel and Terzis sought to show superior results with perineurial repair over epineurial repair in rabbit sciatic nerves by means of an elegant series of measurements, including quantitative ultramicroscopy and electrophysiology. Although a slight advantage was suggested with perineurial repair, there were no statistically significant differences in the results from the two types of repair.

Cabaud and co-workers have recently compared epineurial and perineurial nerve repair techniques in severed ulnar nerves in cats. Their careful objective and subjective measurements showed no statistically significant differences between the two groups.

In summary, although the concept of funicular approximation by means of perineurial repair is theoretically attractive and several studies suggest that funicular repair produces better results than epineurial repair, there is no statistically significant evidence to support this as yet.

Clinically the funicular method of repair can be used at the time of acute injuries. To identify corresponding funiculi, one notes their diameter and location within the nerve. A binocular loupe can be used, but an operating microscope allows more precise technique. The funiculi are reapproximated with one to four 10-0 to 12-0 nylon sutures. Funiculi toward the center of the nerve require fewer sutures.

Hakstian recommended the use of electrophysiological techniques to aid in funicular orientation in acute injuries. It is possible to produce motor responses with electrical stimulation of the distal nerve stump for up to 4 days after injury. Stimulation of the proximal stump elicits subjective sensations from the patient as long as the cells of origin in the dorsal root ganglia are intact. Thus, better pairing of predominantly motor and sensory funiculi can theoretically be achieved at the time of repair. No controlled studies demonstrating this, however, have been reported.

Because the funicular pattern remains constant over only 0.25 to 5 mm of nerve length, some authors have condemned secondary funicular repair. However, even secondary funicular repair allows more axons to regenerate into funiculi and results in less loss of axons into connective tissue than conventional epineurial repair.

Millesi's results (see p. 289) using funicular repair technique and nerve grafting are so outstanding that some type of funicular repair appears to be the method of choice for secondary nerve repair. For secondary funicular repair the nerve ends are resected as described previously (p. 278) for secondary epineurial repair, and then individual funiculi are united. The gap created by resection frequently necessitates mobilization of the nerve for 8 to 10 cm proximally and distally; at times epineprial sutures of 6-0 silk are necessary to relieve tension on the funicular repair. If stay sutures are required to relieve tension, a nerve graft (p. 281) is probably indicated.

### With loss of a major portion of nerve length

Even during primary repair of a laceration produced by a very sharp instrument, the nerve ends are separated by 1 to 2 cm. The gap can become considerable when neuroma is resected and immense at the time of secondary nerve repair after an untidy injury.

*Mobilization.* The most commonly used technique to overcome a gap between the ends of a nerve is proximal and distal mobilization of the nerve. Sunderland, Seddon, and others have stated that proximal and distal mobilization for virtually any distance will not impair the resulting nerve repair. Smith demonstrated, however, that mobilization for greater than 8 cm resulted in significant devascularization of the nerve. Lundborg found that mobilization of the sciatic nerve in rabbits for greater than 7 cm caused significant impairment of the microcirculation of the nerve. He did not, however, demonstrate that mobilization altered nerve function after nerve repair. Kline and others studied nerve action potentials and electromyograms following treatment of tibial nerve injuries in monkeys. They studied crushed nerves and severed and repaired nerves. At the time of injury, one nerve was completely mobilized while the opposite nerve was not mobilized. There was no ultimate difference in return of nerve action potentials or electromyograms. If mobilization for more than 8 cm is accomplished, the mobilized nerve may act as a graft and be vascularized from its bed. No one has proved that mobilization alone impairs the results of nerve repair, however.

*Stretching.* A second common technique to overcome a gap is traction on the nerve. Smith found that acute traction produced little evidence of change in the nerve, but Highet showed that prolonged traction leads to distal scarring and fibrosis. The combination of stretching and nerve division led to significant impairment of blood flow in the rabbit's tibial nerve. Thus, mobilization of a nerve combined with nerve repair impairs circulation in the proximal and distal nerve segments. Scarring and fibrosis will usually impair regeneration of the nerve. At times a repair under even mild tension will actually disrupt.

*Joint flexion.* Hyperflexion of a joint allows the nerve to bridge the joint. A relative increase in nerve length is obtained by this technique. In many war injuries, acute flexion of the elbow was used to overcome large gaps in the median and ulnar nerves. Recent evidence suggests that hyperflexion of the joints leads to the same distal scarring and impediment to return of nerve function that follow constant tension on the repair. Impairment of regeneration occurs regardless of how slowly the joint is returned to its extended position. Hyperflexion in the elderly person may lead to permanent flexion contractures. Thus, flexion of no more than 30 degrees at any one joint is probably all that is desirable. If flexion greater than 30 degrees is needed to obtain apposition of the nerve ends, then other techniques (see following) should be used.

*Nerve transposition.* Transposition of the nerve to gain a relative increase in length has been used most commonly for ulnar nerve injuries. The nerve is moved from its normal position (posterior to the medial epicondyle of the humerus) to the subcutaneous tissues anterior to the elbow. This does not seem to lead to any dysfunction of the ulnar nerve.

Sunderland describes overcoming gaps of 5 to 12 cm with satisfactory return of nerve function by a combination of mobilization, stretching, joint flexion, and transposition. The patients described, however, did not have normal return of either sensation or motion. Thus, one cannot help wondering if a better return might have followed a repair in which extensive mobilization and/or stretching were not used.

*Bone shortening.* Shortening of the bone to allow apposition of nerve ends has been reported. Almost all reports involve shortening the humerus by 2 to 6 cm. This technique is rarely indicated except during replantation of an amputated portion of the limb. Occasionally bone shortening can be used if there is an associated nonunion of a fractured humerus.

*Isografts.* After nerve isografts had been condemned for many years, renewed interest in them has developed. Millesi and co-workers in a series of experiments in cats and rabbits evaluated the following: (1) conventional nerve suture, (2) nerve suture following a microsurgical technique and funicular repair, (3) the effect of tension at the suture site, and (4) nerve grafting. He reached the following conclusions:

1. Much of the connective tissue that develops at the site of a nerve repair tends to be peripheral to the sutures in the epinerium.
2. This connective tissue pushes the sutures into the funiculi and decreases the chance of funiculi crossing the suture line.
3. Repair by microsurgical technique gives better results than conventional nerve sutures.
4. The most important factor impairing

nerve regeneration is tension at the suture site.

5. Exact approximation of the funiculi is difficult to achieve by epineurial suture.

6. Axon regeneration and the ultimate result are improved after nerve grafting.

He identified the funiculi in the proximal and distal nerve ends and made an attempt to locate corresponding funiculi. Multiple small diameter (approximately 1 mm) segments of nerve were used as a cable graft. Each segment of nerve graft was sutured to a few funiculi proximally and distally. These grafts could be extremely long, at least 20 cm in length; each was sutured with a single 10-0 suture. The graft was long enough to allow full motion of all joints without placing *any* tension on the anastomosis (Fig. 10-10). Microscopic magnification was used during the entire procedure. The results of his nerve grafting technique in humans are discussed later in this chapter under the heading "Results of Nerve Repair" (p. 284).

*Pedicle grafts.* Pedicle grafting involving the use of the divided nerve or a portion of an adjacent intact nerve has been tried. Theoretical considerations of the intermixing from one funiculus to another within the course of a nerve and of the relatively small proportion of total nerve volume that is actual nerve elements (Fig. 10-11)

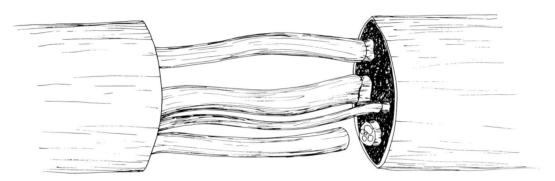

**Fig. 10-10.** Cable isograft showing each cable joining several funiculi.

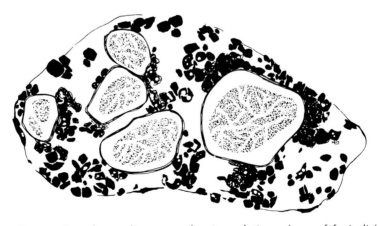

**Fig. 10-11.** Cross-section of a median nerve showing relative volume of funiculi *(stippled)* and adiposed tissue *(black)*.

indicate that these procedures would not be effective. Clinical use has verified the theoretical considerations, and results in the arm have not been satisfactory. McCarty has reported a successful nerve pedicle operation using the common peroneal portion of the sciatic nerve as a graft for the tibial portion of that nerve.

Ney recommended the use of a nerve pedicle graft in irreparable damage of the median and ulnar nerves in the forearm. Barnes and Strange each expanded this suggestion. The procedure is applicable only when there is simultaneous injury to the median and ulnar nerves. The nerve pedicle graft is the entire adjacent nerve. In this procedure the ulnar nerve is sacrificed to restore continuity of the median nerve. The proximal ends of the two nerves are anastomosed, and the ulnar nerve is partially divided (preserving its longitudinal blood supply). The distance from the partial division to the anastomosis is equal to the original gap between the ends of the median nerve. Finally, after 4 to 6 weeks, the ulnar nerve is redivided at the site of the original partial transection and sutured to the distal end of the median nerve (Fig. 10-12). Seddon and Brookes have each reported success using this technique. Their results are presented in the section "Results of Nerve Repair."

## Immobilization

The classically recommended period of immobilization is 4 weeks. Healing rabbit sciatic nerves reach preinjury tensile strength 4 weeks after wounding. In Mukherjee's study of immediately repaired nerves, the limbs were not immobilized. This experimental situation may not be comparable to the clinical resection of neuroma and secondary repair. No clinical study comparing periods of immobilization has been reported. Millesi allows unrestricted motion beginning 10 days after nerve grafting. It may be that immobilization for a full 4 weeks is not required.

If a large gap has been overcome by mo-

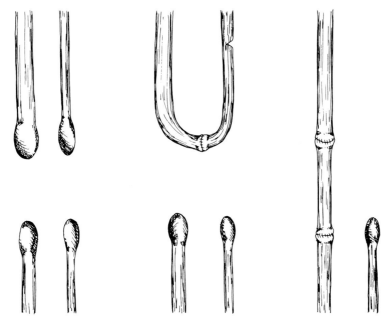

**Fig. 10-12.** From left to right, stages in nerve pedicle grafting using a segment of an adjacent divided nerve (ulnar) to replace a segment of another divided nerve (median).

bilizing the nerve or flexing the joints, Seddon recommends placing radiopaque markers on either side of the anastomosis. Radiographs are taken immediately post-operatively to indicate the relationship between the two markers. After remobilization of the joints has occurred, further radiographs are taken. If the markers have separated by several centimeters, then disruption of the nerve repair is present, and reexploration of the nerve is indicated.

## RESULTS OF NERVE REPAIR
### General factors influencing results

Many factors influence results following nerve repair, but in general they can be divided into two groups. The first group includes those factors over which the surgeon has no control: (1) etiology of the injury, (2) injury to associated structures, (3) the level of the injury, (4) the type of nerve injured, and (5) the age of the patient. In the second group are factors over which the surgeon has some control: the type of repair that is used (that is, primary, secondary, funicular, epineurial, etc.) and the interval between wounding and repair.

*Factors not under the surgeon's control*

*Etiology of the injury.* All authors agree that injuries associated with loss of a substantial portion of the length of the nerve will result in a poor ultimate return of nerve function. Loss of nerve substance is usually due to gunshot wounds or avulsion injuries from farm or industrial equipment. The retrograde changes in the cell body are more severe after gunshot wounds than after sharply incised wounds. Finally, injury to associated structures is more common with gunshot wounds or avulsive injuries.

*Associated injury.* The presence of associated injury to the bone or major vessels usually adversely affects the results following peripheral nerve repair. A few authors have stated that major artery injury did not influence the results of nerve repair. Certainly, associated injury to the nerve

bed causing decreased number of small vessels and increased fibrous tissue has been shown to impair the results of nerve repair.

Repair and healing of associated injury to tendons, muscles, bones, and skin may delay the repair of a nerve. Joints may stiffen because of lack of normal tendon function or because of unsatisfactory position of the bones (see Chapter 12). The thumb may become stiff and adducted because of injury in the web space; even when normal median nerve function returns, palmar abduction might be impossible.

*Level of the injury.* The level of the injury has been said to be important in determining results of nerve repair. The important factor appears to be the proximity of the nerve injury site to the parent cell body, with more proximal injuries resulting in greater retrograde disturbances, which may or may not recover fully. The distance between the regenerating axon tip and denervated end organs is also a factor in successful nerve repair. An injury of the median nerve just superior to where it supplies the flexor digitorum profundus of the index and long fingers may be followed by excellent return of function in these muscles, but no return of function in the muscles of the thenar eminence. This phenomenon may well be related to the volume of cell cytoplasm that is lost because of the injury. Much more cytoplasm is lost from an injury in the brachial plexus than from an injury of the digital nerve at the level of the metacarpophalangeal joint. The neuron may be unable to regenerate large volumes of axoplasm. In addition, there is the important relationship between the interval from injury to repair and the ultimate quality of function, as is mentioned later (p. 285). Obviously, the more proximal the injury, the greater the delay in ultimate reinnervation; thus, after an injury in the brachial plexus, the intrinsic muscles of the hand may undergo irreversible changes despite regeneration at a maximal rate.

*Type of nerve injured.* Many authors

have suggested that the results of nerve repair are much better in a pure sensory or a pure motor nerve. Theoretical considerations related to the intermixing of axons within funiculi support these observations. Most authors report that repair of digital nerves yields better sensory return than repair of median or ulnar nerves. The level of injury and other factors may also explain the more satisfactory results after digital nerve repair.

Although there is some intermixing between funiculi, the majority of any single funiculus is made up of either sensory or motor axons. This anatomical fact adds to the theoretical advantages of funicular suture.

*Age of the patient.* All clinical and experimental evidence strongly indicates that the younger individual has a much better result following nerve repair than the older individual. This is true whether one considers chimpanzees or humans. The percentage of good results of nerve repair begins decreasing almost from birth, but after about 15 years of age the percentage stabilizes. Insufficient reports of nerve repair in very old persons are available to prove or disprove the theory that "nerve repair past the age of 50 is always unsatisfactory." Occasionally excellent return of function is reported in persons 40 or 50 years of age.

As mentioned previously, many factors that affect the results of nerve repair are interrelated. Younger patients usually have more supple joints and soft tissue distal to the level of nerve injury; these factors alone would increase the chance of return of normal function after nerve injury. Also, children can adapt an intact motor unit to replace one that has been lost much more readily than adults. The young patient can reorient himself with great ease to a new sensory pattern following incomplete return of sensation.

*Factors under the surgeon's control*

*Type of repair.* An improved result may follow funicular repair (p. 278). Likewise,

there is good experimental and some clinical evidence that a poorly performed repair with inaccurate apposition of the nerve ends will lead to a greater percentage of unsatisfactory results. Extensive mobilization of the nerve may be followed by satisfactory return, but it will probably lead to less satisfactory return than if extensive mobilization is not required.

*Interval between wounding and repair.* Finally, the interval between injury and repair is important. Repair beyond 3 years has never been reported to be associated with any significant return of muscle function. Theoretically, changes in the distal nerve (shrinkage, loss of volume) should lead to poorer results if repair is delayed for 3 months after injury. In studies on nerve injuries during World War II, there was a steady decline in the percentage of satisfactory recovery of motor function beginning about 3 weeks after injury. There is little correlation between the degree of return of sensory function and the interval between wounding and nerve repair. Again, many factors are interrelated; nerve repair may be delayed because of severe associated injuries.

## Methods of evaluating results

Testing for return of motor and sensory function is described in Chapter 13. Motor strength of any muscle is usually classified on the basis of voluntary power as shown in Table 10-1. A better classification of nerve recovery is based on the Medical

**Table 10-1.** Grading of muscle power

| Grade | Extent of muscle power |
|-------|------------------------|
| 0 | No contraction |
| 1 | Trace of contraction |
| 2 | Active movement with gravity eliminated |
| 3 | Active movement against gravity |
| 4 | Active movement against gravity and resistance |
| 5 | Normal power |

**Table 10-2.** Classification of motor recovery

| Grade | Extent of motor recovery |
|-------|--------------------------|
| M0 | No contraction |
| M1 | Return of preceptible contraction in the proximal muscles |
| M2 | Return of perceptible contraction in both proximal and distal muscles |
| M3 | Return of function in both proximal and distal muscles to such a degree that all important muscles are sufficiently powerful to act against resistance |
| M4 | Return of function as in M3 with the addition that all synergic and independent movements are possible |
| M5 | Complete recovery |

**Table 10-3.** Classification of sensory recovery

| Grade | Extent of sensory recovery |
|-------|----------------------------|
| S0 | Absence of sensibility in the autonomous area |
| S1 | Recovery of deep cutaneous pain sensibility within the autonomous area of the nerve |
| S2 | Return of some degree of superficial cutaneous pain and tactile sensibility within the autonomous area of the nerve |
| S3 | Return of superficial cutaneous pain and tactile sensibility throughout the autonomous area with disappearance of any previous overresponse |
| S3+ | Return of sensibility as in S3 with the addition of some recovery of two-point discrimination within the autonomous area |
| S4 | Complete recovery |

Research Council's standards and should be uniformly adopted. Classifications of motor recovery and sensory recovery are shown in Tables 10-2 and 10-3, respectively.

**Clinical reports of nerve repairs**

We have analyzed the results of nerve repair reported since World War II. We have classified the results by level of injury and nerve involved (Tables 10-4 to 10-7).

The first group of patients is taken from the Medical Research Council report. These are primarily young men who sustained gunshot or fragment wounds during the war. As noted previously this combination of factors would undoubtedly bias the results (Tables 10-4 and 10-5).

Larsen reported on 17 radial nerve lacerations in the arm, 11 radial nerve lacerations in the forearm, 142 digital nerve lacerations, 88 median nerve lacerations, and 78 ulnar nerve lacerations. One fourth of his patients were under 14 years of age. Fifty-seven percent of the nerve injuries were caused by sharp laceration, and the remainder were associated with some crushing and contusion of tissue. Epineurial repair with 6-0 or 7-0 silk was used. Primary

and secondary repair were both accomplished in about 50% of the patients. The joints were immobilized 10 degrees short of full flexion, and immobilization was continued for 4 weeks. The results are recorded in Tables 10-4 to 10-7.

In 1961 Stromberg and co-workers reported on 59 median, 45 ulnar, and 59 digital nerve injuries; primary repair was utilized in only 27 of the patients. They evaluated their results only on the basis of sensory return and used a modification of the classic sweat test. It was noted that almost all patients said that their hand function was satisfactory. The best results, as always, were in children. They did not give the details of suturing technique or period of immobilization (Tables 10-4, 10-5, and 10-7).

In 1961 Flynn and Flynn reported the result of nerve repair in 40 median and 40 ulnar nerve injuries. The return of sensory function was evaluated primarily by the sweat test; however, in addition light

**Table 10-4.** Results of median nerve repair

| Source | Wrist level | | | | Forearm level | | | |
|---|---|---|---|---|---|---|---|---|
| | Motor | | Sensory | | Motor | | Sensory | |
| | Total nerves | Nerves with M3 or better function | Total nerves | Nerves with S3 or better function | Total nerves | Nerves with M3 or better function | Total nerves | Nerves with S3 or better function |
| Medical Research Council | 158 | 63 | 145 | 16 | | | | |
| Larsen | 78 | 47 | 78 | 56 | 14 | 5 | 14 | 6 |
| Stromberg | | | 46 | 44 | | | | |
| Flynn | 40 | 20 | 40 | 20 | | | | |
| McEwan | | | | | | | | |
|    Children | 26 | 24 | 28 | 26 | | | | |
|    Adults | 15 | 9 | 18 | 12 | | | | |
| Onne | | | 32 | 18 | | | | |
| Sakellariades | 58 | 29 | 62 | 35 | 7 | 2 | 7 | 0 |
| Boswick | | | 32 | 27 | | | | |
| Seddon | 52 | 34 | 53 | 13 | | | | |
| Total | 427 | 226 (53%) | 534 | 267 (50%) | 21 | 7 (33%) | 21 | 6 (29%) |
|    Millesi (nerve grafting) | 7 | 4 | 4 | 4 | 24 | 19 | 34 | 33 |

**Table 10-5.** Results of ulnar nerve repair

| Source | Wrist level | | | | Forearm level | | | |
|---|---|---|---|---|---|---|---|---|
| | Motor | | Sensory | | Motor | | Sensory | |
| | Total nerves | Nerves with M4 or better function | Total nerves | Nerves with S3 or better function | Total nerves | Nerves with M4 or better function | Total nerves | Nerves with S3 or better function |
| Medical Research Council | 93 | 15 | 155 | 59 | | | | |
| Larsen | 62 | 0 | 62 | 39 | 18 | 0 | 18 | 6 |
| Stromberg | | | 32 | 28 | | | | |
| Flynn | 40 | 4 | 40 | 8 | | | | |
| McEwan | | | | | | | | |
|    Children | 24 | 17 | 22 | 22 | | | | |
|    Adults | 22 | 5 | 25 | 21 | | | | |
| Onne | | | 17 | 13 | | | | |
| Sakellariades | 68 | 30 | 70 | 33 | 18 | 6 | 18 | 8 |
| Boswick | | | 24 | 21 | | | | |
| Seddon | 60 | 21 | 57 | 39 | | | | |
| Total | 369 | 92 (25%) | 504 | 283 (56%) | 36 | 6 (17%) | 36 | 14 (39%) |
|    Millesi (nerve grafting) | 3 | 1 | 3 | 3 | 36 | 18 | 36 | 30 |

**Table 10-6.** Results of radial nerve repair

| Source | Motor | | Sensory | |
|---|---|---|---|---|
| | Total nerves | Nerves with M3 or better function | Total nerves | Nerves with S3 or better function |
| Larsen | 22 | 14 | 23 | 15 |
| Sakellariades | 7 | 6 | | |
| Seddon | 67 | 53 | | |
| Total | 96 | 73 (76%) | 23 | 15 (65%) |
| Millesi (nerve grafting) | 13 | 12 | | |

**Table 10-7.** Results of digital nerve repair

| Source | Total nerves | Nerves with S3 or better function | Nerves with S3+ or better function |
|---|---|---|---|
| Larsen | 142 | 136 | 92 |
| Stromberg | 59 | 59 | 5 |
| Onne | 22 | 12 | 8 |
| Boswick | 23 | 20 | 3 |
| Seddon | 21 | 18 | 9 |
| Total | 267 | 245 (92%) | 117 (48%) |
| Buncke (micro repair) | 20 | 17 | 12 |

touch sensibility, pin-prick sensibility, and two-point discrimination were noted. The technique of repair was not mentioned, but the hand was immobilized for 4 weeks in 30 degrees of flexion (Tables 10-4 and 10-5).

McEwan reported the results of repair of 39 median and 31 ulnar nerve injuries in children and 30 median and 41 ulnar nerve injuries in adults. In both adults and children, the majority of the injuries were caused by sharp lacerations. Primary repair with epineurial sutures of 7-0 silk was accomplished in all tidy wounds. The results in children were much better than in adults (Tables 10-4 and 10-5) and in tidy wounds than in untidy wounds. The results were slightly better after primary repair.

Onne extensively evaluated the recovery of sensation after primary and secondary epineurial nerve repair in 32 median, 17 ulnar, and 22 digital nerves. Postoperative follow-up was very complete. The return of two-point discrimination in millimeters was roughly proportional to the age in years up to about 20 years of age; after 20 years of age, return of two-point discrimination to less than 15 mm was rare following median and ulnar nerve injury. Good return of two-point discrimination after digital nerve sutures was recorded up to about 50 years of age. There was no difference in results of primary and secondary nerve repair (Tables 10-4, 10-5, and 10-7).

Sakellariades reported on 172 injured median, ulnar, and radial nerves; 67% of the injuries were caused by sharp lacerations. Approximately one fourth of the patients were children. Better results were obtained in children and patients with sharp injuries and minimal or no loss of nerve length. He did not give the details of his suturing technique or period of immobilization. He found that the results of secondary repair were slightly better than primary repair. We have utilized the t-test to analyze his results, and using the 5% level to reject the null hypothesis, we have found that there is no significant difference in the results of primary and secondary nerve repair. The results are given in Tables 10-4 and 10-6.

Boswick and others reported on 23 digital, 37 median, 30 ulnar, and 3 radial nerve repairs. The damaged nerves were repaired with 6-0 silk epineurial stitches, and the hand was immobilized for 3 weeks. Only 3 patients having digital, 3 patients having median, and 4 patients having ulnar nerve repair had return of two-point discrimination. However, the authors did not state exactly what the minimum separation of the two points was in order to have return of two-point discrimination. Results were better in children. Patient evaluation of a "good" result occurred in 81% of the digital, 77% of the median, 79% of the ulnar, and 27% of the combined median-ulnar nerve injuries. The patients' beliefs emphasize that although results are not satisfactory by objective criteria, the result may be subjectively satisfactory. Boswick's results are given in Tables 10-4, 10-5, and 10-7.

In 1972 Seddon reported the results of repair of 53 median and 60 ulnar nerve injuries at the wrist and of 67 radial nerve injuries and 21 digital nerve injuries. Both primary and secondary repairs were carried out; the results appeared better for primary suture of digital nerves and equivocal for other nerves. If one compares S3 or better function, the results were not significantly better after primary repair of digital nerves (Tables 10-4 to 10-7).

Buncke has reported the results of repair of 20 digital nerves using a microscope and fascicular repair with 8 to 10 sutures of 10-0 nylon. Included in his 20 cases were 2 digital nerves repaired with a nerve graft. There were 12 sharp and 8 crushing injuries, and 7 primary and 13 secondary repairs. The hands were immobilized for only 2 weeks with the digit in flexion. He measured the return of two-point discrimination. Although accurate comparison is difficult, his results are the best reported for sensory return following digital nerve repair (Table 10-7).

Brookes and Seddon have each reported results following nerve pedicle grafting of the ulnar nerve to the median nerve. They had a combined total of 18 patients, and in all patients light touch sensation and motor function of the thenar muscles were recorded. In at least eight of the patients, some element of two-point discrimination returned, and independent synergic or normal function of the thenar muscles was present. In view of Millesi's results (following) the present usefulness of this procedure is unclear.

Millesi has reported the clinical use of cable nerve grafting. His technique involves the following: (1) use of an operating microscope, (2) dissection of groups of fasciculi beginning well proximal or well distal to the neuroma, (3) transection with scissors of groups of fasciculi either proximal or distal to any fibrosis, (4) use of a small diameter donor nerve, usually the sural, (5) identification of corresponding fasciculi by their pattern, and (6) suturing segments of the donor nerve to groups of three or four fasciculi using a single 10-0 nylon stitch in the epineurium of the graft and the perineurium of one fasciculus. If the nerve is partially transected, the intact fasciculi are preserved, and segments of graft are used to join the divided fasciculi (inlay graft). Active exercises begin 10 days after grafting. The contraindications to grafting were the following: (1) If the gaps in the nerve were equal to or less than 2 cm and the nerve could be anastomosed without tension with the joints in extension, direct fascicular repair was used; (2) if gaps in the ulnar nerve were up to 4 cm, the nerve was transposed to a position anterior to the elbow; and (3) if the nerve injury was associated with nonunion of a fracture, the bone was shortened to allow end-to-end approximation of the nerve. The original and a subsequent report by Millesi and co-workers concerned 38 median, 39 ulnar, and 13 radial nerve grafting procedures in patients followed for a minimum of 2 years. The results are shown in Tables 10-4, 10-5, and 10-6. The results appear outstanding;

indeed, if one eliminates persons under 12 years of age from his study, the results are statistically significantly better than anyone else has reported. Nerve grafting has been used in too few children to allow statistical analysis.

## SUMMARY

Using conventional nerve repair, one has about a 50% chance of producing grade M3 (Table 10-3) or better motor function and grade S3 (Table 10-3) or better sensory function following repair of a median nerve injury at the wrist and about a 30% chance of producing the same results after median nerve repair in the forearm.

Because ulnar nerve motor function is relatively more important than ulnar sensory function, Seddon originally categorized those patients having ulnar motor function as grade M4; we have continued this classification. About 25% of the patients have grade M4 or better motor function following repair of ulnar nerve injuries at the wrist and about 17% have a comparable result following repair of ulnar nerve injuries in the forearm and arm. About 55% of the patients recover grade S3 or better sensory function after repair of ulnar nerve injuries at the wrist, and about 40% have a comparable result following ulnar nerve injuries in the forearm or arm.

Following radial nerve repair, about 65% of the patients have grade S3 or better sensory return, and about 75% of the patients have grade M3 or better motor nerve function.

The results of digital nerve repair were much better than results of median or ulnar nerve repair. The patient has about a 90% chance of gaining S3 or better sensory return and about a 50% chance of gaining S3 plus return of sensory function.

## BIBLIOGRAPHY

Barnes, R.: Traction injuries of the brachial plexus in adults, J. Bone Joint Surg. 31B:10, 1949.

Bora, F. W.: Peripheral nerve repair in cats; the fascicular stitch, J. Bone Joint Surg. 49A:659, 1957.

Bora, F. W., Pleasure, E. D., and Didizian, N. A.: A study of nerve regeneration and neuroma formation after nerve suture by various techniques, J. Hand Surg. 1:138, 1976.

Boswick, J. A., Jr., Schneewind, J., and Stromberg, W., Jr.: Evaluation of peripheral nerve repairs below elbow, Arch. Surg. 90:50, 1965.

Brooks, D.: The place of nerve-grafting in orthopaedic surgery, J. Bone Joint Surg. 37A:299, 1955.

Brown, P. W.: Factors influencing the success of the surgical repair of peripheral nerves, Surg. Clin. North Am. 52:1137, 1972.

Buncke, Harry J.: Digital nerve repairs, Surg. Clin. North Am. 52:1267, 1972.

Cabaud, H. E., Rodkey, D. V. M., McCarroll, H. R., and others: Epineurial and perineurial fascicular nerve repairs; a critical comparison, J. Hand Surg. 1:131, 1976.

Edshage, S., and Wittenstrom, E.: A new method for evaluating sensory function in finger tips. Presented at American Society for Surgery of the Hand, January, 1973.

Field, J. H.: Peripheral nerve suturing using a nerve miter box to trim the ends, Plast. Reconstr. Surg. 44:605, 1969.

Flynn, J. E., and Flynn, W. F.: Median and ulnar nerve injuries; a long range study with evaluation of the ninhydrin test, sensory and motor returns, Ann. Surg. 156:1002, 1961.

Goto, Y.: Experimental study of nerve autografting by funicular suture, Arch. Jap. Chir. 36:478, 1967.

Grabb, W. C., Bement, S. L., Koepke, G. H., and others: Comparison of methods of peripheral nerve suturing in monkeys, Plast. Reconstr. Surg. 46:31, 1970.

Hakstian, R. W.: Funicular orientation by direct stimulation, J. Bone Joint Surg. 50A:1178, 1968.

Highet, W. B.: Traction injuries to the lateral popliteal nerve and traction injuries to peripheral nerves after suture, Br. J. Surg. 30:212, 1942.

Khodadad, G.: Microsurgical techniques in repair of peripheral nerves, Surg. Clin. North Am. 52:1157, 1972.

Kline, D. G., and Hackett, E. R.: Reappraisal of timing for exploration of civilian peripheral nerve injuries, Surgery 78:54, 1975.

Kline, D. G., Hackett, E. R., Davis, G. D., and Myers, M. B.: Effect of mobilization on the blood supply and regeneration of injured nerves, J. Surg. Res. 12:254, 1972.

Laing, P. G.: The timing of definitive nerve repair, Surg. Clin. North Am. 40:363, 1960.

Langley, J. N., and Hasmimoto, M.: On the suture of separate nerve bundles in a nerve trunk and on internal nerve plexuses, J. Physiol. **51**:318, 1917.

Larsen, R. D., and Posch, J. L.: Nerve injuries in the upper extremity, Arch. Surg. **77**:469, 1958.

Lundborg, G.: Structure and function of the intra-neural microvessels as related to trauma, edema formation, and nerve function, J. Bone Joint Surg. **57A**:938, 1975.

McCarty, C. S.: Two-stage autograft for repair of extensive damage to sciatic nerve, J. Neurosurg. **8**:319, 1951.

McEwan, L. E.: Median and ulnar nerve injuries, Aust. N.Z. J. Surg. **32**:89, 1961.

Millesi, H., Meissl, G., and Berger, A.: The inter-fascicular nerve-grafting of the median and ulnar nerves, J. Bone Joint Surg. **54A**:727, 1972.

Millesi, H., Meissl, G., and Berger, A.: Further experience with interfascicular grafting of the median, ulnar, and radial nerves, J. Bone Joint Surg. **58A**:209, 1976.

Mukherjee, S. R.: Tensile strength of nerves during healing, Br. J. Surg. **41**:192, 1953-54.

Ney, K. W.: Technique of nerve surgery in the medical department of the United States Army in the World War: Surgery, Vol. 11, Part I, Section 3—Neurosurgery, Washington, D.C., 1927, U.S. Government Printing Office.

Onne, L.: Recovery of sensibility and sudomotor activity in the hand after nerve suture, Acta Chir. Scand. (Suppl.) **300**:5, 1962.

Orgel, M. G., and Terzis, J. K.: Epineurial vs. perineurial repair, Plast. Reconstr. Surg. **60**:80, 1977.

Sakellarides, H.: A follow-up study of 172 periph-eral nerve injuries in the upper extremity in civilians, J. Bone Joint Surg. **44A**:140, 1962.

Seddon, H.: Surgical disorders of the peripheral nerves, London, 1972, The Williams & Wilkins Co.

Smith, J. W.: Microsurgery of peripheral nerves, Plast. Reconstr. Surg. **33**:317, 1964.

Smith, J. W.: Factors influencing nerve repair, Arch. Surg. **93**:433, 1966.

Strange, F. G.: Case report on pedicle nerve graft, Br. J. Surg. **37**:331, 1950.

Stromberg, W. B., Jr., McFarlane, R. M., Bell, J. L., and others: Injury of the median and ulnar nerves, J. Bone Joint Surg. **43A**:717, 1961.

Sunderland, S.: Nerves and nerve injuries, London, 1972, Churchill Livingstone.

# CHAPTER 11

# Restoration of tendon continuity

Techniques for the management of acute tendon lacerations include: (1) primary or delayed tenorrhaphy, (2) skin closure and secondary tendon grafting, (3) insertion of a Silastic rod anticipating subsequent tendon grafting, (4) tenodesis or arthrodesis, (5) primary tendon grafting, and (6) primary tendon transfer. Of these, the first two methods are used most frequently. Insertion of a Silastic rod at the time of original injury is used infrequently; secondary insertion of a Silastic rod is advocated if extensive scarring from the initial injury is anticipated. The indications for primary tenodesis or arthrodesis will be discussed in detail. Primary tendon grafting and tendon transfer are rarely indicated. A systematic appraisal of the patient, the techniques available for managing the patient's particular problem, and a comparison of the results obtained by the various techniques of treatment of lacerated tendons will be presented. It is anticipated that this will allow a rational approach to the common problems encountered in tendon injuries.

## APPRAISAL OF THE PATIENT AND THE INJURY

Even though it may seem superfluous when a patient has a severe injury, a thorough inquiry into the mechanics of the injury—the how, when, where, and why—is obligatory. Information about prior treatment must be obtained. If the injury was job-related, the type of machine and the circumstances of the injury should be noted. This information may aid in developing measures to improve job safety and in evaluating the patient's particular injury. The physical surroundings of the patient, for example, dirt, chemicals, and metal shavings at the time of the injury should be described. If at all possible, the position of the hand when the injury occurred should be noted. If the fingers or wrist are in extension, the tendon injury will usually lie directly beneath the skin wound. If the fingers or wrist are flexed, the tendon injury will usually lie proximal to the skin wound; this displacement occurs on both surfaces of the hand and forearm but is more noticeable on the volar surface. The dominant hand should be noted. Information about the general health of the patient should, of course, be obtained. Information about the patient's occupation and hobbies may be helpful in selecting the simplest and quickest method of management. A satisfactory range of motion for the ring finger of a laborer may be quite different from a satisfactory range of motion for the ring finger of a violinist.

## Examination of the injured hand

The initial examination requires a series of simple clinical tests, which are exercises in applied anatomy. This examination must be done by the operating surgeon himself. A very unpleasant and unsatisfactory situation to both the surgeon and the patient may arise if the surgeon relies upon someone else's preoperative evaluation. The location of the skin injury provides insight into which underlying structures might be injured. Observation of the hand and the wrist can provide nearly as much information as a detailed dynamic examination. One should strive to sharpen his powers of observation until this is possible.

Two general principles are important in evaluating the possibility of tendon injury. First, a specific movement may be decreased or absent even while the involved tendon is intact. There are several explanations for this. Motion of the tendon may cause pain because of movement of surrounding injured structures. The patient may not understand what movement is desired. This can be demonstrated by the examiner, and the patient can produce the desired movement with his uninvolved hand. Nerve injuries may prevent the patient from accomplishing the desired motion even though the tendon is intact. The second and seemingly contradictory principle is that some motion may be present despite severe injury to the tendon. This can happen for a variety of reasons. Several tendons may produce the same motion; for example, the long flexors can flex the wrist, the metacarpophalangeal, proximal interphalangeal, and distal interphalangeal joints; laceration of the prime flexors of these joints may be masked by this overplay. When the tendons become anatomically independent, a specific test will usually allow determination of whether the tendon is intact. Communicans connecting adjacent tendons may provide motion in several fingers through a single intact tendon. These communicans are usually present on the dorsum of the hand but very rarely on the volar surface.

*Specific tests for tendon continuity.* The first test for tendon continuity is undisturbed observation of the injured hand. If a flexor digitorum profundus tendon is cut, the finger lies extended from its normal position only if its companion sublimis is divided (Fig. 11-1). If the flexor digitorum profundus is divided and the companion sublimis is intact, only the distal interphalangeal joint will assume an extended posture. When the sublimis is divided and the profundus is intact, the finger will assume a normal posture. These characteristic postures become more noticeable when the wrist is dorsiflexed. Conversely,

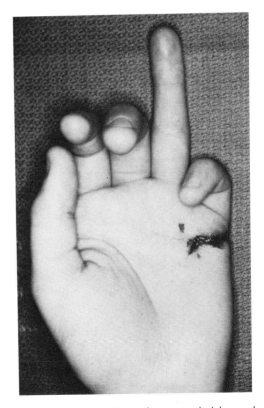

**Fig. 11-1.** The ring finger lies extended beyond its natural position because of division of both the flexor digitorum superficialis and flexor digitorum profundus. Deformity would be exaggerated by dorsiflexion of the wrist. A typical tidy wound.

division of the extensor tendon allows the digit to lie more flexed than the uninjured digits, and volar flexion of the wrist exaggerates the asymmetry.

The second test is to determine the amount of resting tension in the fingers. The resistance to passive extension is compared in injured and uninjured fingers. The amount of resistance to passive flexion when the extensor tendons are lacerated is variable; thus, the test is less useful. A combination of observation, passive motion, and resistance to passive motion is the only method of indirectly assessing tendon injury in the unconscious patient.

Some of the muscle tendon units have very short tendons; however, the effects of transection of the muscle itself will be described because these muscles may be divided by lacerations in the forearm and hand.

*Volar surface.* To discuss levels of tendon laceration and evaluating results, the hand and forearm have been divided into five zones (Fig. 11-2). About 70% of the tendon lacerations are located in zones 1 and 2. Accurate testing for division of the flexor digitorum sublimis and/or the flexor digitorum profundus in these areas is of great clinical importance. If there is no active flexion at either the proximal or distal interphalangeal joint, then both the flexor digitorum sublimis and the flexor digitorum profundus have been divided. If the patient is unable to flex the distal interphalangeal joint, the flexor digitorum profundus has been divided. If the patient is unable to fully flex the proximal interphalangeal joint of the long, ring, or little fingers while the remaining fingers are held in extension by the examiner, then the flexor digitorum sublimis to that finger is divided. This test is less helpful in the index finger, since the flexor digitorum profundus may be more independent of the profundus group. In fact, in some individuals all of the profundus tendons may be functionally independent. The lack of active motion at the

interphalangeal joint of the thumb indicates that the flexor pollicis longus has been divided. However, if the thumb metacarpophalangeal joint is held in extension, the intrinsic muscles of the thumb can produce enough flexion of the distal phalanx to confuse the novice.

If the flexor pollicis longus is intact, function of the flexor pollicis brevis must be tested by direct palpation at its insertion into the radial sesamoid bone. It is very difficult to separate the function of the opponens pollicis and the abductor pollicis brevis. Specific examination for the integrity of these muscles should be carried out in all lacerations involving the thenar emi-

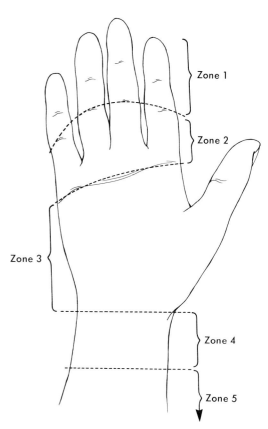

**Fig. 11-2.** Palmar view of the hand and wrist to show the zones into which the hand has been divided for purposes of discussion.

nence. Integrity of the adductor pollicis is indicated by the ability of the patient to ulnarly adduct the thumb without producing flexion of the interphalangeal joint (Fig. 11-3). Continuity of the abductor digiti minimi and the first dorsal interosseous can be determined by having the patient abduct the little finger and the index finger respectively while the muscle bellies are palpated directly.

One can palpate the tendon of the flexor carpi radialis by having the patient simultaneously radially deviate and flex the wrist against resistance. The integrity of the flexor carpi ulnaris is evaluated by palpation of the tendon during simultaneous flexion and ulnar deviation of the wrist against resistance. Continuity of the palmaris longus is demonstrated by having the patient flex the wrist approximately 10 degrees and oppose the thumb and little finger lightly while simultaneously trying to move the little finger and thumb out of opposition (Fig. 11-4). The muscle belly and tendon of the brachioradialis can be palpated along the radial border of the forearm during elbow flexion against resistance. The remaining intrinsic muscles of the hand cannot be examined directly.

*Dorsal surface.* On the dorsal surface of the hand and forearm approximately 20% of extensor tendon lacerations occur in zone 1, 50% in zone 2, and 20% in zone 3; the other two zones share the re-

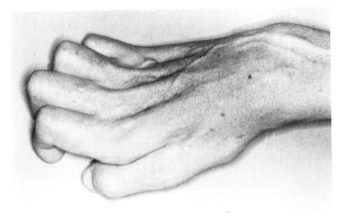

**Fig. 11-3.** Inability to abduct the thumb against the index finger without producing flexion of the interphalangeal joint (Froment's sign).

**Fig. 11-4.** The maneuver to demonstrate the palmaris longus tendon.

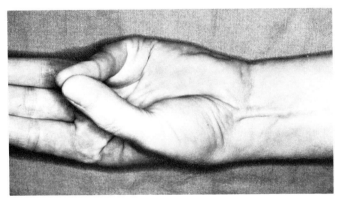

mainder (Fig. 11-5). Thus, about 70% of tendon lacerations on both the dorsal and volar surfaces of the hand and forearm are located in zones 1 and 2. Lacerations over the middle phalanx and at the distal interphalangeal joint are associated with loss of active extension of the distal interphalangeal joint. Tendon division at the level of the proximal interphalangeal joint may be difficult to detect, but weakness of extension of that joint can be detected. The true boutonnière deformity is almost never seen acutely (Fig. 11-6). Division of the extensor digitorum communis over the metacarpophalangeal joint eliminates extension of the metacarpophalangeal joint when the inter-

phalangeal joints are flexed. If the interphalangeal joints are allowed to extend, the extensor apparatus may allow some extension at the metacarpophalangeal joint. Laceration of the independent extensors of the index and little fingers becomes obvious when the long and ring fingers are flexed and the patient is asked to extend the index and little fingers. Division of the extensor pollicis longus will usually eliminate active extension at the interphalangeal joint of the thumb. Weak extension of the interphalangeal joint of the thumb may be produced by the insertion of the adductor pollicis into the extensor hood of the thumb. Lacerations of the extensor digitorum com-

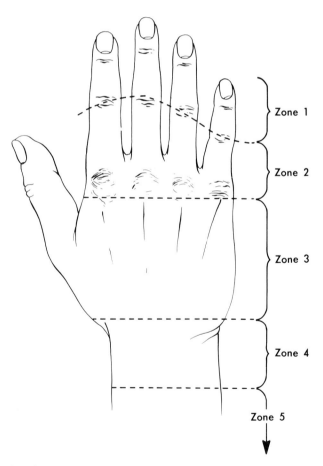

**Fig. 11-5.** The dorsal view of the hand and wrist showing the zones into which the hand has been divided for purposes of discussion.

munis over the dorsum of the hand and at the wrist result in a lack of active extension at the metacarpophalangeal joint against resistance. The tendon of the abductor pollicis longus can be palpated in the anatomical snuff box as the patient radially abducts the thumb with the metacarpophalangeal and interphalangeal joints held in extension. The extensor pollicis brevis can be examined by the same maneuver while the interphalangeal joint of the thumb is held in flexion. At times it is quite difficult to separate the tendons of the extensor pollicis brevis and the abductor pollicis longus by palpation.

It is difficult to examine separately the extensor carpi radialis longus and brevis tendons, but both can be palpated during dorsiflexion and radial deviation of the hand. The extensor carpi ulnaris can be palpated at the ulnar border of the wrist as the hand is deviated ulnarward and dorsiflexed. Continuity of the supinator is indicated by the patient's ability to strongly supinate the forearm while the elbow is held in extension.

Tests of hand function requiring patient cooperation are very difficult in young children or inebriated individuals. Observation of the posture at rest and during gross movement often reveals the extent of injury. Exploration of the wound in the operating room while the patient is anesthetized and the arm rendered bloodless is required in some patients to determine the extent of injury.

### Indications and contraindications for primary repair of tendon lacerations

In general, wounds can be classified as either tidy or untidy (Figs. 11-1 and 11-7). A typical tidy wound is one inflicted by a clean sharp object that produces a minimum of concomitant injury, for example, the wound incurred by a housewife who lacerates a tendon on a broken glass. An untidy wound is associated with a crushing injury that forces foreign material into the tissues, for example, the wound caused by a punch press covered with oil and grease. A gray area exists between the two extremes. Tidy wounds can be considered for primary repair of the injured structures, but untidy wounds must be converted to tidy wounds before one can proceed with a plan of definitive repair.

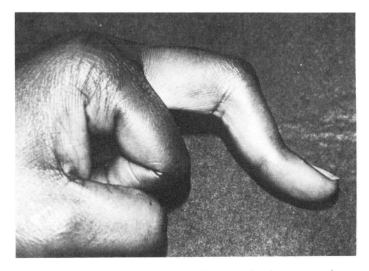

**Fig. 11-6.** A classic boutonnière or buttonhole deformity after laceration of extensor tendon over proximal interphalangeal joint.

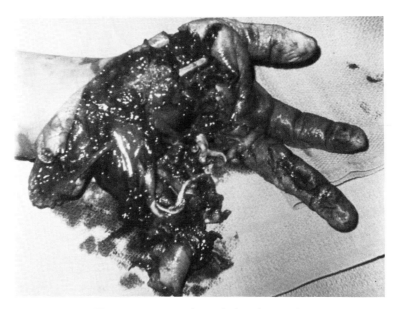

**Fig. 11-7.** A typical untidy hand wound.

There has not been a well-controlled study to correlate the incidence of infection with the interval between wounding and tendon repair. Most authors have been unable to demonstrate any relationship between the interval from wounding to repair and the incidence of postoperative wound infection. Usually repair can be safely accomplished up to 12 hours after wounding. More recently the concept of delayed primary repair has been championed. This involves closing the skin wound, treating the patient with systemic antibiotics, and performing a definitive repair after several days. There are obvious advantages to this approach, but, again, it has not been proved to be the most effective technique.

*Indications for primary repair.* Tendon lacerations within the hand and forearm, except on the volar surface between the distal palmar crease and the flexion crease of the proximal interphalangeal joint (zone 2) (Fig. 11-2), should be repaired primarily unless specific contraindications are present. Evidence in recent years has indicated that even in zone 2, lacerations can be repaired

primarily, and excellent results have been accomplished by surgeons whose practice is limited principally to hand surgery and who have had extensive experience in tendon repair. Primary tendon repair in zone 2 may be indicated in patients of all ages for some, but not all, surgeons.

In children under 8 (and possibly all those under 12), primary tendon repair should be performed regardless of the site of the laceration. Similarly, patients over the age of 50 should undergo primary tendon repair. These statements are based on the functional results that will be presented subsequently (p. 314).

*Contraindications to primary repair.* All agree that either obvious infection or gross contamination is an absolute contraindication to primary tendon repair regardless of the site of the laceration. In fact, closure of such contaminated wounds is not advised. Human bite injuries are a classic example; these injuries most frequently involve the metacarpophalangeal joints of the ring and little fingers. Delayed primary repair of the tendons may be utilized in

## GENERAL TECHNIQUES OF TENDON REPAIR

Frequently the tendon ends are not readily visible through the laceration site, and greater exposure must be obtained by enlargement of the wound with proximal and distal extensions of the lacerations (Fig. 11-8). One should not compromise the repair simply because exposure is inadequate. When the wound is enlarged, the flexion creases should not be crossed at right angles, but the incisions should be modified to allow optimum exposure and prevent contracture across a flexion crease. Occasionally the traumatic wound provides adequate exposure; that is, the tendon ends can be seen during flexion of the joints of the hand or wrist. Similarly, extension of the same joints frequently exposes the cut ends of extensor tendons. For lacerations in zone 2, if the proximal end of the tendon is not visible in the wound, a 2-cm transverse incision at the distal palmar crease overlying the course of the tendon will allow retraction of the proximal end of the tendon into the wound (Fig. 11-9). After the proximal suture is accomplished, a Silastic rod is passed through the proximal opening of the fibro-osseous tunnel and out the distal laceration site. The suture is passed through the Silastic rod, and the rod is extracted distally. This technique allows adequate exposure for completing the anastomosis and replaces the tendon in its normal position.

The search for the ideal suture for tendon repair continues. Experimental studies reveal a considerable variation in the inflammatory reaction around suture materials. The most severe inflammatory reaction occurs around the catgut suture, whereas the least severe reaction is observed when monofilament steel is utilized. (See the following list.)

REACTION TO SUTURES FROM GREATEST TO LEAST

Catgut, plain
Catgut, chromicized

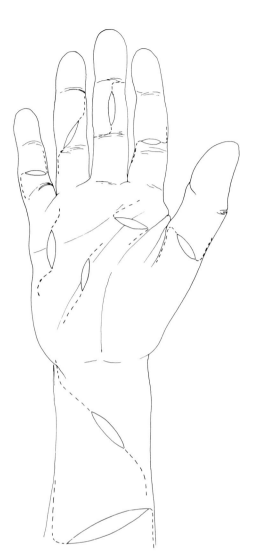

**Fig. 11-8.** Appropriate extensions of lacerations in order to obtain greater exposure.

this situation. In the extremely untidy wound, primary repair of any structure, except possibly the skin, is contraindicated.

Care of a hand injury in a patient with concomitant life-threatening injuries (for example, crushed chest, intra-abdominal hemorrhage, brain damage), should be placed in proper prospective. As soon as these more life-threatening injuries have been stabilized, the injured hand can be treated.

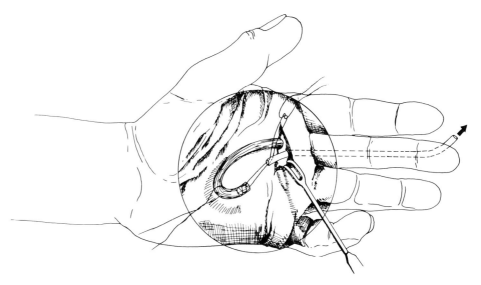

**Fig. 11-9.** A Silastic rod has been passed through the digital sheath to allow passage of the proximal cut end of the tendon into the original wound.

Silk
Cotton
Polyester
Polyglycolic acid
Polypropylene
Nylon
Monofilament steel

The tensile strength or knot-pull breaking strength of sutures varies widely. Cotton and catgut are the weakest, whereas monofilament steel is the strongest. (See the following list.)

**KNOT-PULL BREAKING STRENGTH FROM LEAST TO GREATEST**

Cotton
Catgut
Silk
Polypropylene
Nylon
Polyglycolic acid
Polyester
Monofilament steel

Consequently, monofilament steel has gained wide acceptance. Steel is difficult to use, however, primarily because of its tendency to kink. Monofilament nylon, braided polyester, polypropylene, and Tef-

lon-coated Dacron all have their champions. Results of clinical studies comparing the use of wire and other suture materials have been equivocal.

**Flexor tendon repair**

Although a wide variety of techniques are available, the Bunnell buried or permanent stitch (Fig. 11-10) and the double right-angle stitch (Fig. 11-11) are the most popular. The buried or permanent version of the Bunnell stitch is usually accomplished with a double-armed monofilament steel suture; the needles have tapered ends. There is no reason to grasp a tendon end with a hemostat. Even though it appears clumsy, the tendon ends can be managed easily with moistened fingers. Occasionally the tendon must be transfixed utilizing a straight needle in the wound. However, transfixion creates adhesions and should be done only when absolutely necessary, not simply for convenience. Beginning 1.5 cm from the end of the tendon, the needle is passed transversely through the tendon. Both needles are reinserted to cross the tendon at a 45-degree angle. This is re-

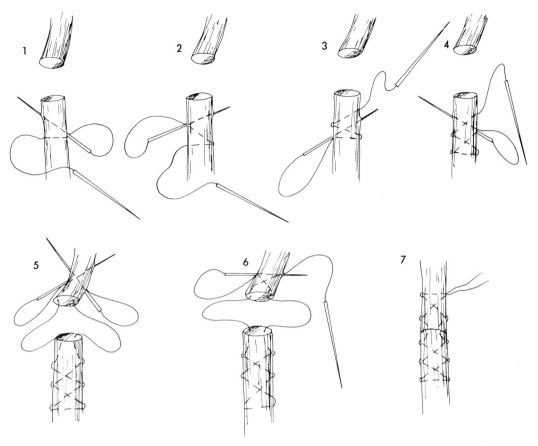

**Fig. 11-10.** The Bunnell buried or crisscross suture (see text for details; see also Fig. 11-22).

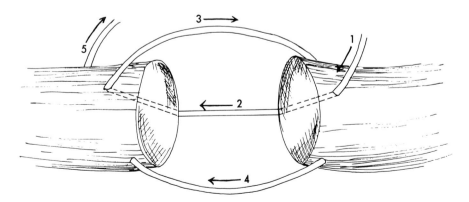

**Fig. 11-11.** The double right-angle suture. The numbers indicate the steps in its insertion.

peated once or twice before the needles are inserted almost parallel with the tendon to exit on the border of the free end of the tendon. The distal part of the anastomosis is accomplished by inserting the needles just inside the free edge of the tendon end and bringing the needles out 5 mm from the cut end. The crisscrossing suture is continued for at least two crosses. To allow approximation of the cut ends, the tendon ends are coapted while the sutures are on *opposite* sides of the tendon. Finally, one suture end is held taut while the other is passed transversely across the tendon. The suture is tied snugly to produce an accordion effect on the tendon ends. After the tendon anastomosis is returned to its original bed, the involved finger is put through a range of motion and the tendon anastomosis observed to confirm that the tendon ends are snugly approximated. If a gap appears between the tendon ends, the anastomosis must be taken down and repeated. Repeat suturing is not very satisfactory and can be avoided by paying attention to de-

tails. When wire suture is employed, the buried Bunnell stitch can be used anywhere on the flexor surface except in zone 2. The distinct angular motion of the tendons in zone 2 tends to produce fracture of wire sutures. If a synthetic suture is used, the buried Bunnell stitch can be used anywhere on the flexor surface. Usually 3-0 or 4-0 is used for finger flexor tendons, and 2-0 or 3-0 suture is used for the wrist flexor tendon ends.

Lacerations in zone 1 that leave less than 1.5 cm of distal tendon stump can be treated by advancement and reinsertion of the tendon into the bony distal phalanx (Fig. 11-12). A pullout wire is looped around the double-armed wire suture, and a Bunnell stitch is inserted in the proximal tendon end. The periosteum of the distal phalanx is elevated at the insertion of the profundus tendon, and a drill hole is placed through the phalanx to exit through the nail. A straight Keith needle is placed in the drill hole, and the suture ends are threaded through the needle for advance-

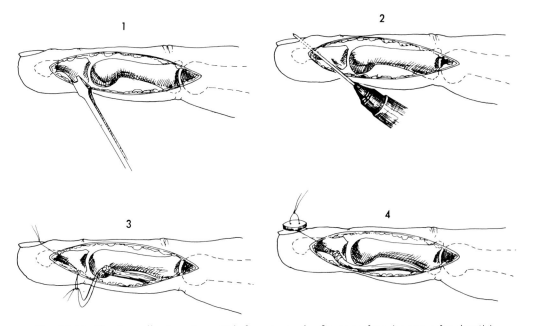

**Fig. 11-12.** The Bunnell reinsertion stitch for use on the flexor surface (see text for details).

ment. The suture ends are tied over a button on the nailbed. Again the anastomosis site must be inspected to ensure against soft tissue interposition or failure to snugly approximate the tendon end to the raw bony surface. After 3 weeks the suture is divided beneath the button and pulled out with the proximal pullout wire. The use of synthetic suture material makes the incorporation of a pullout suture superfluous. When one of the synthetic sutures is cut beneath the button, the suture is easily extracted by pulling on the remaining end.

The Bunnell pullout stitch (Fig. 11-13) can be used to circumvent the fracturing of the buried Bunnell stitch in zone 2 repairs and to avoid leaving permanent suture material in the hand or forearm. A pullout wire is looped around the double-armed suture. The crisscross technique is used in the proximal end of the tendon. In the distal tendon segment, a variety of techniques have been used, including a single cross or simply passing the sutures through a length of tendon substance. The distal ends of the suture are brought through the skin and tied over a button. After 3 to 4 weeks the suture tied over the button is divided and the entire suture extracted by pulling on the proximal pullout

wire. Unfortunately, snug approximation of the tendon ends is not accomplished, and the anastomosis can separate. As a consequence, the Bunnell pullout stitch has not gained wide popularity.

To overcome the proximal pull of the muscle bellies, Verdan developed a technique of blocking proximal tendon gliding. The tendon ends are repaired with four simple sutures of 6-0 silk after the digital sheath is widely resected. To prevent disruption of this anastomosis, a 0.7-mm stainless steel wire is passed transversely through the skin and the digital sheath to impale the tendon proximal to the anastomosis. In a similar maneuver a second needle is placed distal to the anastomosis (see Fig. 4-15). If the anastomosis is so far distal that the distal wire cannot gain adequate purchase, the distal interphalangeal joint is immobilized in flexion with a transarticular Kirschner wire. This technique can be used for injuries in zones 1 and 2. An external dressing augments immobilization. The transfixion wires are removed after 3 weeks.

Kleinert recommends an end-to-end anastomosis utilizing synthetic suture material. A buried 5-0 Bunnell suture is used for the tendon anastomosis. In addition, a 6-0 running suture repairs the periphery of the

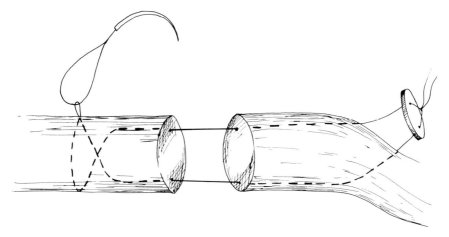

**Fig. 11-13.** The Bunnell pullout suture. The sutures may be passed through the distal tendon for variable distances.

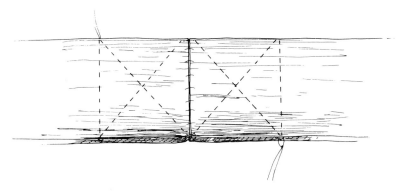

**Fig. 11-14.** Kleinert technique, using a modified Bunnell and a running stitch.

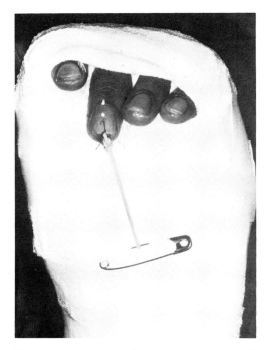

**Fig. 11-15.** Young and Harmon traction technique to allow protected early active motion.

tendon ends (Fig. 11-14). Postoperatively, dynamic splinting of the injured finger by a rubber band attached to the nail is used, as originally described by Young and Harmon in 1960 (Fig. 11-15).

Another technique for repair in zone 2 is a modified Mason stitch (Fig. 11-16). This stitch was intended to have sufficient strength to allow early active motion. In experimental tests the suture ruptured or pulled out in a significant number of trials. Clinical experience has not been sufficient to allow adequate assessment.

Tsuge has introduced a new intratendon suture technique. His technique usually requires more time than the Bunnell technique. An assistant must retract the edges of the longitudinal opening in the tendon while the sutures are inserted. Tsuge reported satisfactory tendon gliding using his technique. No other authors have reported using Tsuge's technique.

Simple horizontal mattress stitches allow rapid approximation of tendon ends and can be used in zone 3 (Fig. 11-17). The double right-angle stitch is also useful in zone 3. It is inserted using a single-arm suture and passing the suture from superficial to deep through the proximal tendon, from deep to superficial through the distal tendon, then from side to side through the proximal tendon and side to side through the distal tendon (Fig. 11-11). One must be certain that the central cores of the tendon are snugly approximated. When sutures are placed only through the periphery of the tendon, disruption may occur because the cores of the tendons are not approximated and the dead space becomes filled with a hematoma.

No one has reported a comparative study of different suture techniques in patients. Several authors have evaluated tensile

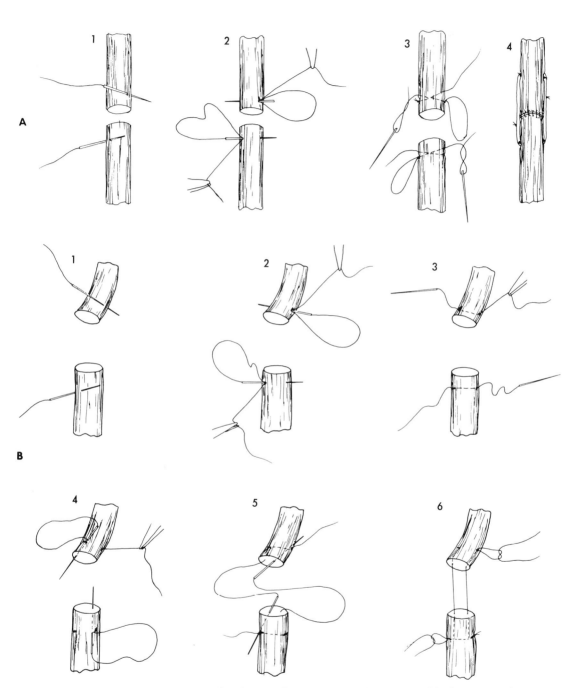

**Fig. 11-16. A,** Mason's original technique for suturing tendons. **B,** Modified Mason technique (Kessler), developed to allow early active motion (see text for details).

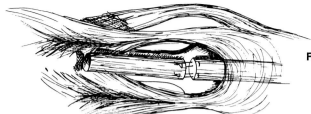

**Fig. 11-17.** Horizontal mattress suture.

**Fig. 11-18.** Figure-8 technique.

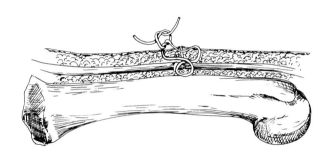

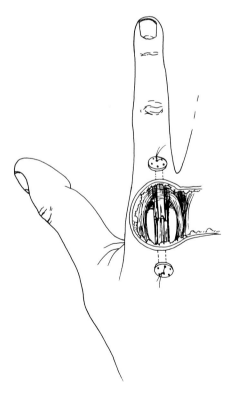

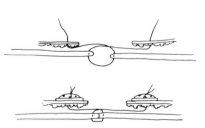

**Fig. 11-19.** Far-near–near-far technique.

strength of various tendon repairs. We compared tendon gliding after different suture techniques. Using the chicken as an experimental animal, we compared the Bunnell, Kleinert, modified Mason-Allen, and Tsuge repairs. There were no significant differences in tensile strength, scar deformation, or actual tendon gliding.

### Extensor tendon repair

The Bunnell buried stitch described previously (p. 300) (Fig. 11-10) can be used

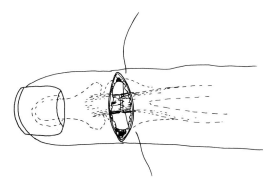

**Fig. 11-20.** Roll stitch. Stitch enters and leaves through intact skin and is designed to be removed.

in zones 4 and 5 and the proximal portion of zone 3 of the extensor surface. In the distal portion of zone 3 and in zones 1 and 2, Bunnell advocated a figure-8 stitch (Fig. 11-18) to approximate the tendon ends and the skin simultaneously. Occasionally, inadequate coaptation of the tendon ends is obtained with this suture. A far-near-far stitch (Fig. 11-19) that is tied over buttons can be used in this area. It is inserted by passing the sutures through the skin over the proximal tendon, then from superficial to deep through the distal tendon, then deep to superficial through the proximal tendon, and then out the skin over the distal tendon. Two sutures are used and tied over a button (Fig. 11-19). A simple over-and-over running stitch, also called the roll stitch (Fig. 11-20), is useful for approximating the extensor tendons in zones 1, 2, and 3. Occasionally the insertion of the extensor tendon into the distal phalanx will require reattachment to the pony phalanx (Fig. 11-21). The presence of a bone chip in the avulsed tendon greatly simplifies this procedure, because the tendon at this level is so thin that sutures

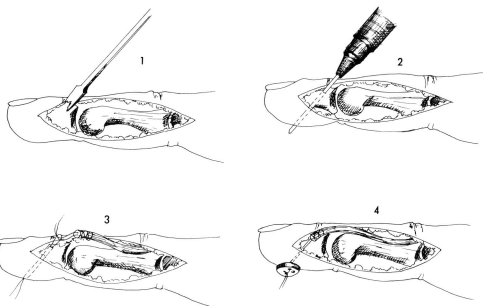

**Fig. 11-21.** Reinsertion technique for the extensor tendon (see text for details).

readily pull out of the end. The presence of the bony chip gives substance to the tendon, making suture retention more reliable.

### PRIMARY REPAIR OF FLEXOR TENDONS OF THE FINGERS AND THUMB

Most authors have recommended that primarily repaired completely lacerated flexor tendons be immobilized for 21 days. The joints upon which a particular tendon acts are immobilized in about 30 degrees of flexion. This immobilization was recommended for lacerations in all zones. Kleinert, Duran, Emery, and others have advocated active or passive motion beginning a few days after surgery. No author has reported the effects of early motion applied randomly, nor has anyone used statistical analysis. Using the chicken as an experimental animal, we attempted to determine when the completely lacerated flexor tendon should be mobilized. In primarily repaired completely lacerated chicken flexor tendons, mobilization 11 days after injury resulted in significantly greater tensile strength than mobilization at 0, 3, 7, or 21 days. No change in tendon motion could be demonstrated in the mobilized tendons. Only if mobilization was begun 3 days after injury was the rupture rate increased. The only evidence for immobilizing tendons for 21 days is anecdotal. We have started a clinical trial beginning mobilization 11 days after injury.

### Flexor tendon repairs in zone 1

Tendon lacerations or avulsions of the tendon at its insertion in zone 1 involve only the profundus tendon and should be treated by either direct suture of the tendon ends using Bunnell's buried technique (Fig. 11-10), Bunnell's pullout wire technique (Fig. 11-13), Verdan's technique (see Fig. 4-15), or Kleinert's technique (Fig. 11-14). If the laceration lies within 1.5 cm of the insertion of the profundus tendon, the proximal tendon end can be advanced and reimplanted into the bony phalanx using Bunnell's reinsertion technique (Fig. 11-12). When an advancement procedure is indicated, it provides the best results. Similar techniques can be utilized in the thumb. In all techniques requiring direct suture of the tendon ends, the portion of the fibrous sheath overlying the normal range of excursion of the anastomasis is excised.

Rigg advocates transferring a slip of the sublimis tendon to the distal severed profundus tendon. His patients obtained either some active flexion or a tenodesis effect. Nine patients obtained 11 degrees of active flexion; however, the average loss of extension was about 25 degrees. His technique is conceptually interesting but has not been generally accepted.

### Flexor tendon repairs in zone 2

For years many have advocated that primary management of lacerations of the flexor digitorum profundus alone or in combination with the flexor digitorum sublimis should be by simple closure of the skin followed by tendon grafting as a secondary procedure. Although Kleinert and Verdan have reported excellent results from primary repair (Fig. 11-22), it should be

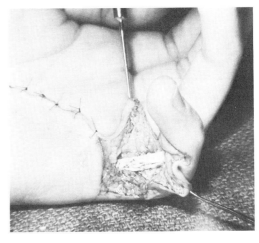

**Fig. 11-22.** Primary repair of flexor sublimis and profundus tendons in zone 2.

noted that from 20% to 40% of the patients require a secondary tenolysis in order to gain these results.

A primary tenodesis (Fig. 11-23) of the distal interphalangeal joint has been advocated when only the flexor digitorum profundus has been divided. Certainly tenodesis will allow an earlier return to work than either primary repair or secondary tendon grafting of lacerations in this area. The tenodesis may eventually elongate and necessitate an arthrodesis (Fig. 11-24) of the distal interphalangeal joint. Preoperatively, the advantages and disadvantages of tenodesis must be discussed with the patient. Evaluation of the patient's desires and needs may help determine whether active motion at the distal interphalangeal joint is of special importance.

In the first type of tenodesis (Fig. 11-23, A), the distal stump of the profundus

tendon should reach the shaft of the middle phalanx. The distal interphalangeal joint is held in 30 to 40 degrees of flexion with a transarticular Kirschner wire. A Bunnell pullout wire suture is placed in the proximal end of the distal tendon stump. The periosteum is removed from the volar surface of the middle phalanx, and two drill holes are drilled in the middle phalanx passing from the volar to the dorsal surface. The ends of the suture are passed through these drill holes, and the suture is tied over a button on the dorsum of the finger. The pullout wire suture is removed at 3 weeks, and the Kirschner wire is removed after 5 to 6 weeks.

If insufficient distal tendon remains (certainly one should have entertained an advancement procedure), an arthrodesis of the distal interphalangeal joint may be indicated. The proximal and distal bone ends on either side of the joint are resected in

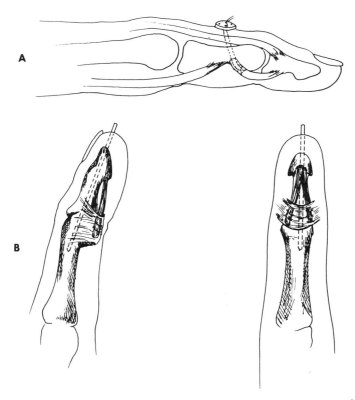

**Fig. 11-23.** Two techniques for tenodesis. Technique in **A** requires greater tendon length.

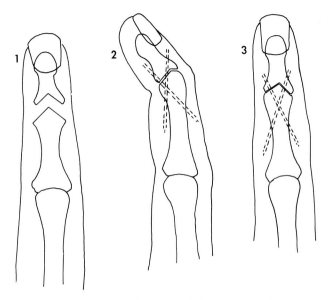

**Fig. 11-24.** Technique for arthrodesis of distal interphalangeal joint.

the shape of a V. The joint is placed in 30 to 40 degrees of flexion and immobilized with transarticular Kirschner wires (Fig. 11-24). The results of primary repair and secondary tendon grafts are compared in the subsequent section.

### Flexor tendon repairs in zone 3

When repairing flexor tendons in zone 3, one should take great care to develop as favorable a bed for the tendon anastomosis as possible. As the wound is enlarged, the skin flaps are reflected from the palmar fascia so that a thick layer of fat is left attached to the skin. The palmar fascia forms compartments for the flexor tendons, and these rigid fascial structures must be excised to prevent the formation of nonyielding adhesions. After the anastomosis is complete, its bed is formed by the lumbrical muscle laterally, the fatty tissues of the palm dorsally, and the subcutaneous tissue volarly.

When only the profundus tendon is lacerated, it should be repaired primarily with the classic Bunnell stitch (Fig. 11-10). Lacerations of both the profundus and superficialis tendons in adults should be treated by resection of the superficialis tendon and repair of the profundus tendon. In children both the flexor digitorum superficialis and flexor digitorum profundus tendon can be repaired. Division of the superficialis tendon alone may go unrecognized, but, if recognized, should be repaired.

### Flexor tendon repairs in zone 4

Deep lacerations involving the ligaments forming the carpal tunnel result in extremely dense scar formation. Every effort should be made to displace the anastomosis away from the ligamentous injuries. Flexion of the metacarpophalangeal joints and the wrist is of value in displacing the anastomosis.

When the flexor digitorum superficialis and the flexor digitorum profundus tendons are divided, the flexor digitorum superficialis tendon to the index finger, the digitorum profundus tendons, and the flexor pollicis longus are repaired in adults. However, in children all divided tendons may be repaired. If only the flexor digitorum superficialis tendons are divided, they are repaired. Occasionally only the flexor digitorum profundus tendons are divided and, of course, they should be repaired. All tendons at this level can be repaired utilizing the buried Bunnell stitch (Fig. 11-10), the pullout Bunnell stitch (Fig. 11-13), or the double right-angle stitch (Fig. 11-11). In all cases resection of the overlying flexor retinaculum is required.

### Flexor tendon repairs in zone 5

Primary repair for all combinations of tendon lacerations is indicated in zone 5. If the tendons, musculotendinous junction, or muscles are not repaired, scar will bridge the gap but leave the muscle tendon unit longer than normal, considerably reducing its functional capacities.

Repair by the techniques used in zone 4 is satisfactory. When lacerations involve the muscle bellies, these should be repaired with great care to maintain function and strength.

### Treatment of partial tendon lacerations

Most authors have recommended that partial tendon lacerations be sutured. We have shown that suturing partial tendon lacerations in chickens decreases both the tensile strength and gliding. Also, immobilizing partial tendon lacerations in chickens causes decreased tensile strength and gliding. Furthermore, 6 to 7 days after injury is the ideal time to begin mobilization of the partial tendon laceration in chickens. To confirm our experimental data, we treated 17 patients with 20 partial flexor tendon lacerations by not suturing the tendon and by early mobilization of the digit. Patients were allowed only gentle active motion. These partial tendon lacerations varied from 25% to 95% of the cross-sectional area. Sixteen of the patients obtained excellent function of the digit, and one obtained good function. None of the partial tendon lacerations ruptured, and no patient developed trigger finger. We believe that partial flexor tendon lacerations should not be sutured and that mobilization

of the injured digit begin 6 to 7 days after the injury in cooperative patients.

### Primary insertion of Silastic spacer

In six reported patients either a Silastic tendon graft or a simple Silastic rod has been implanted as a primary procedure. Van der Meulen sutured the Silastic rod to the distal end of the flexor digitorum profundus but did not suture the proximal end. Nicolle anastomosed the Silastic tendon to the distal end of the flexor digitorum profundus at the fingertip and the proximal end to the same tendon in the midpalm. In all cases, autogenous tendon grafting was performed after 2 to 3 months. The active range of motion in four of these patients varied from 60% to 91% of normal, and the active range of motion in two is unknown. Nicolle felt that the results with primary insertion of the Silastic tendon were slightly poorer than those in which the Silastic tendon graft was inserted secondarily (followed ultimately by an autogenous tendon graft done at a third operation).

### Primary flexor tendon grafting

Flynn reported eleven cases of primary tendon grafting with good (fingertip touched palm) or fair (fingertip flexed to within 1½ inches of palm, and 45 degrees of active flexion at each interphalangeal joint) results. He recommended a more extensive evaluation of primary tendon grafting.

Harrison has reported the results of both primary and delayed primary (7 to 14 days after injury) tendon grafting. He has reviewed his results with 30 primary and 30 delayed primary flexor tendon grafts. He utilizes a nylon figure-8 stitch placed in the distal end of the tendon graft to attach it to the distal remaining flexor digitorum profundus stump. The proximal anastomosis is carried out by placing the figure-8 stitch in the proximal end of the flexor digitorum profundus and a separate figure-8 stitch in the proximal end of the tendon graft. Finally, these two sutures are tied together. He utilized both palmaris longus and extensor digitorum longus tendons for tendon grafts. A discussion of the results of his technique is given on p. 321.

Three cases of primary tendon grafting for injuries of the flexor pollicis longus overlying the shaft of the metacarpal have been reported. The details of anastomoses were not given. The authors stated that postoperative motion was satisfactory in all cases but did not give the actual range of motion of the individual joints.

## PRIMARY REPAIR OF PROPER FLEXORS OF THE RADIOCARPAL JOINT

Isolated injuries of the proper flexors of the radiocarpal joint should be repaired. In particular, an intact flexor carpi ulnaris is of vital importance to the person who must use a hammer. Repair is with a buried Bunnell stitch (Fig. 11-10) (using 2-0 or 3-0 suture material), and the wrist is held in a position of approximately 30 degrees flexion for a period of 5 weeks. The fingers are allowed to have active motion throughout the 5 weeks.

## PRIMARY REPAIR OF EXTENSOR TENDONS OF THE FINGERS AND THUMB

As with the flexor tendons, the extensor tendons have been divided into zones for discussion purposes (Fig. 11-5).

### Extensor tendon injuries in zone 1

Open lacerations of tendons in zone 1 produce the mallet finger deformity and are treated by primary suture. Permanent sutures of silk, nylon, polyester, and so forth, placed in a horizontal mattress fashion are suitable (Fig. 11-17). Stainless steel wire can be used but should not be left in place permanently, since it frequently causes irritation of the skin. A continuous over-and-over pullout roll stitch works satisfactorily (Fig. 11-20). If insufficient distal stump remains for an anastomosis, the tendon

should be reinserted by the pullout wire technique (Fig. 11-21). In general, tendon suture in this area only approximates the tendon ends, and immobilization is relied upon to maintain this approximation. A smooth Kirschner wire crossing the interphalangeal joint provides excellent immobilization while tendon healing is taking place. Kirschner wire immobilization is required for 5 to 6 weeks, after which an external splint is used for 2 to 3 weeks. Forceful active movement is avoided until 7 to 8 weeks after repair. Maximal recovery of motion may require a year.

When the joint is extensively damaged and tendon substance is lost, primary arthrodesis (Fig. 11-24) is indicated. The joints should be arthrodesed as follows: index finger, 15 degrees flexion; long finger, 20 degrees flexion; ring finger, 30 degrees flexion; and little finger, 30 degrees flexion. Closed disruptions of the extensor tendon in the absence of bony fracture should be treated by transarticular Kirschner wire fixation of the distal interphalangeal joint in slight hyperextension or by splinting with an external volar splint in slight hyperextension for at least 6 weeks (Fig. 11-25). If the deformity begins recurring after the splint or wire has been removed, additional immobilization for 3 to 4 weeks is required.

### Extensor tendon injuries in zone 2

Lacerations over the proximal interphalangeal joint predispose to the development of the classic boutonnière deformity (Fig. 11-6). However, this deformity is rarely observed immediately after an injury. The location of the wound and its apparent depth and weakness in extension are indications for exploration of the wound.

Acute closed injuries are treated by transarticular Kirschner wire fixation or external splinting of the proximal interphalangeal joint in full extension. The pin enters the midlateral line of the middle phalanx, and the end is left protruding. If Kirsch-

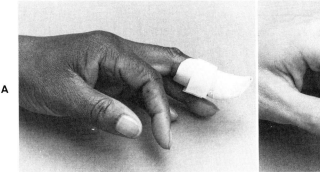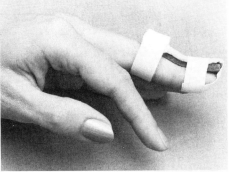

**Fig. 11-25.** Volar splint, **A,** and dorsal splint, **B,** used interchangeably for external immobilization of a mallet finger. A volar splint is used when dorsal skin wounds are present. A dorsal splint is used in patients who require more use of their fingertip pulp for daily activities. They may be used interchangeably, particularly if one kind or the other is poorly tolerated, for example, pressure changes.

ner wire fixation is used, the distal interphalangeal joint remains free, and early flexion is encouraged.

Open lacerations require the same immobilization of the proximal interphalangeal joint. In addition, the tendon is repaired with a continuous pullout wire (roll) (Fig. 11-22), interrupted (Fig. 11-19), or near-far–far-near (Fig. 11-21) stitch. Partial lacerations and lacerations involving one of the lateral bands are repaired with interrupted sutures. Partial lacerations are detected only by wound exploration. If these lacerations are unrepaired, delayed rupture may occur. Delayed ruptures are treated as closed injuries (as mentioned in the preceding paragraph).

Internal fixation is maintained for 5 weeks, and an external splint is worn for an additional 2 weeks. After the splint is removed, active extension of the proximal interphalangeal joint is encouraged, and the distal interphalangeal joint flexion is continued with manual support of the proximal interphalangeal joint. Active flexion of the proximal interphalangeal joint is begun 8 weeks after injury. Maximal recovery may take 1 year. In patients over 50 years of age, internal and external

splinting is used for 1 week less than the time previously mentioned.

Injury at the level of the metacarpophalangeal joint will produce weakness or complete absence of extension of the proximal phalanx. The tendon can be repaired with a horizontal mattress (Fig. 11-19), roll (Fig. 11-22) or near-far–far-near (Fig. 11-21) stitch. The wrist joint is splinted in 30 to 40 degrees of dorsiflexion, the metacarpophalangeal joint is splinted at 0 degrees, and the proximal and distal interphalangeal joints are splinted in 30 to 40 degrees of flexion. Active motion is again begun after 4 weeks, but strenuous active motion is withheld until 8 weeks after repair.

**Extensor tendon injuries in zone 3**

Lacerations in zone 3 are usually difficult to detect due to interconnection (communications) between the various extensor tendons and the presence of the proper digital extensors for the index and little fingers. However, weakness is evident in the involved finger when it is compared with the uninvolved fingers or the fingers on the uninjured hand. Repairs utilizing buried Bunnell (Fig. 11-10), pullout Bunnell (Fig. 11-13), horizontal mattress (Fig. 11-19), or near-far–far-near (Fig. 11-21) stitches all yield satisfactory results. Immobilization and remobilization are as described for zone 2.

### Extensor tendon injuries in zones 4 and 5

Tendon repair in zones 4 and 5 is accomplished with a Bunnell buried (Fig. 11-10) or pullout stitch (Fig. 11-13). The extensor retinaculum overlying the range of motion of the tendon anastomosis should be excised, but some remnant of the extensor retinaculum must be preserved to prevent dorsal bow-stringing. The amplitude of motion at this point is so slight that usually a portion of the retinaculum can be preserved. Lacerations of the tendons, musculotendinous junction, or muscle in the distal forearm should be repaired primarily, because the muscle will retract and scar in the retracted position if repair is delayed. Lacerations of the muscle should be treated by repair of the fascia, and the muscle belly should be treated with permanent horizontal mattress sutures. The wrist is splinted in 30 to 40 degrees of dorsiflexion, the metacarpophalangeal joints in 45 degrees of flexion, and the interphalangeal joints in 30 to 40 degrees of flexion for a period of 4 weeks. Active extension is encouraged and must return before full flexion is allowed.

### PRIMARY REPAIR OF PROPER EXTENSORS OF THE RADIOCARPAL JOINT

To obtain adequate exposure of the tendon ends, it may be necessary to enlarge the wound proximally or distally. The tendons are repaired with a Bunnell buried stitch (Fig. 11-10) of 2-0 or 3-0 suture material. If digital extensors have been injured, splinting is the same as noted for extensor zones 4 and 5. If the finger or thumb extensors have not been lacerated, they are allowed active motion with the wrist held in 30 to 40 degrees of dorsi-

flexion. Lacerations of the muscle substance or at the musculotendinous junction should be repaired by horizontal mattress stitches.

### RESULTS OF PRIMARY TENDON REPAIR
#### Results of primary repair of flexor tendons

The following is an analysis of virtually all the series of primary repair of tendon lacerations published in English since 1940. It is difficult to find one classification system that will allow a uniform comparison of results. Some authors measure the number of degrees of active flexion following repair, whereas others measure the distance between the pulp and the distal palmar crease during full flexion. Even among those who measure the distance between the pulp and the distal palmar crease, there is variance as to what constitutes an excellent, good, or fair result. Modification of the method proposed by Verdan for "evaluation of fingers subjected to reconstructive tendon surgery" seems to be the most accurate. This involves measuring the active range of motion at all three joints involved in the digit and comparing this active range of motion with the same digit in the uninjured hand.

The Clinical Assessment Committee of the American Society for Surgery of the Hand has recommended that all reports be classified in terms of total active motion. This figure is obtained by measuring the active flexion of each finger at the distal interphalangeal, proximal interphalangeal, and metacarpophalangeal joints. The lack of full extension in degrees at each joint is also measured. Total active motion is thus the difference between the sum of active flexion at each joint and the sum of the lack of extension at each joint.

Miller, in one of the earliest series, analyzed the results of primary repair in 300 patients. The tendons were sutured with the Mason stitch, and the hands were immobilized for approximately 3 weeks. An excellent result was a return to the preoperative status; a good result signified

80% restoration of normal function; and a fair result indicated 50% restoration of normal function. For comparison, the excellent results have been put into a single excellent-good category. His results are given in Table 11-1.

Posch reported the results after repair of 241 flexor tendon lacerations. These repairs were cared for by many different surgeons under the supervision of a few surgeons. The Mason stitch was utilized, and the patients' hands were immobilized for 3 weeks. The results were classified using the criteria of Miller. The results are shown in Table 11-1.

Siler reported the results of primary repair of 65 flexor tendons. He used the Mason buried stitch (Fig. 11-16, *A*) and immobilized the tendons for 3 weeks. A classification of results similar to that outlined by Miller was used. His results are shown in Table 11-1.

In 1950 and again in 1951, Rank and Wakefield reported a series of 137 repairs of flexor tendons. In general, secondary tendon grafting was carried out for injuries within zone 2, and the results are not included in this analysis. A Bunnell pullout (Fig. 11-13) or buried (Fig. 11-10) stitch of wire or silk suture was used. The hands were immobilized for 3 weeks postoperatively. The method of evaluation of the results is not clear but apparently is based on a comparison with normal function. A good result was one in which the patient had 90% to 100% of normal flexion and the fingertip reached the palm; a moderate result was 50% to 80% of normal flexion, and a poor result was less than 50% of normal flexion. The moderate group is considered fair in our Table 11-1.

Jennings reported the results of repair of 46 flexor tendons utilizing the barbed suture, in 1952 and 1955. He did not give details about the period of immobilization. His results were classified on the basis of measurements from the distal palmar crease to the fingertip. Flexion to within

1 inch of the distal palmar crease was considered a good result; flexion to within 2 inches was classified a fair result, and the remainder were classified poor results (Table 11-1).

Flynn reported 346 flexor tendon injuries that were treated in a city hospital by surgeons, many of whom had little training in hand surgery. The tendons were usually sutured with the buried Bunnell stitch (Fig. 11-10) using silk, but on occasion the pullout wire technique (Fig. 11-13) was used. The results were roughly equal in the two suture categories. The period of postoperative immobilization was not reported. He classified a good result as one in which the patient could touch the palm and a fair result as one in which the patient could bring the fingertip to within 1½ inches of the palm and could achieve 45 degrees of flexion at each interphalangeal joint (Table 11-1).

Kyle and Eyre-Brook reported results in 57 consecutive cases of repair of flexor tendon injuries in the hand. Flexor tendon grafting was carried out for those injuries within zone 2. The repair was accomplished by the Bunnell buried wire technique (Fig. 11-10), and the hands were immobilized for 3 weeks. Results were classified as excellent if the fingertip to palmar crease distance was ½ inch or less, and fair if the distance between the palmar crease and the pulp was ½ to 1¼ inches. The remaining cases were considered poor results.

Van't Hof used the Bunnell pullout stitch (Fig. 11-13) and steel suture. The hands were immobilized for about 3 weeks postoperatively. Results were classified in the terms described by Boyes, but we have reclassified the results using ½ inch or less fingertip to distal palmar crease distance as excellent to good and ½ inch to 1½ inches fingertip to distal palmar crease distance as fair results. In the thumb, an excellent or good result was considered to be obtained when 75% of normal func-

**Table 11-1.** Results of primary repair of flexor tendons

| | | Miller | Posch | Siler | Rank | Jennings | Flynn | Kyle | Van't Hof | Kelly | Lindsay | McCash | Madsen | Salvi | Jensen | Winston | Suzuki | Green | Urbaniak | Total |
|---|---|---|---|---|---|---|---|---|---|---|---|---|---|---|---|---|---|---|---|---|
| Zone 1 | Excellent-good | 2 | | 2 | 6 | | | | 7 | 5 | | | 1 | | 21 | 13 | | | | 60 |
| | Fair | | | 13 | | | | | 3 | 5 | | | 3 | | 4 | 5 | | | | 34 |
| | Poor | | | 1 | | | | | 1 | 4 | | | 2 | | 5 | 5 | | | | 19 |
| Zone 2 | Excellent-good | 32 | 10 | 1 | 6 | {25 | 14 | 2 | 6 | 42 | 6 | 4 | 34 | 14 | 16 | 28 | 3 | 31 | | 260 |
| | Fair | | 10 | 13 | 1 | | 29 | 1 | 3 | 25 | 20 | 5 | 5 | 6 | 4 | 4 | 2 | 10 | | 174 |
| | Poor | 15 | 6 | 2 | | 7 | 46 | | 7 | 34 | 5 | 2 | 4 | 2 | 4 | 4 | 3 | 7 | | 148 |
| Zone 3 | Excellent-good | 10 | 3 | 9 | 3 | 13 | 9 | | 3 | 10 | | 5 | | | | 21 | | | | 99 |
| | Fair | 1 | | 12 | | | 4 | | 2 | 4 | | 5 | | | | 4 | | | | 34 |
| | Poor | | 4 | 3 | | | 6 | | 1 | 6 | | 1 | | | | 2 | | | | 26 |
| Zone 4 | Excellent-good | 17 | 25 | | | | 60 | | 3 | 20 | | | | | | 22 | | | | 137 |
| | Fair | | 6 | | | | 28 | | 2 | 9 | | | | | | 0 | | | | 45 |
| | Poor | 1 | 3 | | | | 16 | | 1 | | | | | | | 1 | | | | 22 |
| Thumb | Excellent-good | 8 | 8 | 3 | 14 | | 16 | | 4 | 25 | | | | | 11 | | | | 14 | 107 |
| | Fair | | 4 | 6 | 4 | | 7 | 2 | 11 | 9 | | | | | 10 | | | | 12 | 57 |
| | Poor | 1 | | 2 | 2 | | 6 | | 8 | 6 | | | | | 7 | | | | 4 | 27 |
| | | | | | | | | | | | | | | | | | | | | 1249 |

tion resulted, and a fair result when 50% to 75% of normal flexion resulted (Table 11-1).

Kelly reported the results of primary repair of 275 flexor tendons. In general a buried Bunnell stitch (Fig. 11-10) utilizing monofilament wire was used. The hands were immobilized postoperatively for approximately 3 weeks. Results were evaluated using essentially the technique described by Flynn (p. 315) (Table 11-1).

Lindsay reported a series of 31 primary or delayed primary repairs in zone 2 on children 2 to 14. These repairs were done either by himself or under his direct supervision. The repairs were usually accomplished by a Bunnell buried suture (Fig. 11-10). He mentions the use of a barbed suture but does not give details of the construction of the suture. The hands were immobilized for 4 weeks postoperatively. His results were classified according to the method reported by Boyes, but we have reclassified his results as we did for Van't Hof (p. 315) (Table 11-1).

McCash (Table 11-1) reported the results of 22 primary repairs and 8 delayed primary repairs. He inserted tendon grafts for the majority of zone 2 injuries. The tendons were sutured utilizing either the Bunnell reinsertion stitch (Fig. 11-12), the buried Bunnell stitch (Fig. 11-10), or the figure-8 stitch tied over a distal button. The tendons were immobilized for 3 weeks. He does not give the method of classification but divided results into very good, good, and poor.

Madsen reported a series of 53 flexor tendon injuries repaired by delayed primary suture within the digital sheath. Verdan's technique was used (see Fig. 4-15). The hands were immobilized for 3 weeks. A good result was obtained if the finger touched the palm; a fair result if the fingertip came within 1.5 to 3 cm of the palm. All other results were considered poor (Table 11-1).

Salvi reported 22 cases of flexor tendon division in the digital sheath treated by delayed primary suture utilizing Verdan's technique (see Fig. 4-15). Results were classified as follows: very good if the pulp touched the palm not more than 2.5 cm from the distal palmar crease, good if the pulp touched the palm more than 2.5 cm from the distal palmar crease, and medium if the pulp did not touch the palm but was within 2.5 cm of the palm. His very good and good results we have classified as excellent-good and his medium results as fair (Table 11-1).

Chang and associates have reported on avulsion injuries of the long flexor tendons. These of course were zone 1 injuries. They are differentiated from lacerations in that they are closed injuries. Early diagnosis was missed in 85% of the patients; however, if the diagnosis was made early and tendon advancement could be performed, all patients obtained good results. If tendon grafting was required, only 55% of the patients obtained good and excellent results, 5% fair results, and 25% poor results.

Jensen and Weilby reported the results of primary tendon suture in the thumb and fingers utilizing a modified Bunnell stitch using wire sutures, or the Bunnell reinsertion technique. They resected the tendon sheaths and immobilized the digits for 3 weeks. We have reclassified their results, combining the excellent and good categories (Table 11-1).

Winston has reported his results of treatment of injuries to the flexor tendons. He used a Bunnell stitch of silk sutures and removed the tendon sheath. He maintained 3 weeks of postoperative immobilization. His results are given in Table 11-1.

Suzuki has attempted direct tendon repair in a most difficult group of patients. These were patients who developed severe scarring and inadequate tendon gliding following a repair in zone 2. Instead of the usual flexor tendon grafting or Silastic rod insertion followed by flexor tendon grafting, he performed direct end-to-end repair and wrapped the repair with a free graft of fascia. A modified Bunnell stitch of 3-0 nylon was used, and the fingers were immobilized for 4 weeks. His results have been reclassified slightly and are shown in Table 11-1.

Green and Niebauer performed primary and secondary flexor tendon repairs in no man's land (zone 2). A Bunnell pullout stitch of wire or nylon was used, and the fingers were immobilized for 3 weeks. The results of their treatment are given in Table 11-1.

Urbaniak and Goldner reported on primary repair, delayed primary repair, and reinsertion techniques in lacerations of the flexor pollicis longus. They obtained excellent results in approximately 50% of their patients (Table 11-1). We have reclassified their fair results as poor and their good as fair based upon the criteria given on p. 320.

McFarlane compared flexor tendon grafting and primary flexor tendon repair in 100 cases. His method of analysis does not allow easy conversion to a classification similar to those reported by others. He reports no significant difference between the results of primary repair and those obtained by flexor tendon grafting.

Verdan has championed primary tendon repair. Analysis of the results according to specific zones and in terms of percent return of function has not been reported in the English language literature.

Hauge's results in 318 cases of primary or secondary tendon repair were so unsatisfactory in all flexor zones as to make them incomparable with any other reported results. The same was not true, however, for the results of repair in the extensor region.

Bolton's series of primary tendon repairs was small and seemed highly selected. The results he reported were extraordinarily good.

McKenzie, Carter and Mersheimer,

Young and Harmon, Koch, and Burnham all have reported series of primary repair of flexor tendons; none analyzed his results in a fashion that was convertible to our classification.

Bogdanov summarized the results of repair of tendon injuries from Russia but unfortunately did not classify the injuries as to their exact location. He summarized 702 flexor tendon repairs and said "good" results were obtained in 493 (70%). He reported a personal series of 167 flexor tendon injuries. He states that he obtained 77% good results in all flexor tendon injuries, including 65% good results in zone 2. He did not define a good result.

Kleinert and associates have performed over 360 primary tendon repairs in no man's land. They state that "more than 75% of the patients have obtained good or excellent function." They did not say what percentage had fair or poor function or define their classifications. Thus, it is impossible to compare their results with those of other authors.

Nigst reported on repairs of the flexor pollicis longus. If the laceration was distal to the metacarpophalangeal joint, he frequently used a technique of lengthening the tendon at the wrist and reinserting it. His results are not classified by our system; however, approximately 40% got excellent or good results, 40% fair results, and 20% poor results.

### Results of secondary tendon graft for flexor tendon injuries

Rank and Wakefield reported a series of flexor tendon grafts apparently performed in zone 2 injuries. They used palmaris longus tendon as the graft, sutured the graft distally with silk to the remaining profundus tendon, and made the proximal anastomosis with silk at the level of the lumbrical muscle. Occasionally a Bunnell pullout suture was used. The hands were immobilized for 3 weeks. A good result was classified when 90% to 100% of finger flexion returned and the fingertip reached the palm; a moderate result was 50% to 80% of normal finger flexion, and a poor result was less than 50%. The results are shown in Table 11-2.

Kyle reported tendon grafting using either the palmaris longus or the extensor digitorum longus tendon as the graft. Occasionally, the flexor digitorum sublimis was used as the graft. The proximal anastomosis was achieved by the interwoven method of Pulvertaft or a direct end-to-end anastomosis using a modified Bunnell buried stitch. The distal attachment of the graft was by reinsertion into the bone. The hands were immobilized for 3 weeks. The method of classification of results has been mentioned previously (p. 315), and the results are given in Table 11-2.

In Pulvertaft's reported series of tendon grafts, either the palmaris longus or the extensor digitorum longus to the fourth toe was used. The proximal anastomosis was interwoven. The distal attachment was usually to the remaining portion of profundus tendon with a Bunnell pullout suture; however, reinsertion was occasionally used. He expressed his flexor pollicis longus tendon graft results in percentage of joint movement. These have been reclassified; an excellent or good result implies 80% return of movement; a fair result indicates 50% return of movement, and a poor result less than 50% of normal movement (Table 11-2).

White reported a group of flexor tendon grafts in 1956. The palmaris longus was usually used as the graft. The Bunnell reinsertion technique was used distally, and the Bunnell buried or pullout stitch was used for the proximal anastomosis at the level of the lumbrical muscle. He classifies an excellent result as one in which the patient was able to extend the finger fully to obtain composite flexion at all three finger joints of 200 degrees and to flex the tip to within 1 inch of the distal palmar crease. A good result was that in which the patient was able to bring the fingertip to within 1 inch of the distal palmar crease and to reach composite flexion of 180 degrees. Fair results were considered to be present in patients who were able to flex the fingertip to within 1½ inches of the distal palmar crease and who could reach composite flexion of 150 degrees. The remaining results were considered poor. For the purposes of this study, the excellent and good results have been combined into a single category. The results are shown in Table 11-2.

Bell and associates reported a series of flexor tendon grafts performed on children. Tendon grafts were the extensor digitorum longus tendons. The distal attachment was gained by reinsertion and additional sutures to the remaining flexor digitorum profundus tendon. The proximal anastomosis was by the interwoven technique at the level of the lumbrical muscle. The patient's

**Table 11-2.** Results of tendon grafting

| | | Rank | Kyle | Pulver-taft | White | Bell | Thomp-son | Boyes | Weeks | Ur-baniak | Total |
|---|---|---|---|---|---|---|---|---|---|---|---|
| Zone 2 | Excellent-good | 12 | 10 | 30 | 32 | 21 | 47 | | 15 | | |
| | Fair | 10 | 12 | 46 | 14 | 5 | 18 | 542 | 22 | | 836 |
| | Poor | 2 | 22 | 36 | 21 | 2 | 31 | 65 | 16 | | 195 |
| Thumb | Excellent-good | 6 | | | 15 | | | | | 0 | 112 |
| | Fair | | | | 9 | | | 70 | | 10 | 49 |
| | Poor | 2 | | | 7 | | | 23 | | 17 | 1192 |

hands were immobilized for 3½ weeks. Good results were those in which 75% return of function was evident, and fair results those in which 50% of return of function was present (Table 11-2).

Thompson reported 100 primary and secondary tendon grafts. The techniques used are those described previously for Rank and Wakefield (p. 318). The results were classified by the technique of White (p. 319). The hands were immobilized for 3 weeks, and physical therapy was given. The results are outlined in Table 11-2.

In 1971 Boyes and Stark reported the monumental study of 1,000 flexor tendon grafts. They used a Bunnell reinsertion stitch distally and a proximal anastomosis in the palm using the Bunnell buried stitch. Results were reported using Boyes' classification. Results in thumb tendon grafts were on the basis of percent return of normal function. We have considered that 80% or greater of return of function was an excellent result, 50% to 80% a good result, and less than 50% a poor result. When they reported the results, they excluded some patients because of excess scar or loss of extension postoperatively. These have been included in our classification as poor results since other authors have not excluded such cases (Table 11-2).

We have reported on the rate of functional recovery after flexor tendon grafting with and without prior insertion of a silicone rod. The silicone rods were used in patients who had severe scarring in the digit. If scarring was mild, tendon grafting was performed without inserting a rod. The final total active motion was independent of whether a silicone rod had been inserted. The results are given in Table 11-2.

Urbaniak used tendon grafts for some lacerations of the flexor pollicis longus. The results in his patients are given in Table 11-2. We have reclassified his results based upon the criteria below.

Kilgore and associates have suggested

that a tendon graft should not be used to replace the flexor pollicis longus if the adductor pollicis muscle is functioning. They suggested arthrodesis or tenodesis of the interphalangeal joint. Their data are insufficient to document the effectiveness of tenodesis or arthrodesis.

### Statistical analysis of results of primary repair and tendon grafting for flexor tendon injuries

In order to obtain uniform classification of results, we have considered an excellent or good result as one in which the fingertip came within ½ inch of the distal palmar crease or there was 80% of normal function. A fair result would be one in which the fingertip came within 1¼ to 1½ inch of the distal palmar crease, and the patient had 50% of normal function. The remainder of the results have been considered poor. In the thumb, a result was considered excellent if 80% of normal joint motion was obtained, fair if 50% to 80% of normal joint motion was obtained, and poor in the remainder of the cases.

We have carried out numerous comparisons using the chi square test for statistical significance. We have considered a $p$ value of between 0.01 and 0.05 as significant and a $p$ value of less than 0.01 as highly significant. We have compared the number of excellent or good results with the fair results and with the poor results in the various series and have also placed the excellent, good, and fair results in a single category and compared the combined group with the poor results.

Miller, Posch, Flynn, and Kelly had significantly worse results in zone 2 when these are compared with other zones. The results of Siler, Jensen, and Winston were not significantly different in the various zones. Flynn did not have any significant difference in the results of repair in zones 3 and 4, but Kelly had significantly better results in zone 4. It seems for purposes of discussion that the hand need only be divided into three zones: zone 1, distal to the proximal interphalangeal joint; zone 2, between the proximal interphalangeal joint and an imaginary line connecting the proximal and distal palmar flexion creases; and zone 3, proximal to the imaginary line. The results of repair in zones 3, 4 and 5 (Fig. 11-2) are not consistently different.

The combined results (all authors) of primary repair in zone 2 are significantly worse than the combined results (all authors) after tendon grafting. The differences were highly significant when excellent-good results were compared with fair ones and also with poor ones. The differences were also highly significant when excellent-good and fair results were combined and compared with poor results. Individual author results comparing repair with grafting show a significant difference if the excellent-good results are compared with the fair results. But when excellent-good and fair results are combined and compared with poor results, there is no significant difference. There is a highly significant difference in the results of flexor tendon grafting among the various authors; Rank, Bell, and Boyes have significantly fewer fair and poor results than the other authors. If one compares the best results obtainable there is no significant difference between the results of secondary tendon grafting as reported by Boyes and the results of primary repair as reported by Madsen. Indeed, Madsen's results in zone 2 were significantly better than those produced by tendon grafting as reported by Pulvertaft, White, or Thompson. Boyes reported that results of secondary tendon grafting were much worse in patients older than 50. Bell's results of tendon grafting in children are not significantly better than those Lindsay reported for primary repair in children.

Harrison claimed better results with delayed primary tendon grafting. When the chi square test is used, there is no significant difference between his primary and delayed primary tendon grafts. Indeed, there is no difference between either one of Harrison's two series and the combined results (all authors) of tendon grafts (Table 11-2). Finally, there is no significant difference between Harrison's series of delayed primary tendon grafts, Boyes' secondary tendon grafts, or Madsen's primary repairs.

In summary, the chance of producing a poor or unsatisfactory result after primary repair of a flexor tendon injury in zone 1, 3, and 4, are about 15%. The chance of producing a poor or unsatisfactory result after primary repair of the flexor pollicis longus is about 17%. The chance of producing an unsatisfactory result after primary repair in zone 2 is approximately 28%.

We conclude that in zone 2 injuries in a person under 12, tendon grafts will not produce a better result than primary repair. Furthermore, in persons over 50, the results of both tendon graft and primary repair are unsatisfactory. The disadvantage of additional immobilization and the disability required for a tendon graft are probably not justifiable. In persons between 12 and 50, secondary tendon grafting is probably the method of choice for treatment of tendon lacerations. However, individual surgeons utilizing primary repair in zone 2 can produce results equal or superior to those produced by tendon grafting.

There is no adequate series of repairs of flexor tendon injuries in zone 5 to allow statistical analysis. However, we believe that the results of primary repair are extremely good.

### Results of primary repair of extensor tendon injuries

In 1942 Miller reported the results of repair of 180 extensor tendons. It is unclear exactly what technique of repair was used. The extensor tendons were immobilized for 3 weeks, and then physical therapy was begun. He considered an excellent result one in which the patient had normal function of the finger. A good result was one in which there was a 10 degree loss of extension (he considered this approximately 80% restoration of function). A fair result was one in which there was 45 degrees loss of extension (50% functional impairment). The remainder were poor results. The results are shown in Table 11-3.

In 1953 Flynn reported the results of repair of extensor tendons at the Boston City Hospital. He reported on 84 lacerations of the extensors of the fingers in all zones and 13 repairs of the extensor pollicis longus. The results were classified as good, fair, or poor. The method by which the results were classified into various categories, the duration of the immobilization, and the technique of repair were not described.

Hauge reported the results of primary and secondary suture of 406 extensor tendons. A wide variety of methods of repair were used. The patients' hands were immobilized for 3 weeks. Successful results were classified as those in which approximately complete recovery of tendon func-

tion had been obtained; satisfactory results signified tendon function about half of normal; the remainder were called unsuccessful.

In 1959 Kelly reported the results of treatment of 37 closed and 307 open injuries to the extensor tendons. In zones 3, 4, and 5, repair was by the Bunnell buried stitch of 4-0 multifilament stainless steel wire. The patients' hands were totally immobilized for 4 weeks, and then passive motion was begun. Active motion was begun after 5 weeks. In zone 2 the extensor hood was repaired with 5- monofilament wire, the lateral bands were repaired with 4-0 multifilament wire, and the extensor expansion was repaired with 5-0 nylon sutures. In zone 1, repair was with 4-0 wire mattress stitches. Either the distal interphalangeal joint or both the distal and proximal interphalangeal joints were immobilized with Kirschner wires. The Kirschner wires were left in place for 3 weeks, and then external splints were used for an additional 10 to 14 days. Closed injuries in zone 1 were almost always treated with Kirschner wire immobilization, and results were good or excellent in 19 of 22 cases. Results were classified as

**Table 11-3.** Results of primary repair of extensor tendons

| | | Miller | Flynn | Hauge | Kelly | Dargan | Total |
|---|---|---|---|---|---|---|---|
| Zone 1 | Excellent-good | | 10 | 5 | 9 | (revised) | 24 |
| | Fair | | 4 | 9 | 1 | | 14 |
| | Poor | | 7 | 5 | | | 12 |
| Zone 2 | Excellent-good | | 9 | 123 | 24 | 15 | 171 |
| | Fair | | 4 | 64 | 8 | 5 | 81 |
| | Poor | | 6 | 25 | 3 | 2 | 36 |
| Zone 3 | Excellent-good | 14 | 21 | 37 | | 15 | 87 |
| | Fair | | 9 | 11 | 1 | 5 | 27 |
| | Poor | 1 | 7 | 4 | 3 | 3 | 17 |
| Zone 4 | Excellent-good | 15 | 5 | 30 | 56 | | 106 |
| | Fair | | 2 | 5 | 2 | | 9 |
| | Poor | 2 | | | | | 2 |
| | | | | | | | 586 |

excellent if the patient had not lost more than 5 degrees of motion at each interphalangeal joint, good if the loss was not more than 10 degrees, and poor if the loss of extension was greater than 10 degrees.

In 1969 Dargan reported the results of repair of extensor tendon injuries using a much shorter period of immobilization. The tendons were repaired by simple stitches of 4-0 silk or Teflon. Two weeks after repair, the splint was removed and full use of the hand allowed. Passive exercise was prohibited. He classified an excellent result as one in which there was normal extension and normal flexion; good results were present when there was loss of extension of 15 degrees or less and normal flexion; fair results were those with loss of 15 to 45 degrees of extension and loss of flexion up to 2 cm; poor results had less function than those in the fair category. It is difficult to completely analyze his results since he merely states that good to excellent results were obtained in 90% of the cases. For the purposes of this study, we have reclassified the remaining 10% as poor results.

### Statistical analyses of the results of primary repair of extensor tendon injuries

The chi square test was used for statistical analysis as outlined under the heading "Statistical Analysis of Results of Primary Repair and Tendon Grafting for Flexor Tendon Injuries" (p. 320).

Neither Flynn nor Kelly had significantly different results within the various zones on the dorsum of the hand. Thus, for reporting of results, division of the dorsum of the hand into zones (Fig. 11-5) is arbitrary and probably should be abandoned.

In summary, poor results following primary tendon repair occurred in 13% to 24% of the cases in zone 1, 2, and 3 but in only 2% of the repairs in zone 4. Insufficient numbers are available to predict exactly results of repair in zone 5, but poor results probably occur in 1% to 2%

of the cases. Also, few repairs of the extensor pollicis longus or abductor pollicis longus are reported; however, excellent, good, or fair results are probably obtained in 95% to 99% of the cases. The classic teaching about the period of immobilization for extensor tendons (4 weeks) may not be accurate. Dargan's results with only 2 weeks immobilization are as good as any reported.

### Results of primary repair of proper flexors and extensors of the radiocarpal joint

Too few wrist tendon injuries have been reported to allow statistical analysis; however, our experience and that of most other authors indicate that poor results are produced in only 1% to 2% of the cases.

### BIBLIOGRAPHY

Bell, J. L., and others: Injuries to flexor tendons of the hand in children, J. Bone Joint Surg. **40A:**1220, 1958.

Bogdanov, R. F.: Repair of injuries to the tendons of the hand, Br. Med. J. **2:**1315, 1955.

Bolton, H.: Primary tendon repair, Hand **2:**56, 1970.

Boyes, J. H., and Stark, H. H.: Flexor-tendon grafts in the fingers and thumb, J. Bone Joint Surg. **53A:**1332, 1971.

Burnham, P. J.: Repair of tendon injuries in the hand, Arch. Surg. **78:**316, 1959.

Carter, S. J., and Mersheimer, W. L.: Deferred primary tendon repair results in 27 cases, Ann. Surg. **164:**913, 1966.

Chang, W. H., Thomas, O. J., and White, W. L.: Avulsion injury of the long flexor tendons, Plast. Reconstr. Surg. **50:**260, 1972.

Chong, J. K., Cramer, L. M., and Culf, N. K.: Combined two-stage tenoplasty with silicone rods for multiple flexor tendon injuries in "no-man's-land," J. Trauma **12:**104, 1972.

Dargan, E. L.: Management of extensor tendon injuries of the hand, Surg. Gynecol. Obstet. **128:**1269, 1969.

Elliott, R. A.: Injuries to the extensor mechanism of the hand, Orthop. Clin. North Am. **1:**335, 1970.

Emery, F. E.: Immediate mobilization following flexor tendon repair, J. Trauma **17:**1, 1977.

Everett, W. G.: Suture materials in general surgery, Prog. Surg. **8:**14, 1969.

Flynn, J. E.: Problems with trauma to the hand, J. Bone Joint Surg. **35A:**132, 1953.

Ford, J. C., Smith, J. R., and Carter, J. E.: Primary tendon grafting in injuries of the thumb flexor, South. Med. J. **64**:78, 1971.

Green, W. L., and Niebauer, J. J.: Results of primary and secondary flexor-tendon repairs in no man's land, J. Bone Joint Surg. **56A**:1216, 1974.

Harrison, S. H.: Delayed primary flexor tendon grafts of the fingers, Plast. Reconstr. Surg. **43**:366, 1969.

Hauge, M. F.: The results of tendon suture of the hands; a review of 500 patients, Acta Orthop. Scand. **24**:258, 1954.

Herman, J. B.: Tensile strength and knot security of surgical suture materials, Am. Surg. **37**:209, 1971.

Iselin, F., and Peze, W.: Use of chemically preserved tendon allografts in hand surgery, Hand **8**:167, 1976.

Jennings, E. R., Mansberger, A. R., Jr., Smith, E. P., Jr., and Yeager, G. H.: New technique in primary tendon repair, Surg. Gynecol. Obstet. **95**:597, 1952.

Jennings, E. R., and Yeager, G. H.: Barbwire tendon suture, Arch. Surg. **70**:566, 1955.

Jensen, E. G., and Weilby, A.: Primary tendon suture in the thumb and fingers, Hand **6**:297, 1974.

Kelly, A. P.: Primary tendon repairs; a study of 789 consecutive tendon severances, J. Bone Joint Surg. **41A**:581, 1959.

Kessler, I., and Nissim, F.: Primary repair without immobilization of flexor tendon division within the digital sheath; an experimental and clinical study, Acta Orthop. Scand. **40**:587, 1969.

Kilgore, E. S., Jr., Newmeyer, W. L., Graham, W. P. III, and Brown, L. G.: The dubiousness of grafting the dispensable flexor pollicis longus, Am. J. Surg. **132**:292, 1976.

Kleinert, H. E., and others: Primary repair of flexor tendons in "no man's land," J. Bone Joint Surg. **49A**:577, 1967.

Kleinert, H. E., Kutz, J. E., Atasoy, E., and Storma, A.: Primary repair of flexor tendons, Orthop. Clin. North Am. **4**:865, 1973.

Koch, S. L.: Division of the flexor tendons within the digital sheath, Surg. Gynecol. Obstet. **78**:9, 1944.

Kyle, J. B., and Eyre-Brook, A. L.: The surgical treatment of flexor tendon injuries in the hand; results obtained in a consecutive series of 57 cases, Br. J. Surg. **51**:502, 1954.

Lindsay, W. K.: Direct digital flexor tendon repair, Plast. Reconstr. Surg. **26**:613, 1960.

Madsen, E.: Delayed primary suture of flexor tendons cut in the digital sheath, J. Bone Joint Surg. **52B**:264, 1970.

Mason, M. L.: Primary and secondary tendon suture, Surg. Gynecol. Obstet. **70**:392, 1940.

McCash, C. R.: The immediate repair of flexor tendons, Br. J. Plast. Surg. **14**:53, 1961.

McFarlane, R. M., Lamon, R., and Jarvis, G.: Flexor tendon injuries within the finger, J. Trauma **8**:987, 1968.

McKenzie, A. R.: Function after reconstruction of severed long flexor tendons of the hands; a review of 297 tendons, J. Bone Joint Surg. **49B**:424, 1967.

Miller, H.: Repair of severed tendons of the hand and wrist; statistical analysis of 300 cases, Surg. Gynecol. Obstet. **75**:693, 1942.

Nicolle, M. B.: A silastic tendon prosthesis as an adjunct to flexor tendon grafting; an experimental and clinical evaluation, Br. J. Plast. Surg. **22**:224, 1969.

Nigst, H.: Repair of lesions to the flexor pollicis longus tendon, Reconstr. Surg. Traumatol. **14**:107, 1974.

Posch, J. L.: Primary tendon repair, Surg. Clin. North Am. **28**:1323, 1948.

Potenza, A. D.: Flexor tendon injuries, Orthop. Clin. North Am. **1**:355, 1970.

Pulvertaft, R. G.: Tendon grafts for flexor tendon injuries in the fingers and thumb; a study of technique and results, J. Bone Joint Surg. **38B**:175, 1956.

Rank, B. K., and Wakefield, A. R.: Flexor tendon repair in the hand, Aust. N.Z. J. Surg. **19**:232, 1950.

Rank, B. K., and Wakefield, A. R.: tendon repair in the hand—a supplementary paper, Aust. N.Z. J. Surg. **21**:135, 1951.

Rank, B. K., and Wakefield, A. R.: Surgery of repair as applied to hand injuries, Baltimore, 1970, The Williams & Wilkins Co.

Riggs, B. M.: A simple tendon transfer for the isolated division of the flexor digitorum profundus, Hand **7**:246, 1975.

Salvi, V.: Delayed primary suture in flexor tendon division, Hand **3**:181, 1971.

Shaw, P. C.: A method of flexor tendon suture, J. Bone Joint Surg. **50B**:578, 1968.

Siler, V. E.: Primary tenorrhaphy of the flexor tendons in the hand, J. Bone Joint Surg. **32A**:218, 1950.

Suzuki, K.: Delayed flexor tendon repair in the digital sheath with end-to-end suture and fascial graft, Hand **8**:141, 1976.

Thompson, R. V.: An evaluation of flexor tendon grafting, Br. J. Plast. Surg. **20**:21, 1967.

Tsuge, K., Ikuta, Y., and Matsuishi, Y.: Intratendinous tendon suture in the hand; a new technique, Hand **7**:250, 1975.

Urbaniak, J. R., and Goldner, J. L.: Laceration of

the flexor pollicis longus tendon; delayed repair by advancement, free graft or direct suture, J. Bone Joint Surg. **55A**:1123, 1973.

Van der Meulen, J. C.: Recent advances in flexor tendon repair, Arch. Chir. Neerl. **23**:129, 1971.

Van der Meulen, J. C.: Silastic spaces in tendon grafting, Br. J. Plast. Surg. **24**:166, 1971.

Van't Hof, A., and Heiple, K. G.: Flexor tendon injuries of the fingers and thumb; a comparative study, J. Bone Joint Surg. **40A**:256, 1958.

Verdan, C. E.: Primary repair of flexor tendons, J. Bone Joint Surg. **42A**:647, 1960.

Verdan, C. E.: Primary and secondary repair of flexor and extensor tendon injuries. In Flynn, J. W., editor: Hand surgery, Baltimore, 1966, The Williams & Wilkins Co.

Weeks, P. M., and Wray, R. C.: Rate and extent of functional recovery after flexor tendon graft-ing with and without silicone rod preparation, J. Hand Surg. **1**:174, 1976.

White, W. L.: Secondary restoration of finger flexion by digital tendon grafts, Am. J. Surg. **91**:662, 1956.

Winston, M. E.: The results of treatment of injuries to the flexor tendons, Hand **4**:45, 1972.

Wray, R. C., Holtmann, B., and Weeks, P. M.: Clinical treatment of partial tendon lacerations without suturing and with early motion, Plast. Reconstr. Surg. **59**:40, 1977.

Wray, R. C., Moucharafieh, B., Braitberg, R., and Weeks, P. M.: Effects of mobilization on partially lacerated tendons, Surg. Forum **27**:570, 1976.

Young, R. E., and Harmon, J. M.: Repair of tendon injuries of the hand, Ann. Surg. **151**:562, 1960.

# POSTOPERATIVE MANAGEMENT

# CHAPTER 12
## Management of the stiff hand

### CAUSES

Stiffness in the injured hand results from any of the following conditions, either alone or in combination: edema, scar formation, or muscle contracture. These conditions render the hand stiff by interfering with either joint mobility or power gliding of the musculotendinous unit. The alterations associated with each of these conditions will be discussed.

Edema is the first and most obvious reaction of the hand to injury. It is commonly associated with trauma, infection, or vasomotor abnormalities. Edema is reversible; the degree and rapidity of reversibility determine its deleterious effects. If edema can be controlled early, subsequent scar formation is minimized in comparison with the scar that forms if edema is prolonged and brawny.

A classic example of the reversible effect of edema is the relatively insignificant laceration that results in a swollen hand. After the sutures have been removed, the hand is not exercised properly and is held in a dependent position. Flexion of the metacarpophalangeal joints is limited to about 45 degrees, but interphalangeal joint flexion is greater. This variation in flexion between joints results from the blocking effect of palmar edema on the metacarpo-

phalangeal joints and the fact that tendon gliding is restricted by edema.

In the digital sheaths, the tendons lie free of any mesentery except for small vincula longa and vincula brevia. Gliding occurs by the tendons sliding over each other within the smooth rigid fibro-osseous tunnel, which contains a lubricant. (However, in the palm, gliding is more specialized since a well-developed paratenon encircles the tendon.) The inner layer of this sleeve permits gliding up to the point where an adjacent layer is activated. This layer activation continues until the entire paratenon is gliding. This arrangement permits maximum tendon gliding with a minimum of movement of the outer layer of the paratenon (Fig. 12-1). This provides contact with fixed structures in the vicinity without restriction of gliding.

The effects of edema on tendon gliding can be readily appreciated from this arrangement. As fluid collects in the layered paratenon, tendon gliding is inhibited by the increase in work necessary to effect tendon gliding and the decrease in longitudinal paratenon gliding. Consequently, edema forming after a minor skin wound may restrict tendon gliding even though the joints exhibit a near-normal range of passive motion. Often one is unable to produce

**329**

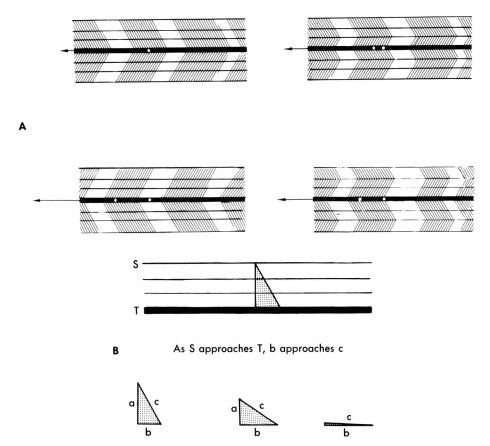

**Fig. 12-1. A,** The mesotenon facilitates flexor tendon gliding while minimizing movement at the periphery of the mesotenon. **B,** The outer layer of the mesotenon indicated as *S,* and the tendon proper as *T.* As the paratenon is more closely applied to the tendon, the distance of the gliding is increased.

full passive extension of the joints because the swollen paratenon restricts gliding of the flexor tendons. If the patient is treated vigorously, the edematous process can be reversed, normal tendon gliding restored, and a full range of active and passive motion regained.

When the edematous process involves the entire hand—its soft tissues, paratenons, and joint capsules—active and passive movements are severely limited. Aggressive treatment must be instituted, or the edematous phase will be supplanted by the cicatrix phase; the severity of the latter response determines the ultimate functional result. Although edema is a reversible process, that is, something we can more or less control, we have almost negligible control of the cicatrical phase. Thus, treatment of the initial edematous phase must be aggressive, frequent, and directed primarily toward reversing the edematous process. This edematous phase is particularly malignant when vasomotor instability is present.

If the edematous stage is not reversed rapidly, the cicatricial stage will become manifest, varying in degree from mild to severe. As a result of their interrelationship, cicatrix can form in any area involved in edema formation. This is a most important concept. Scar forms at the site of injury and at many sites far removed from the injury. A tendon lacerated in the fibro-osseous tunnel may evoke scar formation in the paratenon of the flexor tendons proximal to the wrist. An appreciation of this fact is mandatory for proper management. The formation of scar is particularly disabling in regard to tendon gliding because tendon gliding is impaired no matter what the position of the tendons in relation to joint extension or flexion. However, the degree of joint impairment depends more on the anatomy of the joint, its supporting structures, and the position of the joint when the cicatrix was forming and while it matured. Thus, when the hand experiences cicatrix formation, positioning can help preserve joint function yet have no effect on tendon gliding.

Involvement of muscle at this stage compounds functional loss. Muscle may become involved by internal or external cicatrix formation or by a less well understood phenomenon—myostatic contracture. The degree of functional impairment in the first two forms depends on the extent of muscle necrosis and scar formation. This is particularly evident in Volkmann's ischemic contracture and local ischemic contracture within the hand. These phenomena are associated with obvious muscle necrosis and extensive scar formation. Direct injury to the muscle, for example, in lacerations and crush injuries, may result in significant adhesions between the muscle and the surrounding fixed structures. Myostatic contracture is an entirely different phenomenon and one that occurs much more frequently than is generally appreciated. If tension within a skeletal muscle is completely relieved for several days (as by cutting a flexor tendon and allowing the cut ends to retract until no tension is present in the muscle belly), fixation of the muscle belly at this retracted length occurs. If the muscle is reactivated sufficiently early, the

contracture can be overcome by active and passive exercises. However, if the muscle is allowed to remain in the shortened position for weeks, attempts to restore it immediately to its original length produce structural damage. For this phenomenon to occur, the muscle must be innervated; that is, denervated muscle does not develop a myostatic contracture. The dorsal nerve roots must be sectioned to prevent myostatic contracture. This suggests that the integrity of local reflexes is essential for the development of the contracture. Histologically, there are no changes demonstrable in the muscle fibers, except for a slight decrease in cross striations. Atrophy of disuse is readily distinguished. The functional change in myostatic contracture is assumed to be a change in compliance of the elastin elements within the muscle fibers, thus shortening the muscle's resting length by 10% to 40%.

The role of muscle imbalance is most striking in the injured hand. With a median and ulnar nerve palsy, first web space contractures frequently develop as a result of the muscle imbalance combined with the effects of edema and cicatrix reaction to the initial injury. When the long flexors to a finger are severed, muscle imbalance positions the finger in extension and the cicatricial reaction to injury fixes the joint ligaments, capsules, and tendons in this position.

The management of stiff joints includes evaluation, nonoperative mobilization, and operative mobilization. The salient points of each area are discussed in the following paragraphs.

## EVALUATION

The factors contributing to joint stability can be classified as capsular or extracapsular. The capsular structures are those participating directly in the joint capsule, whereas the extracapsular factors include structures that traverse a joint and contribute to its stability but do not participate directly in the joint capsule. Basically, joints are stiff either in extension or in flexion. The capsular and extracapsular structures contributing to joint stiffness will be discussed according to the position of stiffness of the joint.

### Metacarpophalangeal joint

#### Stiffness in extension

*Capsular factors.* The capsular factors that contribute to stiffness of this joint in extension include: (1) the collateral ligaments, (2) the dorsal capsule, (3) the volar synovial pouch, and (4) articular surface erosions with or without pannus invasion.

COLLATERAL LIGAMENTS. As noted earlier, the collateral ligaments of the metacarpophalangeal joint are eccentrically placed to render these ligaments slack during metacarpophalangeal extension and taut during metacarpophalangeal flexion. An injury can excite the deposition of new collagen around the collateral ligaments in their slack position (metacarpophalangeal joint extension), fixing these ligaments in the shortened position. When flexion of the joint is attempted, the collateral ligaments must change in length by more than 20% as the arc of flexion is described from 0 to 60 degrees. According to the severity of the shortened position of the ligaments, an arc is subtended until the ligament will not permit further flexion. At this point, the volar lip of the proximal phalanx abuts the articular surface of the metacarpal head, and further attempts at flexion result in prying open the metacarpophalangeal joint dorsally (Fig. 12-2). This is evident clinically by the development of a dorsal depression when flexion of the joint is attempted. Recall the articular surface of the metacarpal head. The marked flaring of the volar tubercle of the index and little finger metacarpals increases the degree of collateral ligament length needed to permit full flexion of this joint. The rigidity one

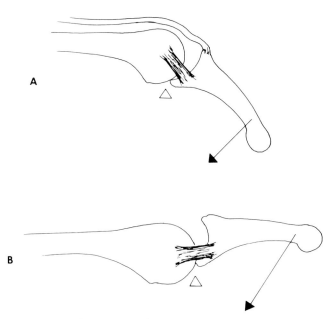

**Fig. 12-2. A,** The tight collateral ligaments allow rotation to 45 degrees, and thereafter the volar lip of the phalanx base pivots against the metacarpal head. **B,** When the collateral ligaments have become rigidly shortened with the metcarpophalangeal joints in hyperextension, attempted rotation forces the base of the proximal phalanx against the metacarpal head.

encounters as he attempts passive flexion of the joint provides an index of the favorability of the scar around the collateral ligaments. Furthermore, the arc of flexion permitted provides an index of the extent of ligament shortening or fixation.

DORSAL CAPSULE. Recall the distinct layer of infratendinous fascia underlying the extensor tendons and bridging the metacarpophalangeal joint to attach to the proximal phalanx. This fascia and the dorsal synovial pouch of the metacarpophalangeal joint may fuse. As scar is deposited around this rigid fascia, the joint becomes fixed in hyperextension. This usually occurs in combination with collateral ligament fixation but may be the prime contributing factor to metacarpophalangeal joint stiffness in extension. On physical examination, this provides a picture similar to collateral ligament shortening except that the dorsal skin depression described earlier is not in evidence. Consequently, an operative approach to the metacarpophalangeal joint fixed in extension by capsular factors requires initial inspection of this dorsal capsule and its excision if any question exists concerning its contribution to joint stiffness. This maneuver will prevent the indiscriminate excision of many normal collateral ligaments.

VOLAR SYNOVIAL POUCH. When the metacarpophalangeal joint is in extension, the leaves of the volar synovial pouch collapse and are coapted. Pannus formation in this collapsed pouch can obliterate the pouch completely. As the proximal phalanx attempts to rotate around the metacarpal head, the normal resiliency of the pouch is absent, and the volar plate is prevented from further rotation by the obliterated pouch. This is particularly evident after collateral ligament and dorsal capsule excision. As the proximal phalanx is rotated around the metacarpal head, the articular surfaces become incongruous when the base of the proximal phalanx approaches the volar pouch. Further flexion is accomplished by the opening of the joint dor-

sally as the proximal phalanx pivots around the obliterated pouch. The state of this pouch can be readily determined during a capsulotomy by inserting a Freer elevator into the pouch and gently defining its confines.

ARTICULAR SURFACE EROSIONS. These are most frequently associated with intra-articular fractures, usually involving the base of the proximal phalanx. As a result of inadequate fracture reduction and prolonged immobilization, pannus formation may become extensive and attach to the fracture site. This attachment may spread to involve normal surrounding cartilage and eventually result in extensive joint destruction and fixation. Prolonged immobilization has been reported to result in extensive pannus formation and resorption of the articular surfaces not maintaining contact. Roentgenographic examination and history provide the clues to this diagnosis.

*Extracapsular factors.* The extracapsular factors that can contribute to stiffness of the metacarpophalangeal joint in extension include: (1) skin contracture, (2) unopposed extension, (3) extensor tendon adhesions, and (4) forearm extensor muscle contractures.

SKIN CONTRACTURE. Inadequate skin coverage of the dorsum of the hand, either from contraction of damaged skin or inadequate replacement of skin loss, can result in fixation of the metacarpophalangeal joints in extension (Fig. 12-3). Occasionally, the skin involvement extends across the wrist, and when metacarpophalangeal joint flexion is attempted, blanching of the skin of the forearm can be observed. The contribution of the skin contracture to metacarpophalangeal joint stiffness is readily apparent on physical examination. However, one is unable to determine the contribution of the capsular factors to this stiffness in extension. This must be determined at the operating table after the skin contracture has been released completely. Then, if the metacarpophalangeal joint cannot be fully flexed, one must be prepared at the operating

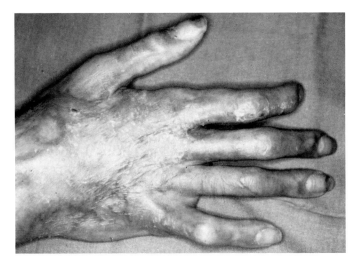

**Fig. 12-3.** Contracture developing in a burn scar fixes the metacarpophalangeal joints in hyperextension.

table to completely evaluate the factors responsible for joint stiffness in extension. It is unjustifiable simply to skin graft the open area and wait until after surgery to fully evaluate the cause of joint stiffness. Replacement of the dorsal skin requires insertion of adequate skin after the joint has been flexed to expose the full extent of tissue loss. When the skin contracture involves the forearm or wrist, these joints are fully flexed after release of the skin contracture. This ensures the insertion of an adequate amount of skin and places the capsular factors of the metacarpophalangeal joint in their most favorable position for subsequent function.

UNOPPOSED EXTENSION. The loss of active flexion at the metacarpophalangeal joints results in a marked muscle imbalance. The extensor units are intact and contract unopposed. Since the extensor tendon provides a slip for insertion into the base of the proximal phalanx, this joint becomes hyperextended even though the proximal and distal interphalangeal joints may be flexed. In this hyperextended position, the capsular factors mentioned earlier can become altered to prevent passive flexion of the metacarpophalangeal joint. This is most

often observed after division of the median and ulnar nerves at the wrist. Obviously, this position should never be allowed to persist. Metacarpophalangeal joint flexion is provided by an external appartus until the motor units and nerve continuity can be reestablished.

EXTENSOR TENDON ADHESIONS. Adhesions around extensor tendons on the dorsum of the hand are evident on clinical examination. When passive flexion of the metacarpophalangeal joint is attempted, blanching of the dorsal skin is noted when the tendon is adherent to the skin. If the tendon is adherent only to the skin, some give will be noted as the skin tents forward to allow a slight improvement in flexion. When the tendon is primarily adherent to the underlying metacarpal, blanching of the skin may not be seen. If these adhesions to bone are dense and nonyielding, a rigid block will be encountered when flexion is attempted; this block does not yield to further pressure. If the tendon adhesions are in the forearm, flexion of the wrist will exaggerate metacarpophalangeal joint extension, whereas extension of the wrist will improve the range of flexion of the metacarpophalangeal joint (Fig. 12-4). Roent-

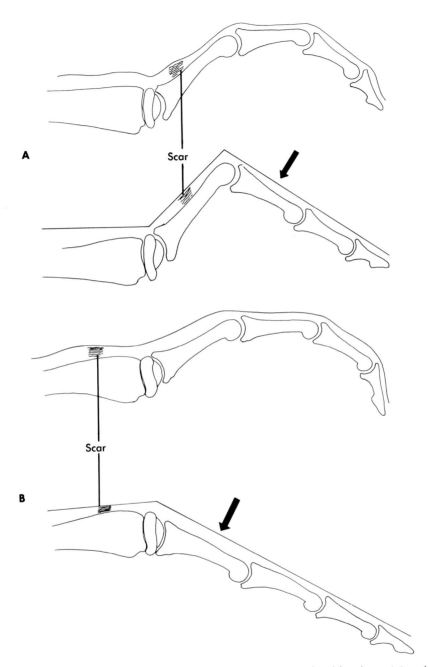

**Fig. 12-4. A,** Scar around the extensor tendons can be localized by determining the effect of position on joint flexion. Scar on the dorsum of the hand limits proximal interphalangeal flexion when the metacarpophalangeal joints are flexed. **B,** Scar proximal to the wrist limits metacarpophalangeal joint flexion when the wrist is flexed but permits metacarpophalangeal joint flexion when the wrist is extended.

genographic examination is important to correlate periosteal callus or fracture callus with the adhesions. Operatively, if release of tendon adhesions in one area does not permit full metacarpophalangeal flexion, one must continue searching for distant adhesions as indicated. If no other extracapsular cause of metacarpophalangeal joint stiffness in extension can be defined, one must systematically evaluate the capsular causes for joint stiffness.

FOREARM MUSCLE CONTRACTURE. Contracture of the extensor muscles may hold the metacarpophalangeal in rigid extension. If the contracture is mild, wrist extension will provide a relative lengthening of the tendons and permit partial or total metacarpophalangeal flexion. Conversely, if the wrist is held in flexion and the metacarpophalangeal in full extension, then gradual passive flexion of the metacarpophalangeal joints will cause the wrist to gradually extend.

### Stiffness in flexion

*Capsular factors.* The capsular factors that can contribute to stiffness of the metacarpophalangeal joints in flexion include fusion of the volar synovial sac and erosion of the articular surfaces with or without fusion.

FUSION OF THE VOLAR SYNOVIAL SAC. When there has been direct trauma to the volar capsule of the metacarpophalangeal joint and the joint is positioned in flexion, scar will rapidly obliterate the volar pouch of the synovial sac. In effect, this fixes the rigid volar plate to the metacarpal and fixes the proximal phalanx in flexion through the volar plate's distal attachment to the proximal phalanx. The vertical fibers of the palmar fascia may contribute to the rigidity of this scar. The history of injury and the method of management provide the diagnostic clues. Frequently, obliteration of this volar sac is associated with injury limited to the extracapsular factors and can contribute to fixation of the joint in flexion.

EROSION OF JOINT SURFACES. This is most often associated with an intraarticular fracture that has not been accurately reduced. The ensuing pannus formation may excite extensive joint erosion and fibrosis with fixation of the metacarpal head and the base of the proximal phalanx. The history of fracture, persistent swelling, pain and tenderness over the joint, and the roentgenographic examination confirm the diagnosis.

*Extracapsular factors.* The extracapsular factors contributing to metacarpophalangeal joint stiffness in flexion include: (1) flexor tendon entrapment, (2) contracture of the forearm musculature, (3) intrinsic muscle contracture, (4) palmar fascia fibrosis, and (5) volar skin loss.

FLEXOR TENDON ENTRAPMENT. Scar around flexor tendons within the palm can prevent extension of the metacarpophalangeal joint. The history usually reveals a tendon laceration and repair in the palm. On physical examination, gradual passive extension of the proximal and distal interphalangeal joints results in gradual flexion of the metacarpophalangeal joint. Flexor tendon entrapment proximal to the wrist is detected by holding the proximal and distal interphalangeal joints in extension and flexing and extending the wrist. As the wrist flexes, the metacarpophalangeal joint will extend. As the wrist extends, the metacarpophalangeal joint will flex.

CONTRACTURE OF THE FOREARM MUSCULATURE. The joints react to passive motion exactly as described for the presence of scar around the flexor tendons above the wrist. Severe contracture, such as Volkmann's ischemic contracture, produces extreme flexion deformity of the digits, yet the wrist is relatively free. Muscle necrosis from direct injury usually affects all muscle groups including the wrist flexors; that is, it involves the more superficial muscles first and each underlying group as encountered. Volkmann's contracture involves the deep muscles primarily and may, in very severe cases, involve the more superficial muscles.

INTRINSIC MUSCLE SHORTENING. Intrinsic muscle shortening or contracture produces flexion at the metacarpophalangeal joint and extension at the proximal and distal interphalangeal joints. The degree of contracture varies from mild to severe. The more severe the contracture, the more exaggerated the metacarpophalangeal joint flexion. The degree of intrinsic tightness can be detected by passively extending the metacarpophalangeal joint to its fullest and attempting passive flexion of the proximal and distal interphalangeal joints (Fig. 12-5). When the intrinsics are contracted, definite resistance to proximal and distal interphalangeal joint flexion is encountered. As the metacarpophalangeal joint is passively flexed, passive flexion of the proximal and distal interphalangeal joints encounters significantly less resistance.

PALMAR FASCIA FIBROSIS. The distal extensions of the palmar fascia bridge the metacarpophalangeal and proximal interphalangeal joints. In Dupuytren's contracture, the proximal interphalangeal joint is more severely involved in a flexion contracture than is the juxtapositioned metacarpophalangeal joint. However, the metacarpophalangeal joint may become severely involved. The diagnosis of Dupuytren's contracture leads to the correct analysis of the cause of the flexion contracture. Occasionally, crush injuries are associated with thickening and contracture of the palmar fascia. As a result, the palm becomes narrower and the metacarpophalangeal joints become flexed. On examination, the hand appears compressed in all planes. The volar skin and fascia are fused, dense, and nonyielding. The hand feels rigid. The history of injury provides the diagnosis.

VOLAR SKIN LOSS. Volar skin loss, as from burns, may produce a flexion contracture of the metacarpophalangeal joints. The contracted skin bridges the metacarpophalangeal joint and through its rigid proximal and distal attachments prevents joint extension. Correction requires replacement with adequate skin. If release of the skin contracture does not provide full passive extension, one must be prepared at the operating table to fully evaluate the cause so that full extension may be gained *before* the graft is inserted.

### Proximal interphalangeal joint

The proximal interphalangeal joints become stiff in flexion much more frequently

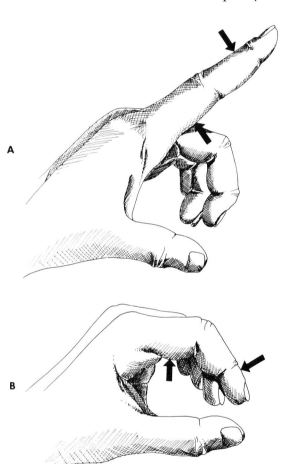

**Fig. 12-5. A,** Contracture of the intrinsic muscles is detected by hyperextending the metacarpophalangeal joint and attempting passive flexion of the proximal and distal interphalangeal joints. **B,** When the metacarpophalangeal joint is flexed, passive flexion of the proximal and distal interphalangeal joints is improved.

than in extension. This is the result of the joint anatomy, particularly with regard to the collateral ligaments and the volar plate.

### Stiffness in extension

*Capsular factors.* The capsular factors that may contribute to stiffness of the proximal interphalangeal joint in extension include: (1) collateral ligament and dorsal joint capsule, and (2) articular surface erosion and pannus formation.

COLLATERAL LIGAMENTS. The dorsal portion of the collateral ligament, a triangular ligament, may become involved in scar formation that includes the dorsal synovial pouch. When the joint is in extension and this pouch has been obliterated and the dorsal portions of the collateral ligaments have become shortened, passive flexion is impossible. The history, a roentgenogram of the joint, and the physical examination aid in the diagnosis. Of course, it is always possible to have a combination of factors, that is, extracapsular and capsular factors, contributing to the stiffness of the joint. In the absence of extracapsular factors and the presence of a normal roentgenogram, stiffness of the proximal interphalangeal joint in extension can be attributed to the dorsal portion of the collateral ligament and synovial capsule.

ARTICULAR SURFACE EROSION. A roentgenogram aids in the diagnosis of this cause of joint stiffness. Usually these changes are associated with an intraarticular fracture that has excited significant pannus formation, articular surface destruction, and eventually, fusion.

*Extracapsular factors.* The extracapsular factors that can be involved in producing stiffness of the proximal interphalangeal joint in extension include: (1) skin contracture, (2) scar about extensor tendons, (3) lateral bands embedded in scar, (4) intrinsic muscle contracture, and (5) shortening of the lumbricales.

SKIN CONTRACTURE. The most common cause of dorsal skin loss predisposing to contracture of the proximal interphalangeal joint in extension is thermal burns. Dorsal skin loss may result from burns actually limited to the dorsum of the hand. Deep second-degree as well as third-degree thermal burns may produce significant contracture (Fig. 12-6). The deep second-degree burn contracts as it heals, particularly when the loose skin of the dorsum of the hand is

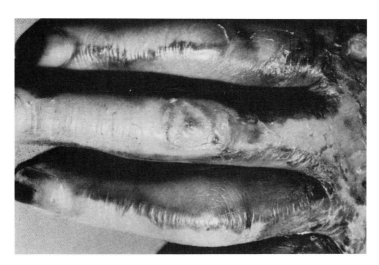

**Fig. 12-6.** The third-degree burn over the dorsum of the proximal interphalangeal joint of the long finger is healing by contraction and epithelialization. The resulting scar will limit joint flexion.

involved. This produces a deficiency of skin. Metacarpophalangeal and proximal interphalangeal joint flexion is restricted by the firm, dense, scarred skin over the dorsum of the hand. Frequently, if the metacarpophalangeal joints are held in extension, the proximal interphalangeal joints can be fully flexed, indicating the absence of capsular changes and defining the culprit as the contracted dorsal skin. This tissue deficiency requires incision or excision of the contracted dorsal skin, full flexion of the metacarpophalangeal and proximal interphalangeal joints, and the insertion of an adequate amount of tissue to permit a full range of joint motion. Less frequently, the dorsal skin of the proximal and middle phalanges is contracted and must be replaced to allow full flexion of the proximal and distal interphalangeal joints. If the wrist is flexed, the amount of skin needed can be decided more accurately. This concept of fully flexing the joints must be appreciated, or insertion of a graft—whether it be free or pedicle—may be inadequate when flexion is attempted (Fig. 12-7). In some cases not only is the dorsal skin involved, but the capsules also are involved.

If possible, this must be determined preoperatively. If not, then this must be determined and corrected at the operating table before the definitive procedure is completed.

SCAR AROUND EXTENSOR TENDONS. This is a frequent occurrence, usually associated with a dorsal injury that may or may not violate the dorsal skin, extensor tendons, or periosteal bone complex. The extensor tendon may become bound in scar at the site of skin injury, yet this does not usually severely limit digital joint flexion. The extensor tendons exhibit such a short amplitude of motion to accomplish full extension and flexion (and the skin usually is loose enough to allow several millimeters of gliding) that flexion and extension are adequate. To produce significant checkreining, the tendon must be embedded in more unyielding scar, for example, a grinding injury that forces coal dust particles into the tissue of the hand. These particles are extremely difficult to remove; in fact, they cannot all be removed. This foreign material excites an extensive and intensive scar reaction that embeds the tendons in scar and binds them to the deep fascia and

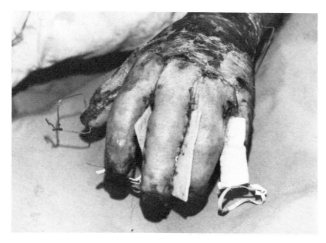

**Fig. 12-7.** A third-degree burn of the dorsum of the hand and fingers. The dorsum has been grafted earlier. The fingers are positioned to ensure insertion of an adequate amount of tissue.

bony metacarpals. This scar readily produces severe checkreining, limiting flexion and extension. The point or area of tendon adherence can be detected by extending the wrist and attempting flexion of the metacarpophalangeal joint. If the metacarpophalangeal joint is stiff in extension, the wrist is flexed to see if this aggravates the extension contracture. If not, then the scar is between the wrist and metacarpophalangeal joint. In this case, when the metacarpophalangeal joint is held in as much flexion as possible, the proximal interphalangeal joint should assume an extended position and offer resistance to passive flexion (Fig. 12-4). As the metacarpophalangeal joint is gradually hyperextended passively, passive and active flexion of the proximal interphalangeal should be improved—at least minimally.

Occasionally the extensor tendon will be bound in scar over the proximal phalanx. This may result from a closed injury that disrupts the periosteum of the proximal phalanx and excites periosteal callus formation (see Fig. 4-25). The extensor tendon over the callus can become firmly adherent to the callus. Attempted passive flexion of the proximal interphalangeal joint meets a nonyielding resistance that is not altered by passive flexion or extension of the wrist or the metacarpophalangeal joint. A more common cause of extensor tendon adherence at the proximal phalanx is in response to fracture callus. Again, the extensor tendon becomes bound in the nonyielding fracture callus, preventing flexion at the proximal interphalangeal joint, no matter what the position of the adjacent joints.

LATERAL BANDS BOUND IN SCAR. If the lateral bands become bound in scar, the proximal interphalangeal joint may be held in the extended position. This is commonly seen after open injury that results in loss of an adjacent digit at least to the level of the metacarpal head. The scar that forms in response to this injury can bind the lateral band and lumbrical muscle to the intermetacarpal ligament. If this fixation occurs with the metacarpophalangeal joint in flexion, the scar can limit proximal interphalangeal joint flexion. This may occur alone or in conjunction with more severe dorsal injuries. We have observed this occurrence only when releasing scar around the extensor tendons, and we have obtained inadequate passive flexion of the proximal interphalangeal joint. In this circumstance, as one attempts passive flexion of the proximal interphalangeal joint, the lateral band becomes taut, yet the extensor tendon is slack. Dissection proximally along the lateral band frees the lumbrical tendon and permits full passive flexion at the proximal interphalangeal joint.

INTRINSIC MUSCLE CONTRACTURE. As the intrinsic muscle shortens, it produces flexion of the metacarpophalangeal joint and extension at the proximal and distal interphalangeal joints. No matter what the cause of intrinsic contracture, the digital joints assume this position. The test for intrinsic tightness requires forced passive extension of the metacarpophalangeal joint in order to exaggerate the effect of the intrinsics on the proximal and distal interphalangeal joints, that is, hyperextension of both joints. With the metacarpophalangeal held in extension, the examiner gently attempts passive flexion at the proximal interphalangeal and distal interphalangeal joints. When the intrinsics are contracted, attempted passive flexion of the proximal and distal interphalangeal joints encounters rigid resistance. For confirmation, the metacarpophalangeal joint is held in flexion, and passive flexion of the proximal and distal interphalangeal joints is again attempted. Under these circumstances, passive flexion is possible, but to a limited extent, since the lateral bands from the contracted interosseous muscles have been relaxed somewhat by flexion of the metacarpophalangeal joint.

SHORTENED LUMBRICALES. Occasionally circumstances arise that produce a relative shortening of the lumbrical muscle, and this may be reflected by significant resistance to flexion at the proximal interphalangeal joint. These circumstances include laceration of the flexor digitorum profundus and sublimis distal to the origin of the lumbrical, and insertion of a flexor tendon graft distal to the origin of the lumbrical that is too long. In both circumstances, the action of the contracting flexor digitorum profundus augments that of the lumbrical, producing a recurvature deformity at the proximal interphalangeal joint. After the history is obtained, the diagnosis is confirmed by acutely flexing the metacarpophalangeal joint and wrist to allow full passive flexion of the proximal interphalangeal joint.

*Stiffness in flexion*

*Capsular factors.* The capsular factors responsible for stiffness of the proximal interphalangeal joints in flexion include: (1) volar plate, (2) accessory collateral ligament, and (3) joint surface erosion with pannus formation adhering to joint surfaces.

VOLAR PLATE. As noted earlier, the volar plate of the proximal interphalangeal joint is a thick, strong, rigid ligament that attaches distally to the volar edge of the base of the middle phalanx and proximally to the laterovolar edges of the proximal phalanx. For flexion of the proximal interphalangeal joint to occur, the ligament must fold upon itself proximally. The loose connective tissue between the two lateral proximal attachments is retracted proximally during joint flexion by the vinculum brevis of the sublimis tendon. With cicatrix formation in this flexed position, the folded attachments of the volar plate become amalgamated. This provides a rigid block to joint extension. In fact, this resistance may be so rigid that simply by feel one can predict that the volar plate is responsible for maintaining the flexion deformity.

ACCESSORY COLLATERAL LIGAMENT. When the proximal interphalangeal joint is held in a continually flexed position for a period

of time, scar may be deposited around the accessory collateral ligaments, which are slack in this position. As joint extension is attempted, resistance is encountered. Involvement of the accessory collateral ligaments usually occurs in conjunction with fixation of the volar plate in flexion. Fibers of the volar portion of the collateral ligament have been observed extending to the volar tubercle of the middle phalanx. While the joint is in flexion, scar in this area may involve these fibers and prevent extension.

JOINT SURFACE EROSION. Erosion of the articular surface with pannus fixation is usually associated with an intraarticular fracture or a long-standing Dupuytren's contracture that has produced a flexion deformity of the joint. Usually a roentgenogram will alert one to the presence of joint erosion. However, the extent and rigidity of the pannus cannot be detected by roentgenograms and should be anticipated from the patient's history. Exuberant pannus formation is usually associated with a long history of pain, swelling, and tenderness in the joint.

By far the most common capsular cause of proximal interphalangeal joint stiffness in flexion is scar amalgamation of the folded proximal portion of the volar plate. Frequently, after release of the volar plate, complete extension is not possible until the volar accessory collateral ligaments have been excised. At the operating table one must continue to search for the cause of stiffness when correction of the initially anticipated cause does not result in complete passive extension of the joint.

*Extracapsular factors.* The extracapsular factors involved in producing stiffness of the proximal interphalangeal joint in flexion include: (1) flexor tendon adhesions, (2) contracture of the forearm musculature, (3) skin involvement, (4) contracture of the oblique retinacular ligament, (5) palmar fascia extension across the proximal interphalangeal joint, and (6) contracture of the fibrous portion of the fibro-osseous tunnel.

FLEXOR TENDON ADHESIONS. Either the profundus or sublimis or both tendons can be involved in proximal adhesions that will restrict proximal interphalangeal joint extension. A laceration at the level of the distal forearm with subsequent repair of the flexor tendons results in an apparent stiffness of the proximal interphalangeal joints (Fig. 12-8). This stiffness can be determined by flexing the wrist and the metacarpophalangeal joints and passively attempting extension of the proximal interphalangeal joints. In this position the restrictive effect of adhesions around the flexor tendons in the forearm will produce minimal effect on proximal interphalangeal joint extension. Similarly, tendon repairs in the palm where the anastomosis is fixed to the palmar tissues by rigid adhesions will have a less restrictive effect on proximal interphalangeal joint extension when the metacarpophalangeal joints are fully flexed. Tendon repairs within the fibro-osseous tunnel frequently adhere and limit proximal interphalangeal joint extension. If the flexor digitorum profundus is the only tendon causing the limitation of proximal interphalangeal joint motion, passive flexion of the distal interphalangeal joint should be accompanied by an improvement in passive extension at the proximal interphalangeal joint, yet full passive extension

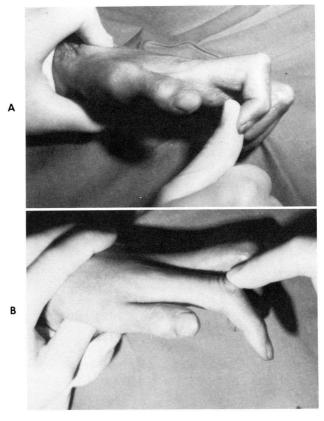

**Fig. 12-8. A,** Flexor tendons repaired in the distal forearm may become embedded in scar and limit extension of the proximal interphalangeal joints when the wrist is in extension. **B,** As the wrist is flexed, the proximal interphalangeal joint extends.

would not usually be gained. Failure to gain improvement in proximal interphalangeal joint extension by this maneuver implies that the flexor digitorum sublimis is stuck in the scar in the flexed position or that the profundus flexor is bound in scar over the middle phalanx. This is a common occurrence when the distal end of the sublimis flexor is not resected far enough distally to avoid its participation in the scar that forms around the profundus flexor anastomosis. Occasionally the sublimis flexor is adhered to the profundus tendon and through this adherence checkreins the proximal interphalangeal joint. If this occurs, the distal interphalangeal joint will be fully movable passively while the proximal interphalangeal is checkreined. In these circumstances, flexion of the wrist and metacarpophalangeal joint will improve extension of the proximal interphalangeal joint.

Fractures of the proximal phalanx involve the periosteum contributing to the fibro-osseous tunnel. Frequently the long flexors become bound in the fracture callus, resulting in checkreining of passive extension at the proximal interphalangeal joint and active flexion at the distal inter-

phalangeal joint when the proximal interphalangeal joint is fully flexed passively (Fig. 12-9).

FOREARM MUSCLE CONTRACTURE. The history, combined with involvement of more than one tendon unit, usually provides the correct diagnosis. Again, wrist and metacarpophalangeal flexion will permit full extension of the proximal interphalangeal joint if only the forearm muscle is involved.

SKIN CONTRACTURE. Skin loss over the flexion creases of the proximal interphalangeal joint and the volar surface of the proximal phalanx may produce a severe contracture of the proximal interphalangeal joint (Fig. 12-10). When considering corrective surgery, one can determine the extent of skin loss by comparing points on the skin of the involved finger with similar points on the uninvolved opposite finger. If after complete excision or release of the scar contracture, complete joint extension is not passively obtained, then the capsular factors contributing to joint stiffness must be defined and corrected before the skin loss is repaired. Frequently, release of the skin contracture does not completely correct the flexion deformity, and capsular factors must be considered

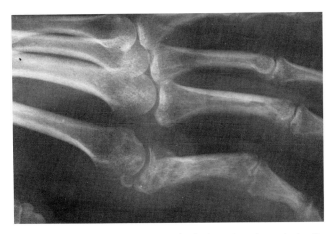

**Fig. 12-9.** Fracture at the base of the proximal phalanx has bound the flexor tendons in scar with the proximal and distal interphalangeal joints flexed. Passive flexion of the proximal interphalangeal joint improves the range of motion in the distal joint.

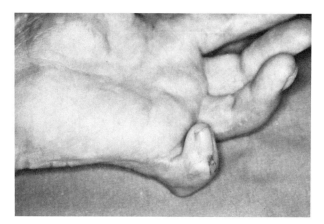

**Fig. 12-10.** Skin contracture on the volar surface of the little finger has produced a marked flexion deformity.

and corrected at the same sitting. This may require release of the volar plate, opening and exposure of the flexor tendons, or even capsulotomy. Thus, the operation that originally was to involve a simple skin grafting procedure now requires pedicle flap coverage. One must be prepared to accurately diagnose and treat these problems at the operating table. Occasionally in the little finger, a band of scar tissue on the ulnar side of the flexor surface can produce significant contracture. One must appreciate the proximal extent of this damaged tissue to allow adequate tissue replacement.

OBLIQUE RETINACULAR LIGAMENT. We have not seen involvement of this ligament to be solely responsible for joint stiffness. It has been a contributing factor when other capsular structures are primarily responsible for stiffness of the proximal interphalangeal in flexion. To appreciate the oblique retinacular ligament contribution, one must identify and preserve the ligament until the primary cause of joint stiffness is corrected. If passive extension of the joint is still not obtained and the oblique retinacular ligament is contracted, it can be detached proximally from the digital sheath. Release of this ligament has not contributed significantly to improved joint extension in our cases.

PALMAR FASCIA EXTENSIONS. Digital extension of the palmar fascia becomes significant in Dupuytren's contracture involving the proximal interphalangeal joints. Bands of palmar fascia apparently extend across the proximal phalanx and proximal interphalangeal joint to unite by dense attachments to the volar plate insertion on the middle phalanx and into the retinacular ligament and flexor tendon sheath. Passive flexion of the metacarpophalangeal joint does not alter the range of passive motion at the proximal interphalangeal joint, because the fibrous bands have extensive attachments along the proximal phalanx and on either side of the proximal interphalangeal joint. This degree of attachment varies with the stage of advancement of Dupuytren's contracture. Early stages demonstrate less severe scarring than the later stages.

FIBRO-OSSEOUS TUNNEL CONTRACTURE. As the anterior part of the fibro-osseous tunnel bridges the proximal interphalangeal joint, it becomes thinned and is formed by the parietal synovium of the digital sheath and a few circular fibrous bands. Injury in this area of the flexor sheath may excite enough scar formation to convert this normally flexible part of the sheath into a thickened nonyielding an-

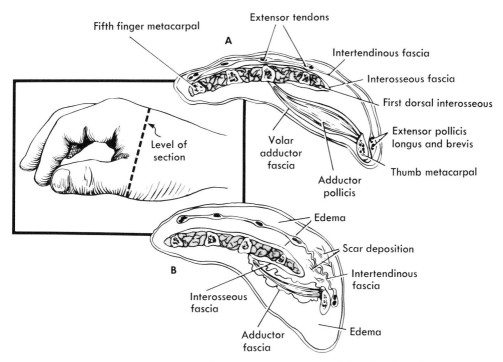

**Fig. 12-11. A,** Fascia interconnects the extensor apparatus of the thumb and common extensors of the fingers by bridging the thumb-index web space. The adductor pollicis muscle is covered by fascia. **B,** Edema on the dorsum of the hand adducts the thumb. Scar formed around the intertendinous fascia and the adductor pollicis fascia holds the thumb in the adducted position.

terior scar. When this occurs in flexion, the scarred sheath interferes with normal joint extension. This is seen as a result of direct trauma to the sheath and in association with Dupuytren's contracture. The extensions of the palmar fascia across the proximal interphalangeal joint become amalgamated with the anterior portion of the fibro-osseous tunnel and thereby severely limit extension. This limitation of passive and active extension occurs no matter what positions the remaining digital joints are in.

**Thumb-index web contracture**

The adductor pollicis muscle is covered on its volar and dorsal surfaces by a fascial layer that is continuous over the free distal border of the muscle. The volar fascia blends into the thenar fascia. The dorsal fascia attaches to the long finger metacarpal where it joins a fascial layer that extends radially over the interosseous muscles to cover the first dorsal interosseous muscle and join the posterior interosseous fascia on the dorsum of the hand beneath the extensor tendons (Fig. 12-11).

The fascia interconnecting the extensor tendons of the fingers spreads radially to cover the first web space and attach to the extensor aponeurosis of the thumb. This bridging fascia covers the fascias of the first dorsal interosseous and adductor muscles and extends distally toward the skin fold of the web space. Here it forms a distinct edge suspended between the common extensor of the index finger and the extensor pollicis longus. The free edge blends into the subcutaneous tissue of the web. The most frequent causes of contracture of the thumb-index web space are local injuries, such as burns or crush injuries, and distant injuries, such as injury of the median and ulnar nerve at the wrist or any injury that excites considerable edema formation.

In the crush injury the injured thumb assumes the adducted position as a result of the tissues' reaction to injury. Edema of the thumb web space does not force the thumb into abduction as one might expect. Rather, the thumb is forced into adduction by the ballooning of the loose dorsal web skin as the thumb web space becomes edematous. With involvement of the entire hand, this process of edema distends the dorsal skin, which in turn pulls the thumb into an adducted position. This reaction to injury leads to a variable degree of scar deposition along the fascial planes, as noted earlier. As this scar is deposited, the thumb is fixed in the adducted position. Scar is also deposited in the dermis and subdermal areas to fix the thumb in an adducted position. This results in an actual loss of skin (Fig. 12-12). Recall the ligaments around the carpometacarpal joint of the thumb. The anterior and posterior oblique ligaments extend between the base of the thumb metacarpal

and the base of the index metacarpal. As the thumb remains in a contracted position, scar is deposited in and around these ligaments, which are lax in the adducted position. This contributes further to the fixed adducted relationship of the thumb-index metacarpals. The adductor pollicis muscle will develop a myostatic contracture if immobilized in the adducted position for an extended period. The superficial head of the first dorsal interosseous muscle may contribute significantly to maintaining this adducted position.

The primary tissue of the first web space involved in burns is the skin. With loss of skin, the reaction to injury causes deposits of fluid anterior and posterior to the extensor tendons. As this fluid accumulates, the skin over the dorsum of the hand is distended, adducting the thumb. As the extensor tendons are elevated from their bed by the edematous reaction, the intertendinous fascia between the finger and thumb extensors becomes taut, contributing further to the contracture. With the eventual reparative processes appearing in the skin wound, fibrogenesis and scar contraction become prominent. As fibrogenesis progresses, scar is deposited between the injured skin and the intertendinous fascia of the web space. Subsequent contracture of the scar results in fixation

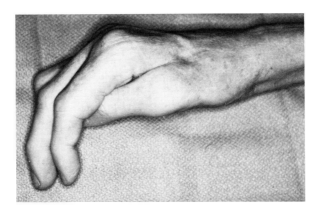

**Fig. 12-12.** The thumb-index web has been completely obliterated. The skin appears to have been resorbed.

of the thumb in an adducted position. To complete the fixation, scar is deposited around the lax anterior and posterior oblique retinacular ligaments bridging from the base of the thumb metacarpal to the index metacarpal. Thus, the injury that began as a skin injury progressed through the edematous process and the reparative process to involve all of the structures bridging the thumb-index web space. After fixation in the adducted position, the adductor pollicis muscle gradually is fixed by scar within its fascia and within the muscle fibers, holding it in the contracted position.

The most frequent nerve injuries associated with development of an adduction contracture of the thumb are division of the median nerve or division of the median and ulnar nerves. When the median nerve is divided, motor function of the recurrent branch that innervates the thenar muscles is lost. Among other actions, these muscles are necessary for abduction of the thumb. Loss of abduction produces a muscle imbalance with the thumb adductors being unopposed. The stage is set for the development of a myostatic contracture of the adductor pollicis. The adductors of the thumb include those innervated by the ulnar nerve and the extensor pollicis longus, which is innervated by the radial nerve. The degree of adduction contracture of the web space developing after a median nerve lesion is minimal compared with that developing after a combined median and ulnar nerve division. Furthermore, the degree of contracture is related to the level of nerve injury; that is, the more proximal the nerve injury, the less severe the contracture. These observations indicate that the more distal lesions involving both nerves are usually associated with a more severe injury of the hand, which results in more edema, more reparative tissue reaction, and a more extended period of immobilization. An injury of the same magnitude that cuts only the sensory half of the median nerve and the entire ulnar nerve should never result in the development of an adduction contracture, because the abductors of the thumb are functioning unopposed by the ulnar-innervated adductor pollicis. When both median and ulnar nerves are cleanly divided more proximally (for example, in the midarm), development of an adduction contracture of the thumb-index web is rare. Again, the reparative process is not as manifest in the hand when the injury is more proximal. Furthermore, complete denervation of the arm results in a flaccid hand that does not develop contracture if the reparative process has been minimal. Spasticity of the thumb adductor can produce an adduction contracture without the reparative process being manifest.

## NONOPERATIVE MOBILIZATION OF STIFF JOINTS
### Evaluation

Nonoperative mobilization of stiff joints requires the following of the physician and the therapist: a firm knowledge of skin, bone, nerve, and tendon healing; an understanding of the capsular and extracapsular factors responsible for normal joint stability; an exposure to the operative procedures in order to visualize the internal arrangement within the hand; and a complete understanding of the factors responsible for the development of stiff joints.

With this background one can approach the nonoperative mobilization of stiff joints. Therapy is directed toward (1) establishing goals for the patient, (2) periodically evaluating therapy methods, (3) controlling the comfort of the hand to allow the patient to participate to his fullest in therapy, (4) providing motivation as needed for the patient, (5) accelerating the rate of scar tissue degradation and remodelling, (6) and reeducating job skills.

*Initial evaluation.* In a review of our first 1,300 patients, 42% complained initial-

MILLIKEN HAND REHABILITATION CENTER    WASHINGTON UNIVERSITY    HAND EVALUATION SHEET

AGE ____ SEX ____ COMPUTER NO. _____ NAME _____

COVERAGE _____ DOMINANT EXTREMITY _____ INJURED EXTREMITY _____

EMPLOYER _____ OCCUPATION _____ DATE OF INJURY _____

NATURE OF INJURY _____

DATES OF SURGICAL PROCEDURES _____

_____

RETURN TO WORK DATE _____ SAME OCCUPATION? _____ NEW OCCUPATION _____

A

| I. FUNCTIONAL ACTIVITY (Y-yes; N-no) | DATE:  EVAL. BY: | | | | DATE:  EVAL. BY: | | | | DATE:  EVAL. BY: | | | |
|---|---|---|---|---|---|---|---|---|---|---|---|---|
| | I | L | R | F | I | L | R | F | I | L | R | F |
| A. KEY PINCH BY DIGIT | | | | | | | | | | | | |
| B. PULP TO PULP PINCH BY DIGIT | | | | | | | | | | | | |
| C. PALMAR FLEXION (CM.)  1. FINGERTIP TO DISTAL CREASE  2. FINGERTIP ⊥ TO PALM | | | | | | | | | | | | |
| D. GROSS GRIP (Kg)  R  L | | | | | | | | | | | | |
| E. PINCH GRIP (LB.)  R  L | | | | | | | | | | | | |
| F. PICK UP PENCIL AND SIGN NAME | | | | | | | | | | | | |
| G. BUTTON THE BUTTON | | | | | | | | | | | | |
| H. OPEN AND CLOSE SAFETY PIN | | | | | | | | | | | | |
| I. USE AN EMPTY DRINKING GLASS | | | | | | | | | | | | |
| II. VOLUME OR CIRCUMFERENCE  MEASUREMENT | | | | | | | | | | | | |
| III. DEXTERITY TESTING (SEC.)  A. PEGS | R  L  R - L  L - R | | | | R  L  R - L  L - R | | | | R  L  R - L  L - R | | | |
| B. PINS AND COLLARS | R  L | | | | R  L | | | | R  L | | | |

**Fig. 12-13. A,** The information on this form provides us with a day-by-day objective evaluation of the patient's progress.

| IV. PAIN DESCRIBE PROBLEMS AND SEVERITY TAKING MEDICATION? | DATE: | DATE: |
|---|---|---|
| V. SENSORY EXAMINATION A. TEMPERATURE AND SHARP-DULL DISCRIMINATION | 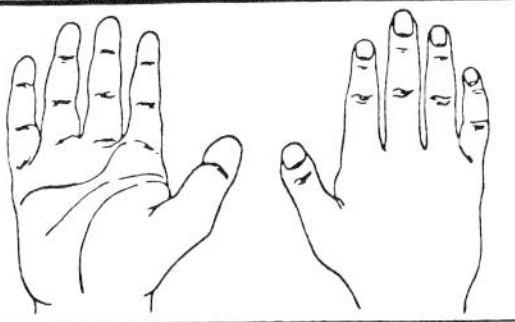 | 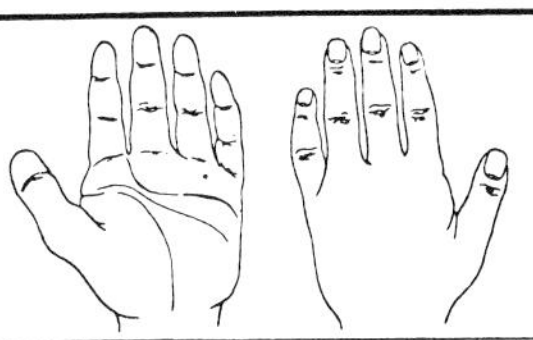 |
| B. STEREOGNOSIS | | |
| C. 2-POINT DISCRIMINATION | T          R I          F L | T          R I          F L |
| D. OTHER SENSORY TESTS CHECK IF DONE | NINHYDRIN SWEAT TEST _____ TEMPERATURE MEASUREMENTS ___ OTHER _____ | NINHYDRIN SWEAT TEST _____ TEMPERATURE MEASUREMENTS ___ OTHER _____ |

VI. JOINT RANGE OF MOTION

**B**

| DATE: | ACT. | PASS. | ACT. | PASS. | ACT. | PASS. | DATE: | ACT. | PASS. | ACT. | PASS. | ACT. | PASS. |
|---|---|---|---|---|---|---|---|---|---|---|---|---|---|
| INDEX: MP EXT. | | | | | | | RING: MP EXT. | | | | | | |
| FLEX. | | | | | | | FLEX. | | | | | | |
| PIP EXT. | | | | | | | PIP EXT. | | | | | | |
| FLEX. | | | | | | | FLEX. | | | | | | |
| DIP EXT. | | | | | | | DIP EXT. | | | | | | |
| FLEX. | | | | | | | FLEX. | | | | | | |
| LONG: MP EXT. | | | | | | | FIFTH: MP EXT. | | | | | | |
| FLEX. | | | | | | | FLEX. | | | | | | |
| PIP EXT. | | | | | | | PIP EXT. | | | | | | |
| FLEX. | | | | | | | FLEX. | | | | | | |
| DIP EXT. | | | | | | | DIP EXT. | | | | | | |
| FLEX. | | | | | | | FLEX. | | | | | | |
| WRIST: EXT. | | | | | | | FOREARM: SUPI. | | | | | | |
| FLEX. | | | | | | | PRO. | | | | | | |
| RADIAL DEV. | | | | | | | | | | | | | |
| ULNAR DEV. | | | | | | | ELBOW: EXT. | | | | | | |
| | | | | | | | FLEX. | | | | | | |
| THUMB: MP EXT. | | | | | | | SHOULDER: | | | | | | |
| FLEX. | | | | | | | FLEX. | | | | | | |
| IP EXT. | | | | | | | ABD. | | | | | | |
| FLEX. | | | | | | | INT. ROT. | | | | | | |
| ABD. | | | | | | | EXT. ROT. | | | | | | |

**Fig. 12-13, cont'd. B,** The active and passive ranges of motion of each joint are measured and recorded during each visit.

ly of stiff joints. The average duration of joint stiffness before we evaluated the patient was 3.42 months. Over 90% had received "therapy." Therapy has acquired a tarnished reputation because of minimal communication between the therapist and the physician. Usually a patient is referred to a therapist after the sutures are removed and the wounds have healed. The therapist may be in the same building, across the street, across town, or even in another town. The point is that there is little or no communication between the physician, the therapist, and the patient. Thus the therapist is proceeding on her own, doing the best job possible. Frequently this therapy may extend for months or even years before the patient finally returns to the doctor, who instructs the patient to stop therapy because it is of no benefit. Or the therapist recognizes the futility of her therapy and finally refers the patient to the physician.

The Hand Rehabilitation Center concept was developed to avoid these problems. Patients are seen at least twice a week by their physician with the therapist present. Treatment plans can be formulated and frequently evaluated. The patient realizes that all this attention and effort are directed toward his recovery and most often responds with much enthusiasm for therapy.

From our experience we have developed an approach to each patient that allows us to avoid the pitfalls previously associated with therapy and to base our treatment plan on an *objective* basis.

The use of an objective basis in therapy eliminates the old subjective approach, that is, "Are you better, worse, or the same?" Most patients want to please you and will say they are better, when in fact there has been little or no progress. Thus, the use of objective measures in our Hand Rehabilitation Center has converted therapy into a science.

*Diagnostic evaluation.* Because we are dealing primarily with stiff joints in this chapter, the evaluation sheet of primary interest is the active and passive range of motion table (Fig. 12-13). Here the patient's entire hand is measured joint by joint, and the active and passive range of motion and the date are recorded. Now we have a baseline, and any subsequent measurements will reflect any change in the patient's status, either improvement or failure to improve.

*Physician's evaluation.* The physician's evaluation is directed toward a general evaluation of the patient's state and his needs. Then the physician must try to determine the cause of the problems in the hand, that is, what is contributing to making the joints stiff. This is an attempt to actually identify the structures responsible for stiffness of the joints (as listed earlier in this chapter). The physician, the patient, and the therapist as a team discuss these findings. The methods for managing stiff joints are discussed with the patient (Fig. 12-14). Treatment is decided based on the physical findings during this evaluation. For example, if there is severe skin contracture preventing movement of the joints, then therapy is a waste of time. The patient must decide whether to leave the hand as it is or undergo surgery to first correct the skin contracture. Similarly, if the joints are rigidly fixed secondary to scar, then therapy is not indicated. With experience, a team will develop a list of contraindications to therapy and will be able to better serve the patient. In our approach, the only choices are: (1) no treatment, (2) therapy, or (3) surgery. The selection of management is obvious in the cases mentioned above, but in the majority of cases the selection of management is not so obvious. The following prognostic evaluation has been developed to aid in proper selection of management.

*Prognostic evaluation.* To determine if therapy can be beneficial, it is given for three half-day sessions over a period of 1 week to those patients for whom surgery is not an obvious selection (Fig. 12-15). Since a baseline was established with our initial measurements, those measurements obtained at the end of the week will indicate if the patient is responding to therapy. Most patients may be placed into one of four groups: Group IV, those who make no progress; Group III, those who make minimal progress; Group II, those who make significant progress; and Group I, those who make remarkable progress (Fig. 12-16). Management decisions are made according to these responses.

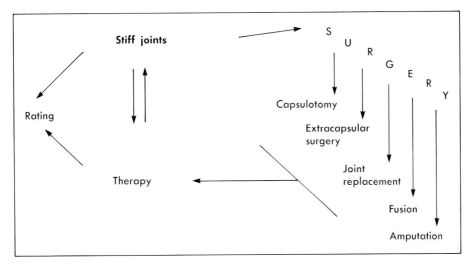

**Fig. 12-14.** The management of stiff joints involves either no treatment, conservative therapy in the Hand Rehabilitation Center, or surgery. The decision is based on the prognostic evaluation.

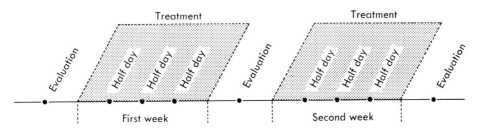

**Fig. 12-15.** The evaluation-treatment plan requires 3 half-days of therapy before reevaluation. An additional 3 half-days may be required according to patient response.

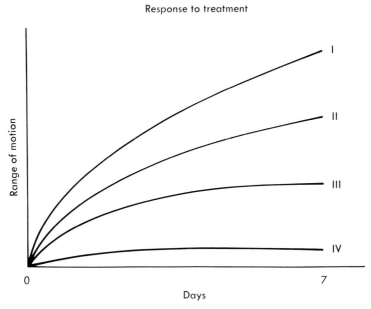

**Fig. 12-16.** The response of most patients to therapy can be described by one of four groupings.

Group IV (no progress). If these patients had been considered candidates for surgery, then either surgery or no further treatment is offered.

Group III (minimal progress). These patients are scheduled for further three half-day sessions over a period of 1 week and then reevaluated.

Group II (significant progress). These patients are scheduled for further therapy during three half-day sessions over a period of 1 week and then reevaluated.

Group I (marked progress). Most of these patients are able to continue their therapy at home or on the job. But we routinely see them for at least one half-day of therapy during the following week and reevaluate them in 1 week.

Thus, at the end of 1 week, all patients have been categorized according to their responses to therapy and can be treated accordingly. This plan for treatment can be accomplished only if the patient's response is recorded in numbers. This provides objective evidence of progress. These recordings can be converted into graphs to better illustrate the rate and extent of the patient's response (Fig. 12-17).

### Treatment

#### Factors impairing treatment

*Pain.* The amount and duration of pain vary considerably among patients with hand injuries. Some patients may have minimal discomfort, whereas in others it is the major problem with their hand. The patient with complaints of moderate

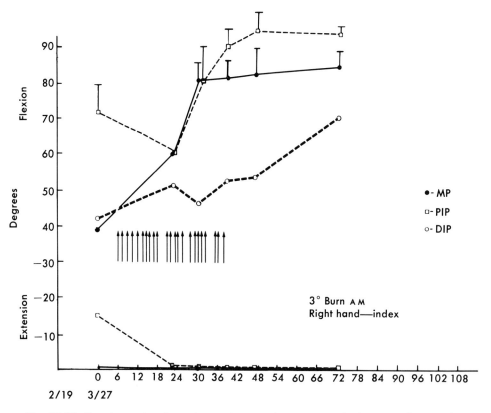

**Fig. 12-17.** The data taken from the evaluation sheets are grafted to provide an indication of the rate and degree of progress. Passive and active ranges are recorded.

to severe discomfort must be thoroughly evaluated by the physician as to the etiology of this pain. For example, movement at a fracture site could be causing the pain. Obviously, the fracture must be properly immobilized before proceeding with therapy. Often we hear complaints: "They kept bending my fingers until they swelled so bad that I can't move any of them now." This represents a failure on the therapist's part to appreciate the proper methods of therapy and recognize the warning signs of too vigorous therapy. Remember a spectrum of tolerance of pain exists as does a spectrum of patients' responses to one method of therapy. Therapeutic modalities that produce heat, such as hot packs, paraffin baths, and whirlpools, frequently relieve pain temporarily. These modalities can be interspersed with other treatment techniques in order to improve circulation and to allow the hand to relax. Occasionally, patients who do not respond to heat may find relief from cold in the form of cold packs wrapped in one layer of toweling. Ice packs produce extreme cold, which is detrimental.

Massage, using gentle motions with firm, constant pressure, is beneficial. If a patient has one particularly painful area, such as a sensitive scar of a painful amputation stump site, tapping with a sponge or the fingertips will frequently help desensitize the area. Another effective method of reducing pain is through the use of activities. Often when a patient is working on a goal-directed task, his attention is diverted, and he is able to work through his pain with a resultant decrease in the pain.

*Edema.* The necessity to control edema is obvious when one reviews the effects of this condition. Swelling around a joint causes stretching of the skin and soft tissue in that area, which in turn produces limited motion. Increased scarring about the joint is the end result of edema. Elevation is the primary treatment for edema.

The patient must be instructed to keep the hand elevated above the shoulder at all times. Elevation of the hand during treatment, massage in a distal to proximal direction, electric compression machines (such as the Jobst Compression Unit), elastic compression garments, and active exercise will all help to eliminate excess fluid in the hand. The use of a string wrap of the fingers and hand will reduce edema significantly.

### Modes of therapy

*Massage.* In order to most effectively apply stress, the hand and the patient must be conditioned to a level that will permit an optimal performance. The use of massage not only applies compressive and distractive forces directly to the scar, but the mechanical rubbing improves the circulation in the part, helps warm the hand, and allows the simultaneous application of oil to dry, thin skin. Thus massage helps to relax the patient, to reduce the edema in the hand, to improve circulation to the hand, and to alter the fibrotic process.

Massage is particularly beneficial in relieving muscle spasm or apprehension in the patient. Massage should precede any dynamic splint since it helps to relax the hand and relieve the tensions within the hand. Another method of warming the hand and improving the circulation is through the application of a paraffin and mineral oil mixture. The mixture is heated to a temperature of about 120° F, and the hand is immersed in the liquid wax and withdrawn after a few seconds. The thin film of wax adhering to the hand is allowed to just lose its shine before the hand is reimmersed. This process of reimmersion is continued until a layer of wax 4 mm thick has developed over the entire hand. Then the hand is covered with towels to help retain the heat of the wax. In the case of a swollen hand, it is kept elevated. After 15 to 20 minutes, the wax is removed and the treatment begun. The application of ice treatment has been recommended by others to decrease spasticity and reduce edema in the hands. Our patients have objected to this quite vigorously, and we have been unable to demonstrate any value of ice therapy.

The therapist now turns attention to the direct application of stress to the scar tissue. This can be accomplished in the following manner: (1) The patient can stress the scar by activating the musculotendinous unit; (2) a dynamic splint can be utilized to stress the scar, or a static splint can be made into a dynamic splint by using an elastic bandage; and (3) direct pressure by massage or bandage may be used. Again, the only clinically proved method of accelerating scar tissue remodelling is the application of stress, either distractive or compressive, to the scar.

*Exercise.* In addition to splinting, the primary method of direct application of stress to the scar tissue is through passive, active, and resisted exercises. Without therapeutic intervention, the scarring process will often cause joint stiffness and tendon adhesions. Therefore, all therapy is directed toward the conversion of unfavorable scar to favorable scar and the transformation of favorable scar to functional scar. Conversion and transformation of this scar occur through the biological processes of degradation and synthesis of collagen. Therapy attempts to accelerate these biological processes. This is accomplished by the following methods: (1) the use of dynamic splinting, (2) direct massage to the area, (3) passive exercise techniques including traction to the joint, joint mobilization, and passive stretching, (4) active exercise, and (5) resisted exercise that is applied through manual resistance, weights, or mechanical resistance. Scar around the tendons is gradually remodelled, and the muscle unit gains strength as evidenced by improved power grip and pinch strength.

Passive movement of the joints alters the restrictive scar around the joints and,

to a lesser extent, the scar around the tendons. Passive stretching is facilitated by applying traction to the joint so that friction between the joint surfaces is decreased. Along with traction, the joint can be mobilized in anterior-posterior, lateral, and rotational glide direction. This type of movement, called physiological movement, makes up what we know as normal joint play, and it is necessary for the performance of anatomical motions such as flexion-extension and abduction-adduction.

During active exercise the tension developed in the musculotendinous unit is transmitted to the offending scar. Tendon gliding is directly affected by the strength of the muscle and the amount of scar adhesions, which restrict tendon motion. Through continued stress on the tendon, the adhesions are remodelled with a resultant increase in active motion. As resistance is added to an exercise, more of the muscle's motor units are activated, and this increases the amount of pull transmitted through the tendon. Thus more stress is applied to the scar.

The respective use of active, passive, and resisted exercise will vary tremendously from one patient to another depending on the amount of pain, joint stiffness, tendon gliding, muscle strength, and wound healing. In each case, the exercise program must be goal-directed and specifically suited to that particular patient.

*Splinting*

PRINCIPLES OF SPLINTING. The therapist designs each splint with a specific goal in mind. Splints may be classified as either static or dynamic. A static splint is nonmovable and maintains the joints in a fixed position. Static splinting includes protective splints and static progressive splints. A protective splint is one that holds the part in a specific position to eliminate reinjury or overstretching. A static progressive splint is fitted while the parts to be splinted are being stretched, and the splint conforms to this forced fixed position. An example

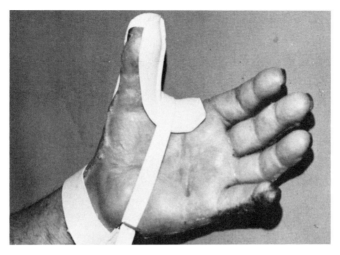

**Fig. 12-18.** The static thumb-index web splint can be converted to a dynamic splint by abducting the thumb as far as possible and preparing the splint, which is positioned with a proximal strap around the wrist.

is spreading the thumb-index web space and fitting a splint to this area (Fig. 12-18). The stresses developed in the tissues are transmitted to the offending scar. As the scar matures and loosens, another splint will be fitted to progressively increase the web space.

A dynamic splint exerts a force on a part by a rubber band in order to increase joint motion. A dynamic splint may also be supportive, as in the case of a radial nerve injury, where the rubber bands help to return the fingers to an extended position and replace the action of the extensor muscles. A dynamic splint consists of a static base to which an outrigger is attached. After the splint and outrigger have been fabricated, a finger loop or sling is fitted around the part to be stressed. A rubber band attached between the sling and the outrigger exerts a dynamic force. The direction and force applied by the rubber band are most important. When the application of stress to effect joint motion is desired, the resultant line of force should form a right angle with the axis of rotation of the joint. In other words, the optimal angle of pull is 90 degrees.

Let us review resultant forces for a moment. When a force (F) is exerted in a particular direction, this force is the resultant of two forces at right angles to one another, $F_1$ and $F_2$ (Fig. 12-19). The greater the angle (a), the larger the force of component $F_1$. Why is this important? If we consider $F_1$ as a significant force (and it can be when dynamic traction is improperly applied), the proximal phalanx is forced against the metacarpal head, producing compression of the articular cartilages. Compression of articular surfaces could lead to cartilage cell destruction, erosions of the articular surfaces, and pannus formation. As a consequence, the application of traction ($F_3$) should be as close to $F_2$ as possible. Ideally, the traction should be applied through balanced traction, one force directly opposing $F_1$ and the second overlapping $F_2$. This would minimize compression of the articular surfaces and concentrate a greater part of the force of traction toward accomplishing joint rotation.

A second concern is that as the proximal phalanx reaches its maximum rotation allowed by the scar, the articular surfaces

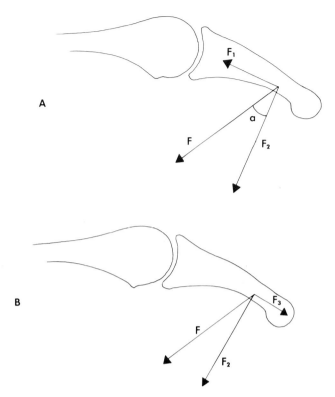

**Fig. 12-19. A,** When a force *(F)* is applied, it is composed of two components: $F_1$ and $F_2$. The greater the angle *(a)*, the larger the component $F_1$, and the smaller angle *(a)*, the smaller the component force $F_1$. **B,** A counterforce *(F_3)* may be applied to counteract the compressive force at the articular surfaces.

become distracted and the volar lip of the proximal phalanx acts as a fulcrum, allowing the dorsal edge of the phalanx to pivot open, much like the turning of the page of a book (Fig. 12-2). This results when the collateral ligaments are considerably shortened or when too great a load is placed on the proximal phalanx too rapidly or when the distance from the joint under treatment is too great. When the collateral ligaments are rigidly shortened and the metacarpophalangeal joints are in hyperextension, dynamic splinting has proved of no value in gaining significant mobilization of the joints. If too great a force is exerted rapidly, the ligaments do not have an opportunity to undergo biological alterations that will allow at least minimal rotation. And finally, the further

away the force is applied from the joint in question, the greater is its mechanical advantage, but unfortunately, the greater are the compressive effects of $F_1$ on the articular surface.

Therefore, a dynamic splint should be constructed so that the force is exerted just distal to the joint being moved. For example, to increase joint motion of the proximal interphalangeal joint, the sling should be placed around the middle phalanx.

How much force should one apply to gain mobilization of a joint? In normally innervated skin, we are limited by the ischemic effects produced by the sling around the fingers. The pressure exerted through this sling cannot exceed the capillary pressure in the cutaneous vessels for an extended period of time, or the skin will be rendered ischemic, and necrosis will ensue. The capillary perfusion pressure of skin in the arterial limb of the capillary loop averages 32 mm Hg, whereas the midpoint and the venous end of the capillary loop exhibit a mean pressure of 20 and 12 mm Hg, respectively. When the major venous vessels to an area are occluded, as by pressure, the pressure in the arterial end of the capillary loop rises to a level of 10 mm Hg above that pressure producing occlusion. Warming the hand produces arterial dilatation resulting in a rise in capillary pressure to 20 to 30 mm Hg. Cooling results in a fall of the capillary pressure. Since capillary pressure varies considerable with manipulation, let us select an average pressure of 30 mm Hg as necessary for perfusion. We can assume that the pull of a well-fitting dynamic splint sling is dissipated over the area covered by the sling. The amplitude of pull is determined by the area of the sling and the required capillary perfusion pressure. A sling that fits the average proximal phalanx measures $20 \times 15$ mm or has 300 mm² of area. Since we can apply 30 mm Hg pressure to each square millimeter, a force of 9,000 mm Hg is possible. This converts to 0.269 lb, which is equivalent to 4.3 oz.

Now, to be able to use this information, one must determine how much force the dynamic splint is generating. Because all rubber bands are different, we place a rubber band in its position on the splint and measure its distance of stretch. This band is transferred to a simple spring-loaded measuring device that permits stretching of the band to the earlier recorded length (as noted when it was on the dynamic splint); and then we directly read the force the band is generating at this length. Use of a linear spring allows direct readings with the apparatus in place. In this manner one can maintain a scientific approach to the application of stress

to the offending scar tissue. As the passive range of motion of the joint improves, the rubber band is changed, its tension is determined and recorded, and so is the duration of time of application. Furthermore, the angle that the force ( F ) makes with this axis of rotation of the joint can be measured directly, and the amount of force producing rotation can be approximated. Clinically, a wide range of tolerance exists. The average person can tolerate 6 oz of force very well for up to 4 hours. The application of a smaller amount of force is tolerated over a much longer period of time. The significance of the amplitude of force will be discussed in Chapter 15.

In the anesthetic hand, it is particularly important to maintain the applied forces below those that will produce ischemic necrosis of the skin. Since the patient's pain pattern is lost, he cannot recognize when excessive pressure is being applied. These patients must be carefully instructed in the application of dynamic splints, the time of actual splinting permitted, and the need to observe the skin for any evidence of circulatory embarrassment.

Now that we are aware of the amount of pressure the skin can tolerate, can we increase the stress on the scar tissue without increasing the pressure of the skin? Recall the thin boy on the long end of the seesaw balancing the stout boy on the short end (Fig. 12-20, A). As the length of the movement arm is increased, the torque created by a given force increases. Thus, the lighter load can produce a torque equal to that of the heavier load if given enough movement arm. Rather than applying the sling to the proximal phalanx, we can apply a cast to the finger (to stabilize the proximal and distal interphalangeal joints) and apply the force to the distal phalanx. Thus, a load of 6 oz applied 1 inch from the metacarpophalangeal joint creates a torque of 6 oz-inches whereas the same load (6 oz) applied 3 inches from the metacarpopha-

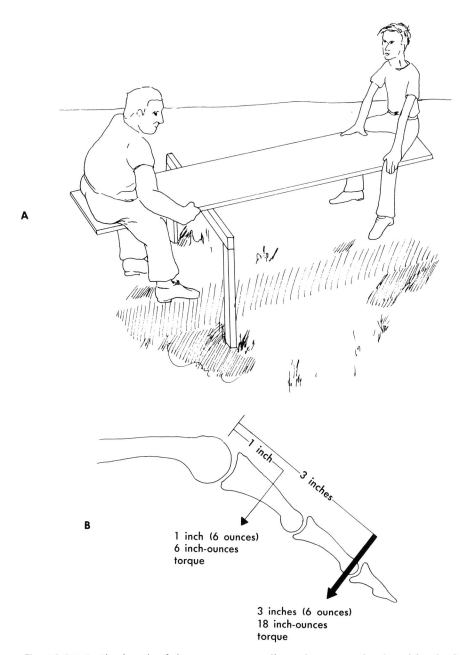

**A**

**B**

1 inch
3 inches

1 inch (6 ounces)
6 inch-ounces
torque

3 inches (6 ounces)
18 inch-ounces
torque

**Fig. 12-20. A,** The length of the moment arm allows the torque developed by the lighter load to equal that of the heavier load. **B,** When the moment arm is lengthened, the same physiological load can be applied but with an increased torque at the axis of rotation of the metacarpophalangeal joint.

langeal joint results in 18 oz-inches of torque at the axis of rotation (Fig. 12-20, B). But remember that the object of dynamic splinting is not to tear scar tissue but to encourage its biological reorganization into a tissue more suitable for joint motion. At this time, we do not know the optimal amount of stress, the optimal length of time of application of stress, or the optimal method of application to bring about the most rapid favorable modification of scar tissue. Only through scientific investigation, beginning with the simple approaches mentioned above, will progress in therapy through a basic understanding of scar tissue remodelling be obtained.

SPLINT CONSTRUCTION. The first step in making a splint is to determine its purpose and then envision its design. Tracing an outline of the hand and then making a paper pattern help to ensure a good fit. Certain anatomical guidelines must be met in designing a splint and making a pattern. Anatomical considerations include following the lines of the hand so that a splint does not restrict motion unnecessarily. Examples are cutting out around the thenar eminence and stopping below the distal palmar crease so that motion of the thumb and metacarpophalangeal joints is not blocked. Bony prominences should be avoided if possible, or care should be taken to see that these areas are properly padded. The part proximal to the joint to which force is applied must be well stabilized by the base or static portion of the splint. However, joints should not be immobilized unnecessarily by a bulky splint. Once a well-fitting pattern has been made, actual construction of the splint is begun.

There are several choices in selecting materials for fabricating a splint, and they fall into two main categories: plaster and thermoplastic materials. Plaster splinting has one disadvantage in that static progressive splints need to be changed often. Thermoplastic materials require use of more equipment and are more expensive, but a close fit can be obtained, and this

method is less time-consuming. A distinct advantage is the ability to modify a thermoplastic splint as the patient changes. Regardless of the splinting material used, a splint is uniquely constructed to fit a particular patient in order to meet a specific goal.

Each splint must be checked frequently to see that it is still accomplishing its purpose and that a proper fit is being maintained. As a patient continues through his course of rehabilitation, several different splints may be indicated to promote maximum hand function. Some of the more common splints will be illustrated and discussed. Basically, dynamic splints can be classified as flexion, extension, or opposition splints.

Flexion splints for the metacarpophalangeal joints can be prepared to include either a volar or dorsal forearm splint. The volar splint covers the forearm and palm to the distal palmar crease to provide stability to the wrist. Either Velcro or buckle straps provide fixation of the splint to the forearm. Unfortunately, when dynamic traction is applied, the splint has a tendency to slip distally, and flexion of the metacarpophalangeal joints is blocked by the displaced edge of the splint. Use of a dorsal splint can avoid this problem (Fig. 12-21). The outrigger is curved

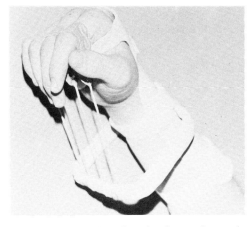

**Fig. 12-21.** Use of a dorsal splint with a volar bar minimizes slippage of the splint distally.

around the forearm onto the volar surface to provide the proper angle with the proximal phalanges. This provides excellent fixation of the outrigger to the splint. The dorsal splint must include a metacarpal bar to ensure stability. The bar is thin and rounded and positioned proximal to the distal palmar crease. After the splint has been completed, dynamic traction is applied. We begin with 4 to 6 oz of force and have the patient wear the splint for 10 to 20 minutes to determine his tolerance. The force is adjusted by changing rubber band size until the patient reports that the splint is tolerable and no evidence of decreased circulation to pressure areas is noted. When the proper force is determined, the patient gradually increases the wearing schedule of the splint during the day. When this is between 4 to 8 hours, the patient generally wears the splint at night so that it does not interfere with hand function. As the patient's tolerance increases and joint motion improves, the force generated by the rubber bands is increased appropriately.

The type of flexion splint prepared for the proximal interphalangeal joints is determined by the state of the metacarpophalangeal joints. If flexion of the latter is normal or nearly normal, a small banding metal splint can be prepared (Fig. 12-22).

Finger loops with rubber bands are attached to the metal band. The splint is simple to prepare, apply, and use. As the proximal interphalangeal joint gains in flexion, the splint may become inadequate because there is not enough distance between the finger sling and the metal band for adequate tension to develop in the rubber band. At this point a strip of rubber surgical glove can be attached to the metal and placed over the dorsum of the middle phalanx. Alternately, a dynamic splint covering the distal phalanx and attaching to the proximal phalanx may be used (Fig. 12-23).

Preparation of extension splints for the metacarpophalangeal joints requires that the wrist be stabilized by a dorsal splint and the outrigger be positioned so that the rubber bands provide force at a right angle to the proximal phalanx. A metacarpal bar and distal forearm straps aid stability.

When extension of the proximal interphalangeal joints must be obtained, the splint outlined previously can be modified so that the splint extends over the metacarpophalangeal joints to the level of the

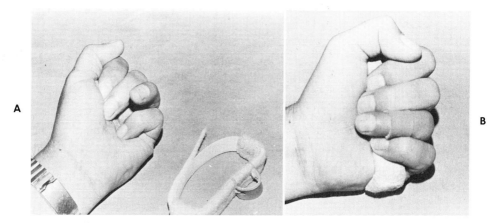

**A**     **B**

Fig. 12-22. **A,** A banding metal splint is helpful to increase proximal interphalangeal joint flexion if metacarpohalangeal joint flexion is at least 60 degrees. **B,** Splint in place.

proximal interphalangeal joints (Fig. 12-24). This area of the splint in contact with the metacarpophalangeal joint and dorsum of the proximal phalanx must be well padded. This arrangement ensures that the force applied to the middle phalanx will be acting primarily on the stiff proximal interphalangeal joint and not forcing a supple metacarpophalangeal joint into hyperextension. When only a single proximal interphalangeal joint is involved, the Wynn-Parry splint is excellent.

The thumb-index web contracture, as with all contractures, is much easier to prevent than to cure. Prevention requires that the surgeon establish a routine pattern that he must observe every time a dressing is applied or reapplied. He must always stop and ask, "What do I want this dressing to accomplish?" Any time there is even a slight trace of an adduction contracture developing, he must place the thumb into the fully abducted position and apply the dressing in such a manner as to maintain this position. Often, if he is not extremely careful, the thumb will be placed in a position of adduction by the application of the dressing—an obvious failure to attend to details.

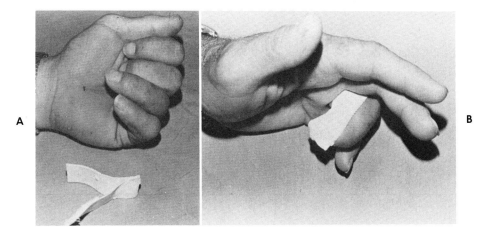

Fig. 12-23. **A**, An elastic band attached with Velcro is used to increase proximal interphalangeal joint flexion. **B**, Splint in place.

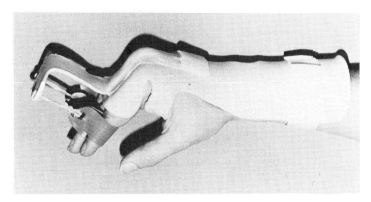

Fig. 12-24. The dorsal outrigger and splint have been modified to aid proximal interphalangeal joint extension without hyperextending the metacarpophalangeal joint.

At each dressing change, the dressing must be reapplied to maintain the position. After the dressing has been discarded, one can use a static or a static progressive splint to maintain abduction as discussed previously.

The dynamic abduction splint can be used as a prophylactic or therapeutic device; it consists of a forearm component that provides stability and serves as an attachment for an outrigger. The outrigger is positioned parallel to the long axis of the thumb. Traction is usually applied by a sleeve encircling the thumb and connecting through rubber bands to the outrigger (Fig. 12-25). Unfortunately, the sleeve is usually positioned distally to gain a greater mechanical advantage, a maneuver that has severe drawbacks. First, the stress is placed primarily on the metacarpophalangeal joint capsule, including the ulnar collateral ligament. Second, the radial side of the proximal phalanx base is wedged against the metacarpal condyle, producing excessive pressure at this point—pressure that could result in destruction of the articular cartilage. And third, only a fraction of the intended dynamic traction force

is delivered to the structures involved in producing or maintaining the contracture, that is, the skin over the dorsum of the web, the intertendinous fascia, the adductor pollicis fascia and fascia of the thenar eminence, and the palmar fascia. In order to accomplish more effective delivery of the dynamic force, traction must be placed directly on the thumb metacarpal. This can be accomplished with skeletal traction (certainly the most efficient) or by modifying the thumb sling to concentrate the pull more on the metacarpal head than the proximal phalanx base (Fig. 12-26).

To obtain skeletal traction, a smooth Kirschner wire is inserted transversely into the thumb metacarpal to enter ulnar to the extensor pollicis longus tendon and exit at the midlateral line of the radial side of the metacarpal head. The entry points of the wire are covered with gauze soaked in Merthiolate. The forearm splint and outrigger are prepared, rubber bands are applied, and the traction is calibrated. Traction may be continuous or intermittent as needed.

Skin traction is much more difficult to apply effectively to the head of the thumb

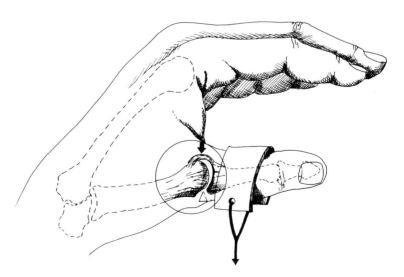

**Fig. 12-25.** A sling around the thumb phalanx will transmit much of the load to the ulnar collateral ligament of the metacarpophalangeal joint.

metacarpal. The usual sling has been modified so that it fits over the metacarpophalangeal joint and increases the delivery of force to the metacarpal, but it is not as effective as skeletal traction. Skin traction is adequate for prophylactic but not for therapeutic measures.

These are but a few of the many types of splints available when one prepares his own splints. Through development of his ability, one can fabricate splints for any problem that may be encountered. Yet remember, the splint is no more than an aid—an aid that must be properly selected, designed, applied, and discarded as the patient's needs dictate. The splint cannot replace the need for physical and occupational therapists who have become experts in the field of hand rehabilitation.

*Combined therapy.* Splinting alone cannot provide adequate treatment for a patient with a hand injury. Splinting must be used in conjunction with a varied exercise program as one part of a comprehensive treatment approach. Once again the importance of frequently recording active and passive joint range of motion must be em-phasized, especially in evaluating the effectiveness of splinting. Specific joint measurements provide a true indication of the patient's progress, that is, the amount of change in relation to time (Fig. 12-17). These numbers may also reveal a decrease in joint range of motion and indicate the need for a splint. Therefore, ongoing evaluation is essential throughout the treatment process, because it provides a means of correlating the stress applied to scarred tissues with the length of application and the biological change in the scar.

Certainly not all, but many patients do require an extra stimulus to begin using their injured hand. Often a patient will carry the hand as though it were not a part of his body. Early in treatment, the therapist evaluates functional skills of daily living. Use of the hand is encouraged in goal-oriented tasks, and often a patient will be involved in a vocational activity. This project can be graded to provide a light to heavy work experience for the injured hand. Knowledge of the patient's occupation allows the therapist to design a program that helps restore the movements

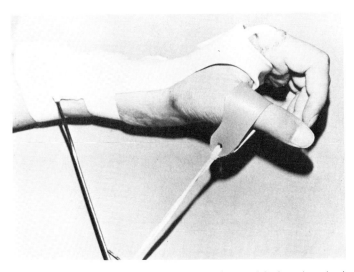

**Fig. 12-26.** The sling around the thumb phalanx can be modified so that the load is placed on the metacarpal head rather than on the ulnar collateral ligament.

and power the patient needs to perform his work tasks.

There are many advantages for a patient being admitted to a rehabilitation center that specializes only in hand problems. The patient sees others with hand injuries, either more or less severe than his own, who are improving and returning to work. This realization creates a totem pole effect that provides hope and encouragement. He gradually realizes that the team's efforts are directed toward attaining his best result in the shortest time possible.

The occupational therapist and the physical therapist work closely with the physician and the patient to provide a comprehensive program. Fundamental to treatment is the patient's understanding of his injury and the important role he must assume in following his prescribed treatment program. Acceptance of his disability coupled with the patient's cooperation and motivation aids in the rehabilitation team's goals of returning each patient to gainful employment and achieving his maximum level of function.

### Specific treatment for stiff joints

*Metacarpophalangeal joints.* Because the metacarpophalangeal joints become stiff in extension, the goal of initial treatment is to increase active and passive flexion of these joints. Exercise and dynamic splinting are the primary means of increasing and maintaining metacarpophalangeal joint flexion. Passive exercise is done by firmly stabilizing the metacarpal before applying force to the proximal phalanx. By utilizing the exercise techniques of joint mobilization and proprioceptive neuromuscular facilitation, which include rhythmic stabilization, contraction-relaxation, and maximal resistance, greater passive range of motion can be achieved. However, it is extremely important to observe the patient's responses and to be aware of his pain tolerance. Each patient will probably experience some varying degree of discomfort during passive exercise, but this should dissipate shortly

after passive stretching. The importance of active exercise must be emphasized, because voluntary motion is essential in maintaining the gains made by passive stretching. During part of each treatment session, patients work independently on a variety of appropriate active exercises, utilizing commercial and custom-made exercise equipment. Each piece of equipment is used to promote a specific goal, which is demonstrated to the patient. Patients are provided with equipment to use at home and are given suggestions on ways to use household items to perform similar active exercises. Resistive exercise also plays an important part in the treatment process. The patient is asked to actively flex and extend his metacarpophalangeal joints against manual resistance and then to hold the extreme of each position against maximal resistance, thereby increasing overall hand strength and endurance.

The patient with stiff metacarpophalangeal joints is fitted with a dynamic metacarpophalangeal flexion splint, which provides an ongoing effect of exercise (Fig. 12-21). The patient is instructed to wear the splint for increasing periods daily until he can wear it comfortably for several hours. He then begins to wear it at night, which allows more spontaneous use of the hand during the day.

*Proximal interphalangeal joints.* As range of motion of the metacarpophalangeal joints improves and is maintained actively, the focus of treatment is directed toward increasing the mobility of the proximal interphalangeal joints. These joints generally become stiff in flexion and often lack several degrees of motion in both extension and flexion. Again, techniques of active, passive, and resistive exercise are employed to increase joint mobility. During passive exercise, the therapist firmly stabilizes the proximal phalanx and then applies slow, firm force on the middle phalanx. Traction may be applied and the joint mobilized to gain more degrees of passive motion. An

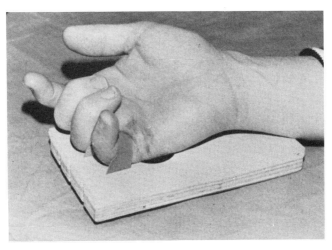

**Fig. 12-27.** Use of a vinyl strap on a slotted board permits independent flexion of proximal and distal interphalangeal joints.

exercise board is used to stabilize the proximal phalanx during active exercise and promote good flexor tendon gliding (Fig. 12-27). The patient's hand is also positioned on this board to work on increasing active distal interphalangeal flexion as well. Another useful piece of equipment can be made by joining two boards at a right angle. The patient pushes his hand into the right angle so that his metacarpophalangeal joints are maintained in 80 to 90 degrees of flexion. He is asked to work on active flexion of his fingers in this position. In addition to specific joint exercise, many resistive activities involving the entire arm are introduced. Prevention of a stiff shoulder, elbow, and wrist is extremely important, and usually this type of active-resistive exercise requires a sustained gross grasp. A wide variety of fine motor tasks that require pinch grip and opposition are also initiated. These activities are goal-oriented and aid in improving dexterity and functional use of the stiff hand.

Dynamic splinting of the proximal interphalangeal joint in extension is accomplished with a Wynn-Parry splint (Fig. 12-28). Dynamic flexion splinting of the proximal interphalangeal joint can be accomplished with the banding metal splint. Usually, the patient continues use of his metacarpophalangeal flexion splint at night and alternates use of the dynamic proximal interphalangeal splints during the day. If necessary, static volar proximal interphalangeal extension splints can be worn in conjunction with the metacarpophalangeal flexion splint at night to maintain proximal interphalangeal joint extension.

Evaluation and observation of the patient's functional use of his involved hand continue throughout the course of treatment. Initially the patient is instructed to use his hand for light, everyday activities. Adaptive devices may be provided to assist the patient in eating and writing if the dominant hand is injured. These should be used on a temporary basis only because all patients are encouraged to use their hands in a normal fashion as soon as possible. Moderately strenuous activities are introduced as the patient improves; often vocational or craft activities are provided. The value of ongoing use of the injured hand in goal-directed activities should not be underestimated.

A general method of management of the stiff hand has been presented, but it must

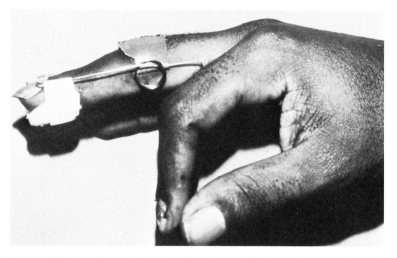

**Fig. 12-28.** Spring wire splint (Wynn-Parry) provides dynamic extension splint.

be modified in order to meet the particular needs of each patient. Once again, the reliability of the patient in following his prescribed treatment program is a large factor in providing effective therapy. Home programs are verbal or written; they are reviewed and updated frequently to ensure that the patient is performing his exercises correctly and that additional ones are added as he progresses. Patient education is a continuous process and is essential in helping the patient understand the nature of his injury and the role he himself must assume in regaining maximum hand function.

***Results of conservative treatment.*** Of the first 1,300 patients treated in the Hand Rehabilitation Center, 546 complained of stiff joints. Complete data were obtained on these patients, providing the basis for evaluation of the results of conservative therapy. The patients had stiff joints for an average of 3.42 months before being seen. Most had received some "therapy." All were treated after being seen in the Hand Rehabilitation Center according to the scheme above.

*Range of motion.* The average range of motion of each finger at the metacarpo-

**Table 12-1.** Results of nonoperative management*

|  | Pretreatment | Posttreatment |
|---|---|---|
| Index |  |  |
| MP | 42° (±14) | 77° (±15) |
| PIP | 42° (±23) | 84° (±26) |
| Long |  |  |
| MP | 43° (±19) | 83° (±16) |
| PIP | 42° (±22) | 76° (±29) |
| Ring |  |  |
| MP | 39° (±20) | 50° (±17) |
| PIP | 40° (±24) | 75° (±29) |
| Little |  |  |
| MP | 33° (±19) | 75° (±20) |
| PIP | 39° (±24) | 71° (±29) |

*The metacarpophalangeal (MP) and proximal interphalangeal (PIP) joints of the finger were measured before treatment and at completion of treatment. Note marked improvement in range of motion after treatment. The numbers in parentheses represent one standard deviation.

phalangeal and proximal interphalangeal joints before treatment and after completion of treatment is presented in Table 12-1. Note the severity of both the metacarpophalangeal and proximal interphalangeal joint stiffness before treatment. At the conclusion of treatment, there had been a

**Table 12-2.** Rehabilitation of stiff hand: duration of treatment

|  | Half-days | Whole days |
|---|---|---|
| Number | 1,572 | 241 |
| Patients | 212 | 212 |
| Average per patient | 7.4 | 1.1 |

**Table 12-3.** Conservative treatment of stiff joints*

|  | No. fingers | Disability (%) | |
|---|---|---|---|
|  |  | Pretreatment | Posttreatment |
| Index |  |  |  |
| MP and PIP | 95 | 55 | 16 |
| PIP | 20 | 35 | 10 |
| Long |  |  |  |
| MP and PIP | 86 | 54 | 18 |
| PIP | 29 | 35 | 15 |
| Ring |  |  |  |
| MP and PIP | 81 | 56 | 35 |
| PIP | 29 | 36 | 15 |
| Little |  |  |  |
| MP and PIP | 74 | 58 | 24 |
| PIP | 39 | 36 | 17 |

*The average disability per joint and finger was calculated before and after treatment.

marked improvement in all fingers and all joints. However, the ring finger had not improved to the same extent as the other fingers.

*Duration of treatment.* Treatment is not given by the hour. Patients are either treated for a half- or a whole day. When we reviewed our patients, we found that the average patient was treated a total of 7.4 half-days and 1.1 whole days (Table 12-2). Recall that the management plan is based on 6 half-days of therapy over a 2-week period. Thus the average patient was treated only 1.4 half-days and 1.1 whole days beyond the period of evaluation and treatment.

*Physical impairment prevented.* The patients have been rated according to workmen's compensation laws, and their physical impairment was determined before and after conservative therapy (Table 12-3). This was converted into weeks of disability, and the total for 546 patients was 12,122 weeks. Since the payment for disability varies among states, the actual savings will vary according to state. Presently, in Illinoiis the payment is $231 per week, whereas in Missouri it is $95 per week. Thus in Illinois the total savings in disability in 546 patients was $2,800.182. The savings in disability was $5,128 per patient.

*Cost of therapy.* A total of 546 patients required 4,048 half-days of therapy and 600 whole days of therapy. At a charge of $25 per half-day and $40 per whole day, the total cost of therapy was $125,580. Thus the cost per patient was $231. The savings in patient cost, that is, the savings in disability minus the cost of patient care, was $2,674,602 for 546 patients!

## OPERATIVE MOBILIZATION OF STIFF JOINTS

When the decision has been made that nonoperative therapy is no longer beneficial, operative therapy must be considered. The indications will be discussed in detail in the final chapter. Only the operative techniques will be discussed in this section.

### Metacarpophangeal joint

*Dorsal approach.* The anesthesized arm is rendered bloodless by a pneumatic tourniquet. The extensor tendons are exposed by four straight longitudinal incisions over the metacarpals. These tendons are divided longitudinally over the metacarpophalangeal joint for 3 cm (Fig. 12-29). The divided extensor hood is retracted. If the dorsal capsule of the joint is involved, it will be thickened, whitish, and rigid. This capsule and the attachments of the extensor tendon to the base of the

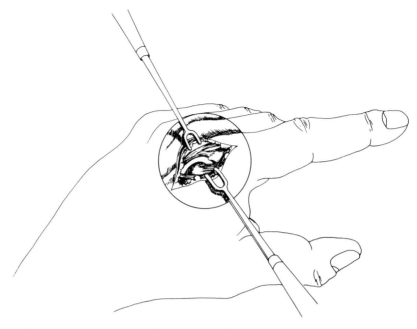

**Fig. 12-29.** The dorsal approach (by Howard) allows direct visualization of the dorsal joint capsule and the collateral ligaments after the extensor tendons have been split longitudinally.

proximal phalanx are excised. If the synovium is not involved, it appears as a thin filmy layer of pliable tissue. If the dorsal joint capsule requires excision, flexion is tested. If flexion is still limited, a Freer elevator is gently inserted between the articular surfaces to probe the volar synovial pouch. The dorsal portion of the collateral ligament is excised. The volar portion of the ligament and the accessory collateral ligament are preserved. Any adhesions that may have formed between the cord portion of the collateral ligament and the head of the metacarpal are freed. Pressure against the base of the proximal phalanx will rotate the proximal phalanx into flexion beneath the head of the metacarpal. Occasionally the finger will snap into full flexion and snap out as extension from full flexion is initiated. This results from remaining strands of the proper collateral ligaments being stretched over the flaring volar radial tubercles as discussed

earlier. This snapping may be eliminated by excision of the offending fibers of the collateral ligament. When the collateral ligament is severely thickened and shortened, the cordlike portion of the ligament should be removed near the tubercle on either side of the head of the metacarpal and a segment excised. The remainder of the accessory collateral ligament is preserved, to prevent ulnar drift of the fingers. One must also take care to preserve the attachment of the interosseous tendon into the base of the phalanx just distal to the attachment of the collateral ligament.

If the phalanx does not rotate into flexion beneath the head of the metacarpal, a curved periosteal elevator should be inserted around the head of the metacarpal to recreate the volar pouch beneath the head of the metacarpal. In long-standing cases, this pouch becomes obliterated as the volar plate becomes adherent to the metacarpal head.

Excursion of the extensor tendons over the dorsum of the hand should be verified. If these tendons are not gliding freely, they should be explored and the adhesions divided over the dorsum of the hand and, if necessary, over the dorsum of the wrist and into the forearm. Furthermore, the extensor hood may require tenolysis on either side of the metacarpophalangeal joint.

The extensor tendon is closed with a running suture of 4-0 stainless steel wire. When the contracture has been severe or the hand extensively injured initially, the metacarpophalangeal joints are flexed 90 degrees and held in position by transarticular Kirschner wires. Otherwise, the wires are omitted and the metacarpophalangeal joints dressed in flexion. The pressure dressing is left in place for 72 hours; then it is removed and a volar plaster splint applied so that one may begin rubber band traction by leather loops around the proximal phalanges. When wires are used, they are left in place for 10 to 14 days; then dynamic splinting is instituted. The dorsal approach provides excellent exposure of the dorsal capsule and the collateral ligaments. However, it does present the following disadvantages:

1. If skin is deficient (even by a small amount), the joints must be immobilized in hyperextension to permit wound closure and healing. This is most evident when a transverse incision has been made.
2. When a longitudinal skin incision is used, minimal tissue deficiency may cause herniation of the metacarpophalangeal joint through the incision if the digit is immobilized in flexion.
3. The longitudinal incision in the extensor tendon may be ruptured by the metacarpal head if the extensor is checkreined by a proximal scar.
4. Attempts at early joint mobilization strain the dorsal incision; the ensuing pain curtails the patient's enthusiasm.

5. If extensor tendon grafts have to be used at later date, the dorsal approach introduces more scarring in the area where tendon gliding is required.

For these reasons a volar approach has been developed.

***Volar approach.*** The arm is rendered bloodless with a pneumatic arm cuff. Longitudinal incisions 2 cm long begin at the free edge of the palmar web spaces and extend proximally on the palm between the metacarpal heads. The ulnar collateral ligament of the little finger is exposed through a midlateral line incision, as is the radial collateral ligament of the index finger. The neurovascular bundles are retracted to expose the edge of the lateral band, which is traced proximally to the level of the metacarpophalangeal joint (Fig. 12-30). The insertion of the interosseous muscle into the proximal phalanx is identified and preserved. The lateral band is retracted to expose the collateral ligament. The collateral ligament insertion is detached and a section of the ligament excised. The "fan" portion of the collateral ligament is preserved.

Division of the ulnar collateral ligament produces a slight radial deviation of the digits during flexion, varying with the tautness of the remaining radial collateral ligaments. This deviation becomes minimal after several months. If the radial collateral ligament is so contracted as to prevent flexion of the metacarpophalangeal joint, access to this ligament in the long ring, and little fingers is readily obtained through the previous incisions. The index will require a radial midlateral incision for exposure.

If the extensor tendons are bound in scar, access to the scar can be readily obtained by sliding the scissors beneath the dorsal hood and proximally beneath the extensor tendon. An avenue for exploration of the volar synovial pouch is readily available.

After adequate joint mobilization has been obtained, only skin sutures are required for

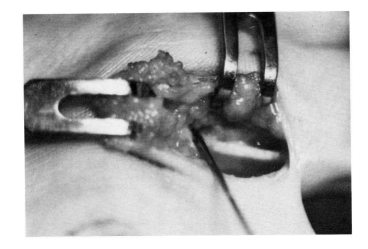

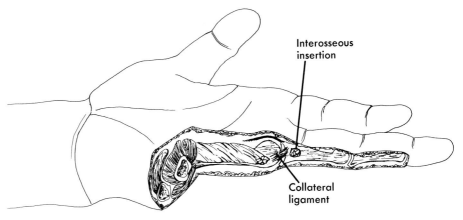

Interosseous
insertion

Collateral
ligament

**Fig. 12-30.** The volar approach does not permit the degree of visualization possible through a dorsal approach but avoids the disadvantages of the dorsal approach.

closure. The hand is completely immobilized for 72 hours. The range of motion after 72 hours determines whether dynamic splints will be employed.

*Management after capsulotomy of the metacarpophalangeal joint.* The patient is generally fitted with a dorsal splint with a metacarpophalangeal flexion outrigger (Fig. 12-21). The splint is extended on the radial aspect at the web space to include a metacarpal bar that is fitted across the palm of the hand below the distal palmar crease. A snugly fitting metacarpal bar preserves the palmar arch, eliminates slippage of the splint, and provides a secure fit when force

is applied with rubber bands and finger loops. Usually a light force (4 to 6 oz) is sufficient to maintain metacarpophalangeal flexion. The patient wears the splint for 10 to 20 minutes during the initial treatment session to ensure a proper fit and to make certain that the force exerted by the rubber bands is tolerable. The patient is then instructed to wear the splint as much as possible but to remove it several times daily for exercise. As the patient heals more completely, stronger force (6 to 10 oz) may be applied, if necessary, to maintain metacarpophalangeal flexion.

Whenever possible, the patient is seen

for therapy 2 to 5 half-days during the next few weeks. Passive exercise to increase joint motion includes the techniques of passive stretching, joint mobilization, and proprioceptive neuromuscular facilitation (rhythmic stabilization, maximal resistance, and contract-relax). In the latter, the patient moves the joint to the point where pain or tendon limits further motion. The therapist gives resistance to the antagonist muscle, and the patient is asked to hold an isometric contraction against this resistance. Then he is told to relax completely, and passive motion is initiated toward the limited range. The process is repeated frequently, and the patient is then asked to actively hold the acquired position.

The importance of active exercise to maintain gains achieved passively must be emphasized. These are often exercises that a patient can perform independently after initial instruction and supervision. Simple exercise equipment to encourage gross grasp and palmar flexion is used to provide goal-directed treatment. When swelling is present, these exercises are performed in an elevated position, and the patient is instructed in edema-reducing techniques.

As healing progresses, exercises that require a combination of metacarpophalangeal and proximal interphalangeal joint flexion are initiated to apply stress to the tight extensor mechanism, as well as to increase finger flexion. Metacarpophalangeal joint flexion is emphasized, but generally flexion and extension exercises are alternated so that the joint does not become stiff in either direction. Active finger extension can be accomplished effectively by asking the patient to extend his fingers and distal palm over the edge of the table at the distal palmar crease. The patient performs active finger extension while using his opposite hand to massage any scars on the dorsum of the hand. This is especially important when the capsulotomy is done from a dorsal approach, because the incision may adhere to the extensor tendons.

When further healing occurs and tenderness decreases, more vigorous exercises are introduced. Passive stretch is applied with greater force, and more resistive exercises are included in the treatment program. Sustained grasp activities are utilized to increase overall hand strength and endurance.

### Proximal interphalangeal joint

*Fixed in extension.* After the anesthetized arm has been rendered bloodless with a pneumatic tourniquet, the proximal interphalangeal joint is exposed through a dorsal incision. The skin flaps are reflected to expose Cleland's ligaments bilaterally. An oblique retinacular ligament is often identified extending from the volar surface of the proximal phalanx through Cleland's ligament and over the proximal interphalangeal joint to insert into the extensor tendon. This retinacular ligament is elevated and retracted to expose the collateral ligaments of the joint. At this point one quickly reviews his preoperative diagnosis regarding the cause of this joint's stiffness. If the joint is stiff because of collateral ligament tightness, the dorsal one third to one half of the collateral ligaments is excised. The dorsal joint capsule is opened, and care is taken to preserve the central slip insertion of the extensor hood into the middle phalanx. Occasionally, after this maneuver one realizes that the extensor apparatus is adherent dorsally, inhibiting flexion. The edge of the lateral band is identified and a Freer elevator inserted and advanced in a proximal direction beneath the extensor apparatus. The extensor apparatus is gently freed from the dorsal surface of the proximal phalanx. If the hood is adherent, flexion of the proximal interphalangeal joint with the metacarpophalangeal joint in extension should be improved. Now the lateral bands are observed. If they are taut enough to prevent flexion, they can be released by excision of a triangle of lateral band tissue distal to the interosseous hood. Only after one has assured himself that none of the extracapsular factors have gone unchecked should the offending part of the collateral ligaments be removed. One must persist until the exact etiology of the joint stiffness is identified and corrected.

The wound is closed, and the joint is placed in 45 degrees flexion. At 48 hours postoperatively, the dressings are discarded, and the patient is begun on active and passive exercises; then a dynamic forearm-palmar splint is prepared and applied. A second outrigger on the splint allows use of the splint as a dynamic extension and flexion splint. The proximal interphalangeal joint must not be allowed to become ankylosed. Alternating the dynamic action can keep the joint mobile during the period of fibrous tissue deposition and organization. To wait 5 to 7 days to begin dynamic splinting significantly reduces the chances of obtaining a mobile joint.

*Fixed in flexion.* The operative procedure used when a joint is held in flexion is quite different from the procedure used when the joint is held in extension. After the anesthetized arm is rendered ischemic with a pneumatic cuff, the skin is opened through a dorsal incision over the joint. As the skin flaps are reflected, Cleland's ligaments and the oblique retinacular ligaments are identified. Cleland's ligaments are opened to allow access to the volar compartment. The oblique retinacular ligaments are usually contracted and require division. The fibro-osseous tunnel is carefully opened at its reflection onto the periosteum of the proximal phalanx. The periosteum is incised and elevated over the distal third of the proximal phalanx with a Freer elevator (Fig. 12-31). This frees the bony attachments of the volar plate to the proximal phalanx. As one tries to extend the proximal interphalangeal joint, the elevated periosteum

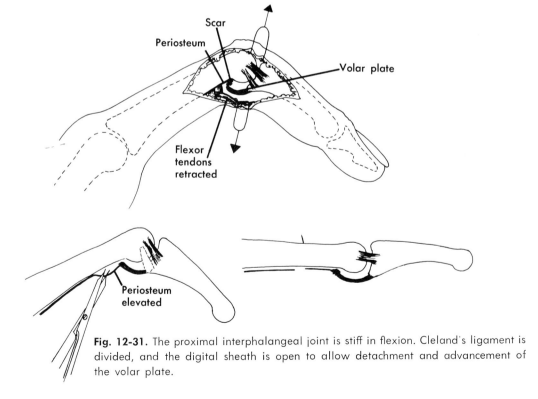

**Fig. 12-31.** The proximal interphalangeal joint is stiff in flexion. Cleland's ligament is divided, and the digital sheath is open to allow detachment and advancement of the volar plate.

becomes taut through the pull of the attached volar plate. Dividing the periosteum as far proximal as possible permits the volar plate to slide forward as the joint is extended and still provide cover for the joint. The most volar fibers of the collateral ligaments usually require division to permit complete extension. Do not hyperextend the joint or fix it in hyperextension. As the joint is extended to a neutral position, a thin smooth Kirschner wire is placed across the joint. Since the visceral synovial layer of the flexor tendons is protected, scarring around these tendons will not be a problem. The wounds are closed. At 10 days postoperatively the Kirschner wire is removed and a forearm-palmar splint prepared to provide dynamic splinting of the proximal interphalangeal joint in flexion and extension. Close observation of the patient is necessary to prevent the recurrence of the flexion contracture. Dynamic splinting is mandatory.

*Management after capsulotomy of the proximal interphalangeal joint.* The patient is usually fitted with a static finger extension splint following removal of the pin. If several proximal interphalangeal joints are released on the same hand, a forearm splint, which extends from the proximal phalanges and crosses the wrist, is fabricated. Metacarpophalangeal joints are held in some degree of flexion, and this part of the splint is well padded (Fig. 12-24). Rubber bands, with light tension, are attached to an extension outrigger to maintain the extended position of the proximal joints. The patient wears the proximal interphalangeal extension splint as much as possible during next few days but removes it often to perform exercises.

Initially proximal interphalangeal joint flexion is increased through active and passive exercise; extension is emphasized and maintained by use of the splint. In 3 to 4 days following pin removal, the patient is fitted with a dynamic proximal interphalangeal joint flexion splint (Fig. 12-22). He is instructed to alternate use of the flexion and extension splints during the day and use the static extension splint at night.

As further healing takes place, the patient may also be fitted with a Wynn-Parry extension splint to wear during the day, because it provides dynamic proximal interphalangeal joint extension. In the case of more than one involved digit, rubber band tension on the previously described dynamic splint will be increased. When a single finger is involved, dynamic proximal interphalangeal joint extension and flexion splints are alternated during the day, and static proximal interphalangeal joint extension splints are worn at night.

Patients are initially fitted with an elastic finger stocking to decrease edema in the digit. An infant blood pressure cuff is used during treatment to apply intermittent pressure and further decrease swelling. As edema decreases and proximal interphalangeal joint flexion and extension improve, the patient may be fitted with an elastic splint (Fig. 12-23). This aids in gaining increased distal interphalangeal joint flexion, while maintaining proximal interphalangeal joint flexion.

The patient is involved in an exercise program similar to the one described in the previous section, but with emphasis on the proximal and distal interphalangeal joints. An exercise board is especially useful here, because it assists the patient in isolating proximal or distal interphalangeal joint flexion. These are provided for each patient to augment his home program. During finger flexion exercises, it is important for the patient to maintain wrist extension, actively or passively, so that the flexor tendons are working through their optimal range. As range of motion at each individual joint improves, treatment is directed at increasing total finger flexion, gross grasp, and functional use of the entire hand.

Both metacarpophalangeal and proximal interphalangeal joint capsulotomy patients are instructed in home exercise programs that are reviewed often and updated as the patient progresses. The use of splints, including application and wearing schedule, is explained as each splint is introduced. Initially, these patients are encouraged to begin using the postsurgical hand for light, everyday activities. This progresses to moderately heavy tasks and more dexterous activities as hand function improves. Avocational and craft activities, such as gardening, woodworking, or leatherwork, which require the use of hand tools, may be introduced to increase use of the hand in ongoing activity. Eventually strenuous, heavy work activities are initiated in order to prepare the patient for return to work.

### Results of operative management of stiff metacarpophalangeal and proximal interphalangeal joints

Of the 526 patients seen in the Hand Rehabilitation Center, 50 did not respond to conservative therapy and have undergone surgical release of the stiff joint (capsulotomy). In these 50 patients there were 54 stiff metacarpophalangeal joints and 60 stiff proximal interphalangeal joints—a total of 114 stiff joints. A number of different etiological agents were associated with the development of stiff joints, and the patients have been further subdivided to reflect these categories (Table 12-4).

The results were expressed as follows for the metacarpophalangeal joint: excellent, 70 to 90 degrees; good, 50 to 70 degrees; and poor, less than 50 degrees. The results were expressed as follows for the proximal interphalangeal joint: excellent, 80 to 110 degrees; good, 60 to 80 degrees; and poor less than 60 degrees.

The results from capsulotomy according to joint and etiological agent are presented in Table 12-5. When expressed in this manner, one can better appreciate the etiological agents that are most frequently associated with excellent, good, and poor results. For example, one can expect satis-

**Table 12-4.** Capsulotomy categories*

| Category | No. MP joints | No. PIP joints | No. patients |
|---|---|---|---|
| Crush injury without skin disruption | 4 | 5 | 3 |
| Closed fracture or dislocation of involved finger | 1 | 6 | 6 |
| Laceration or avulsion of skin | 0 | 9 | 5 |
| Crush, skin disrupture, fracture of involved finger or amputation | 22 | 15 | 12 |
| Distant fracture | 1 | 1 | 2 |
| Ulnar and/or median nerve laceration (forearm or wrist level) | 10 | 11 | 7 |
| Brachial plexus injury | 5 | 0 | 2 |
| Rheumatoid arthritis | 0 | 4 | 1 |
| Burns with loss of extensor tendons | 10 | 2 | 5 |
| Laceration tendons—local | 1 | 3 | 4 |
| Dupuytren's contracture | 0 | 2 | 2 |
| Scleroderma | 0 | 2 | 1 |
| Totals | 54 | 60 | 50 |

*This table illustrates the multiple etiologies associated with stiff joints.

factory results when performing a capsulotomy in a finger in which stiffness developed secondary to a closed fracture or dislocation of the involved finger. Conversely, the results from capsulotomy in stiff finger joints associated with ulnar and median nerve laceration at the wrist are

**Table 12-5.** Capsulotomy results*

| Category | Excellent | | Good | | Poor | |
|---|---|---|---|---|---|---|
| | MP | PIP | MP | PIP | MP | PIP |
| Crush injury without skin disruption | 2 | 0 | 1 | 5 | 1 | 0 |
| Closed fracture or dislocation of involved finger | 1 | 6 | — | — | — | — |
| Laceration or avulsion of skin—distant | — | 3 | — | 1 | — | 5 |
| Crush, skin disrupture, fracture of involved finger, or amputation | 12 | 3 | 3 | 5 | 7 | 7 |
| Distant fracture | 1 | 1 | — | — | — | — |
| Ulnar and/or median nerve laceration (forearm or wrist level) | 5 | 2 | 1 | — | 4 | 9 |
| Brachial plexus injury | — | — | 4 | — | 1 | — |
| Rheumatoid arthritis | — | 1 | — | 3 | — | — |
| Burns with loss of extensor tendons | 1 | — | 3 | 1 | 6 | 1 |
| Laceration tendons—local | 1 | 3 | — | — | — | — |
| Dupuytren's contracture | — | — | — | 1 | — | 1 |
| Scleroderma | — | — | — | — | — | 2 |
| Totals | 23 | 19 | 12 | 16 | 19 | 25 |

*The operative results of capsulotomy according to etiology reveal the need for a large experience before conclusions regarding effectiveness can be made.

not as satisfactory as in some other groups. As our experience increases and we are able to enter enough numbers to be significant, then projection of results preoperatively should be possible.

Another factor of significance is the duration of stiffness before surgery. In the metacarpophalangeal joint, if the capsulotomy was performed within 6 months of injury, the results tend to be excellent or good. If the surgery is performed after 6 months of injury, the results are more evenly distributed between the excellent and poor groups. In the proximal interphalangeal joint, the results are not so encouraging. In those operated on within 6 months of injury, there are more poor than excellent results. If operated on over 6 months after injury, the excellent and poor results are about equal with fewer good results than either excellent or poor. Again, continued experience will allow significant numbers to be developed. However, it is obvious that taken as a group, capsulotomy of the metacarpophalangeal

joint converts 35 of 54 patients to excellent or good results. In the proximal interphalangeal joint, 35 of 60 patients were converted to excellent or good results. Thus, we can predict that in general, a patient has a 65% chance of getting an excellent to good result after metacarpophalangeal capsulotomy and a 59% chance after proximal interphalangeal capsulotomy.

### Thumb-index web contracture

***Conservative management.*** Preventing an adduction is as important as preventing the development of stiff metacarpophalangeal and proximal interphalangeal joints. Routinely, we are concerned about the digital joints and often forget or pay less attention to the thumb-index web until it becomes contracted. Thus, the first step in prevention is cognizance of the problem. Again, measurements are important. A clear plastic goniometer is used; its center is placed over the articulation of the first and second metacarpals. One arm of the goniometer is aligned with the index metacarpal, the other arm with the thumb metacarpal.

Prevention is accomplished by patient education, exercise, and splinting. A diagram of the thumb-index web space is helpful in explaining the mechanism of development to the patient. Preventive measures are discussed, and the patient participates actively in prevention of contracture.

The application of force through exercise or splinting is required to prevent and treat thumb-index web space contractures. This force is always applied at or proximal to the level of the metacarpophalangeal joints of the thumb and index finger. Force applied to the proximal phalanx of the thumb can cause attenuation of the ulnar collateral ligament of the metacarpophalangeal joint of the thumb. Proper application of force by the therapist, the patient, and the splinting devices is required to prevent an untoward reaction of the web space tissues. The tendency to grasp the easily accessible phalanges of the thumb instead of the metacarpal must be avoided.

It is important to instruct patients to use proper exercise techniques as well as to explain the potential disability that results from the adduction contracture.

Therapy is directed toward achieving and maintaining maximum range of motion and strength of the thumb. Multiple techniques are employed to provide increase in motion. Passive manual stretching is performed by applying traction on the thumb metacarpal in the direction of extension, abduction, and opposition. Passive stretching is assisted by massaging the web as the thumb is abducted. Cardboard cones can be used for passive stretching. The narrow end of the cone is placed tightly between the heads of the first and second metacarpals. The patient slides the cone down toward its wider end, gradually increasing the distance between the heads of the metacarpals. Plastic tumblers can be used in a similar fashion and can even be weighted to provide graduated re-

sistance as they are grasped and lifted.

Active exercises are important in maintaining gains made by passive stretching and by encouraging functional use of the hand. Active exercises include: (1) making a large circle with both thumbs (for the patient to compare range), (2) touching the thumb to the portion of the distal palmar crease below the fifth digit, and (3) pinching the thumb against each fingertip (forcing the thumb into full opposition to reach the ulnar digits). Resistive exercise can be accomplished by having the patient pinch a piece of material between the thumb and each finger while pulling on the material with the other hand The use of a pinch gauge allows the patient to see his progress.

If the patient has not yet developed a fixed contracture, a static night splint is usually sufficient to maintain maximum web space when combined with a vigorous exercise program. A splint made of low-temperature thermoplastic material has been beneficial for patients who have median or median-ulnar nerve injuries, direct trauma to the web space area, edema resulting from injury, or immobilization of the hand. A series of static splints can be fabricated to maintain gains in motion.

In order to achieve the optimum fit of the static thumb-index web space splint, several factors need to be remembered. Since the metacarpophalangeal joints of the fingers tend to become stiff in extension, the splint must not prevent full flexion of the metacarpophalangeal joint of the index finger. If the dorsal portion of this splint is extended around to the long finger metacarpal, it will help maintain the thumb in opposition. During fabrication of the splint, the therapist must apply force between the metacarpals. The webbing strap secures the splint for night wear and holds it tightly in the web space. The fit of the splint must be checked and adjusted as it becomes loose.

A dynamic splint is difficult to construct because the metacarpals are not easily accessible for finger loop attachment. A modified version of the basic dorsal plaster cockup splint with opposition outrigger described by DeVore is used. A special thumb-shaped finger loop is made to protect the metacarpophalangeal joint of the thumb and its ulnar collateral ligament. The thumb loop is made of moleskin or leather. The moleskin loop is adhered directly to the skin to prevent the loop from slipping. The leather loop is used on patients with poorly healed skin or skin that is prone to break down.

The same dorsal splint can be combined very effectively with another type of finger loop. The U-shaped finger loop fits closely along the ulnar side of the first metacarpal (Fig. 12-26). The metacarpal bar stabilizes the second metacarpal, allowing force to be applied against the heavy fascia surrounding these structures. This clamp-type loop is made from a piece of spring wire bent to fit snugly along the patient's first metacarpal. The wire must be well padded with moleskin, and the ends of the device may need to be stabilized against the splint with Velcro. Holes are punched into the moleskin at the level of the metacarpophalangeal joint and reinforced with eyelets on either side of the spring wire. Rubber bands are applied at or proximal to the level of the metacarpophalangeal joint of the thumb on both sides and attached to the outrigger. This type of splint has been used successfully on patients who have had deepening and/or release of web space contractures, traumatic injuries to the thumb or median-ulnar nerves, or crushing injuries to the palm of the hand. This splint would not be appropriate for patients with fragile skin.

**Results of conservative treatment.** Thirty-one patients with significant injuries to the thumb-index web space are included in the study. Their average age was 39. There were seven females and 24 males. The average time between initial and final evaluation was 198 days.

Active thumb abduction improved in 29 but was unchanged in 2. The mean increase in active range of motion was 10 degrees for all patients; the mean increase in passive range of motion was 9 degrees, with 25 patients improving and 6 remaining unchanged.

It is impossible to determine in how many other patients the development of a thumb-index web contracture was prevented by the methods of treatment outlined above.

**Operative reconstruction of the thumb-index web space.** A fixed adduction contracture will not improve from rehabilitation alone, but exercise and splinting will keep the contracture from becoming worse. The only effective treatment of a fixed contracture is surgical release. Patients generally begin therapy 1 to 2 weeks after surgery to maintain the surgical gains. Exercises similar to those used to prevent the deformity are employed even more vigorously.

The surgeon must determine the exciting cause leading to development of the contracture and, through examination, determine the relative contribution of each of the factors involved in maintaining the adduction contracture. When skin is lost, the operative procedure must be designed to replace the needed skin. The variety of techniques described for tissue replacement may be somewhat confusing but can be sorted according to the tissue replacement needs. When the contracture primarily involves the skin and is limited to the free edge of the web space, the use of the Z-plasty may be adequate. The gain in length and depth from a Z-plasty is not adequate to compensate significant tissue loss. An advancement flap from the volar surface has been advocated. This requires free grafting along the index finger or the thumb—a situation that leads to significant contracture, particularly in the thumb-index web space. Replacement of significant web space tissue loss can be gained with a distant pedicle flap. This procedure requires attachment of the hand to the donor area for 2 to 3 weeks and a second procedure for flap division. To circumvent this multiple stage procedure, local pedicles from the dorsum of the hand have been advocated. This requires free grafting of the donor site over the dorsum of the hand; the pedicle tissue provides excellent coverage for the web space. This latter procedure will be described in detail.

Under tourniquet ischemia, the dorsal pedicle flap is incised along the line of the free edge of the web space that crosses the metacarpophalangeal joint level of the index finger (Fig. 12-32). The incision is gently curved proximally to the level of the long finger metacarpal base. The veins within the flap are elevated in a plane dorsal to the supratendinous fascia. Elevation of the flap exposes the contents of the web space. If the thumb cannot be fully abducted after elevation of the skin flap—and it usually cannot—the intertendinous fascia between the extensor pollicis longus and the finger extensors is excised back to the axis of rotation of the thumb carpometacarpal joint. This maneuver generally improves abduction but not completely. The thenar and palmar fascial attachments

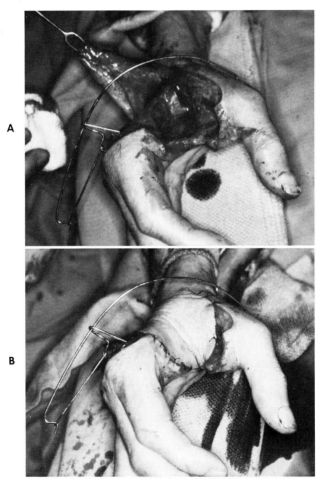

**Fig. 12-32. A,** An operative view of hand shown in Fig. 12-12. The outrigger (described by Littler) maintains the thumb in full abduction. **B,** A dorsal skin flap has been rotated into the restored web space.

to the volar skin of the web are detached by undermining the skin. The fascia covering both sides of the adductor pollicis muscle is excised the width of the muscle. Division of the palmar fascia attachments to the thenar fascia can result in a slightly improved range of motion. If the web is still significantly contracted and the abductor muscle appears normal, the anterior and posterior oblique ligaments between the thumb and index metacarpals are divided. When the fascia and ligaments around the base of the thumb metacarpal are released, care must be taken to avoid damage to the radial artery. Recall its pathway from its subcutaneous location at the wrist. The vessel curves dorsally beneath the abductor pollicis longus, the extensor pollicis brevis, and the extensor pollicis longus tendons to turn volarward before passing between the thumb and index metacarpal origin of the first dorsal interosseous muscle. Here it divides into a deep palmar arch branch and a princeps pollicis artery.

When the primary cause for development of this contracture is muscle necrosis and scarring, the adductor insertion into the sesamoid bone can be detached to achieve full abduction. Instead of completely detaching the transverse head of the adductor, its most distal fibers can be gradually divided until complete release is obtained.

After complete release of the contracture, the position of full abduction must be maintained. Direct pinning of the index-thumb metacarpal has been suggested. Littler has proposed a device that will maintain the thumb in the fully abducted position during the period of healing. One Kirschner wire is inserted into the thumb metacarpal and fashioned as indicated. A second wire is placed in the index metacarpal and fashioned so that its spring provides constant pressure on the thumb metacarpal. After one obtains the particular type of immobilization rig he desires, the pedicle flap is rotated into the web space and sutured loosely in place

to ensure an excess of pedicle tissue in the web. The tourniquet is released and major bleeding controlled. The only spot where major bleeding can be a nuisance is where the radial artery enters the first dorsal interosseous muscle. This must be controlled. If a hematoma is allowed to develop in the newly created web space, scarring will be extensively and will noticeably interfere with function. A full-thickness graft is inserted into the donor area and immobilized with a stent and the usual hand dressing extending to the midforearm. Dressing change is delayed for 2 weeks. The splint is discarded 3 to 4 weeks after surgery, and a static splint is provided.

Palmar contracture may develop in a transverse plane after a crush injury. The reaction to injury results in scar deposition and ultimate contraction about the palmar fascia. The metacarpals are forced together, closing the interdigital web spaces and bringing the phalanges into direct side-to-side contact. This produces a tight, narrow hand. The thumb-index web is usually involved and may be completely obliterated. This web can be reconstructed as noted previously, but an approach to the tightly contracted hand has not been forthcoming. Certainly the process involves at least the palmar skin and fascia, the volar and dorsal fascia covering the interosseous muscles, and the intermetacarpal ligaments. Such an extensive involvement explains the lack of adequate treatment at the present time.

**BIBLIOGRAPHY**

Curtis, R. M.: Capsulectomy of the interphalangeal joints of the fingers, J. Bone Joint Surg. **36A:**1219, 1954.

Devore, G.: Hand splints, Chapel Hill, Hand Rehabilitation Center, University of North Carolina.

Howard, L. D.: Cited by Bunnell, S.: Surgery of the hand, ed. 2, Philadelphia, 1948, J. B. Lippincott Co.

Weeks, P. M.: Volar approach for metacarpophalangeal joint capsulotomy, Plast. Reconstr. Surg. **46:**473, 1970.

# CHAPTER 13

# Problems of nerve regeneration

Stated simply, repair of a completely transected nerve can result in either adequate or inadequate functional recovery. The criteria one uses in evaluating the adequacy of nerve regeneration and the methods of treatment available when the return of function is inadequate will be discussed. Major causalgia, minor causalgia (sympathetic dystrophy), and painful neuromas are also sequelae of disordered regeneration of peripheral nerves. These three conditions occur almost exclusively after injury to a nerve that is not repaired. The pathogenesis, incidence, signs and symptoms, and treatment of major causalgia, minor causalgia and painful neuromas will be discussed in detail.

## FAILURE OF RETURN OF FUNCTION AFTER NERVE REPAIR

The criteria for nerve regeneration along the nerve trunk are an advancing Tinel's sign and distal progress of measurable nerve-evoked potentials. The criterion for functional return is the recovery of both sensory and motor function in end organs. Since nerve regeneration precedes functional return, our examination during the early weeks or months after nerve repair is primarily limited to the position of Tinel's sign or the more cumbersome measurements of nerve-evoked potentials.

## Rate of nerve regeneration

*Tinel's sign.* Although Tinel's sign is indicative only of regenerating sensory axons, it is a useful clinical guide to nerve regeneration, because most peripheral nerve trunks contain a mixture of motor and sensory nerve fibers. The level of nerve repair should always be noted in relationship to a fixed landmark that is well defined, so that on subsequent examinations a definite point of reference is used. Use of the bony prominences does not permit as much accuracy of measurement as does the interphalangeal joint or the distal palmar crease. Knowledge of the exact level of repair allows early accurate evaluation of the movement of Tinel's sign and prediction of the interval between repair and the first sign of return of motor or sensory function.

Tinel's sign is present when paresthesias are produced by percussion over the nerve at the advancing edge of the regenerating axons. Percussion is carried out beginning at the level of nerve repair, and paresthesias seeming to radiate into the area supplied by the nerve are usually produced. If no paresthesias are produced, percussion is continued proximally over the course of the nerve to a level at which paresthesias are produced. If paresthesias are produced at the level of the nerve repair, one percusses distally and records the most distal point at which the paresthesias are perceived. This distal point should be recorded at the time of the first dressing change (usually about 3 weeks from the time of surgical repair). Thereafter, the level at which Tinel's sign is elicited should be recorded monthly.

Recording the distance of advancement over an interval of time allows establishment of the rate of nerve regeneration. Experimentally, regenerating axons crossing a nerve anastomosis are evident in approximately 7 days. The period of delay in humans has not been recorded. Clinical observations of Tinel's sign suggest that the axoplasm is delayed at the site of the anastomosis for 1 to 2 weeks. The degree of scarring present between the nerve stumps and the exactness of alignment of the nerve trunks determine the period of delay in axoplasm successfully crossing the anastomosis. Tinel's sign usually moves distally from 0.5 mm to 2.5 mm per day; the average is approximately 1 mm per day.

*Nerve-evoked potentials.* The rate of nerve regeneration can also be evaluated by means of evoked nerve action potentials. This technique introduces a recording needle electrode percutaneously near the nerve trunk proximal to the site of injury. The nerve is stimulated with a cutaneous contact electrode at various points distal to the injury. The point at which a response can no longer be elicited is assumed to represent the most distal progress of nerve regeneration. Subsequent examinations determine the presence of nerve regeneration if there is progressive distal movement of the point at which a response is no longer elicited.

### Testing for return of motor function

Motor function is determined by a manual muscle test. The results are recorded on a standard form, such as the one illustrated in Fig. 13-1. It is difficult to perform an accurate muscle test on the small muscles of the hand, because several muscles may act together to perform a movement, making it difficult to isolate an individual muscle. One must also be careful that the muscle being tested is indeed performing the task, for example, the flexor pollicis longus produces a motion similar to but not identical to opposition.

### Testing for return of sensory function

The tests used for evaluating sensory function are illustrated in Fig. 13-2. The ninhydrin sweat test and wrinkle test are objective measurements. The remainder are subjective and require patient cooperation and understanding of what responses are expected. The patient and examiner should be comfortable and relaxed, and the hand to be tested should be warm. The atmosphere should be relatively quiet with as few distractions as possible, because the patient will need to concentrate.

*Ninhydrin sweat test.* The fingers are cleaned with acetone, and the patient sits for ½ hour generating sweat. The fingers are then carefully placed on a clean piece of paper and outlined with a pencil. The paper is sprayed with ninhydrin, a solution that reacts with the amino acids in sweat and leaves the paper pink in those areas where sweat has formed.

*Wrinkle test.* The patient submerges his hand in a tub of 108° F water for ½ hour. When the hand is withdrawn, the areas of innervation are compared with denervated areas. The amount of wrinkling varies greatly from one patient to another. Testing both hands is recommended in order to establish a more accurate normal for a particular patient. The results are recorded on a scale from 3 (normal for that patient) to 0 (no wrinkling) on both radial and ulnar aspects of all digits.

*Vibration.* The first two items under the heading "Legend" in Fig. 13-2 refer to testing vibration using two tuning forks, one vibrating at 30 cycles per second (cps) and the other at 256 cps. The tuning fork is vibrated over the pads of the fingers.

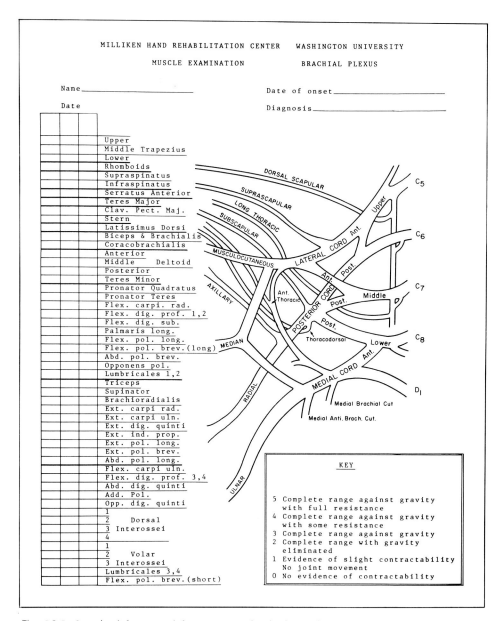

**Fig. 13-1.** Standard form used for testing individual muscles of upper limb. If both upper limbs are involved, a separate form is used for each.

The examiner must be careful to have the tuning fork just barely touching but not pressing on the finger, since the latter may be testing constant pressure rather than vibration. The hand should be well supported. The patient must be instructed to be certain to feel the sensation on the palmar aspect of the digit and not through to the dorsum.

*Moving touch.* Referred to as light movement and heavy movement in Fig. 13-2, this test uses a cotton swab to test light movement, and the examiner's finger, with some pressure applied, to test heavy move-

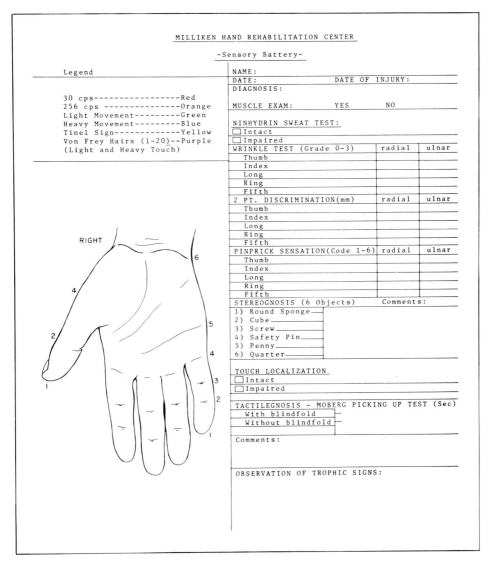

**Fig. 13-2.** Standard form used for recording results of sensory testing. A separate form with a mirror image of the hand diagram is used for the opposite hand.

ment. Each digit is tested from proximal to distal.

**Constant touch.** Von Frey hairs are used for this test.

The tests for vibration, moving touch, constant touch, and Tinel's sign are carefully mapped out on the hand diagram in Fig. 13-2, using different colored pencils for each test.

**Two-point discrimination.** This tests the patient's ability to discriminate two points from one. The points of blunt calipers graded in millimeters are applied longitudinally to both the radial and the ulnar sides of the palmar surface of the digit. The patient, with eyes closed, is asked to state whether he feels two points or one. The calipers are initially set at a distance of greater than 15 mm. The distance is decreased until the patient states he is able to feel only one point. The test should first be demonstrated in an area of normal sensation. The patient should respond correctly 7 out of 10 times. The normal value is usually 2 to 6 mm.

*Pinprick sensation.* The patient is asked to identify between sharp or dull using a safety pin. The level is recorded on the chart using the numbers on the diagram to indicate the areas of the hand.

*Stereognosis.* The patient, with eyes closed, is asked to identify each of the objects listed (Fig. 13-2) by shape and texture as each is placed in his hand. The fashion with which the patient handles each object should be noted; that is, is he using the denervated part of the hand?

*Touch localization.* The examiner touches a spot on the patient's hand and the patient, with eyes closed, is asked to come as close as possible to the same spot using his other hand.

*Moberg picking up test.* A box containing 20 different items of varying shapes and sizes is emptied on a table. The patient is instructed to pick up each item and place it in the box. The test is timed and performed first with the patient's eyes open, then blindfolded. The times are recorded, and the manner in which the patient handles the items or attempts to find them while blindfolded is also described.

## SECONDARY OPERATIONS FOR FAILED NERVE REPAIRS
### Indications

Determining which patients should undergo secondary operation and when is an area of controversy associated with peripheral nerve injury. Theoretically, if the axons advance at 1 mm per day and if one knew the exact level of the nerve repair and the exact level where the muscular branch to a given muscle lay, one could calculate the interval between nerve repair and the return of motor function. Sunder-

land has carefully calculated the distances in 20 individuals between various fixed points and the points where branches of the nerve first innervate a given muscle. The variation at times between the shortest distance to the first branch supplying a given muscle in one individual and the greatest distance to the first branch in another individual might be as much as 10 cm. This would allow at least a 3½ month normal variation in the time to reinnervation, given a perfect nerve repair.

The latent period does depend on the distance between the repair and the muscle and sensory nerve ending to be innervated. Clinically, the interval between nerve suture and the first sign of motor recovery may vary from 3 to 10 months. An acceptable maximum interval between nerve repair and the first return of some motor function is about 8 months for lesions at the elbow or in the forearm for the median, radial, and ulnar nerves and about 5 months for lesions at the level of the wrist for the median and ulnar nerves.

When there is a question of the adequacy of nerve repair, the nerve should be reexplored within 2 to 4 weeks after the wound has healed. If the primary repair or secondary repair is felt to be adequate, the indications for reexploration are based on three considerations: (1) suspected disruption of the suture line, (2) lack of distal progression of Tinel's sign, and (3) lack of return of satisfactory nerve function. The temporal interrelationships of these three considerations allow their division into early, intermediate, and late with respect to the time of nerve repair. The earliest consideration, disruption of the suture line, would be suspected during the first few weeks after nerve repair. If the patient's splint is inadvertently removed or broken and he complains of severe pain localized at the site of nerve repair, it almost invariably indicates disruption of the anastomosis. The attachment of radiopaque markers to the nerve stumps at the time of definitive anastomosis allows subsequent roentgenographic verification of the integrity of the anastomosis.

The second consideration, occurring intermediately after nerve repair, is the advancing Tinel sign. The presence of Tinel's sign progressing distally at the rate of 1 mm per day is only suggestive evidence that adequate motor or sensory return of function will follow. However, the failure of Tinel's sign to progress beyond the level of nerve repair arouses grave concern about the possibility of adequate nerve function. Occasional exceptions to this rule have been reported in the literature; that is, adequate function has been regained even though no Tinel sign was evident during the period of axon regeneration.

In general, reexploration of the nerve repair is indicated if satisfactory sensory and motor function has not returned by 8 months after repair of median, ulnar, and radial nerve injuries in the forearm and by 5 months after median and ulnar nerve repairs at the wrist. Return of function in both proximal and distal muscles to such a degree that all important muscles are sufficiently powerful to act against resistance is grade M3 motor recovery. Return of superficial cutaneous pain and tactile sensibility throughout the autonomous area with disappearance of any previous overresponse is grade S3 sensory recovery. It is impossible to state exactly what level of sensory or motor return is satisfactory, but reexploration of the repaired nerve would not be indicated if: (1) one obtains M3 (see Table 10-2) or better motor return and S3 (see Table 10-3) or better sensory return following repair of a nerve injury at the wrist, and (2) M2 or better motor return and S2 or better sensory return following nerve repair in the forearm. Reexploration is not indicated in these cases, because one would have less than a 50% chance of attaining such levels after reexploration.

In the final analysis, the indication for reexploration of an already repaired nerve injury should be based on the degree of functional impairment that the patient is experiencing in his day-to-day activities. Some patients accept a less than perfect result and perform their jobs quite satisfactorily; for example, some can function with minimal ulnar motor function and only protective sensibility over the ulnar nerve distribution. These same disabilities in other patients may be severely handicapping. If the degree of return of sensory and motor function is unsatisfactory, then an operative procedure may be indicated.

The operative procedures available to correct failure of return of function after nerve repair include: (1) resection of the nerve anastomosis and reanastomosis, with or without a nerve graft, (2) conventional neurolysis, (3) internal neurolysis, (4) transfer of a neurovascular island pedicle flap, and (5) tendon transfers. The neurovascular island flap will aid in the restoration of sensory function without affecting motor function, and conversely, the use of tendon transfers will compensate for the absence of tendon function without affecting sensory function.

The use of a nerve stimulator at the second operative procedure may be helpful. After the site of nerve anastomosis is visualized, the nerve stimulator is applied proximal to the site of repair. If definite muscle contraction is obtained, no further procedure is carried out and the wound is closed. If nerve stimulation evokes no muscle contraction and there is minimal neuroma formation but moderate scarring encircling the nerve, a neurolysis is indicated. If a definite neuroma is present, reanastomosis or nerve grafting should be chosen. Unfortunately, evaluation of the degree of scarring and neuroma formation is subjective.

### Reanastomosis or nerve grafting

Classically, resection of the neuroma and reanastomosis with epineurial sutures was the accepted treatment in selected cases when the initial nerve anastomosis resulted in unsatisfactory nerve function. Experimental and clinical studies indicate that resection of neuroma and funicular repair will provide even more satisfactory results than the classic procedure. Yet the best results are those obtained by nerve grafting. If these results can be duplicated by other surgeons, nerve grafting should become the standard procedure when resection of a neuroma is indicated (p. 281).

### Neurolysis

There are two methods of accomplishing a neurolysis. One is the conventional neurolysis that involves freeing the nerve at the level of the epineurium from the surrounding scar tissue. The other is an internal neurolysis in which scar is removed from around the individual funiculi. In the conventional neurolysis, fine scissors or scalpel dissection is used, and the nerve is separated from surrounding scar tissue. Dissection is begun 3 to 4 cm proximal to the anastomosis and continued to the anastomosis. Then dissection is begun 3 to 4 cm distal to the anastomosis and continued proximally to the anastomosis. Care should be taken to preserve all the neural branches and the longitudinal blood supply to the nerve. Bleeding can be controlled most accurately with a bipolar cautery, and dissection is much more accurate if an operating microscope is used. Dissection is continued until all the scar is removed.

Internal neurolysis involves removal of the scar tissue constricting the individual fasciculi. Actually, minimal scar tissue is removed, but the individual fasciculi are dissected. The procedure is best accomplished with an operating microscope or binocular loupe. Dissection is begun 3 to 4 cm proximal to the anastomosis and continued to the anastomosis. Then dissection is begun 3 to 4 cm distal to the

anastomosis and continued proximally. Jewelers' forceps and fine scissors are needed for dissection. Unfortunately, some of the finer interfunicular communications are divided. Dissection is continued until the larger funiculi are completely dissected. The injection of saline into the connective tissue between the funiculi may aid the dissection.

However, there is yet very little objective experimental or clinical evidence to support the effectiveness of neurolysis. No one has reported a series of neurolyses with entirely adequate preoperative and postoperative documentation of function. Omer reported on neurolysis in 50 patients who had gunshot wounds, fractures, contusions, or lacerations as their original injuries. Thirty of these patients were said to have obtained clinical function after neurolysis; but in 12 of these, function returned within the time range for spontaneous recovery to have occurred. Thus, he felt that neurolysis was successful in only 36% of his patients. Other cases are cited in which dramatic improvement of nerve function immediately followed neurolysis. The only method by which one can obtain accurate information about the effectiveness of neurolysis is to continually plot the rate of return of nerve function. One must demonstrate a plateau in the rate of return and then a new rise in the rate of return of nerve function following neurolysis. The increased rate of return should be much faster than the rate of axon growth. If a series of cases meeting the above criteria could be collected, more exact indications for and contraindications against neurolysis might be established.

### Neurovascular island pedicle flap

The neurovascular island flap was designed to aid in restoration of sensibility to an area in which the sensory nerves had sustained irrevocable damage. By this procedure a section of skin (usually from the ulnar aspect of the middle or ring finger), based on its neurovascular supply, is transferred to the insensitive area. The recipient sites are the areas most often immobilized in pinch, that is, the ulnovolar pad of the thumb and the radiovolar pad of the index finger. Details of the procedure are described in Chapter 8. Other neurovascular island flaps include: (1) a flap of radially innervated skin from the dorsum of the index finger, which is transferred to the thumb; and (2) a flap developed from adjacent surfaces of the ring and middle fingers, which includes the interdigital web, two digital arteries, and two digital nerves. The disadvantages of these island flaps are:

1. Return of useful two-point discrimination (less than 15 mm) takes place in only 6% of the patients undergoing transfer of an island pedicle flap containing a median nerve branch and in 64% of the patients undergoing transfer of an island flap including a radial sensory nerve branch.
2. Sensory reorientation occurs infrequently; that is, the transferred island still feels "like the ring finger."

Markley suggests that some failures of digital neurovascular island flaps to provide useful sensibility may be due to both the small size of the flap with resultant loss of multiple fine nerve branches and the use of a donor flap site proximal to the fingertip where discrimination is normally not so accurate. He recommends use of donor tissue that includes the utmost tip of the digit and is large enough to have sufficient attached subcutaneous tissue to preserve small terminal nerve branches and end organs.

### Tendon transfers to restore motor function

If the nerve damage is irrevocable, tendon transfers may be required to restore function to the hand. The transferred motor function is rarely if ever normal. To evaluate an extremity in which one is considering tendon transfers, one simply lists the assets and the liabilities. The assets are the functioning motor units available in the arm, forearm, and hand. The liabilities are the functional actions necessary to regain function in the extremity. When the liabilities far exceed the assets, one must consider joint fusions (except the wrist) and tenodesis procedures (including the Zancolli procedure for the metacarpophalangeal joints). The variety of tendon transfers available are beyond the scope of this text. Yet one must remember to design the operative procedures for the patient in question, remembering his particular assets and liabilities.

### NONOPERATIVE TREATMENT

The methods of splinting and sensory reeducation presented here are not all-inclusive treatment possibilities, because there is such a variance in deficits and degrees of functional recovery seen with peripheral nerve injuries. The success of treatment depends largely on the creative approach developed by the therapist and on the cooperation of the patient. The following methods of treatment are examples of those currently in use in our Hand Rehabilitation Center.

Patients are usually seen in the Hand Rehabilitation Center 3 weeks after nerve repair. An initial hand evaluation, including muscle test (Fig. 13-1) and sensory battery (Fig. 13-2), is completed during the first treatment session and repeated at appropriate intervals. Based on results of these tests, treatment objectives are established.

The initial treatment program consists of early intervention to reduce edema and scar formation. During treatment the hand is elevated, and scar-softening techniques are initiated. The patient is instructed in passive range of motion of the digits and encouraged to involve his arm and hand in goal-directed activities. Strengthening of uninvolved muscles begins at this time. Depending on the patient's needs, he is supplied with appropriate adaptive equipment that will help improve self-care skills.

Early in treatment, the results of sensory loss, such as insensibility and trophic changes of the skin, are discussed with the patient. He is alerted to the problems and cautioned to use the uninvolved hand and visual cues to reduce the possibility of further injury. Sensory reeducation is initiated when protective sensation is present.

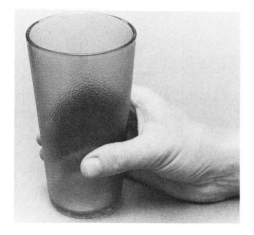

**Fig. 13-3.** The hand in the "position of function," grasping an object. Note the approximately 30 degrees of flexion at the metacarpophalangeal joints.

## Splinting

During the period of motor nerve regeneration, prevention of secondary problems by early intervention and splinting provides optimum care. The purpose of acute splinting with nerve injuries is to correct a muscle imbalance or to maintain the hand in a position of function in order to prevent deformity (Fig. 13-3). Although splinting may be used in the permanent treatment of injuries where no further return of nerve function is expected, the emphasis here is on the temporary treatment of acute injuries by splinting to prevent secondary deformities that may occur during the period of denervation.

The selection of a splint depends on many factors, including the level and severity of injury. The following splints have been found useful and are discussed in reference to certain diagnostic categories.

*Radial nerve injury.* The patient with wrist drop due to radial nerve injury (Fig. 13-4) is fitted with a dynamic supportive splint (Fig. 13-5). The tabs and rubber bands on the outrigger help extend the fingers and replace the action of the nonfunctioning extensor muscles. Depending on the patient's function and need to use the hand, a static cockup splint may suffice to prevent deformity (Fig. 13-6). The

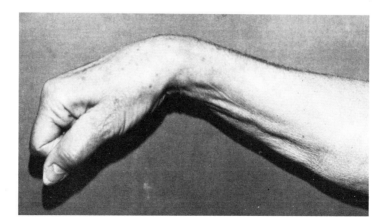

**Fig. 13-4.** Typical wrist drop deformity due to radial nerve injury.

cockup splint is less bulky than a dynamic splint and provides free finger movement.

***Ulnar nerve injury.*** The patient with ulnar nerve injury develops clawing of the fourth and fifth digits (Fig. 13-7). A resting hand splint maintains the hand in a functional position and prevents further hyperextension of the fourth and fifth metacarpophalangeal joints (Fig. 13-8). Fig. 13-9 illustrates a soft leather splint fabricated for clawhand deformity. The finger tabs block hyperextension of the meta-carpophalangeal joints and enable the normal long extensors to fully extend the proximal and distal interphalangeal joints.

***Combined median and ulnar nerve injury.*** Patients with injury to both median and ulnar nerves present a multitude of problems, particularly because they usually have additional injuries as well, most often lacerated flexor tendons. One splint commonly used in the presence of median and ulnar nerve injury combined with repaired lacerations of most or all flexor

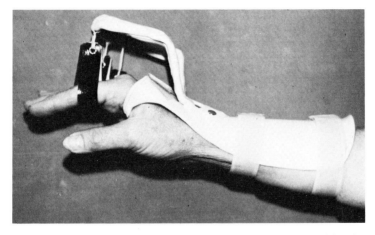

**Fig. 13-5.** Dynamic splint used in radial nerve injury. The tabs and rubber bands on the outrigger help replace the action of nonfunctioning extensor muscles.

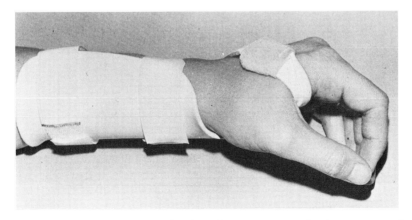

**Fig. 13-6.** Static cockup splint provides free finger movement in the presence of radial nerve injury.

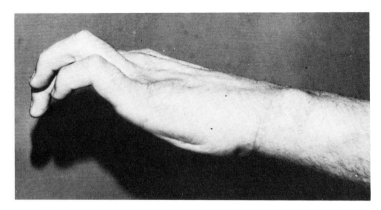

**Fig. 13-7.** Clawing of the fourth and fifth digits due to ulnar nerve injury (note scar at wrist).

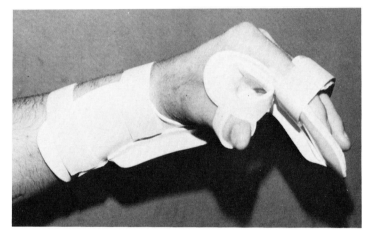

**Fig. 13-8.** Resting hand splint maintains hand in functional position and prevents further hyperextension of metacarpophalangeal joints with ulnar nerve injury.

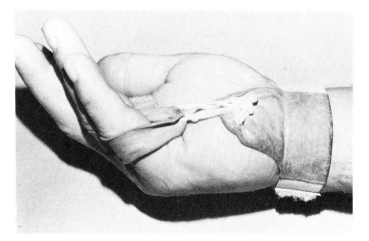

**Fig. 13-9.** Dynamic splint used in ulnar nerve injury. The finger tabs block hyperextension of metacarpophalangeal joints while allowing normal extension of proximal and distal interphalangeal joints.

tendons at the wrist level is illustrated in Fig. 13-10. The goal of this dynamic splint is to increase stress on the scar around the flexor tendons and thereby achieve full finger extension. (It should be noted that this is the only instance in which metacarpophalangeal joints are splinted in extension.) Patients with combined median and ulnar nerve injury are also frequently fitted with a static splint to maintain the thumb-index web space. The static splint is usually worn only at night, whereas the dynamic splint is worn during the daytime.

**Sensory reeducation**

Preliminary information indicates that intensive sensory reeducation may aid restoration of sensory function of the part in question. The important factors involved in sensory reeducation are the following:

1. The patient correlates stimuli from various objects with direct visualization of the objects; eventually visual assistance is eliminated (patient blind-

folded), and the objects are recognized by the stimuli they evoke in the injured part.
2. The educational process must be conducted in an environment suitable for undisturbed study.
3. The patient must be motivated to carry out simple repetitive exercises at home.

The sequence of regeneration of sensory modalities is: (1) pain, (2) vibration at 30 cps, (3) moving touch, (4) constant touch, and (5) vibration at 256 cps. Early phase sensory reeducation can be initiated when the patient is able to appreciate moving touch or perceive vibrations of 30 cps, and then only if the patient does not display hyperparesthesia. Hypersensitivity must be decreased before any sensory reeducation can begin. This is best accomplished by letting the patient stroke his own hand from proximal to distal, using cotton wool first, then progressing to felt and other coarser materials. Following this, sensory

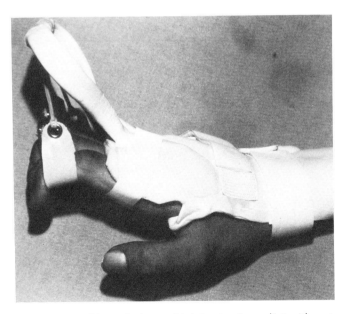

**Fig. 13-10.** Dynamic proximal interphalangeal joint extension splint with metacarpophalangeal joints held in extension. Splint stresses tendon scar tissue in combined median and ulnar nerve injury with tendon lacerations at wrist level.

reeducation can begin. First, moving touch is demonstrated to the patient; that is, moving touch with a pencil eraser is correlated visually with the sensory stimulus it produces. Identifying numbers 1, 3, 6, and 9 written on the tips of the fingers is a good exercise. Washers varying in size from large to small can be rolled up and down the finger. Gradually, the pencil eraser and washers are replaced by cotton, wool, or other very light materials.

Reeducation to the sensation of constant touch is begun when the patient can perceive vibrations of 256 cps. First, the object is felt with the uninjured hand; second, the object is felt with the injured hand while the object is visualized; finally, the object is felt with the injured hand while the eyes are closed. The objects may also be handled in pairs, one in each hand.

After the patient can clearly identify moving touch and constant touch, late phase sensory reeducation training is begun to allow improvement in two-point discrimination. Beginning with large hex nuts or washers, the patient relearns which feelings are associated with various stimuli. Again, the hex nuts and washers are handled first with eyes open, then without the aid of visual reference. The size of the hex nuts and washers is gradually reduced, thus requiring finer discrimination. The patient may also teach himself to identify various coins, based on the sensations associated with the various coins, for example, if the edges of the coin are smooth or rough.

Sensory reeducation sessions can be conducted several times daily, but each session must be brief (15 to 20 minutes) because of the intense concentration required. These sessions are usually continued for a period of weeks or months. Through these techniques, improvement in sensory function has been obtained even after long periods of denervation (years) before sensory reeducation.

## CAUSALGIA

Pain is the central feature of the symptom complex known as causalgia. The term causalgia literally means "burning pain" and was introduced by Mitchell in 1867. Early reports emphasized the burning pain in a limb subsequent to penetrating wounds involving peripheral nerve injury. Later reports included descriptions of the pain as throbbing, bursting, clamping, stabbing, tearing, or gnawing. Aggravation of the pain by physical and emotional stimuli became an important feature of causalgia, in addition to the disabling severity of the pain.

More recently the syndrome of causalgia has come to include also lesser degrees of essentially the same symptom complex, variously referred to as Sudeck's atrophy, sympathetic dystrophy, reflex dystrophy, posttraumatic painful osteoporosis, shoulder-hand syndrome, and so on. The symptom complex still involves disabling pain as the central feature occurring in the distal part of a limb, presumably after injury involving a peripheral nerve. Partial nerve lesions are thought to be the causative factor, but cases of causalgia after complete nerve division have also been reported. Some authors have differentiated between a major and minor form of causalgia. Major causalgia includes a severe symptom complex following penetrating high-velocity wounds that involve a peripheral nerve, most commonly the median nerve in the arm. Minor causalgia includes a lesser symptom complex associated with lesser, often closed, injuries, such as a crush, sprain, or fracture.

The true incidence of causalgia is essentially unknown, owing at least in part to the fact that it is probably not always correctly diagnosed. The time of onset of symptoms can be determined from pooled data of several authors who have reported their series of patients with causalgia: 50% of patients developed symptoms within 24 hours after wounding; another 22% developed symptoms between the first and seventh day after wounding, while the remainder (28%) developed symptoms after 1 week had passed. Of the latter group, there were several patients in whom there was a delay of up to 2 months after injury.

The symptom complex of causalgia usually also includes trophic, vasomotor, and sudomotor changes of the painful part. Initial vasodilatation is followed by vasoconstriction, then subsequent atrophy.

Thus, the appearance of the affected limb may demonstrate the following, depending somewhat on the duration of the illness: (1) edema, (2) erythema or mottled cyanosis of thin, shiny skin, (3) profuse or decreased sweating, (4) increased warmth, although it may be cooler than the normal limb, (5) decrease in volume of subcutaneous tissue with spindle-shaped fingertips, and (6) muscle atrophy (Figs. 13-11 and 13-12). The arm may be held away from

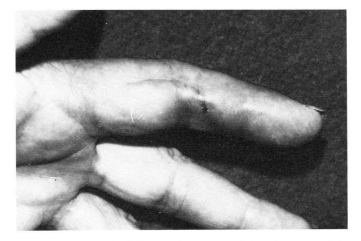

Fig. 13-11. Sympathetic dystrophy following laceration of digital nerve and flexor digitorum profundus. The index finger from the level of the proximal interphalangeal joint distally was moist and violaceous in contrast to the appearance of long fingers. Symptoms temporarily relieved by sympathetic block.

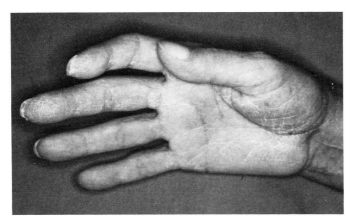

Fig. 13-12. Sympathetic dystrophy following fracture of wrist. Note the extremely dry skin and the changes in the nails.

the body with the elbow in 90 degrees flexion, the wrist nearly neutral, the metacarpophalangeal joints extended, and the thumb in slight palmar and ulnar abduction. The patient may have a protective covering over the limb, such as a towel, and may resist the examiner's efforts to touch the painful part. The joints of the affected part may be stiff, depending on the duration of symptoms. Roentgenological examination shows osteoporosis in 30% to 50% of patients, probably caused by disuse. Such patients are often misdiagnosed as having anxiety neuroses and related disorders of mental effect, particularly since emotional stimuli often precipitate or exacerbate symptoms.

The mechanism of the pathogenesis of causalgia is unknown. Some of the postulated mechanisms include vasospasm in the area of pain, conduction of painful stimuli by sympathetic nerve fibers, and short-circuiting between sympathetic and sensory nerve fibers within the injured nerve.

The short-circuiting theory, as proposed by Doupe and colleagues, is currently most accepted. This theory proposes that causalgia results from cross-stimulation or short-circuiting between efferent sympathetic fibers and afferent sensory fibers. The short-circuiting is thought to result from injury severe enough to break down myelin, thus allowing impulses to pass directly between adjacent nerves. Cross-stimulation can occur between motor and sensory fibers in an injured or compressed nerve in cats (Grant and Richards), but cross-stimulation between sympathetic and sensory fibers has not been demonstrated. Indirect evidence supporting the cross-stimulation theory is the reproduction of causalgia by stimulation of the sympathetic chain (Walker and Nulsen).

This theory further states that the pain from short-circuiting can arise from two mechanisms. Stimuli arising in efferent sympathetic fibers can cross the short-circuit and pass either orthodromically (centripetally, centrally) or antidromically (centrifugally, peripherally). Stimuli passing orthodromically through sensory nerve fibers are interpreted directly as pain. Antidromic impulses may also cause pain in the area supplied by the stimulated sensory nerve and areas supplied by adjacent intact nerves (Lewis).

The pain produced by stimulation of the distal end of a divided nerve is probably due to release of a vasodilator substance, neurokinin. Neurokinin obtained by nerve stimulation will cause burning pain and vasodilatation if injected into an uninjured area.

Based on Doupe's theory, either interruption of the antidromic sympathetic stimulation or removal of the area of short-circuiting should result in cure of causalgia. Sympathetic block will produce remission in 80% to 90% of patients. Resection of the injured portion of the nerve has not relieved symptoms in the majority of patients, however. If nerve resection fails, the adequacy of resection must be questioned. No one knows the exact location or length of nerve involved in short-circuiting. If two nerves are injured, both would have to be resected. Because neither resection of injured nerve nor sympathectomy will cure all cases, other mechanisms of pain production are probably in operation.

**Treatment**

Some patients with causalgia have undergone a spontaneous and complete regression of symptoms. Yet in others, causalgia may persist for many years, as long as 10 to 20 years after injury.

A variety of procedures have been used to treat causalgia. Only sympathetic nerve block and sympathectomy (chemical and surgical sympathectomy, respectively) have consistently produced relief of symptoms in approximately 80% of patients with causalgia of the arm.

Most authors recommend sympathetic block of the stellate ganglion as a diagnostic and therapeutic maneuver in cases of suspected causalgia. The pain may be completely and permanently relieved after one or several sympathetic blocks. If the pain relief from sympathetic block is only temporary, preganglionic surgical sympathectomy is indicated. In a series of 194 patients Slessor and colleagues reported 81% excellent, 14% good, and 5% poor results after sympathectomy for upper limb major causalgia. Kleinert and colleagues reported that 50% of patients with sympathetic dystrophy limited to the upper limb will improve with physical therapy and phenothiazine drug administration. Of the other 50% who did not respond to physical and drug therapy, about 80% were improved by sympathetic nerve block. About 80% of those failing to respond to stellate ganglion block were cured by surgical sympathectomy.

If surgical sympathectomy is reserved for those patients in whom chemical sympathectomy has been effective, it will cure over 90% of patients. Surgical sympathectomy may also be used in patients in whom sympathectic block was ineffective, but both surgeon and patient should understand that the chances of cure are low. If sympathectomy fails to relieve pain, a sweat test should be done to assess the completeness of the sympathectomy. Sympathectomy may be effective in patients whose symptoms have been present for only a few weeks or for many years. Sympathectomy may relieve the severe pain of causalgia, but occasional other lesser pains and paresthesias will persist.

Recurrence of symptoms after surgical sympathectomy has been reported, either spontaneously or as a result of new trauma. Regrowth of sympathetic fibers in a widespread pattern has been demonstrated.

Patients with causalgia whose joints have stiffened and whose muscles have atrophied from disuse present a special problem. When they undergo successful sympathetic nerve block, our patients are seen in the Hand Rehabilitation Center immediately following the injection. They are seen there for frequent (daily) half-day sessions until improved function can be maintained. The goal of therapy at this time is to promote motion of the entire arm with special emphasis on functional use of the hand. This includes active and passive exercise to improve joint mobility. Relaxation methods such as vibration, deep massage, tapping, and other modalities are used to decrease pain. Elevation of the arm during exercise and at rest is encouraged to decrease swelling. Dynamic and static splinting are sometimes indicated in the presence of some residual joint stiffness. Patients are encouraged to use their hands in a normal manner and to eliminate substitution patterns that have developed as a result of painful joints. Patients are instructed in a home program of active and active-resistive exercises for the shoulder, elbow, wrist, and hand. The home program is updated as progress occurs. When symptoms have diminished significantly, a resistive, strengthening program is introduced. Static splints initially worn at night to maintain range of motion gained during the day are discarded. Dynamic splints are now worn at night only, enabling the patient to involve his hand in functional activities throughout the day. The patient is often able to return to work at this time.

## PAINFUL NEUROMA

Neuroma formation following nerve injury has been described in Chapter 3. By definition, a neuroma occurs each time a peripheral nerve is divided. Painful neuromas are the exception rather than the rule. They are most likely to occur along divided distal sensory nerves, such as the digital nerves and the dorsal sensory branch of the radial nerve.

Various treatments have been proposed to alleviate the problem of painful neuromas; none has been consistently successful. Some of the methods employed are:

(1) proximal crushing or ligation of the nerve trunk, (2) resection of the neuroma and suturing the nerve end closed, (3) resection of the neuroma and allowing the proximal nerve end to retract into a sleeve of epineurial tissue, (4) coagulation of the nerve end by heating or freezing, (5) implanting the nerve end in bone, (6) capping the nerve end, and (7) chemical alteration of the nerve end with a sclerosing agent, such as formaldehyde or gentian violet.

Implanting the nerve end in bone has been advocated since 1943 and is theoretically attractive. However, the surgical technique can be difficult. In some cases bone has regenerated to seal off the drill hole, and a new neuroma has developed just superficial to the regenerated bone. Several early advocates have since abandoned the procedure.

Sunderland feels that the best method is probably a combination of proximal nerve ligation and chemical coagulation of the nerve end. But clinical proof for this is lacking. The use of chemicals to coagulate nerve ends, widely used in Europe, has not gained popularity in the United States.

Swanson and colleagues evaluated silicone capping of amputated sciatic and tibial nerves in rabbits. They found that neuroma formation was prevented with a cap length-diameter ratio of 5:1 (minimum) to 10:1 (maximum). The same group reported on the use of silicone caps in 18 patients (with a total of 38 upper limb nerves capped), 17 of whom underwent secondary surgery for the specific purpose of relieving disabling neuroma pain. Fifteen patients were relieved of their preoperative complaints; two patients developed causalgia; one patient had recurrent symptoms in one of four nerves capped and was subsequently relieved by reoperation and recapping.

Smith and Gomez reported percutaneous local injection of painful neuromas with triamcinolone acetonide. They injected 34 posttraumatic and postoperative neuromas of the hand and wrist by infiltrating the surrounding tissues, rather than the nerve end or neuroma itself. A single injection completely relieved the tenderness or paresthesias of 15 neuromas in 11 patients. Symptoms in another nine neuromas in seven patients were relieved after multiple injections. In nine neuromas in five patients there was no relief of symptoms. Seven patients (14 neuromas) had an initial complaint of pain in addition to tenderness or paresthesias; only one of these patients had reduction of pain after steroid injection. One neuroma in each of three patients was not injected; symptoms did not resolve in the uninjected neuromas. Saline injection of neuromas was not used as a control.

Grant advocated a method of dealing with painful neuromas that involved initial injection of the neuroma with a local anesthetic agent. If symptoms were relieved, the neuroma was resected. If symptoms recurred after resection, repetitious percussion or continual massage of the neuroma was undertaken, first with the aid of local anesthesia, then without it.

Desensitization of a painful neuroma by nonsurgical means is a routine part of treatment in the Hand Rehabilitation Center. Treatment can be initiated as soon as the site of injury begins to heal and the patient is able to participate in a program of sensory bombardment. Pain tolerance varies from patient to patient, so the program of desensitization is altered to accommodate each patient's pain threshold. Treatment begins with gentle massage, proceeding to deep pressure massage over the painful area. Gentle tapping of an amputation stump on a soft surface is initiated early. Tapping progresses to a harder surface such as a table top, and the patient is encouraged to increase the force of tapping. At the same time, the patient begins rubbing the sensitive area over a piece of soft material and advances to a rough, textured surface.

Another method of desensitization is the use of vibration directly over the area. Patients are instructed to perform this routine daily, 50 to 100 times each hour. Most patients who are reliable in following this method of desensitization report a significant decrease in hypersensitivity.

## BIBLIOGRAPHY

Barnes, R.: The role of sympathectomy in the treatment of causalgia, J. Bone Joint Surg. **35B:** 172, 1953.

Barnes, R.: Causalgia; a review of 48 cases, Med. Res. Counc. Spec. Rep. Ser. **282:**156, 1954.

Chapman, L. F., Ramos, A. O., Goodell, H., and Wolff, H. G.: Neurohumoral features of afferent fibers in man, Arch. Neurol. **4:**617, 1961.

Dellon, A. L., Curtis, R. M., and Edgerton, M. T.: Evaluating recovery of sensation in the hand following nerve injury, Johns Hopkins Med. J. **130:**235, 1972.

Dellon, A. L., Curtis, R. M., and Edgerton, M. T.: Reeducation of sensation in the hand after nerve injury and repair, Plast. Reconstr. Surg. **53:**297, 1974.

Denmark, A.: An example of symptoms resembling tic douloureux produced by a wound in the radial nerve, Med. Chir. Trans. **4:**48, 1813.

Doupe, J., Cullen, C. H., and Chance, G. Q.: Post-traumatic pain and the causalgic syndrome, J. Neurol. Neurosurg. Psychiatry **7:**33, 1944.

Drucker, W., and others: Pathogenesis of post-traumatic sympathetic dystrophy, Am. J. Surg. **97:**454, 1959.

Echlin, F., Owens, F. M., Jr., and Wells, W. L.: Observations on "major" and "minor" causalgia, Arch. Neurol. Psychiatry **62:**183, 1949.

Evans, J. A.: Reflex sympathetic dystrophy; report on 57 cases, Ann. Intern. Med. **26:**417, 1947.

Freeman, N. E.: Treatment of causalgia arising from gunshot wounds of peripheral nerves, Surgery **22:**68, 1947.

Grant, G. H.: Methods of treatment of neuromata of the hand, J. Bone Joint Surg. **33A:**841, 1951.

Guttmann, L., and Medawar, P. B.: The chemical inhibition of fibre regeneration and neuroma formation in peripheral nerves, J. Neurol. Psychiatry **5:**130, 1942.

Hardy, W. G., and others: The problem of minor and major causalgia, Am. J. Surg. **95:**545, 1958.

Homans, J.: Minor causalgia following injuries and wounds, Ann. Surg. **113:**932, 1941.

Kirklin, J. W., Chenoweth, A. I., and Murphy, F.: Causalgia; a review of its characteristics, diagnosis and treatment, Surgery **21:**321, 1947.

Kleinert, H. E., and others: Post-traumatic sympathetic dystrophy, presentation to American Society for Surgery of the Hand, January 1972.

Lewis, T.: Pain, New York, 1942, The Macmillan Co.

Markley, J. M.: Preservation of close two-point discrimination in the interdigital transfer of neurovascular island flaps, Plast. Reconstr. Surg. **59:**812, 1977.

Mayfield, F. H.: Reflex dystrophies of the hand (the causalgic states). In Flynn, J. E., editor: Hand surgery, ed. 2, Baltimore, 1975, The Williams & Wilkins Co.

Mitchell, S. W., and others: Gunshot wounds and other injuries of nerves, Philadelphia, 1864, J. B. Lippincott Co.

Nathan, P. W.: On the pathogenesis of causalgia in peripheral nerve injuries, Brain **70:**145, 1947.

Omer, G. E.: Injuries to nerves of the upper extremity, J. Bone Joint Surg. **56A:**1615, 1974.

Omer, G., and Thomas, S.: Treatment of causalgia; review of cases at Brooke General Hospital, Tex. Med. **67:**93, 1971.

Owens, J .C.: Causalgia, Am. Surg. **23:**636, 1957.

Rasmussen, T. B., and Freedman, H.: Treatment of causalgia, J. Neurosurg. **3:**165, 1946.

Richards, R. L.: Causalgia, Arch. Neurol. **16:**339, 1967.

Schumacher, H. B., and others: Causalgia, Surg. Gynecol. Obstet. **86:**452, 1948.

Seddon, H.: Surgical disorders of the peripheral nerves, ed. 2, Edinburgh, 1975, Churchill Livingstone.

Slessor, A. J.: Causalgia; a review of 22 cases, Edinburgh Med. J. **55:**563, 1948.

Smith, J. R., and Gomez, N. H.: Local injection therapy of neuromata of the hand with triamcinolone acetonide, J. Bone Joint Surg. **52A:** 71, 1970.

Spiegel, I. J., and Melowski, J. L.: Causalgia, J.A.M.A. **127:**9, 1945.

Sunderland, S.: Nerves and nerve injuries, Edinburgh, 1972, Churchill Livingstone.

Sunderland, S., and Kelly, M.: The painful sequelae of injuries to peripheral nerves, Aust. N.Z. J. Surg. **18:**75, 1948.

Swanson, A. B., Boeve, N. R., and Lumsden, R. M.: The prevention and treatment of amputation neuromata by silicone capping, J. Hand Surg. **2:**70, 1977.

Toumey, J. W.: Occurrence and management of reflex sympathetic dystrophy (causalgia of the extremities), J. Bone Joint Surg. **30A:**883, 1948.

Ulmer, J. L., and Mayfield, F. H.: Causalgia, Surg. Gynec. Obstet. **83:**789, 1946.

Walker, A. E., and Nulsen, F.: Electrical stimulation of the upper thoracic portion of the sympathetic chain in man, Arch. Neurol. Psychiatry **59:**559, 1948.

White, J. C., and others: Causalgia following gunshot injuries of nerves, Ann. Surg. **128:**161, 1948.

Wirth, F. P., Jr., and Rutherford, R. B.: A civilian experience with causalgia, Arch. Surg. **100:**633, 1970.

Zalis, A. W., Rodriquez, A. A., Oester, Y. T., and Mains, D. B.: Evaluation of nerve regeneration by means of nerve evoked potentials, J. Bone Joint Surg. **54A:**1246, 1972.

# CHAPTER 14

# Restoration of tendon gliding

The restoration of tendon gliding after primary repair of a severed tendon depends on the patient's ability to biochemically modify the scar that forms in response to the injury. This scar must be modified to form loose, filmy adhesions. Of course, the patient is not totally responsible for the result he obtains from a tendon repair. The milieu in which scar forms about a repaired tendon is determined by several factors: (1) the extent of tissue damage resulting from the injury, (2) the handling of the tissues by the individual performing the surgical repair, and (3) the response of these tissues to postoperative therapy. Our ability to control the extent of tissue damage resulting from the injury is limited by the extent of débridement permissible. The latter two factors are determined by the expertise of the surgeon and the therapist, respectively. In every patient with a repaired tendon, the surgeon's and the therapist's manipulation of the tissues can determine the environment in which scar forms about the tendon and under ideal circumstances can produce an environment that will take full advantage of the patient's ability to favorably alter his scar tissue response. Therapy can be good or bad. The poorly informed, overly aggressive therapist can convert an ideal situation in a hand into an unfavorable situation to which the patient reacts by forming more undesirable scar. This is frequently signalled by the development of pain, swelling, or redness in the hand in response to therapy.

In this chapter we will present the current methods of management, the historical basis for development of these methods, and the results of management according to these methods. Postoperative therapy has received little attention in the past, and apparent advances are being suggested with increased frequency. Only scientific evaluation of these methods will prove their effectiveness.

## POSTOPERATIVE MANAGEMENT AFTER PRIMARY TENDON REPAIR

Restoration of tendon gliding after tendon repair or tendon grafting is frequently less satisfactory if specific postoperative therapy is not used. Postoperative therapy includes active and passive range of motion exercises and dynamic and static splinting. Obtaining as much passive motion as possible is of prime importance, because the range of passive motion obtained defines the upper limit for the range of active motion that can be realized. In our discussion of the management of the stiff hand (Chapter 12), we have presented the techniques of exercising and splinting to obtain as much passive motion as possible. These techniques should be reviewed when reading this chapter; either alone or in combination, they are useful in restoring tendon gliding after tendon repair or grafting. Young children are an exception to the rule; they may obtain a satisfactory range of motion without any specific postoperative treatment. The results of tendon surgery in children are almost uniformly good. The reasons for the better results in young children are incompletely defined but certainly involve their ability to favorably modify scar tissue. This is fortunate, because young children are not very cooperative about wearing splints or performing specific exercises.

For more than 30 years, management after primary repair of a divided flexor tendon has been based on the writings of Mason and Allen (1941). In recent years newer techniques have been introduced and are rapidly gaining in popularity. Basically the methods of postoperative management include: (1) early motion and (2) delayed motion. These methods can be further divided into whether they include active and passive exercises either in combination or alone. To provide better insight into the development of the methods of postoperative management, the concept of delayed motion will be presented first, followed by the more recent concept of early motion.

**Delayed motion**

Mason and Allen (1941) defined the course of events in the experimental animal after primary tendon suture and immobilization. The animals were divided into four groups depending on the period of immobilization of the leg, the length of time the leg was exercised, and the manner in which it was exercised after termination of the immobilization. In group I, observations were made on tendons taken from a leg held rigidly in plaster for periods

varying from 2 to 35 days. In group II, animals were immobilized for 3 weeks and then allowed free use of the extremity for 1 to 6 weeeks. In group III, the animals that inadvertently removed their casts were studied. In group IV, a plaster and metal splint was applied to allow restricted movement after 1 week of rigid immobilization.

Study of the tensile strength gain in group I revealed the following. At 2 days, the tendon tensile strength was very low, and it became even lower by the third to fifth day after suturing. Softening of the tendon ends markedly reduced the effectiveness of the tendon sutures. On the fifth day, the holding power of the tendon and its tensile strength began to rise. A cuff of surrounding tissue attached to the site of tendon repair was evident by 10 days. This cuff of restrictive tissues reverted to gliding tissue sometime between the fourteenth and the twenty-first day. Grossly, tendon repairs immobilized for 28 to 35 days were well healed. The peritendinous tissues had become loose and filmy, readily permitting unrestricted tendon gliding. A reconstituted digital sheath was evident at 5 weeks. If mobilization was begun at 21 days, the tendon ends were larger and more bulbous than in the immobilized tendons. Furthermore, a greater separation of the tendon ends at the repair site was noted. In animals that were allowed mobilization before 21 days, the rate of tendon repair rupture and extent of fibrous tissue reaction was much greater than in those immobilized for at least 21 days.

Mason and Allen wanted to determine if there is a certain phase in tendon healing when use and motion are actually harmful and another phase when they are beneficial—exactly when we are still trying to determine today! To do this, they compared the tensile strength of completely immobilized tendons with that of tendons subjected to restricted and unrestricted motion. At 14 to 16 days, all three groups had similar tensile strengths. After 14 to 16 days, the tensile strength increased rapidly in those tendons subjected to some degree of stress (motion).

They concluded that it was unwise to initiate motion during the time that both the tensile strength and the suture-holding power of the tendon were dropping. Furthermore, they suggested that motion should not be allowed before the tenth day and probably not before the fourteenth day. These conclusions were based on the observations that: (1) early active unrestricted motion leads to the production of a marked tissue reaction and adhesion formation, and (2) restricted motion can be started safely at the end of 2 weeks.

The recommendations of Mason and Allen have been slightly modified through years of clinical experience, and now the delayed motion techniques include the following: (1) Tendon suture is immobilized for 21 days; and (2) restricted exercises are begun at 21 days, and the amplitude and vigor of exercise are gradually increased until unrestricted use is allowed 8 weeks after suture.

***Techniques of therapy.*** No active or passive motion of the involved digit is permitted during the first 3 weeks. On the twenty-first day, the dressing is removed, and an initial evaluation is completed. Only gentle, active motion is allowed at this time, and some evaluation items are deferred, such as measurement of gross grip strength and passive extension of the injured finger. At 6 to 7 weeks, when the tendon repair is stronger, all evaluation items are performed.

The following exercises are begun on the twenty-first day: (1) gentle, active proximal interphalangeal flexion with the metacarpophalangeal joint held in as much extension as possible using gentle positioning; (2) gentle, active distal interphalangeal flexion with the metacarpophalangeal and proximal interphalangeal joints stabilized in their relaxed position; (3) passive

flexion of metacarpophalangeal, proximal interphalangeal, and distal interphalangeal joints; (4) active and passive flexion exercises of uninvolved digits, as well as gentle, active extension; and (5) gentle, active flexion and extension of the wrist. Patients are instructed in the importance of scar massage to reduce adherence of the skin to the underlying tendon repair. Massage is accomplished with slow, firm pressure to the scar without forcing the finger into extension.

The patient is fitted with a dorsal protective splint to hold the digit in a relaxed position and to prevent sudden extension (Fig. 14-1). Velcro straps are attached just below the crease of the proximal interphalangeal joint and below the crease of the distal interphalangeal joint so that the patient is able to actively flex his distal interphalangeal joint with both straps in place. By undoing the distal strap, he can also work on increasing active proximal interphalangeal flexion with the proximal phalanx stabilized. The splint allows the patient to work on individual joint motion

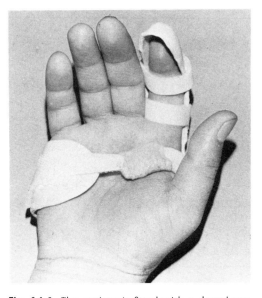

**Fig. 14-1.** The patient is fitted with a dorsal protective splint to prevent sudden digital hyperextension.

and to use his other fingers freely without fear of extending the injured finger and rupturing the tendon repair.

Patients are seen two to three times weekly for treatment following tendon repair. They perform the exercises outlined above, as well as scar massage. They are instructed to begin using their injured hand with the splint in place for light, everyday activities. They are encouraged to exercise for 10-minute periods several times daily. The work-rest concept of exercise is utilized in order to avoid putting undue stress on the tendon repair.

During the fifth and sixth week after tendon repair, the patient continues to work on increasing active proximal and distal interphalangeal joint flexion, with the metacarpophalangeal joint held in increasing increments of extension. He is provided with an exercise board to help isolate specific motion at each joint and thereby promote increased tendon gliding. More repetitions of each exercise are performed, and gross flexion and extension exercises of the entire hand are begun. Passive proximal and distal interphalangeal joint extension exercises of the entire hand are begun. The therapist holds both the metacarpophalangeal and distal interphalangeal joints in flexion while passively extending the proximal interphalangeal joint. Both the metacarpophalangeal and proximal interphalangeal joints are held in flexion while the distal interphalangeal joint is passively extended. Scar massage is more vigorous, and use of the protective splint is decreased.

During the seventh and eighth week, more active extension of the finger is encouraged, and resistance is applied to active flexion. Resistance increases the stress on the scar through active muscle contraction, and the patient is asked to hold the extreme of both flexion and extension for a few seconds to further increase stress on the tendon adhesions. As the patient gains increased flexion with the metacarpophalangeal joint held in exten-

sion, the metacarpophalangeal joint is gradually stabilized in greater degrees of flexion to further promote tendon gliding and to increase full flexion of the digit. A right-angle exercise board is used to hold the metacarpophalangeal joint in 90 degrees flexion while the patient works on active finger flexion. To add stress to the adhesions, massage is now done in a distal direction as the patient actively flexes the finger and in a proximal direction as the patient extends the finger. The patient should now be able to perform everyday activities with the injured hand, but he is cautioned against any strenuous exercise.

Patients who have limited proximal and distal interphalangeal extension are fitted with a dynamic splint. Increased extension can be gained by the use of the dorsal outrigger splint with rubber band traction or a Wynn-Parry spring splint. The dynamic force applied by either splint is low initially, and it is gradually increased according to the patient's ability to wear the splint for longer periods of time as determined by his tissues' reaction.

During the ninth and tenth week, the treatment program is more varied, and activities involving the use of the entire hand are begun. The exercises are more resistive and incorporate the use of specific exercise equipment, such as thermoplast, hand grippers, and weights. Resistance is graded with each exercise activity, and the goal is to increase overall hand strength in preparation for return to work.

*Results.* The results of primary flexor tendon repair combined with delayed motion postoperatively are summarized in Table 11-1. Briefly from the composite tabulation, 76% of primary flexor tendon repairs for injuries in zone 2 are rated as fair to excellent. The remaining 24% are poor results.

**Early passive motion**

Young and Harmon (1960) reasoned that voluntary and involuntary spasms and muscle contractions pulling against a suture line result in repeated trauma to the suture line with frequent partial or complete tearing of the repair. They devised a method of repair to minimize this problem. The severed tendon was repaired with a running suture of 5-0 chromic catgut. A silk suture was placed through the tip of the fingernail and tied to a rubber band (Fig. 14-2). The rubber band was gently pulled until the finger rested in partial flexion, then it was secured to a wrist band of adhesive tape. No other dressings were used. On the first postoperative day, the patient began gentle passive extension of the injured finger. As the finger was released, the rubber band brought it back into flexion. Passive motion was increased day by day, until full motion was accomplished by 3 weeks. No *active* motion was permitted until the end of the third week when the rubber band was removed.

Harmon and Young reported on 103 patients who sustained laceration of the flexor tendons only. They classified their results according to whether or not permanent disability awards were made to the patients by the Industrial Commission of the State of Ohio. Of 103 patients, 101 patients received no awards for disability.

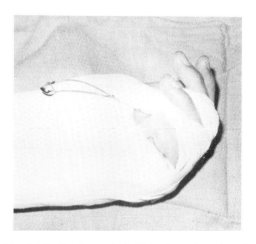

**Fig. 14-2.** The finger is held in the relaxed position by a nylon suture passed through the nail and attached to the dressing through a rubber band.

Only two patients presented enough restriction of motion to receive compensation!

Encouraged by the report of Harmon and Young, Duran and Houser studied their techniques both experimentally and in the clinical setting. Recently they presented their perfected technique for management of patients with repaired flexor tendons in zones 2 and 3 of the hand. Their method of management is described below in detail.

In the operating room, after the tendon repair is complete, the wrist is placed in 20 degrees flexion, and the metacarpophalangeal joint of the finger is maintained in its normal balanced position. Under direct vision, the distal phalanx is extended until the tendon repair glides 3 to 5 mm. This moves the flexor digitorum profundus repair away from the fixed structures that may have been damaged in the area and away from the repair of the flexor digitorum superficialis. The amount of distal phalanx extension required to provide 3 to 5 mm of tendon gliding is recorded.

Next, the middle phalanx is extended until both tendon repairs glide 3 to 5 mm distally. This moves both tendon repairs away from the damaged fixed structures at the site of the injuries.

A dorsal splint extending distally to the level of the metacarpophalangeal joints is used for wrist immobilization, with the wrist maintained in 20 degrees flexion. A removable wedge of sponge beneath the hand may be helpful in managing the thumb and index finger, because the flexed wrist places them in considerable extension at the distal joint, creating difficulty with the extension exercises. During exercises, the wedge is removed, and the wrist is placed in a neutral position. The wedge is replaced after passive exercises are completed. This is not a problem in the long, ring, and little fingers.

At the end of the operative procedure, a hole is placed in the free border of the nail, and a nylon suture is placed through it, tied, and connected to a rubber band that is secured with a safety pin to the volar aspect of the forearm dressing under light tension.

Exercises are started *immediately*, the first having been carried out under direct vision of the tendon repair at the time of surgery. Exercises are performed in the morning and evening with six to eight motions for each tendon every session. Between exercises the fingers are covered securely with stockinett. Uninvolved fingers are gently passively exercised at each session. Training of the patient or parents is considered essential to the success of the procedure.

Controlled *passive* motion alone is continued for 4½ weeks. The dorsal splint is removed, and the rubber band is attached to a wrist band. Passive motion exercises are continued even after gentle active extension exercises are begun. One week later, the wrist band and nail suture are removed. Active flexion is begun and increased with supervision. Active extension motion is gradually increased. The anastomosis is protected for 2 additional weeks as active exercises continue. Occasionally it is necessary to use a dynamic

splint to correct a proximal interphalangeal joint contracture. If splinting is necessary, it is begun 6 weeks after tendon repair. For the next 2 weeks, it is used gently and is gradually increased as needed.

The method of early mobilization used at the Hand Rehabilitation Center is based on the method described above by Duran and Houser. Some modifications of their method have become necessary and are presented below.

The patient is seen in the Hand Rehabilitation Center within the first 24 to 48 hours following tendon repair. The dressing applied during surgery is removed, and the patient is fitted with a dorsal protective splint (Fig. 14-3). This splint holds the wrist in 20 to 30 degrees flexion, the metacarpophalangeal joints in 90 degrees flexion, the proximal and distal interphalangeal joints of the uninvolved fingers in extension, and the injured finger in flexion at all joints; and it allows free movement of the thumb. The splint is worn at all times during the next 4½ weeks except for occasional removal during therapy sessions to soak the hand and to clean the splint.

Positioning of the injured finger to per-

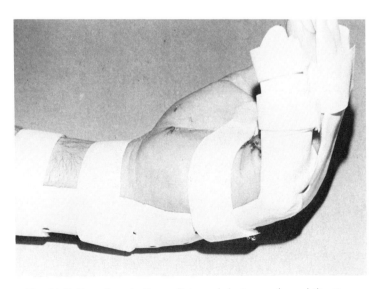

**Fig. 14-3.** Dorsal protective splint used during early mobilization.

form controlled passive extension exercises is done in two ways. In the first, the portion of the splint fitted over the injured finger allows 20 to 25 degrees passive extension at both the proximal and distal interphalangeal joints. Between exercise sessions, a foam wedge is placed between the splint and the involved finger to maintain a flexed position. Velcro straps hold the finger and the wedge in place and prevent active flexion (Fig. 14-4). The second method includes the use of a clothing hook glued to the fingernail. A rubber band is attached to the hook and to the wrist strap, which holds the splint in place. Both ways of positioning the finger with repaired flexor tendons have been satisfactory. Velcro straps hold the uninvolved fingers in place and prevent any active flexion of these digits (Fig. 14-5).

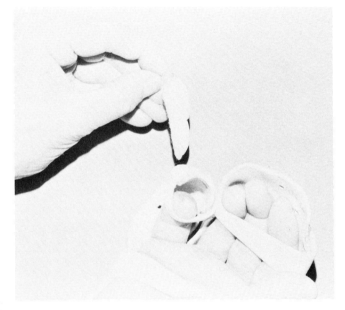

**Fig. 14-4.** Injured little finger positioned with foam wedge.

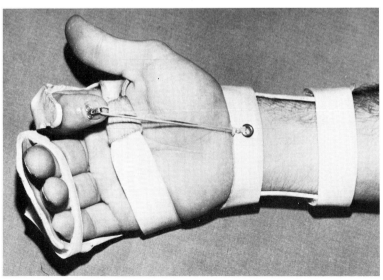

**Fig. 14-5.** Injured index finger positioned with dorsal protective splint and rubber band traction.

According to Duran and Houser, 3 to 5 mm of extension of the tendon repair in a passive exercise program is sufficient to prevent firm adherence of a repaired flexor tendon in zones 2 and 3 of the hand. The patients are seen frequently during the first week, and they perform one set of exercises with the therapist. This helps to ensure that they are properly instructed and able to carry out the exercises independently each day. When both the patient and the therapist are confident, the patient assumes full responsibility for the exercises, but the patient continues to be seen at regular intervals during the next 4½ weeks.

In the first method, exercises are done by removing the foam wedge, and the distal interphalangeal joint is extended to the limit of the splint six to eight times. Next the proximal interphalangeal joint is extended six to eight times while the middle phalanx is held. Passive flexion of the digit is done several times to prevent joint stiffness. Then the wedge and straps are replaced. In the second method, the rubber band remains attached, but the finger is again extended at the distal and proximal interphalangeal joints to the limits of the splint six to eight times. Passive flexion exercises of the finger are performed, and the finger resumes its original position in slight flexion as determined by the tension of the rubber band. In both instances, the uninvolved fingers are passively exercised at each session.

At 4½ to 5½ weeks, the hand remains positioned in the splint, but active extension exercises replace controlled passive motion. The patient is also allowed to actively flex and extend the uninvolved digits during the two exercise sessions per day.

At 5½ weeks, the dorsal splint is reduced in size to resemble the dorsal protective splint shown in Fig. 14-1. The patient wears this splint at all times for 1 additional week. Gentle, active flexion exercises of the injured finger are begun and increased with supervision. The treatment program now follows the one outlined previously for immobilized tendon repairs.

The success of either method requires maximum cooperation from the patient in following his prescribed treatment program. However, the qualitative and quantitative characteristics of the scar around the tendons are important in determining the ultimate results. But when all other factors are equal, the degree of self-motivation becomes the primary determinant of the effectiveness of any exercise program aimed at the restoration of normal tendon gliding.

Duran and Houser reported on flexor tendon repairs in 30 fingers and four thumbs of 32 patients.

Measurements in degrees of flexion at each joint of the finger (distal interphalangeal, proximal interphalangeal, and metacarpophalangeal) was made, and a second measurement of the proximal interphalangeal joint was made. These were added together. Loss of extension in the same joints was subtracted from the total. These measurements were compared with those of the same finger of the normal hand.

In tendons repaired in zone 2, there were eleven cases whose average range of motion was 89% of normal. Four patients with tendon ruptures offset some excellent results and thus reduced the overall result. Twenty-seven of 34 digits (four thumbs and 30 fingers) in 32 patients studied were graded as 83% to 100% of normal range of motion. Three fingers were graded as 79% to 83% of normal range of motion. The remaining four fingers represented the tendon ruptures. In two fingers, ruptures occurred early in the study when therapy was not as controlled as desired. Rupture occurred in a third case, an uncooperative child who was not a candidate for this method of management. The fourth finger was ruptured by heavy exercise at 6 weeks after repair.

Kleinert modified the method of Young

and Harmon as follows. The tendon repair is accomplished with a single crisscross suture that approximates the tendon ends and a circumferential suture that seals the tendon edges. The repaired tendon is protected with a dynamic splint constructed at the end of the operative procedure. A dorsal plaster splint is applied with the wrist in flexion and the finger in extension. Dynamic rubber band traction is applied to the fingernail, holding the finger in flexion but permitting full active extension. The flexor muscle relaxes during finger extension. When flexion is attempted, the stretched rubber band immediately flexes the finger, reducing tension on the site of tendon repair and the likelihood of rupture if the flexor muscle contracts.

Splints and sutures are removed after 3 weeks. Limited active exercise is permitted for the next 7 to 10 days. Then to regain maximum function, subsequent active and passive exercises are carried out by the patient under the physician's supervision. Dynamic splints aid in overcoming flexion contractures. It is only by the persistence and insistence of the physician that satisfactory results are obtained. Early poor results can become good-excellent results with exercises and splinting.

Kleinert reported that 87% of the patients obtained good to excellent results. Equally good results were obtained when the profundus alone was severed and when both the profundus and the superficialis were severed.

### Early active motion

No control studies are available today regarding the use and effectiveness of early active motion.

## OPERATIVE PROCEDURES WHEN TENDON GLIDING IS UNSATISFACTORY

The patient determines when he has an unsatisfactory result. If he is able to function well in his job and is satisfied with the result, even though it may not be perfect, then the result is adequate. If he is unable to function adequately, and an unsatisfactory result has been obtained, the surgeon is faced with several decisions. The first is: how long does one wait to be sure a result is going to remain unsatisfactory? We will discuss this in depth in Chapter 15. After we have decided that the patient has an inadequate result, we must determine what is causing the failure of the tendon to glide. If the limiting factor is stiff joints, then the method of therapy to improve passive joint motion must be instituted (see Chapter 12). If passive limitation of active motion is due to unyielding adhesions about the tendon repair, the surgeon has several choices of treatment. The operative procedures available for the restoration of tendon gliding include: (1) tenolysis, (2) repair of the disrupted anastomosis, (3) insertion of a Silastic rod and subsequent tendon grafting, (4) secondary or tertiary tendon grafting, (5) tenodesis, (6) arthrodesis, and (7) amputation. Tenolysis is the most frequently employed procedure, and repair of a disrupted anastomosis is the second most frequent. The insertion of a Silastic rod aids in the preparation of a pseudosheath, thus providing a better bed for a subsequent tendon graft. The combination of Silastic rod insertion and subsequent tendon grafting is preferred to direct secondary or tertiary tendon grafting. Better results are produced by the combination of procedures. Tenodesis or arthrodesis is used more frequently at the distal interphalangeal than at the proximal interphalangeal or metacarpophalangeal joint. When the flexor sublimis tendon is functioning, fixation of the distal interphalangeal joint allows excellent function in flexion and good function in extension. Function in either flexion or extension is severely compromised when either the proximal interphalangeal or the metacarpophalangeal joint is arthrodesed. Amputation is reserved for consideration in cases refractory to all nonoperative and operative procedures.

## Tenolysis

The primary indications for tenolysis after tendon repair and failure of postoperative measures to restore tendon gliding over a period of months are: (1) The passive range of joint motion exceeds the active range of joint motion, and (2) the active range of joint motion is insufficient to meet the patient's requirement. Satisfactory skin coverage (that is, skin and subcutaneous tissue), skeletal stability, adequate joint function, and at least protective sensation are needed before tenolysis is undertaken.

Because the results of tendon repair are least satisfactory in flexor zone 2 (the area between the distal palmar crease and the proximal interphalangeal joint crease; see Fig. 11-2), the patient undergoing tenolysis has usually had either a primary repair or a tendon graft inserted after an injury in zone 2. He exhibits a fair result when the fingertip can be actively flexed to between ½ inch and 1½ inches of the distal palmar crease or a poor result when the fingertip cannot be actively flexed to within 1½ inches of the distal palmar crease. However, tenolysis may be used after laceration of flexor or extensor tendons at any level.

Tenolysis after extensor tendon injuries is uncommon because of the excellent results produced from extensor tendon repair (see Table 11-3). The most common sites of extensor tenolysis are in zone 2 (dorsum of the finger) and zone 3 (hand) (see Fig. 11-5).

It is important to determine as accurately as possible the level of the most significant adhesions that are preventing gliding. (The maneuvers that aid in localizing these adhesions are presented in Chapter 11.) Furthermore, one must realize that the adhesions are always more extensive than preoperative examination implies. Thus, one must be prepared to explore the entire length of the tendon at the time of surgery. We do not consider the tenolysis procedure to be a minor operation. It is performed in the operating suite, with the arm under local anesthesia and the field rendered bloodless by the pneumatic tourniquet.

The ideal interval between primary tendon repair or primary tendon grafting and secondary tendon grafting or tenolysis is unknown. Verdan states that if a satisfactory range of motion is not obtained, tenolysis should be performed 3 months after primary repair of flexor zone 2 injuries. Kleinert, Boyes, and Pulvertaft have all recommended waiting 6 months before performing a tenolysis. The reasons for the delay are apparently twofold: (1) Tendon function may improve spontaneously up to 6 months after tendon repair, and (2) tendon grafts have ruptured if tenolysis is done 3 or 4 months postoperatively. Rupture of tendon graft did not occur if the tenolysis was delayed for 6 months, but the minimal safe interval between tendon grafting and tenolysis is unknown. Early identification of those persons who are going to require tenolysis may be possible using techniques that are discussed in Chapter 15.

We have performed a controlled randomized experiment to determine the ideal time for tenolysis. The chicken was used as the experimental animal, because our previous work has allowed extrapolation from experimental work in chickens to clinical work with patients. We evaluated the effectiveness of tenolysis at 1, 3, 6, 12, 16, and 24 weeks after primary tendon repair, using three criteria for measurement: the rate of rupture, the tensile strength of the repair site, and the blood supply to the tendons undergoing tenolysis. Tenolysis performed at 1 and 3 weeks after primary tendon repair led to a higher rupture rate and markedly weakened the tendon repairs. Furthermore, the blood supply of the tendon was decreased by this procedure at this time. By 6 weeks, the effects on the blood supply were variable. By 12 weeks, the tenolysis actually resulted in an increased blood supply to the tenolysed tendon and did not materially affect its tensile strength. Similar results are found at 16 weeks. By 24 weeks, the effects of tenolysis on the blood supply were again variable. In the experimental animals, tenolysis at 12 weeks after primary tendon repair does not weaken the tendons and actually results in an increased blood supply to the tendon. Others authors have shown that tenolysis at 10 weeks results in improvement of tendon gliding. At

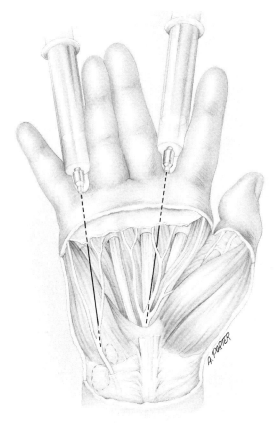

**Fig. 14-6.** The median nerve may be anesthetized at the wrist by depositing local anesthesia through a long spinal needle inserted along the proper digital nerve in the web space and passing the needle proximal to the level of the wrist. The ulnar nerve is blocked by following the common digital nerve to the little finger subcutaneously to the level of the hook of the hammate.

present the timing of tenolysis is largely based on subjective criteria.

***Technique.*** The procedure can be carried out with the patient under general anesthesia, regional block, or local anesthesia (Fig. 14-6). Local anesthesia is preferable, because it permits instant evaluation of the effectiveness of the tenolysis by active motion of the digit by the patient. Supplementing the local anesthesia with intravenous narcotics or tranquilizers allows greater patient comfort. If general anesthesia or axillary block anesthesia is used, the adequacy of the tenolysis can be judged only by traction upon the appropriate tendon proximal to the tenolysis or by electrical stimulation of the involved muscle. Active voluntary muscle contraction is much more accurate than either proximal traction or electrical stimulation. Paralysis from ischemia produced by the tourniquet usually develops in about 30 minutes. Thus, the tourniquet must be deflated, and circulation to the muscles must be restored before motion produced by voluntary contraction or muscle stimulation can be evaluated.

If the tenolysis is performed after a simple primary repair, the site of the repair should be exposed first through an appropriate incision (Fig. 14-7). The tendon is detached from surrounding structures by sharp dissection. The range of motion is evaluated by having the patient actively flex the finger. If an unsatisfactory range of motion is evident, traction is placed on the tendon by a broad round instrument (Hager dilator), and its distal freedom is determined. If the tendon is free distally, all the joints distal to the site of traction will flex. If full flexion is not obtained, exposure of the distal course of the tendon is required. As the tendon is pulled up by the instrument, one can evaluate the gliding of the tendon proximal to the test site. If free proximal gliding is not obtained, the incision must be extended proximally to expose the site of adhesions. One must obtain

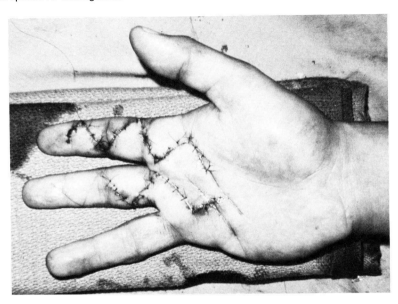

**Fig. 14-7.** This patient had undergone primary repair of the flexor tendons at the mid-proximal phalanx level. The zigzag incisions provide excellent exposure of the repair site and of adhesions along the course of the tendons.

freedom of tendon gliding as complete as possible without totally severing the blood supply to the tendon. Care must be taken to preserve a pulley mechanism. Tenolysis should be continued until the active range of motion is equal to the passive range of motion. Tendon strippers are not helpful and may actually damage the tendon or surrounding structures. All adhesions must be divided under direct vision.

If tenolysis is done following failure of a tendon graft, the tendon graft may require exposure throughout its entire length. Mid-lateral or zigzag incisions are used in the digit. The zigzag incision has the advantage of greater exposure, but it has the disadvantage of crisscrossing the tendon in three locations. These incisions may be directly extended into the palm, or separate palmar incisions over the course of the tendons may be made. Again, careful sharp dissection and division of only the rigid adhesions under direct vision are the proper techniques. Adequate hemostasis is extremely important. After the wound is closed but while the digit is still anesthetized, a help-

ful psychological ploy is to allow the patient to see the range of motion he can produce (Fig. 14-8). This maneuver convinces the patient that a given range of motion is obtainable in the postoperative period. Most patients will expend extreme effort to reach a goal they know is obtainable. Application of hydrocortisone into the wound before closure has been advocated to reduce the recurrence of adhesions, yet the effectiveness of topical steroids in preventing adhesions has not been proved. Active range of motion exercises are begun 24 hours after surgery. Early active exercises are particularly important in obtaining a satisfactory result after tenolysis. Occasionally, dynamic splints may aid in the restoration of extension.

***Postoperative therapy.*** Patients are referred to the Hand Rehabilitation Center 24 hours after surgery, and active range of motion exercises are begun. Active metacarpophalangeal, proximal interphalangeal, and distal interphalangeal flexion and extension exercises are performed frequently

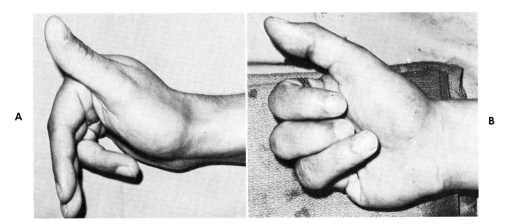

**Fig. 14-8. A,** Preoperatively there is no active flexion at the proximal or distal interphalangeal joints of the index and long fingers. **B,** At the operating table, the patient is shown the degree of flexion he has obtained immediately by tenolysis.

to prevent adhesions from re-forming and again restricting tendon gliding. Patient education is essential in order for each patient to realize the importance of continuing to exercise throughout the day. Patients are instructed to keep their hands elevated initially in order to reduce edema. An elastic finger stocking made from an ace wrap is used at night and whenever the patient is not exercising. This single finger pressure garment helps reduce edema, and it applies direct pressure to the incision. An inflatable finger cuff is also used to further eliminate swelling and to apply pressure on the scar tissue during the treatment session. Cold packs can be applied intermittently to reduce the inflammatory response to exercise. Gentle, passive exercise is indicated to prevent joint stiffness. Dynamic splinting is also initiated if the patient displays limited motion in flexion or extension of any joint. When the incision is healed and the sutures are removed, scar massage is begun. As the patient progresses and his tolerance improves, more vigorous and resistive exercises are added to increase hand strength. The overall goal of therapy is to maintain good tendon gliding and to promote maximum functional use of the hand.

**Table 14-1.** Incidence of tenolysis and amputation after primary tendon repair

| Author | Cases | Tenolyses | Amputations |
|---|---|---|---|
| Kyle | 9 | 2 | |
| Kelly | 185 | 8 | 8 |
| McCash | 22 | 1 | |
| McKenzie | 45 | 5 | 2 |
| Madsen | 53 | | 2 |
| Green | 71 | 4 | |
| Tsuge | 33 | 2 | |
| Totals | 418 | 22 | 12 |
| Percentages | | 5% | 4% |

**Results.** As can be seen from Tables 14-1 and 14-2, the reported incidence of tenolysis has varied widely. Tenolysis has been performed in 4% to 22% of the patients having primary tendon repair and in 2% to 27% of the patients having secondary tendon grafting. An average 5% of the patients have had tenolysis after tendon repair, and 11% of the patients have had tenolysis after tendon grafting.

Kyle recommended tenolysis if the range of motion was not satisfactory for the patient; tenolysis was performed on 8 patients after tendon grafting and on 2 patients after simple repair of a lacerated tendon.

**Table 14-2.** Incidence of tenolysis and
amputation after tendon grafting

| Author | Cases | Tenolyses | Amputa-tions |
|---|---|---|---|
| Kyle | 48 | 10 | 6 |
| Kelly | 71 | 10 | 3 |
| McCash | 33 | 9 | |
| Fetrow | 374 | 91 | 5 |
| Thompson | 100 | 5 | 5 |
| Boyes | 607 | 14 | 3 |
| Totals | 1,233 | 139 | 22 |
| Percentages | | 11% | 2% |

The total number of patients with tendon
lacerations was not given. Tenolysis was
performed on 12 tendons; 10 of the tenolyses were performed after tendon grafting
and 2 after primary tendon repair. Eight of
the tenolyses were performed after simple
secondary tendon grafting, and 2 were successful; one of the 2 tenolyses performed
following primary tendon repair was
successful. The other 2 tenolyses were performed after tertiary tendon grafting;
neither was successful. The need for complete visualization of the entire tendon
graft was emphasized.

Kelly reported on the indications for
and the effectiveness of tenolysis after both
primary repair and tendon grafting. He
is the only author to report the incidences
of tenolyses in the various areas of the
hand. In zone 2 (see Fig. 11-1) there were
134 tendon repairs and 4 tenolyses were
performed; 6 tendon grafts were performed
after failure of repairs in this area. In zone
3 there were 4 secondary tenolyses and 2
seondary tendon grafts in a total of 22
tendon repairs. The reason for the higher
incidence of tenolysis in zone 3 injuries is
unclear. In 71 patients treated with tendon
grafting (usually in zone 2 injuries) there
were 10 secondary tenolyses. Four of these
10 patients had improvement of function
following tenolysis, but the degree of improvement was not noted.

McCash reported one tenolysis out of
22 primary tendon repairs and 9 tenolyses
out of a total of 33 secondary tendon repairs and secondary tendon grafts.

Fetrow (1969) published the most extensive paper concerning tenolysis. He reported on 220 flexor and extensor tenolyses
in 134 patients; 24 patients had tenolysis
performed more than one time on a given
tendon, and 31 patients had simultaneous
tenolysis of two or more tendons. Ninety-
one tenolyses were required following 374
flexor tendon grafts (24%). Almost all the
tendon grafts were performed secondarily
for treatment of tendon lacerations in flexor
zone 2. Follow-up was obtained on 68 of the
tenolyses that were performed after flexor
tendon grafting. A good or excellent result
was classified as one in which the fingertip
flexed to within ½ inch of the palm; a fair
result was classified as one in which the
fingertip flexed to between ½ inch and 1½
inches of the palm, and the remainder were
classified as poor results. The results of the
68 tenolyses were:
1. Eighteen patients had an improvement in range of motion that was insufficient to change the classification.
2. Seventeen patients had their result
improved from the fair category to
the good or excellent category.
3. Eight patients had improvement sufficient to change the final result from
the poor category to the good or excellent category.
4. Five patients were improved enough
to change their final classification
from the poor category to the fair
category.
5. Twenty patients had either no improvement or an actual decrease in
function.

Thus, 26% of the patients were improved;
44% of the patients were greatly improved; and 30% of the patients were unchanged or made worse by tenolysis following flexor tendon grafting.

Seventy-two tenolyses were performed

after primary repair of flexor tendon lacerations, but the total number of primary flexor tendon repairs from which these 72 were selected was not noted. The primary repairs were performed for injuries in zones other than zone 2. Follow-up information could be obtained for 39 of the tenolyses. The results were:

1. Eleven patients had improved function but insufficient improvement to reclassify the final result.
2. Seventeen patients were improved sufficiently to change their final result from the fair to the good or excellent category.
3. Two patients were improved sufficiently to change their final result from the poor to the good or excellent category.
4. Six patients were improved sufficiently to change their final result from the poor to the fair category.
5. Three patients were either unimproved or made worse by the procedure.

Thus, 28% of the patients were improved; 64% were greatly improved; and 8% were unchanged or made worse from tenolysis following primary flexor tendon repair. Tenolysis after primary tendon repair or secondary tendon grafting seems to be very beneficial in selected patients.

Twelve patients had tenolyses of their extensor tendons; there was improvement in extension in 10 of these 12 patients postoperatively.

Tenolysis was performed to relieve adhesions that had developed after infection; all 8 patients having flexor tenolysis following infection were improved; 5 of the 7 patients having extensor tenolysis following infection were improved.

Three of 8 patients having flexor tenolysis to relieve adhesions associated with metacarpal or phalangeal fractures were improved; all 3 patients having extensor tenolysis to free adhesions from carpal or phalangeal fractures were improved.

Some of the other indications for tenolysis were: postoperative adhesions following tendon transfer, adhesions developing after crush injury, adhesions caused by gunshot wounds, and adhesions developing after operative correction of congenital anomalies. In this mixed group, 15 patients were improved, 1 was not improved, and 2 were worse. Cortisone was given daily for 2 weeks to 31 (51 tenolyses) of the 134 patients; there was no significant difference in the results in patients given cortisone and those not given cortisone.

Thompson reported the performance of 5 tenolyses following 100 flexor tendon grafts; 2 patients were improved following the tenolyses. He believed that other patients would have been improved by tenolyses, but the patients either refused surgery or did not return for follow-up.

Madsen reported on 53 flexor tendon injuries that occurred within the digital sheath; all were repaired primarily. The results of repair were outstanding. Two patients had amputations for treatment of an unsatisfactory result, but no tenolyses were reported.

In 607 flexor tendon grafts reported by Boyes, 8 of 14 patients undergoing tenolysis were improved. Fusion of the distal interphalangeal joint was performed in 6 other patients.

Green reported on 71 flexor tendon lacerations that underwent primary and secondary repair in zone 2. Four of these patients required secondary tenolysis, but did not report performing any amputations. Tsuge suggested a new intratendon suture technique for repair of flexor tendons. Two tenolyses were performed primarily, and he did not mention the need for amputation.

Several authors emphasize that tenolysis will be needed more often if tendon injury is associated with joint, bone, nerve, or severe skin injury than if the tendon injury is an isolated problem. Certainly this seems reasonable, because the degree of scarring is more severe.

### Repair of a disrupted anastomosis

The diagnosis of a ruptured anastomosis is usually obvious. The patient frequently notes a brief episode of pain or discomfort at the site of tendon disruption. Loss of the tenodesis effect is noted after disruption of a repair. Most disruptions occur in the second or third postoperative week. If a simple tendon repair disrupts after surgery, rerepair will produce a satisfactory result in the majority of cases. In the 607 tendon grafts, Boyes reported 14 repair ruptures. Tendon graft function in 11 of these 14 ruptures was salvaged by repair of the disruption.

Any patient who has a disrupted anastomosis and undergoes a secondary repair or a flexor tendon graft is understandably more apprehensive when therapy is initiated. The treatment procedure closely follows the one outlined for immobilized primary tendon repairs. However, these patients need greater reassurance and very careful instruction in their home program. Passive exercise and scar massage are important aspects of treatment, because each surgical procedure produces additional scarring.

The patients we have seen with ruptured anastomoses several weeks after tendon repair have often reported that after having used their hand continuously during a strenuous activity, they noticed that their finger would not bend. Therefore, the work-rest concept of exercise or activity is especially emphasized with these patients, in order to prevent fatigue of the tendon and subsequent rupture.

### Insertion of Silastic rods and subsequent tendon grafting

Mayer and Ransohoff (1936) demonstrated that a new sheath (pseudosheath) formed around celloidin tubes placed in scarred tendon beds. Milgram (1945) used stainless steel implants to induce pseudosheath formation. Tendon grafts were to be inserted through the pseudosheaths. The pseudosheath was believed to decrease the development of adhesions after tendon grafting. Because both celloidin and stainless steel implants are rigid, stiffness of the fingers developed during the period of implantation. The joint stiffness was so severe that the potential benefits of the pseudosheath could not be realized. Hunter (1965) expanded the concept of pseudosheath formation but utilized a reinforced flexible silicone rubber prosthesis. His original attempts were directed toward development of a permanent artificial tendon. However, disruptions at the points of attachment of the artificial tendon led to at least temporary abandonment of the concept. He demonstrated that a more adequate pseudosheath was formed if the silicone rod actually moved. He developed the following procedure: (1) forming the pseudosheath by a Dacron reinforced Silastic prosthesis attached distally, (2) improving the pseudosheath by passive motion of the distally attached Silastic prosthesis, and (3) subsequent tendon grafting.

*Technique of rod insertion.* A midlateral line incision or a zigzag is made from the midportion of the distal segment to the proximal crease of the proximal segment. The entire scar is excised. Pulleys are maintained if possible. If new pulleys have to be reconstructed, this is accomplished with a Dacron graft or a tendon woven into the periosteum of the phalanx. This distal end of the rod is sutured beneath the profundus tendon at its insertion into the distal phalanx. The rod is passed through the pulleys. A Blair fascia passer is inserted from the finger through the palm, through the carpal tunnel, and through the skin of the distal forearm to a point approximately 5 cm proximal to the distal wrist crease. A suture is attached to the tip of the Blair fascia passer and retracted into the finger. The proximal end of the rod is tied to the suture and pulled through the palm, the carpal tunnel, and into the distal forearm. The rod is brought up through the skin and cut, allowing it to retract to the level of the musculotendinous junction of the profundi. Hunter recommends leaving the proximal end of the Silastic rod free in the distal forearm. Nicolle has developed a Silastic prosthesis that is sutured distally to the stump of the flexor profundus tendon and proximally to the flexor profundus tendon in the midpalm. If the proximal anastomosis is not accomplished, the adequacy of motion can be estimated by placing tension on the proximal end of the Silastic rod. Proximal tension should allow flexion of the fingertip to the palm or a passive range of motion equal to the preoperative passive range of motion. In Nicolle's technique, the length of the prosthesis should be appropriate to position the fingertip in slightly greater flexion than that of its neighbors.

*Postoperative management.* The dressing is discarded approximately 7 days after surgery. The primary goal of treatment at this time is to increase and maintain the passive mobility of all joints. This is accomplished by several methods, and the patient is seen one to two times weekly until it is apparent that he will be able to maintain the desired range of motion at the metacarpophalangeal and interphalangeal joints.

The therapist utilizes passive exercise and joint mobilization techniques to increase passive flexion. The patient is shown how to bend his finger passively as part of his home program. Active-resistive extension exercises are done to prevent joint contractures. The patient is fitted with a dynamic proximal interphalangeal joint flexion splint initially. As motion at this joint improves, the patient is fitted with an elastic distal interphalangeal joint flexion splint. If limitation in extension at either joint is noted, the patient is also fitted with a Wynn-Parry spring extension splint.

The patient is encouraged to use his hand in a normal manner as soon as possible. A small Velcro splint is used to attach the finger without flexor tendons to the next finger, in order to protect it from reinjury and to prevent it from getting in the patient's way. This increases his ability to use his hand functionally, while it provides continuous passive exercise to the joints of the injured finger. With the use of this splint, many patients are able to return to some type of employment during the period before flexor tendon grafting.

The most common complication of Silastic rod insertion reported by Hunter was synovitis. The synovitis was characterized by pain in the fingertip, swelling along the course of the tendon, and swelling and erythema in the forearm. The synovitis was thought to be caused by excessive early motion or buckling of the prosthesis. Other authors have also reported synovitis developing after insertion of a Silastic rod; extrusion of the prosthesis occurred in one case. Synovitis may lead to adhesions within the new pseudosheath. When wound infections have developed, removal of the prosthesis is necessary to eliminate the infection. When the wounds are completely healed, and there is no evidence of synovitis, and the scars have matured to the state of becoming soft, and supple joints have been obtained, one can then proceed with removal of the rod and insertion of a flexor tendon graft. In our personal series of 29 rod insertions, the duration of rod implant before flexor tendon grafting ranged from 70 to 168 days. When the percentage of recovery is plotted against the duration of rod implant, there is no significant difference in the final functional result if the rod has been in place anytime between 70 to 168 days (Fig. 14-9). Because of these data, we proceed with tendon grafting as soon as the wounds have met the criteria established above.

*Tendon grafting after rod insertion.* A midlateral line incision is made through the previous incision site at the level of the distal phalanx for approximately 3 cm. This exposes the insertion of the flexor profundus

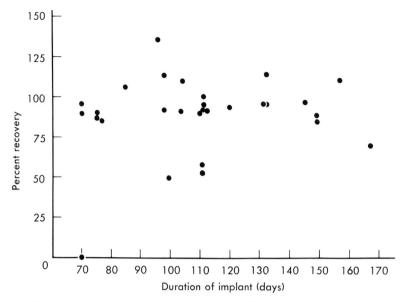

**Fig. 14-9.** The duration of rod implant from 70 to 168 days had no influence on the percent recovery of total active motion at 1 year.

tendon and the rod that has been sutured to its undersurface. A second longitudinal or transverse incision is made in the distal forearm just proximal to the proximal wrist crease. The rod is removed and a tendon graft is obtained. The plantaris tendon is the tendon of choice, because we prefer to accomplish our proximal tendon repair in the distal forearm. The palmaris tendon is not usually long enough to permit spanning the palm. If the tendon graft and the profundus tendons are of nearly equal caliber, a Bunnell suture is used. If not, a Pulvertaft suture is used. The distal end of the tendon graft is attached to the terminal phalanx. The longitudinal forearm incision is closed with a Z-plasty.

*Management after flexor tendon grafting.* All digits are maintained in a large compressive hand dressing in the position of function but with the wrist in a neutral position for 3 weeks. No active or passive motion is permitted during this time. After 3 weeks of complete immobilization, the dressing and sutures are removed.

During the first week after dressing removal, the following exercises are begun: (1) passive flexion of the metacarpophalangeal and the proximal and distal interphalangeal joints, (2) gentle active proximal interphalangeal joint flexion with the metacarpophalangeal joint stabilized in the amount of extension attainable through very gentle positioning, (3) gentle active distal interphalangeal joint flexion with the metacarpophalangeal and proximal interphalangeal joints stabilized in their relaxed position, (4) massage of the fingers and hand without forcing the fingers into extension, and (5) massage of the palmar or wrist scar in a proximal to distal direction during active finger flexion.

During the second through the fourth weeks when the patient is performing exercises 2 and 3 above, the metacarpophalangeal and proximal interphalangeal joints are stabilized in gradually increasing amounts of extension. By the fifth week, resistance is applied to these flexion exercises. During this time, the massage, as described above, is applied with increasing force. These basic exercises are continued until the patient has reached full recovery. Additional exercises are added as indicated below.

During the second week of rehabilitation, gentle passive extension of the proximal interphalangeal joint is obtained with the metacarpophalangeal and distal interphalangeal joints flexed. Similarly, the distal interphalangeal joint is extended with the metacarpophalangeal and proximal interphalangeal joints flexed. Active flexion of the proximal and distal interphalangeal joints with the metacarpophalangeal joint stabilized in flexion is initiated.

During the third week, gentle passive extension of both the proximal and distal interphalangeal joints is encouraged, with the metacarpophalangeal joint first in flexion, then in increasing amounts of extension. Active extension of the fingers is encouraged.

All patients are encouraged to exercise frequently during the day for periods of 5 to 20 minutes per hour.

Patients are fitted initially with a static dorsal protective splint to hold the digit in flexion and prevent extension. With the splint in place, the patient can continue to work on active flexion and move his other fingers freely. Within 2 weeks after dressing removal, this splint is discarded.

Within 4 weeks after removal of the dressing, individual patient problems begin to appear. Often passive extension of the proximal and distal interphalangeal joints is not possible. Dynamic splinting of these joints is begun when indicated during the fourth week after dressing removal. Dynamic force is applied through the use of a rubber band in an outrigger hand splint or with piano wire in a spring-type finger extension splint. Dynamic splinting does not exceed 7 to 8 oz of pull with a rubber band splint, or 9 to 10 oz with a piano wire splint. Patients are encouraged to use their hands gradually for functional

**Table 14-3.** Results reported by Hunter for flexor tendon reconstruction in patients who had previous tendon surgery

| Result | Number |
|---|---|
| Excellent-good | 20 |
| Fair | 9 |
| Poor | 6 |

activities and to perform daily activities as soon as they can tolerate them.

***Results.*** Hunter reported results in patients who had had previous tendon surgery (Table 14-3); results are classified using the criteria given previously. He did not state the level of all original injuries, but many occurred in zone 2. These results are significantly better than the average results following primary repair in zone 2 injuries (see Table 11-1). There is no significant difference between Hunter's results and Boyes' results for this entire series of tendon grafts or between Hunter's and Madsen's results in primary repairs in zone 2 injuries. If one considers only patients who have had previous tendon surgery, there is no significant difference in the number of poor results reported by Hunter and the number reported by Boyes. However, the number of excellent or good results reported by Hunter is significantly higher than that reported by Boyes.

In our personal series of 29 Silastic rod insertions followed by rod removal and flexor tendon grafting, 62% obtained fair to excellent results and 38% poor results (Table 14-4). All patients were followed for at least 52 weeks. One patient was considered a graft failure because of extensive scar. He regained only 99 degrees of total active motion and is included in the statistical analysis. One patient sustained a disruption of the insertion of the tendon graft into the distal phalanx on the twenty-fifth day after surgery. This was reattached 2 days later. At 52 weeks he had regained 240 degrees of total active

**Table 14-4.** Extent of functional recovery* and recovery of total active motion at 52 weeks after flexor tendon grafting following rod insertion

| Result | Percent |
|---|---|
| *Functional recovery* | |
| Excellent | 28 |
| (< 1.2 cm) | |
| Fair | 34 |
| (> 1.2 < 3.5 cm) | |
| Poor | 38 |
| (> 3.5 cm) | |
| *Total active motion* | |
| Excellent | 38 |
| (220° to 270°) | |
| Fair | 38 |
| (180° to 220°) | |
| Poor | 24 |
| (< 180°) | |

*Pulp to distal palmar crease distance.

motion in the finger. One rod became exposed and required removal. The rod was reinserted after the skin wound had been healed for 3 months, and the patient gained 188 degrees of total active motion at 52 weeks.

### Summary of results

*Six weeks after tendon grafting.* The average patient had regained 100% of his preoperative gross grip strength and 134 degrees of total active motion, which was 66% of the total active motion he would have at 1 year.

*Twelve weeks after tendon grafting.* The average patient had regained 120% of his preoperative gross grip strength and 147 degrees of total active motion, which was 72% of the total motion he would have at 1 year.

*Twenty-two weeks after tendon grafting.* The average patient had regained 130% of his preoperative gross grip strength and 182 degrees of total active motion, which was 90% of the total active motion he would have at 1 year.

*Fifty-two weeks after tendon grafting.* The average patient had regained 162% of

preoperative gross grip strength and 202 degrees of total active motion.

Of the total passive motion obtained before tendon grafting, 90% was realized as active motion 1 year after grafting.

### Tendon grafting after a primary repair or previous tendon graft

If primary repair or primary or secondary tendon grafting fails to produce an adequate result, a tendon grafting procedure can still be accomplished; however, insertion of a Silastic rod and subsequent tendon grafting are more commonly employed than direct insertion of a tendon graft.

*Technique.* Tendon grafting is carried out by exposing the normal course of the tendon through a midlateral or volar zigzag incision and either a separate incision in the palm or continuation of the digital incision. The damaged tendon and synovial sheath are removed, but the fibrous pulleys are retained if at all possible. If the pulleys cannot be retained, they are reconstructed with a segment of tendon. The plantaris tendon provides an ideal graft, but the palmaris longus and the extensor digitorum longus tendons are available if needed. The tendon is attached distally with the Bunnell reinsertion stitch (see Fig. 11-12) and proximally with the Bunnell buried stitch (see Fig. 11-10); either wire or polyester sutures can be used. The proximal repair can be at the level of the lumbrical muscle or in the wrist. The length of the graft is chosen to pull the injured fingertip into slightly more flexion than its normal resting position. An additional method (modified from Curtis) to determine the length of the graft is as follows:

1. While the profundus muscle is not under tension, the relationship between the cut end of the tendon and a fixed point is determined.
2. Maximal tension is placed on the cut end of the tendon, and the new relationship between the cut end and the fixed point is noted.

3. The distance the cut end was moved is recorded; this should be at least 35 mm.
4. The proximal repair between the tendon graft and the profundus tendon is made.
5. With the wrist neutral and the digit extended, the point on the graft opposite the future site of the distal repair is marked.
6. Traction is placed on the tendon graft until the marked point moves a distance equal to that recorded in step 3. If the original distance (step 3) was less than 35 mm, the finger joints should be flexed to obtain an apparent motion of 35 mm.
7. The point on the tendon graft now lying opposite the future site of the distal anastomosis is the final distal end of the tendon graft.
8. Excess tendon graft is removed.
9. The distal repair is completed.

***Postoperative management.*** Postoperatively, the tendon graft after previous tendon surgery is managed the same way as the tendon graft after rod removal. This has been described earlier and will not be repeated here.

***Results.*** Boyes reported on 139 tendon injuries that were treated by primary tendon repair or tendon grafting and resulted in an unsatisfactory range of motion. Only 35% of patients who had an unsatisfactory result after previous tendon surgery had an excellent or good result following secondary or tertiary tendon grafting. Sixty-four percent of patients who did not have major scarring in their fingers had a good or excellent result following secondary tendon grafting. Thus, results of tendon grafting in patients with previous tendon surgery were significantly worse than the results in patients who did not have scarring of their fingers.

Kyle reported on nine patients who had a previous tendon graft or primary repair and who underwent secondary or tertiary

**Table 14-5.** Extent of functional recovery* and recovery of total active motion at 52 weeks after flexor tendon grafting

| Result | Percent |
|---|---|
| *Functional recovery* | |
| Excellent | 29 |
| (< 1.2 cm) | |
| Fair | 50 |
| (> 1.2 < 3.5 cm) | |
| Poor | 21 |
| (> 3.5 cm) | |
| *Total active motion* | |
| Excellent | 46 |
| (220° to 270°) | |
| Fair | 38 |
| (180° to 220°) | |
| Poor | 25 |
| (< 180°) | |

*Pulp to distal palmar crease distance.

tendon grafting; all nine of these patients had a poor result; one had an amputation. Other factors that were found to impair the results of tendon grafting were joint damage, joint stiffness, bilateral digital nerve injury, and patient age of greater than 40 years.

In our personal series of 21 flexor tendon grafts done as a result of injury to both flexor tendons in zone 2, 79% obtained a fair to excellent result, and 21% obtained a poor result (Table 14-5). Measurement of the passive and active range of motion of each joint, total active motion of each finger, distance of digital pulp to distal palmar crease during flexion, gross grip, and pinch strength was obtained before operating and at 4, 6, 8, 10, 12, 16, 20, 22, 24, 28, 34, and 52 weeks after grafting. Of the 21 patients, one was lost to follow-up 6 weeks after flexor tendon grafting. This patient was considered to be a poor result and was assigned zero movement of the proximal and distal interphalangeal joints in our statistical analysis. All of the remaining patients were followed for a period of at least 1 year. No infections or tendon disruptions occurred.

*Summary of results*

*Six weeks after tendon grafting.* The average patient had regained 50% of his preoperative gross grip strength and 115 degrees of total active motion, which was 50% of the motion he would obtain at 1 year.

*Twelve weeks after tendon grafting.* The average patient had regained 66% of his preoperative gross grip strength and 176 degrees of total active motion, which was 77% of the motion he would have at 1 year.

*Twenty-two weeks after tendon grafting.* The average patient had regained 150% of his preoperative gross grip strength and 196 degrees of total active motion, which was 86% of the total active motion he would have at 1 year.

*Fifty-two weeks after tendon grafting.* The average patient had regained 160% of preoperative gross grip strength and 227 degrees of total active motion.

Of the total passive motion obtained before tendon grafting, 91% is regained by 1 year after grafting. The results of tendon grafting in patients with uncomplicated injuries is discussed in Chapter 11.

Composite tendon allografts have been proposed for patients in whom primary repair and/or flexor tendon grafting has failed. In experimental animals, the gross and microscopic appearances of allografts and autografts are similar. Allografts in patients have been done so rarely that evaluation is difficult.

## Arthrodesis, tenodesis, and amputation

If splinting, active range of motion exercises, and tenolysis have failed to produce a satisfactory range of motion, and the finger is detracting from the overall function of the hand, an arthrodesis, tenodesis, or amputation may be indicated.

Arthrodesis and tenodesis are more useful when an inadequate range of motion is present in the distal interphalangeal joint than when present in the proximal interphalangeal or metacarpophalangeal joint. The technique of arthrodesis and tenodesis is described in Chapter 11. If the patient has a normal functioning sublimis tendon and tendon repair or grafting has failed to produce an adequate range of motion of the distal interphalangeal joint, arthrodesis or tenodesis will produce a satisfactory result in the majority of the patients. If the patient is unable to flex the proximal interphalangeal joint, he usually has insufficient motion to strongly flex the metacarpophalangeal joint. If sufficient range of motion of the metacarpophalangeal joint remains, the proximal interphalangeal joints should be arthrodesed in a position functional for the patient's needs. In some patients this is 40 to 50 degrees flexion, whereas in others it is less. A trial period with a light splint or a Kirschner wire to immobilize the joint can be informative before definitive surgery. The combination of insufficient flexion strength at the metacarpophalangeal joint and lack of an ideal functional position of the proximal interphalangeal joint limits the usefulness of proximal interphalangeal joint fusion after failure of tendon repair or grafting. Amputation is usually indicated. Boyes reported that 1% of patients undergoing tendon grafting ultimately require distal interphalangeal arthrodesis.

About 4% of patients having primary repair of a tendon laceration will ultimately require amputation, and from 1% to 12%, of patients with an average of about 2%, will require an amputation after tendon grafting (Table 14-1).

*Technique of amputation.* Amputation of the index finger is accomplished through the incisions shown in Fig. 14-10; the bone is transected approximately 2 cm distal to the carpometacarpal joint. After the incisions are made, attention is turned to the dorsal aspect. Traction is placed on the extensor tendon, and it is divided at the proximal end of the incision. If branches of the radial nerve can be identi-

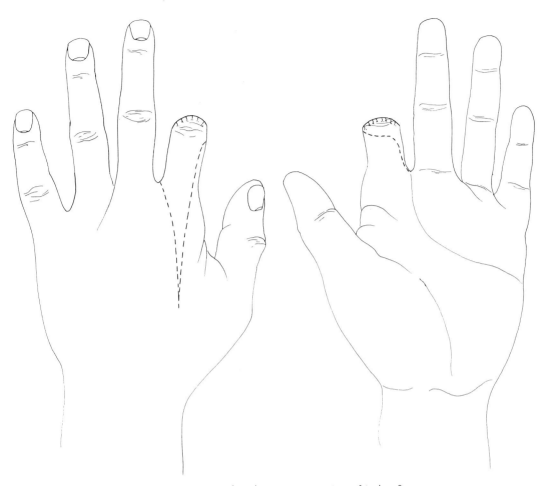

**Fig. 14-10.** Incisions for elective amputation of index finger.

fied, they are divided 1 to 2 cm proximal to the level of the incision. The first dorsal interosseous muscle is detached from its insertion and protected. The branch of the digital nerve to the radial aspect in the index finger is transected and buried in the interosseous muscles. All muscles are stripped from the metacarpal. Care is taken to preserve the common digital nerve that supplies the ulnar aspect of the index finger and the radial aspect of the long finger. The branch to the radial aspect of the index finger is divided just distal to the bifurcation of the common digital nerve into the two proper digital nerves. Traction is placed on the flexor tendon, and the tendon is divided at the level

of the proximal extent of the incision. The transverse metacarpal ligament is divided. The bone is divided 2 cm distal to the carpometacarpal joint. The bone is bevelled beginning proximally on the radial aspect and extending distally on the ulnar aspect of the metacarpal. The index metacarpal and the skin between the incisions are removed. The tendinous insertion of the first dorsal interosseous muscle is reattached to the interosseous insertion in the base of the proximal phalanx of the long finger. After the tourniquet is released and the bleeding is controlled by elevation and cautery, the skin is closed in the usual fashion.

Amputation of the little finger is accomplished through an incision similar to the one used for the index finger, following a technique similar to the one described previously. The insertion of the abductor digiti minimi is transferred to the proximal phalanx of the ring finger.

Amputation of the long or ring finger results in an open space (amputation gap) between the remaining fingers. The primary disability from the amputation gap is inability to hold small objects in the palm without dropping them. Occasionally scissoring and overlapping of the remaining fingers may occur if they are fully flexed. If the functional ability of the hand is impaired by the presence of the gap, two techniques have been developed to decrease the size of the amputation gap: (1) The

border finger can be transferred toward the midline of the hand, or (2) extensive soft tissue resection may permit juxtaposition of the remaining fingers.

The incisions for transposition of the index finger are shown in Fig. 14-11. The skin included in the incisions is removed and the third metacarpal exposed from its dorsal aspect. Traction is placed on the extensor tendon, and the tendon is divided at the proximal end of the incision. The third metacarpal is divided approximately 4 cm proximal to the metacarpophalangeal joint. The digital nerves to the long finger are divided near the midportion of the metacarpal. Traction is placed on the flexor tendons, and they are transected. The third metacarpal and the interosseous

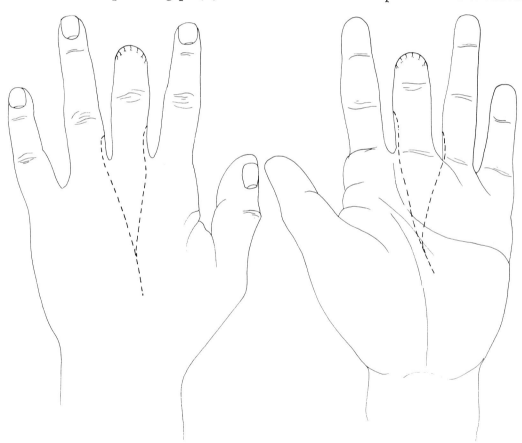

**Fig. 14-11.** Incisions for transposition of index finger at the time of amputation of the middle finger.

muscles to the long finger are removed. The flexor and extensor tendons of the index are retracted, and the second metacarpal is divided at the same level as the third metacarpal. The intrinic muscles to the index finger are partially dissected free at their insertions. The remaining portions of the second metacarpal are bevelled from proximally on the radial aspect to distally on the ulnar aspect. A bone graft from the substance of the third metacarpal may or may not be used. Longitudinal Kirschner wires across the junction of the second and third metacarpals and a transverse Kirschner wire through the distal end of all the metacarpals aid in stabilization.

Transposition of the little finger is ac-complished by a technique similar to that used for the index finger.

The incision for soft tissue correction of the amputation gap is shown in Fig. 14-12. All the skin between the two inci-sions is removed. The transverse carpal ligament is divided at the level of the skin incisions. Traction is placed on the extensor tendon, and it is divided at the level of the proximal end of the incision. The metacarpal is transected about 1 cm distal to the carpometacarpal joint. Trac-tion is placed on the flexor tendon, and it is divided at the proximal extent of the incision. The digital nerves to the injured finger are divided at the midmetacarpal level. The transverse carpal ligament is

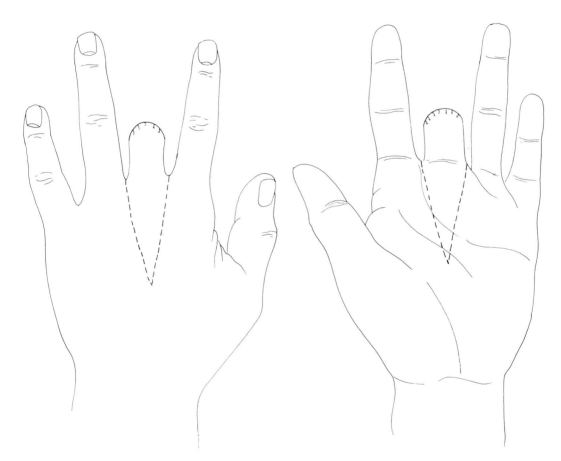

**Fig. 14-12.** Incisions for soft tissue correction of amputation gap.

carefully reconstructed and the skin closed. Butler has reported satisfactory cosmetic and functional results in 17 hands; our experience has been that the amputation gap partially recurred following this soft tissue resection.

*Therapy after amputation.* Treatment following amputation of a finger due to a failed flexor tendon repair is aimed at restoring maximum function of the rest of the hand. Phantom pain is explained, and the patient uses his hand in a variety of goal-directed activities and exercises to aid in adjustment to the absence of the digit and to increase the functional use of the hand.

## BIBLIOGRAPHY

Boyes, J. H.: Flexor tendon grafts in the fingers and thumb, J. Bone Joint Surg. 32A:489, 1950.

Boyes, J. H.: Bunnell's surgery of the hand, Philadelphia, 1970, J. B. Lippincott Co.

Boyes, J. H., and Stark, H. H.: Flexor-tendon grafts in the fingers and thumb, J. Bone Joint Surg. 53A:1332, 1971.

Brooks, D. M.: Problems of restoration of tendon movements after repair and grafts, Proc. R. Soc. Med. 63:67, 1970.

Bruner, J. M.: Problems of postoperative position and motion in surgery of the hand, J. Bone Joint Surg. 35:355, 1953.

Butler, B.: Soft tissue management of the amputation gap, presentation to the American Society for Surgery of the Hand, February, 1973.

Carstam, J.: The effect of cortisone on the formation of tendon adhesions and no tendon healing; an experimental investigation in the rabbit, Acta Chir. Scand. 182(suppl.):5, 1953.

Chacha, P.: Free autologous composite tendon grafts for division of both flexor tendons within the digital sheath of the hand, J. Bone Joint Surg. 56A:960, 1974.

Chong, J. K., Cramer, L. M., and Culf, N. K.: Combined two-stage tenoplasty with silicone rods for multiple flexor tendon injuries in "no-man's land," J. Trauma 12:104, 1972.

Curtis, R. M., and Hoopes, J. E.: Injuries of the hand. In Ballinger, W., editor: The management of trauma, Philadelphia, 1968, W. B. Saunders Co.

Duran, R. J., and Houser, R. G.: A preliminary report in the use of controlled passive motion following flexor tendon repair in zones 2 and 3 of the hand. In American Academy of Orthopaedic Surgeons, editors: Symposium on tendon

surgery in the hand, St. Louis, 1975, The C. V. Mosby Co.

Fetrow, K. O.: Tenolysis in the hand and wrist, J. Bone Surg. 49A:667, 1967.

Green, W. L., and Niebauer, J. J.: Results of primary and secondary flexor-tendon repairs in no-man's land, J. Bone Joint Surg. 56A:1217, 1974.

Hunter, J. M.: Artificial tendons; early development and application, Am. J. Surg. 109:325, 1965.

Hunter, J. M., and Salisbury, R. E.: Flexor-tendon reconstruction in severely damaged hands, J. Bone Joint Surg. 53A:829, 1971.

Hurst, L. N., McCain, W. G., and Lindsay, W. K.: Results of tenolysis, Plast. Reconstr. Surg. 52:171, 1973.

Kelly, A. P.: Primary tendon repairs, J. Bone Joint Surg. 41A:581, 1959.

Kleinert, H. E., and others: Primary repair of laceration flexor tendons in "no-man's land," J. Bone Joint Surg. 49A:477, 1967.

Kleinert, H. E., and Meares, A.: In quest of the solution to severed flexor tendons, Clin. Orthop. 104:23, 1974.

Kline, D. G., and Hackett, E. R.: Reappraisal of timing for expression of civilian peripheral nerve injuries, Surgery 78:54, 1975.

Kline, D. G., Hackett, E. R., Davis, G. D., and Meyers, M. B.: Effects of mobilization on the blood supply and regeneration of injured nerves, J. Surg. Res. 12:254, 1972.

Kyle, J. B., and Eyre-Brook, A. L.: The surgical treatment of flexor tendon injuries in the hand; results obtained in a consecutive series of 57 cases, Br. J. Surg. 41:502, 1954.

Lindsay, W. K., and McDougall, E. P.: Direct digital flexor tendon repair, Plast. Reconstr. Surg. 26:613, 1960.

Lundborg, G.: Structure and function of the intraneural microvessels as related to trauma, edema formation, and nerve function, J. Bone Joint Surg. 57A:938, 1975.

Madsen, E.: Delayed primary suture of flexor tendons cut in the digital sheath, J. Bone Joint Surg. 52B:264, 1970.

Mason, M., and Allen, H.: An experimental study of tensile strength, Ann. Surg. 113:424, 1941.

Mayer, L., and Ransohoff, N.: Reconstruction of the digital tendon sheath; a contribution to the physiological method of repair of damaged finger tendons, J. Bone Joint Surg. 18:607, 1936.

McCash, C. R.: The immediate repair of flexor tendons, Br. J. Plast. Surg. 14:53, 1961.

McKenzie, A R.: Function after reconstruction of severed long flexor tendons of the hand, J. Bone Joint Surg. 49B:424, 1967.

Milford, L.: The hand, St. Louis, 1971, The C. V. Mosby Co.

Milgram, J. E.: Transplantation of tendons through performed gliding channels, Bull. Hosp. Joint Dis. **21**:250, 1960.

Millesi, H., Meissl, G., and Berger, A.: Further experience with interfascicular grafting of median, ulnar and radial nerves, J. Bone Joint Surg. **58A**:209, 1976.

Miu, T. K.: Transplantation of preserved composite tendon allografts, J. Bone Joint Surg. **47A**:65, 1975.

Nicolle, F. V.: A silastic tendon prosthesis as an adjunct to flexor tendon grafting; an experimental and clinical evaluation, Br. J. Plast. Surg. **22**:224, 1969.

Omer, G. E.: Injuries to nerves of the upper extremity, J. Bone Joint Surg. **56A**:1615, 1974.

Parry, C. B. W.: Rehabilitation of the hand, London, 1966, Butterworth & Co. Ltd.

Pulvertaft, R. G.: Tendon grafts for flexor tendon injuries in the fingers and thumb, J. Bone Joint Surg. **38B**:175, 1956.

Reynolds, B., Wray, R. C., Jr., and Weeks, P. M.: Should an incompletely severed tendon be sutured? Plast. Reconstr. Surg. **57**:36, 1976.

Thompson, R. V.: An evaluation of flexor tendon grafting, Br. J. Plast. Surg. **20**:21, 1967.

Tsuge, K., Ikuta, Y., and Matsuishi, Y.: Intratendinous tendon suture in the hand, a new technique, Hand **7**:250, 1975.

Van der Meulen, J. C.: Silastic spacers in tendon grafting, Br. J. Plast. Surg. **24**:166, 1971.

Verdan, C. E.: Primary and secondary repair of flexor and extensor tendon injuries. In Flynn, J. W., editor: Hand surgery, Baltimore, 1966, The Williams & Wilkins Co.

Weeks, P. M., and Wray, R. C.: The rate of functional recovery after flexor tendon grafting with or without silicone rod preparation, J. Hand Surg. **1**:174, 1974.

Wray, R. C., Ollinger, H., and Weeks, P. M.: Effects of mobilization on tensile strength of partial tendon lacerations, Surg. Forum **26**:557, 1975.

Young, R. E., and Harmon, J. M.: Repair of tendon injuries of the hand, Ann. Surg. **151**:562, 1960.

Zalis, A. W., Rodriquez, A. A., Oester, Y. T., and Mains, D. B.: Evaluation of nerve regeneration by means of nerve evoked potentials, J. Bone Joint Surg. **54A**:1246, 1972.

# CHAPTER 15

# Operate, rehabilitate, or rate

The decision to operate, rehabilitate, or rate is based primarily on clinical experience. The object in this chapter is to present methods of evaluation that aid in making this decision without relying completely on clinical experience. To arrive at the proper decision as one examines the patient, one must evaluate the hand in terms of its functional capacity. Determination of functional capacity requires evaluation of the following: (1) adequate tissue coverage, (2) nerve regeneration, (3) tendon gliding as reflected by active joint motion, and (4) the ability to perform the tasks essential to the patient's job. Clinical examination allows one to determine the adequacy of skin coverage; however, only by frequent examinations can one determine both quantitatively and qualitatively the changes that the scar is undergoing around joints, tendons, and skin grafts. These observations must be converted to numbers to allow an objective approach to the problems of scar remodelling. For ease of discussion the problems are separated, but frequently a patient presents problems involving more than one system.

## EVALUATION OF TISSUE COVERAGE

The adequacy of skin replacement can be determined by answering the following

questions: (1) Does the new skin inhibit tendon gliding? (2) Does it inhibit joint motion? (3) Does it provide adequate coverage and tactile function?

### Inhibition of tendon gliding

Grafted skin may inhibit tendon gliding because of the scar that forms between the skin and the underlying tendons. This may be either at the site of interface of the graft and the tendon (as with a free graft) or at the periphery of the graft-recipient site junction (as with a pedicle graft). The point of skin attachment can be detected by a variety of maneuvers. For example, when a flexor tendon is caught in scar at the dermal interface of a wound, attempts to activate tendon gliding result in blanching of the skin in the area of skin-scar-tendon fixation (Fig. 15-1). When this is not immediately evident, the joints distal to the point of scar attachment are passively flexed, and the patient is asked to pull as hard as possible on the involved flexor tendon. Flexion of these distal joints releases all of the pull of the long flexors on the distal joints and concentrates the stress on the site of the adhesions. The tension created by the scar pulling on the skin causes the skin to blanch, thus localizing the point of skin attachment. Similarly, scar attachment over the dorsum of the hand can be localized,

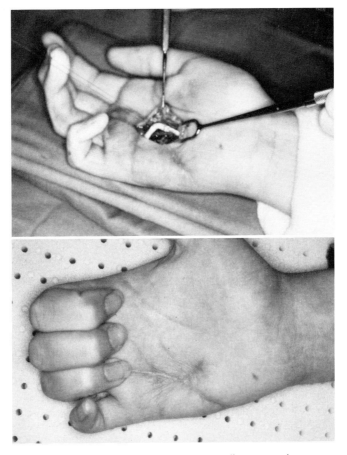

**Fig. 15-1.** The scar around the tendon anastomosis is adherent to the scar participating in the healing of the skin wound.

but here the joints distal to the site of scar have to be extended. When there is significant inhibition of tendon gliding by scar, one must be prepared to evaluate the potential of the scar to improve. Suggested methods for evaluation of this potential will be discussed with tendon gliding.

When free grafts have been placed over improperly prepared beds (for example, tendons, bones, and fascia), one must determine the potential for the contracted skin graft to undergo functional improvement. Certainly, the individual with extensive clinical experience can accurately judge the degree of improvement one can

expect under such circumstances. Yet this judgment is not always available, and a method for determining the tissues' potential for improvement is desirable.

**Inhibition of joint motion**

Visual examination usually reveals the extent of tissue loss by scarring or graft contraction over a flexion crease. This can be accurately determined by marking the proximal and distal extents of the scar and transposing these markings (maintaining their actual positions) onto the opposite uninvolved finger. The extent of contraction in the scarred area will be evidenced by the amount of tissue included between the markings on the normal finger. When a large discrepancy is evident, the contracture must be released and new skin introduced. When there is evidence for potential increase in the compliance of minimal to moderate skin losses, the improvement in the passive range of joint motion can be used to adequately document and evaluate the changes. Again, accurate and frequent assessments of passive joint motion allow one to determine when the scar has realized its potential for improvement; that is, the change in joint motion reaches a plateau, and thereafter only minimal improvement is observed. Clinical judgment gained through extensive clinical practice can allow one to determine those joints that obviously require surgical correction of the flexion contracture. Yet the striking improvement in tissue compliance gained by dynamic splinting—as reported from the Galveston Burn Center—indicates that conservative management has a greater range of application than has been appreciated. Of course, if one has had the opportunity to manage the case in question from the time of injury, he is provided with a much greater insight into the state of the recipient site.

Occasionally dorsal scar proximal to a flexion crease will limit flexion of the juxtaposed joint. The dorsum of the hand is particularly prone to develop significant contracture because of the laxity of this skin. The decision to replace or add skin is determined by the extent of tissue lost and the ability of the scarred tissues to undergo favorable biological alteration to permit full joint flexion. Adherence to the old adage of waiting until the healed scar has matured to replace and add new tissues can be of questionable value. Certainly the tissues will undergo remodelling, and there will be some improvement, even if ever so slight. But at the same time, the joint ligaments can become fixed in an undesirable position (for example, metacarpophalangeal joint extension), a condition that can require surgical destruction of the ligaments that provide metacarpophalangeal joint stability. One can save many subsequent capsulectomies if the need for tissue replacement is recognized early and treated promptly and adequately. This decision can be postponed somewhat longer in children, because their tissues are particularly capable of undergoing extensive remodelling and restoration to a functional state, thereby permitting normal joint motion.

### Inadequate tactile function

Moberg suggests that a two-point discrimination of less than 15 mm is functional. When the two-point discrimination is greater than 15 mm, what does one do? Nonoperative treatment could include sensory reeducation, which will be discussed later in this chapter. The earlier discussion of wound coverage revealed that the only neurovascular flaps that routinely maintain two-point discrimination below 15 mm are the local advancement flaps in which nerve continuity is maintained and distant flaps that are innervated by a sensory branch of the radial nerve. If one contemplates replacement of tissues with an innervated flap, the flap that includes the radial nerve is the choice for the thumb, and the local advancement flap is appropriate for the thumb and fingers. These flaps maintain two-point discriminatory ability better than any of the innervated flaps in use today. Yet when a denervated pedicle flap covers a finger—as for an avulsion of the skin of the finger—an island flap is the only flap that can provide tissue durable enough for function even though its two-point discrimination function may become less than that desired. Avulsion of the skin of a finger usually includes loss of the neurovascular bundles. Consequently, there are no digital nerves to invade a free graft and provide sensitivity.

Use of the innervated local advancement

flaps or the radial sensory flap should be considered for coverage only when the ulnovolar pad of the thumb and the radiovolar pad of the index and possibly the long finger are denervated, and restoration of nerve continuity to these areas is not feasible. If the index and long fingers are missing, then sensory coverage for the fingers used in pinch should be considered.

Included under evaluation of tactile function is the phenomenon of hyperesthesia in a grafted area. This is important in the areas of the thumb and finger pads utilized in pinch. Generally, the problems with hyperesthesia can be classified into those with neuromas beneath the graft, those where the graft covers bone directly, making the bone easily palpable and frequently subjected to trauma, and those where neither of these two conditions is present. When neuromas are involved, as determined by history and physical examination, a number of methods have been suggested for their control. The use of Silastic caps has been extremely effective in Tauras' cases. In our cases, use of these caps has been associated with a high incidence of recurrent hyperesthesia. Our experience has shown that effective management of the painful neuroma involves tracing the nerve proximally for several centimeters and transposing the neuroma into the bony phalanx. Care must be taken to position the neuroma within the medullary cavity. Others have reported this method as being ineffective.

Hypersensitivity may be associated with a skin graft applied directly on bone, for example, a guillotine amputation through a distal phalanx covered with a graft. At least three methods of treatment are available: (1) The graft may be excised and a local advancement flap utilized for coverage; (2) the graft may be excised and a local or distant denervated flap utilized; or (3) the patient may gently tap the sensitive tip until the pain threshold is elevated to a point where the fingertip is only minimally sensitive. This last procedure has been effective in only a small percentage of patients. Obviously, the use of the local advancement flap is most desirable when feasible. In the third type of hypersensitivity, no neuroma is detectable and no bone is exposed. The fingertip is simply sensitive. We have been unable to improve these patients and have rated them for sensory and functional loss of the finger. When the management of hypersensitivity is considered, it is important to discuss thoroughly the procedures and costs involved, the time required, and the fact that the procedure—no matter which is chosen—can fail. In our experience, when the problem has been present for a year or more, treatment has been followed by a high recurrence rate.

## EVALUATION OF NERVE REGENERATION

After a nerve has been severed and repaired, how can one evaluate the success of the repair without waiting an extended period of time to determine the ultimate functional result? This becomes particularly important when a patient is referred for follow-up care after a nerve repair. When a pure motor or a mixed nerve is involved, the anatomical pattern of muscle innervation has been used to determine if recovery is occurring and the rate of recovery. This is done by recording the times at which different muscles show the first signs of voluntary contraction and correlating the time intervals with the approximate lengths of the different nerve branches. But when the median nerve is cut in the midforearm area and a repair has been accomplished, is there any way to determine if the repair is adequate, or do we have to wait until sensory and motor function can be tested to make a judgment? First, we note how long before the axons begin to regenerate and cross the repair site. Many reports are available, but they include time spans of only 3 to 138 days. The average time is 30 to 60 days.

Tinel's sign is one method of evaluating nerve regeneration. By gently tapping along the course of the involved nerve, one can elicit the phenomenon that the patient describes as "pin and needles," "numbness in the involved finger," and "electricity shooting into the involved fingers." One begins at the distal extent of the nerve trunk (the distal phalanx level for the median and ulnar nerves) and taps gently along the nerve trunk while progressing proximally. When the phenomenon is elicited, the examiner marks the spot and repeats the test. When the level of regeneration is firmly established, its position is measured from the end of the finger and recorded with the date of examination. Unfortunately, this test does not tell us how many axons have successfully traversed the anastomosis site to enter the distal stump. The only indication of the success, and this by no means a quantitative measure, is the speed of advancement across the anastomosis and the degree of sensitivity elicited at the site of anastomosis even as Tinel's sign continues its distal advancement. Frequent observations reveal the rate of advancement of Tinel's sign.

Tinel's sign has been considered to be a significant indicator of regeneration but has recently fallen into disfavor. Even a few misdirected fibers can produce the tingling sensation associated with Tinel's sign. On occasion, Tinel's sign has been absent even though regeneration was occurring. Furthermore, Tinel's sign has been noted to be progressing in an acceptable fashion, even though reoperation revealed a severed nerve with separation of the glioma and neuroma. Woodhall noted that at least 75% of the nerve lesions that required resection and suture were associated with a properly advancing Tinel sign.

However, Henderson (1948) reported his experience treating over 400 nerve injuries in prisoner-of-war hospitals in Germany from 1940 to 1945. About 60 nerve repairs were performed, but others were prohibited. This provided an opportunity to correlate clinical findings with subsequent operative findings when surgery was permitted. He believes that Tinel's sign is of value if interpreted according to Tinel's original description. The following is the result of Henderson's observation. After a nerve injury, a latent period of 2 to 3 weeks elapses before new axon outgrowth occurs. Many axon sprouts are evident, but only one matures and migrates distally in each sheath. The first few inches of advancing axons are unmyelinated and sensitive to percussion. As the axons mature, they are myelinated, and the sensitivity persists only at the leading edge of the unmyelinated axons. The number of fibers present in the nerve trunk can be distinguished from the number that have escaped at the nerve repair site by comparing the strength of the sensations induced by percussion. If interpreted in this manner, Henderson believes the test is more helpful than any other method of assessing the amount of regeneration taking place before motor or sensory recovery occurs.

On the basis of Tinel's sign, he placed patients into four groups. In group I, no regeneration occurred, and Tinel's sign did not advance beyond the site of nerve injury. In group II, minimal regeneration occurred, with only a few fibers crossing the injury site to enter the distal sheaths. Tinel's sign at the neuroma site was strong and remained strong, even though a weak advancing Tinel sign was noted. The persistently strong neuroma response at the site of injury or repair was felt to be a more important prognostic sign than the weak peripheral response. In group III, partial regeneration occurred. The advancing Tinel sign was either strong or weak, but waves of advancing axons were evident as noted by multiple areas of greater sensitivity along the nerve trunk (Fig. 15-2). Thus, new fibers are continually leaving the neuroma to progress distally. The de-

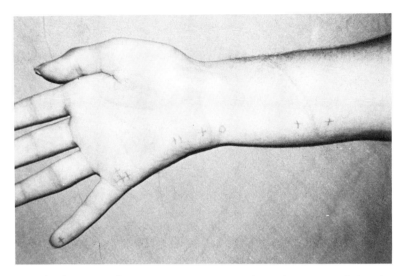

**Fig. 15-2.** Multiple areas of sensitivity are present along the course of the ulnar nerve.

cision to reoperate depends on an estimate of the proportion of fibers in the first wave and how much recovery the surgeon thinks will take place. In group IV, complete regeneration is indicated by a strongly advancing Tinel sign. Tenderness at the site of repair is strong, but within 6 months it has fully disappeared. In summary, Henderson suggests that Tinel's sign is of no value within the first 2 months. After 2 months, one can begin grouping patients as described above. However, this grouping cannot be confirmed until 3 or 4 months after injury or repair. A strongly advancing Tinel sign provides no information as to whether or not the regenerating fibers are in the proper distal sheaths. A strong peripheral response simply means that many fibers are growing distally.

**Evaluation of motor recovery**

Because the nerves have an orderly management of innervation of specific muscles, one can record when different muscles show the first signs of voluntary contraction and correlate the time intervals with the approximate lengths of the different nerve branches. This will reveal progressive reinnervation, if the nerves are regenerating at an acceptable qualitative manner.

In group I and possibly group II, the decision to reoperate is straightforward. In group III, arrival at a decision is more difficult. Other factors must be brought into focus to aid in decision making. These include: (1) the circumstances of repair, (2) the type of injury, (3) the time between injury and surgery, and (4) the expertise of the surgeon.

What is the maximum period that repair can be delayed and satisfactory recovery can occur following delayed nerve suture? Nerve repair is justified as long as the axons possess the capacity to regenerate, the distal stump has not collapsed into a tube of scar, and the denervated tissues are in good condition.

Human nerves retain the capacity to regenerate for at least 1 and possibly 2 years. The endoneurial tube can collapse and shrink but still provide a conduit for a regenerating nerve from 12 to 24 months. However, the distal stump may shrink to approximately 50% of the size of the proximal stump. Peripheral muscles have the capacity to completely recover functionally even if denervation has been complete for 1 year. Zachary (1954) has suggested that sensory recovery may still be possible by nerve repair for 2 to 3 years after injury, whereas motor recovery is possible up to 18 months after injury. Furthermore, he reports that a low median nerve lesion that was unrepaired until 2½ years after the injury resulted in useful return of abduction to the thumb after repair.

Even though a range of values is available regarding nerve regeneration, maintenance of endoneurial tube integrity, and survival of peripheral muscle and sensory organs, it is evident that repair performed within at least 1 and sometimes 2 years after injury can be expected to provide good functional results.

For purposes of this discussion, observation for 4 to 6 months does not seem unreasonable when one is presented with a patient who has undergone primary nerve repair by a reputable surgeon. Thus the decision in the early follow-up care is based on the circumstances, the type of injury, the time between injury and surgery, and the expertise of the surgeon.

If a patient falls into group II suggested by Henderson, and if his nerve was repaired in the emergency room by a surgeon who is not considered to be expert at nerve repairs, then reoperation is indicated. Any combination of the above conditions that suggests less than optimum repair of the nerve in a patient in group II or III strongly indicates that reoperation is necessary.

Zalis and colleagues have described the use of nerve-evoked potentials in evaluating nerve regeneration during the period after nerve repair but before function is regained distally. Five patients were referred several months after initial nerve repair. Electromyograms at initial examination revealed denervation of the muscles.

Serial examinations revealed early signs of regeneration, such as evoked muscle potentials after nerve stimulation and nascent motor units under voluntary con-

trol. Nerve potential recordings were obtained by placing two needle electrodes high in the arm to serve as recording electrodes. A surface electrode was used distally to stimulate the nerve; thus, centripetal recordings were obtained. The stimulating electrode was moved distally from the site of nerve injury, and several recordings were obtained. Serial examinations allow evaluation of the regenerative process, yet they do not indicate how many axons have successfully crossed the suture line and are proceeding distally in the appropriate conduits.

When the nerve to a muscle has been sectioned, most muscles develop a fibrillation phenomenon 14 to 28 days after nerve injury (yet some denervated muscles are electrically silent). This is due to the regular contraction of the individual muscle fibers. Normal muscle that is completely relaxed is electrically silent. Motor unit activity appears before clinical evidence of recovery. After suture of a mixed nerve, the first signs of motor recovery may not be detectable for 3 to 4 months after motor unit action potentials are detected. Thus the detection of action potentials is no guarantee that useful recovery may be expected. The most important change revealed by electromyogram is the evidence of progressive reinnervation with spreading of action potentials to more distal muscles.

### Prognostic evaluation of sensory recovery

Dellon and colleagues studied 12 patients in an attempt to determine the earliest prognostic evaluation of sensory recovery. These studies were based on the observations that group A beta fibers, which mediate the perception of touch, are composed of a mixture of slow- and fast-adapting fibers.

When the epidermis is indented, the fast-adapting fibers discharge a small number of impulses. No further impulses are discharged until the stimulus is removed. Conversely, the slow-adapting fibers respond to stimuli by releasing a rapid sequence of impulses, which is gradually reduced quantitatively until the stimulus is removed. Thus, perception of constant touch cannot be a function of fast-adapting fibers, but it is a function of slow-adapting fibers. However, a moving stimulus excites a continuing response from both types of fibers.

Of the group A beta fibers, the slow-adapting fibers contribute 10% of the total, whereas the fast-adapting fibers contribute 90% of the total.

The fast-adapting fibers may be divided into two groups: those that respond maximally in the range of 2 to 40 cps (group I) and those that respond maximally in the range of 60 to 300 cps (group II). The former are located more superficially in the skin than the latter.

Dellon and associates devised the following evaluation: (1) stroking to evaluate moving touch perception (fast-adapting fibers), (2) applying slight constant pressure (slow-adapting fibers), (3) tuning fork at 30 cps (fast-adapting fibers, group I), (4) tuning fork at 256 cps (fast-adapting fibers, group II), (5) pinprick (to evaluate thinly myelinated group A delta and the nonmyelinated group C fibers), and (6) two-point discrimination.

All patients were examined at 1- to 3-week intervals, depending on the rapidity of their recovery. A constant pattern of sensory recovery in the hands was observed. Return occurred in the following order: first, pinprick pain; second, perception of 30 cps and moving touch; third, perception of constant touch; and fourth, perception of 256 cps. Since pain fibers are the smallest in diameter, they are expected to regenerate more quickly than the larger touch fibers. The fast-adapting group A beta fibers that respond to 30 cps recover earlier than do the fast-adapting fibers that respond to 256 cps. The pacinian corpuscles are considered the paradigm of the fast-adapting receptors. Thus the testing of 256 cps discrimination is testing the regenera-

tion and maturation of the pacinian corpuscles.

In none of the 15 injured nerves tested was two-point discrimination appreciated before the constant-touch stimulus was perceived at the fingertip. However, from these excellent studies, no record is made of the ultimate functional recovery (sensory) or the correlation of the time intervals to the appearance of the responses. Only the order of responses is reported.

### Management during early sensory return

After we are assured that the repair is adequate and axons are progressing to the end organs, we concern ourselves with the extent of recovery of motor power and sensation. Chapter 10 provides standards for reporting motor power and sensation return.

Since less than 2% of the cases with complete transection of the median and ulnar nerves at the wrist recover normal two-point discrimination (3 to 5 mm), Dellon and associates have suggested sensory reeducation in patients with inadequate sensory return. They feel that the reason for the poor results is the failure of the patient to realize his full sensory potential, rather than the failure of the surgeon to achieve an adequate nerve repair. An exercise program was developed, based on the timing of return of the various modalities of cutaneous sensitivity. Reeducation is divided into an early phase and a late phase. The early phase is begun before the perception of moving touch and/or constant touch has been recovered at the distal phalanx. After recovery of these modalities has occurred to the level of the distal phalanx, the late phase of reeducation is begun. The program trains one to improve his discriminatory ability. In the first nine patients, six were entered in the late phase of sensory reeducation program. The two-point discrimination in these patients ranged from 45 to 8 mm before treatment, which lasted 2 to 6 weeks. At the end of the treatment period, two-point discrimination in this group ranged from 2 to 15 mm. These results support the propositions that: (1) there is a time during nerve regeneration when the patient will begin to demonstrate less recovery of functional sensation than he is capable of and (2) specific sensory exercises begun at the appropriate time will help the patient realize this full potential for recovery.

Motor regeneration is better when repair is performed in pure nerves, that is, when all the fibers in the repaired nerve are motor fibers. This can occur only in the motor branch of the ulnar and median nerves that are within the hand and the posterior interosseous branch of the radial nerve and the anterior interosseous branch of the median nerve that are in the forearm. Comparison of motor return in the median, ulnar, and radial nerves, lacerated at a level where they are mixed nerves, reveals that return is best in the radial and poorest in the ulnar. Motor return generally precedes sensory return, because the motor branches are usually proximal to the sensory endings. However, the ulnar nerve's motor branch is only slightly shorter than its sensory branches. Appropriate procedures to restore muscle balance can be undertaken after an adequate period of waiting for motor return. The outstanding results reported by Millesi in obtaining motor return, even in the ulnar nerve in older patients, make reevaluation of our techniques mandatory. According to his results, if a nerve has been repaired under undue tension and the progress of regeneration is minimal, one is justified in resecting the anastomosis and performing the individual funicular repairs with nerve grafts.

## EVALUATION OF TENDON GLIDING AND JOINT MOBILITY

Evaluation of skin coverage and nerve regeneration is based primarily on clinical impression. In the routine evaluation of tendon gliding and joint mobility, one generally waits 6 months to a year to evaluate the functional results and to make a decision regarding the indications for further surgery. This is purely empirical. Is there any way we can make this decision earlier? Since the functional result is based on the biological activity of the offending scar, our attention must be directed to this scar. Through this approach, our experience has led us to the conclusion that these decisions can be made much earlier than previously believed. To allow dissection of the conglomerate problem into its components and analysis of each component, we first assume that the musculotendinous unit is intact functionally and the joints are supple. Failure of the tendons to glide in this case is the result of scar tissue inhibiting the gliding action of the tendons. Stress is the only modality we have available clinically to stimulate the biological processes of scar degradation and reorganization. Thus, our initial evaluation is directed toward determining the immediate mechanical effects of stress on scar, its subsequent biological course, and the intervening changes in mechanical properties as revealed by the changes in response of the scar to stress.

From a correlation of these results one can acquire answers to the following questions: (1) Is this a scar that has the biological potential to undergo favorable remodelling? (2) Is this scar undergoing significant favorable remodelling? (3) Has this scar reached its full potential or capacity for remodelling? Obviously in these cases the decisions regarding whether to operate, rehabilitate, or rate are based on the answers to these questions.

When a patient is seen soon after an injury has been repaired and the wounds are healed (recall that healing of all injuries requires scar formation), we first determine if the resulting scar has the potential to undergo favorable remodelling.

### Evaluation of the initial scar

The only clinical means we have available to stimulate favorable remodelling of scar is the application of stress to the scar. Our clinical skills are at the mercy of the biological processes of collagen degradation, synthesis, and reorganization, for these are what determine the final functional characteristics of the scar. Recall that the favorable scar is one that can undergo remodelling to produce flimsy, nonrestricting adhesions. The unfavorable scar is one with biological characteristics that prevent biological alteration into favorable scar. We have been investigating the response of different scars in different locations in an effort to determine if there is a common denominator that will allow us to predict a favorable scar or an unfavorable scar. The scars tested have been around tendon anastomoses, tendon grafts, stiff joints from intrinsic causes, and skin contractures.

The application of force to a scar allows definition of the scar's mechanical characteristics for correlation with its later biological behavior. First, we must consider the mechanical response of tendon to stress, because applying stress to the scar around a tendon is accomplished by applying stress to the tendon, which in turn transmits the stress to the scar.

The flexor pollicis longus tendon was tested to determine its percent elongation (strain) in response to an increasing load (stress). From the resulting data, a stress-strain curve has been plotted (Fig. 15-3). As the initial small load is applied, a small but significant elongation of the tendon is evident. As the load increases, the percent elongation rapidly decreases until further loading results in breakage of the tendon. Note particularly the size of the loads applied. This stress-strain curve for human tendon can be divided into four distinct zones. The initial zone covers the curve formed by inducing a strain from 0% to 1.5%. Here, there is a considerable increase in length in response to a small increase in stress. The physical change occurring in the tendon during this period is the straightening of the wavy collagen fiber pattern. The second zone

covers the curve representing a change in strain from 1.5% to 3%. In this zone the collagen fibers become polarized and straightened to assume a portion of the stress. In the third zone the strain increases from 3% to 5%. In this zone the entire stress is assumed by the collagen fibers in pure tension. At this point the stress-strain curve forms a straight line. As the strain exceeds 5%, rupture of the collagen fibers becomes evident.

"Creep" measures another significant response: the percent elongation that a structure exhibits when a load is applied and is maintained at a constant level over an extended period of time. When a flexor tendon is subjected to a constant force of $10 \times 10^{6}$ dynes/cm$^2$, the strain increases from 0.950% to 0.985% in 16.6 minutes (an elongation of 0.03%). This creep is a linear function of the log of time, and in the human flexor tendon the amount of creep is exceedingly small.

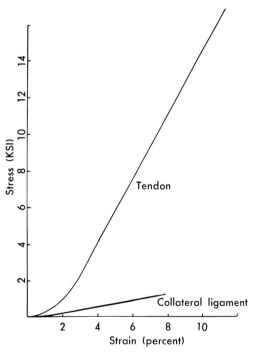

**Fig. 15-3.** The stress-strain curves for tendon and metacarpophalangeal joint ligaments are depicted.

When the collateral ligaments of the metacarpophalangeal joints are subject to an increasing load, the percent elongation observed allows the plotting of its stress-strain curve. The difference in the responses of joint ligament and flexor tendon is evident when plotted on a single chart. The joint ligament exhibits a much greater elongation with a much smaller load than does the flexor tendon—a finding that could have been surmised from the functional requirements of each.

However, when a ligament of predominantly elastic fibers is subjected to a small force, it reaches its functional length so rapidly that an accurate measure of creep cannot be projected for its functional length. As a consequence of these observations, it is evident that when a load is applied to a finger to determine the deformation of scar around the collateral ligaments, the observations relative to creep actually reflect creep in the scar around the ligament. Thus, these observations provide a baseline for the application of stress to a scar through the involved tendon or to the involved joint ligaments. Furthermore, the physiological loads (that is, the loads the skin circulation can tolerate) that we can apply to a finger are far below those that cause tendon elongation; thus, we can assume that the changes seen at lower loads are the result of physical changes within the scar tissue. Normally the loads used are from 4 to 8 oz which, when calculated in terms of torque per cross-sectional area of the tendon, actually approximates only 38 gm/mm² of cross-sectional area. As noted from the stress-strain curve for tendon, a load this small actually results in minimal strain in the tendon. When applied to elastic ligaments, this small load produces a much greater effect, but when applied to the collateral ligaments of a joint, the strain is comparable to that developing in tendon. Thus, we can assume that the strain recorded after the application of a small torque is the result of changes in the scar that is restricting tendon gliding.

From necessity, the data concerning scar (adhesions) that restricts tendon gliding have been derived from the study of scar that is at least 3 weeks old. Since all scars undergo some biological alteration to become either favorable or unfavorable adhesions, can we detect which scar has the potential to form favorable adhesions through its initial response to loading while the scar is still immature? Application of these loads should not be interpreted as "manipulation." Manipulation is the procedure of applying great stress to scar around a joint under general anesthesia in order to rupture the scar and thus allow improved joint motion momentarily. In these cases, the reparative process evoked usually fixes the joint in an even more unfavorable position with greater scar production in response to the new wounds. The application of stress should be directed toward minimizing the reparative response and maximizing the biological reorganizational response. Consequently, the torque applied should be very small.

### Initial response of scar around tendon anastomosis

Initial responses of scar around tendon anastomosis will be illustrated through case discussion. In the first case, the patient had undergone repair of all flexor tendons at the wrist 3 weeks before evaluation of the scar. A torque (load × moment arm) of 550 gm/cm was applied to the long finger profundus. The amount of deformation in the scar was plotted in centimeters against time (Fig. 15-4). After the application of the torque, the scar immediately was deformed 0.26 cm and thereafter assumed a linear increase over the next 36 minutes. During this time, a total increase in scar deformation of 0.7 cm was observed. Two days later a torque of 500 gm/cm was applied, and an instant increase in scar deformation of 0.50 cm was

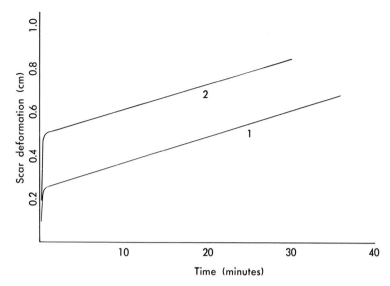

**Fig. 15-4.** The application of a load (1) to the scar around the tendon anastomosis resulted in a gradual deformation of the scar. Two days later (2) this deformation was significantly increased.

observed, which increased linearly to 0.85 cm at 30 minutes. The amount of permanent deformation recorded between these tests was 0.20 cm. This step-by-step increase in permanent deformation associated with the change in compliance of the scar indicates a favorable scar, that is, one that will respond favorably to rehabilitative measures. The subsequent biological behavior of this scar is depicted in Fig. 15-5. Note the rapid increase in the range of joint motion during a period of 5 weeks.

The practical mechanics of applying stress and measuring deformations require that the stress be applied in a direction opposite to what we normally employ in mobilizing scar. That is, scar around the flexor tendons is stressed by the patient contracting the muscle belly and exerting a proximally directed stress on the scar. The application of stress by an external apparatus requires exerting the stress in a distal direction. When performing a tenolysis under local anesthesia, one can appreciate the tremendous force generated by the forearm muscles in flexion. Yet

these forces are momentary and not sustained. Certainly the external forces applied do not approach those generated by the muscles, but the external forces can be constant—a significant feature. Thus, the scar around a flexor tendon is being deformed by forces in extension. Certainly the scar must be yielding in both directions to permit gliding of the tendons during full extension and flexion. This raises the question of positioning after a flexor tendon anastomosis is performed. If the wrist is extended and the fingers are slightly flexed, the application of external force can only accomplish full extension. If the anastomosis is displaced proximally and the joints are flexed, dynamic splinting to full extension would of necessity permit full flexion. This would be feasible only if one can demonstrate that the application of a constant but small force is more beneficial than the intermittent application of a large force for short periods of time—as accomplished by the forearm musculature.

In a second case, 11 weeks after repair

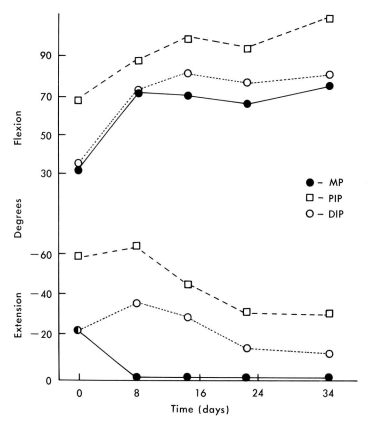

**Fig. 15-5.** The biological behavior of scar tissue over a period of 3 weeks results in a marked alteration of its physical characteristics.

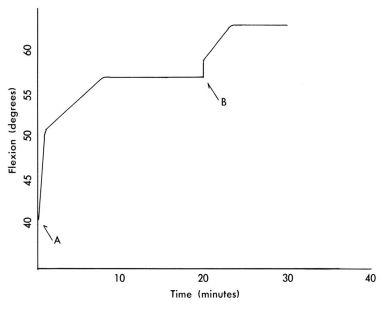

**Fig. 15-6.** The application of a load (A) to the long finger resulted in a marked improvement in joint rotation. At 20 minutes an additional load (B) was applied, which induced further improvement.

of a laceration of the extensor tendons, 430 gm/cm of torque was applied (in flexion) to the long finger. This resulted in a rapid increase in joint flexion from 40 to 51 degrees, followed by a more gradual rise to 57 degrees (Fig. 15-6). At this point the torque was increased to 510 gm/cm. Accompanying this increase in torque was an increase in joint flexion to 62 degrees. Thus, a total increase of 22 degrees in joint flexion was observed over a 30-minute period. The biological behavior of the scar around the extensor tendons is depicted in Fig. 15-7. Within 7 days, full flexion and extension had been obtained.

The deformation response to stress can be correlated directly with the ultimate functional result, which is a reflection of degradation and reorganization of the scar. Yet, if this initial evaluation is not available, one can still predict the biological course of the scar through frequent observations of the changes within the scar as reflected by tendon gliding. The extensive adhesions that form around a flexor tendon graft and the proximal anastomosis can exhibit a spectrum of behavior. Frequently we can pinpoint which area of scar is most unyielding, but the entire extent of the scar is contributing to the in-

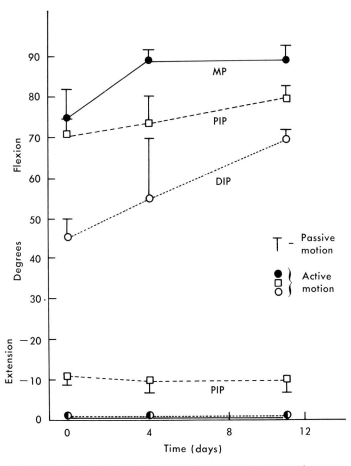

**Fig. 15-7.** The biological behavior of the scar tissue reveals a rapid improvement in joint motion, reflecting a change in the physical characteristics of the scar tissue.

hibition of tendon gliding. Obviously the functional result—as reflected by active range of joint motion—depends on alteration of the entire scar. This can be determined by frequent observations, as noted earlier.

Patient G. R. underwent flexor tendon graft to his ring finger. At 3 weeks post-operatively, the active and passive ranges of joint motion were noted (Fig. 15-8). Within 10 days after beginning therapy, he exhibited 68 degrees active flexion at the distal interphalangeal joint and 89 degrees flexion at the proximal interphalangeal joint. Flexion at the metacarpophalangeal was normal. This rapid change in scar

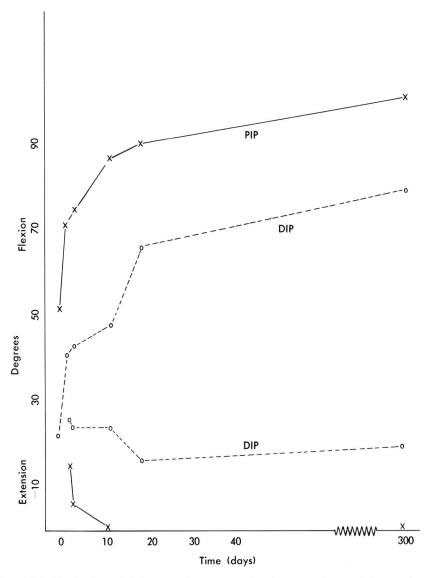

**Fig. 15-8.** The biological behavior of scar around a flexor tendon graft is noted to allow significant improvement within the first 3 weeks after removal of the dressing. This level of improvement was constant over the ensuing 7 weeks.

remodelling and reorganization provides an indication of the final functional result expected. Of course, many patients do not progress at this rate. Yet the rate of change is not the only factor concerned. Finding steady improvement, no matter what the rate, indicates that the patient does not require operative intervention and is too early to rate (Fig. 15-9).

How can one determine if the patient is regaining function at an acceptable rate? We recorded the rate of change of motion after flexor tendon grafting with and without previous rod insertion, and then developed a rate of change for the average patient (Fig. 15-10). The fact that a patient is improving progressively is more important than how he compares with the average patient.

On the other hand, many patients who undergo a flexor tendon graft demonstrate a very small increase in range of motion and reach a plateau that calls for a decision (Fig. 15-11). This decision can be that further surgery is indicated, for example, tenolysis or excision of tendon graft and insertion of Silastic rod, or that a rating can be provided with reasonable certainty that the improvement has reached a maximum. There are many patients whose progress falls between these two extremes. Invariably, one can predict within the first 2 or 3 weeks the eventual improvement in tendon gliding that will oc-

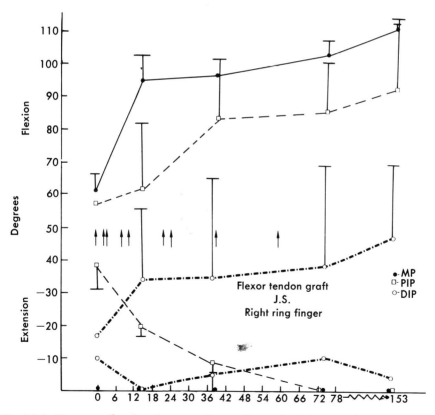

**Fig. 15-9.** Three weeks after flexor tendon grafting, the behavior of the scar around the tendon graft is charted in terms of active and passive joint rotation. The interconnecting lines indicate the level of active motion, whereas the upright *T* indicates passive flexion, and the inverted *T* marks passive extension.

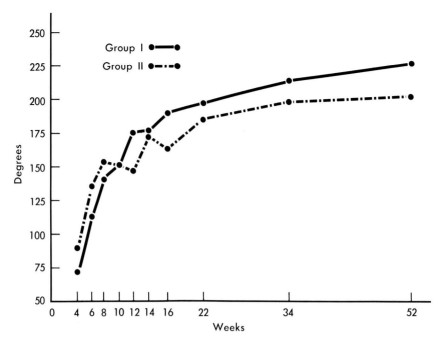

**Fig. 15-10.** The rate of recovery after tendon grafting with prior use of a rod (Group II) and without prior use of a rod (Group I) is depicted above.

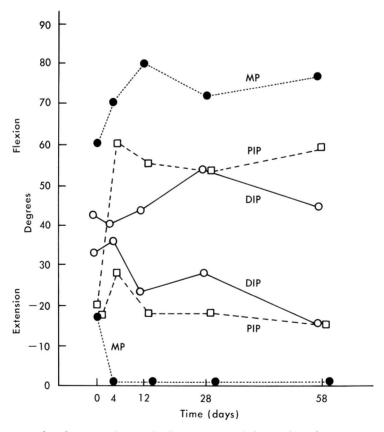

**Fig. 15-11.** After flexor tendon graft, the scar around the graft underwent improvement to a point of plateau and thereafter remained constant. Note the passive range of joint motion.

cur. Only after accumulating extensive data classified according to age, type of injury, severity, and so forth, can a baseline performance be obtained to provide controls for evaluation of any alterations in therapeutic methods. The simple charting of progress or lack thereof is the first step in this direction.

### Initial response of scar around collateral ligaments

To obtain pure cases of collateral ligament involvement is difficult, because there always appears to be some involvement of the dorsal capsule in those who come to surgery. However, in the examples to be presented, the scar is virtually limited to the collateral ligaments. For example, patient L. J. had clinically stiff collateral ligaments of the fifth finger metacarpophalangeal joint. He had sustained an injury to his thumb 8 weeks before these tests, and the metacarpophalangeal joints had become stiffened while in a dressing. A torque of 510 gm/cm was applied, with the joint coming to rest instantly at 50 degrees flexion (Fig. 15-12). A linear in-

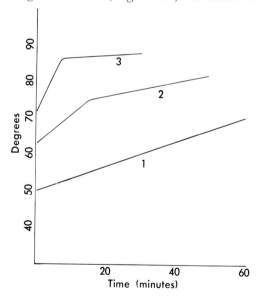

**Fig. 15-12.** The application of a load to the collateral ligament on three different occasions reveals a step-by-step increase in joint rotation over a 2-day period.

crease in joint rotation was observed for 60 minutes during the constant application of this torque. After 60 minutes, the joint exhibited 72 degrees flexion (an increase of 22 degrees flexion in 60 minutes). Two days later, a second loading produced an instant rotation of the joint to 63 degrees flexion. A torque of 520 gm/cm was applied, and over a 12-minute period, a linear increase in joint flexion to 78 degrees was observed; thereafter the increase in joint rotation proceeded at a much lower rate. After 45 minutes, the joint exhibited 82 degrees flexion, a total increase of 19 degrees over a 45-minute period. Two hours later, a third loading of 560 gm/cm produced an instant rise in joint flexion to 71 degrees, followed by a slower linear rise to 84 degrees within 8 minutes; then a new rate of rotation was assumed. After 29 minutes the joint exhibited 88 degrees flexion.

It is assumed that these considerable increases in joint rotation are the result of mechanical alterations within the scar around the collateral ligaments. From these observations one can predict that this patient has a favorable scar around the collateral ligaments, a scar that will respond to rehabilitative measures without operative intervention. Furthermore, improvement will be progressive, and any attempt to rate the patient at this point would be contraindicated. The subsequent changes in metacarpophalangeal joint motion are indicated in Fig. 15-13. Within 3 weeks, the patient had regained a normal range of active and passive metacarpophalangeal joint motion.

Of course, not all scars around collateral ligaments are favorable. The collateral ligaments in a long-standing hyperextension deformity of the metacarpophalangeal joints were evaluated. As the metacarpophalangeal joint was subjected to a constant torque of 453 gm/cm, the joint rotation observed during a period of 152 minutes was less than 5 degrees. The patient underwent intensive therapy for

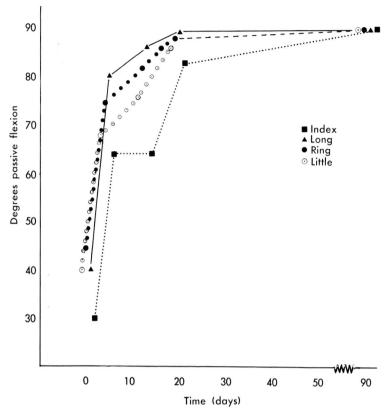

**Fig. 15-13.** Biological activity of the scar around the metacarpophalangeal joint characterized in Fig. 15-12 is presented.

months. When the biological changes in the scar were charted, the scar was definitely unfavorable, a prediction that could have been made from the brief evaluation studies (Fig. 15-14).

### Initial response of scar involving the joint capsule

The intraarticular fracture evokes an inflammatory response that involves all of the structures of the joint capsule. This may lead to fibrosis and inhibition of joint motion. In one case an intraarticular fracture of the metacarpal head resulted in the development of a stiff metacarpophalangeal joint. The scar around the joint was evaluated 3 weeks after the injury. A torque of 540 gm/cm was applied and instantly produced 64 degrees of joint

rotation. A linear increase in joint rotation occurred for 34 minutes, after which a plateau was reached. After the plateau was established, the torque was increased to 640 gm/cm, and within 5 minutes a sharp increase in joint rotation to 84 degrees was observed, after which it levelled off (Fig. 15-15). This indicates a favorable scar.

This use of data provides the application of real numbers to a patient's progress; that is, it provides an objective measure. The response "I think I am getting better" is a subjective observation on which we cannot establish a scientific approach to hand surgery. Recording and interpreting data are essential aids in restoring function. The data can be used to help make the decision to operate—for example, to perform a tenolysis.

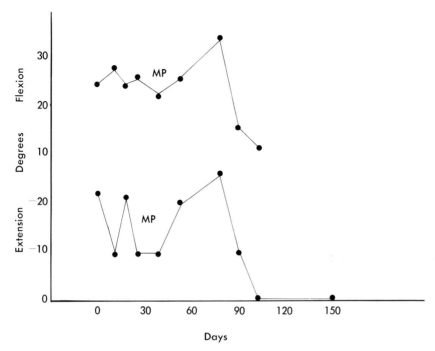

**Fig. 15-14.** The collateral ligaments are rigidly fixed in a shortened position. There is no change in these ligaments despite intensive therapy over a long period of time.

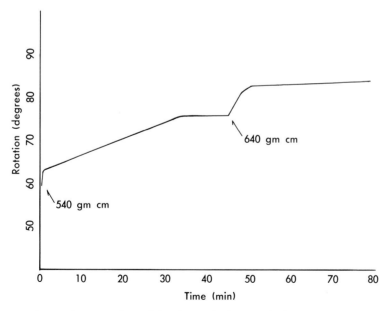

**Fig. 15-15.** The application of small loads resulted in marked improvement in joint flexion within 1 hour.

Thirty days after fracture of the ring and little finger metacarpals, patient N. K. was first seen and begun on therapy directed at restoring passive joint motion and tendon gliding (Fig. 15-16). The flexor tendons were bound in fracture callus at the level of the proximal phalanx. The distal interphalangeal joint exhibited minimal flexion and no improvement. The metacarpophalangeal joint exhibited only slight progress in gaining extension, but flexion was noticeably improved. Because of the apparent lack of progress in distal interphalangeal joint flexion, the decision to perform a tenolysis was made. Three days after the tenolysis, the ranges of active motion of the proximal and distal interphalangeal joints had significantly improved. Again, the simple acquisition of data by frequent observation assists in making a decision regarding further surgery.

## REHABILITATION

From the preceding remarks, we can make the decision on a rational basis whether to operate, rehabilitate, or rate. The following comments apply directly to decisions regarding the restoration of tendon gliding or joint mobility.

From the data just presented, it is evident that a brief initial evaluation of the scar's physical characteristics can provide additional information to aid in decision making. As a consequence, we subject all such cases to the initial evaluation test. This involves the application of various loads to the scar and determination of its deformation. Thereafter, the patient is begun on intensive therapy for at least three half-day sessions, Monday, Wednesday, and Friday. During this time the various rehabilitative procedures outlined in Chapter 12 are utilized. Data regarding joint motion and tendon gliding are

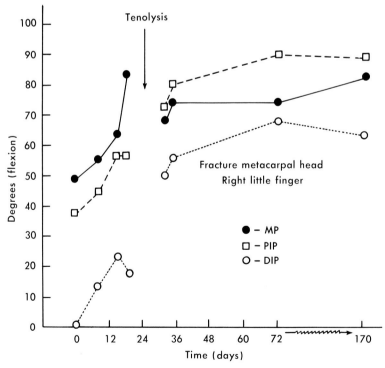

**Fig. 15-16.** Frequent observation and charting help one make decisions regarding selection of rehabilitation, reoperation, or rating.

obtained on Monday and Friday. An evaluation session on Friday afternoon allows review by the therapists, physician, and patient of the patient's response. The plan for therapy is altered as the changes in progress are noted. A second week consisting of three half-day therapy sessions provides additional data, which are reviewed at a second evaluation session.

The patients can be placed into one of four groups, as noted in Chapter 14. If the patient is making progress, therapy is continued either in the Hand Rehabilitation Center or at home. When the patient is no longer improving, the decision to operate or rate is made. This decision is based on the patient's functional needs. In the case of failure of a tendon to glide, the operative choices are as follows: (1) tenolysis, (2) resection of scarred tendon and tendon graft, (3) resection of scarred tendon and insertion of a Silastic rod, anticipating flexor tendon grafting at a later date, (4) joint fusion, or (5) amputation of the part (Fig. 15-17). This decision is based on the surgeon's judgment, as in-

fluenced by his clinical experience and the patient's needs. The latter concern should play the major role in making this decision. If the decision is that operative intervention is not indicated, then the patient's disability can be rated. In the cases where failure of joints to rotate is encountered, the various causes of joint stiffness outlined in Chapter 12 must be reviewed and the causes pinpointed. When the cause of joint stiffness can be corrected by surgery, this fact should be presented to the patient and the implications fully explained. Certainly, the procedure requires only 2 to 3 days of hospitalization, but the patient must be aware of the period of rehabilitation involved before he can return to work. Joint replacement can be considered when the articular surfaces are no longer functional or when extensive scar around the joint has completely embedded the joint capsule. Joint fusion is readily accepted for the distal interphalangeal joint, but for the proximal interphalangeal and metacarpophalangeal joints, in our experience, it has been uniformly unsatisfactory

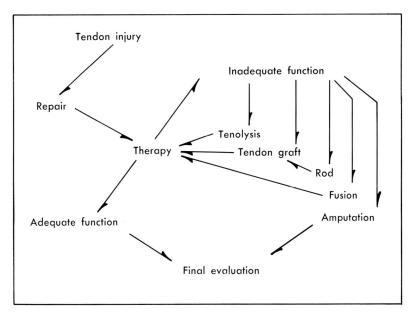

**Fig. 15-17.** All of the possible methods for management of a lacerated tendon are depicted above.

in laborers. Amputation in laborers has usually followed fusion of the metacarpophalangeal or proximal interphalangeal joints.

If the degree of progress after 2 weeks of therapy has been significant, the only decision to make is whether to continue therapy in a hand rehabilitation center or have the patient continue the therapy at home. A number of factors are involved in making this decision, including age, distance from home, motivation, and intensity of therapy required. We encourage patients to assume more responsibility for their rehabilitation, and within the 2-week period the patient can master most of the therapist's techniques. It is important that the patient return for a half-day session each week or every other week for splint adjustments, reevaluation, and reinforcement of the need for him to continue working as intensively at home as he did in the center.

Subsequent evaluation sessions provide recordings of progress that are discussed at meetings of the patient, the therapists, and the physician. When progress has reached a plateau as determined by the patient's data, the decision to operate or rate must be made.

With regard to tendon gliding, the most frequent operative decision is whether or not a tenolysis is indicated. At this stage, when the patient has improved significantly but not fully, we utilize tenolysis frequently. (The results of tenolysis are reviewed in Chapter 13.) If the surgeon decides that tenolysis is not indicated or the patient rejects further surgery, the patient may be rated. Most physicians wait about 12 months from the time of injury to make the routine rating.

With regard to joint mobility, active motion is a function of tendon gliding, and this would have been evaluated previously. Passive joint motion may be a function of tendon gliding or of scar remodelling within the joint. Thus, tenolysis

may be required to improve passive motion of the joint. When passive joint motion is limited by intracapsular scar and the passive range of joint motion has reached a plateau below optimum, the decision to operate or rate must be made. Even though the metacarpophalangeal joints passively flex to 90 degrees when one clinches the fist for grasp, the metacarpophalangeal joints are actively flexed only 75 to 80 degrees. In general, if the patient exhibits 65 degrees of metacarpophalangeal joint flexion, operative intervention is not indicated. Usually, the lack of at least 75 degrees of proximal interphalangeal joint flexion indicates the need for surgery on this joint. If the articular surfaces are functional, the operative procedure is selected as discussed in Chapter 12. Where the articular surfaces have been destroyed, the operative procedure may be arthroplasty, arthrodesis, or insertion of a prosthetic joint. This decision is based on the needs and desires of the patient and the surgeon's experience.

This phase of rehabilitation is directed toward accelerating the favorable modification of scar tissue. A second phase involves assisting the patient in regaining the skills required to perform his job. In cases of severe injury, this phase is directed more toward having the patient learn how to use the hand for any job. The goal for one group is returning the patient to his previous job, whereas for the second group the goal is preparing him for a new job. These techniques are well covered in Wynn's book on rehabilitation of the hand and will not be repeated here.

## RATING

Nothing is more exasperating to the surgeon than attempting to obtain a method of determining a patient's permanent partial disability that is consistent from one area to another. Medically, disability is physical impairment and inability to perform physical functions normally. Legally, disability is a permanent injury to the body for which the patient should or should not be compensated.

The Workmen's Compensation statutes categorize disability as temporary total disability, temporary partial disability, permanent partial disability, or permanent disability. Temporary total disability is the period of time during which the injured patient is totally unable to work. Temporary partial disability is that period when the patient has reached a state of improvement so that he may resume some type of gainful employment. Permanent partial disability applies to permanent damage or to loss of use of some part of the body after maximum improvement has been acquired. Permanent disabilities are expressed in units that allow conversion to a monetary scale. These units are determined by the region of the body involved and the extent of the involvement. The physician is asked to provide his own personal opinion regarding the final rating of disability. Guidelines have been provided through the *Journal of the American Medical Association,* "Guides to the Evaluation of Permanent Impairment—the Extremities and Back," February 15, 1958, and the "Manual for Orthopaedic Surgeons in Evaluating Permanent Physical Impairment," prepared by the American Academy of Orthopaedic Surgeons. The physician's evaluation is limited strictly to a decision on the extent of permanent physical impairment and the resulting loss of permanent physical function. In evaluating the hand, one is concerned basically with amputations, sensory loss, and restrictions of joint motion. The relative value of the digits to the whole hand are: thumb, 40%; index finger, 20%; long finger, 20%; ring finger, 10%; and little finger, 10%. When the metacarpal of a digit is involved, an additional 10% of the hand is added to the digit value.

An amputation through the distal half of the distal phalanx is equivalent to 25% permanent partial disability of the finger,

whereas an amputation through the distal interphalangeal joint is rated as a 50% permanent partial disability of that finger (Fig. 15-18). Any amputation proximal to the distal interphalangeal joint is recorded as 100% disability of the involved finger. Sensory loss is rated as depicted in Fig. 15-19. Note the differences in the radial and ulnar sides of the finger pads. This is calculated only with regard to sensory loss on the palmar surface of the digits or hand.

The restriction of joint motion can be evaluated by measuring loss of motion of the joint in question and consulting the tables prepared in the "Guide to the Evaluation of Permanent Impairment—the Extremities and Back." However, when more than one joint is involved in the same finger, some states require a composite disability rating for the finger. This com-

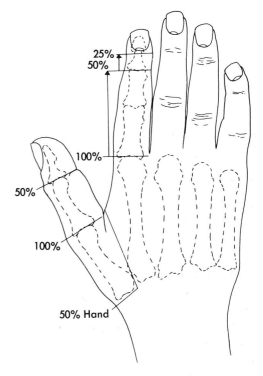

**Fig. 15-18.** The percent of partial permanent physical impairment is correlated with the level of amputation.

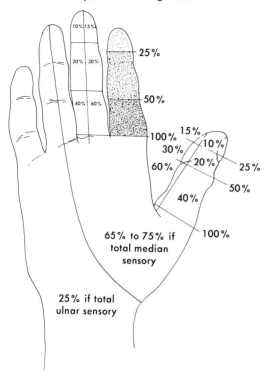

**Fig. 15-19.** The correlation between sensory loss and partial permanent physical impairment is indicated. Note that the radial side of the finger-pads and ulnar side of the thumbpad are considered areas of greatest functional significance.

interphalangeal joint of the index finger is rated as 20% permanent partial disability of the finger as a whole. The whole finger is worth 45 weeks. Thus the rating should be 20% of 45 weeks, or 9.0 weeks. The proximal interphalangeal joint is rated at 30 weeks. To obtain the correct percentage loss at the proximal interphalangeal joint, we solve (% rating) × (30 weeks) = 9.0 weeks. Rewritten, 9.0 weeks ÷ 30 weeks = the percentage rating at the proximal interphalangeal joint level.

Our final evaluation is performed on a chart that we utilize for rating that provides a complete record of the patient's progress to the point of discharge.

### BIBLIOGRAPHY

Dellon, A. L., Curtis, R. M., and Edgerton, M. T.: Evaluating recovery of sensation in the hand following nerve injury, Johns Hopkins Med. J. **130**:236, 1972.

Dellon, A. L., Curtis, R. M., and Edgerton, M. T.: Reeducation of sensation in the hand after nerve injury and repair, Plast. Reconstr. Surg. **53**:297, 1974.

Guides to the evaluation of permanent impairment—the extremities and back, 1958, Journal of the American Medical Association.

Henderson, W. R.: Clinical assessment of peripheral nerve injuries; Tinel's test, Lancet **2**: 801, 1948.

Manual for orthopaedic surgeons in evaluating permanent physical impairment, Chicago, American Academy of Orthopaedic Surgeons.

Millesi, H., Meissl, G., and Berger, A.: The interfascicular nerve-grafting of the median and ulnar nerves, J. Bone Joint Surg. **54A**:727, 1972.

Tauras, A. P., and Frackelton, W. H.: Silicone capping of nerve stumps in the problem of painful neuromas, Surg. Forum **18**:504, 1967.

Woodhall, B., Nulsen, F. E., White, J. C., and Davis, L.: Peripheral nerve regeneration, Washington, D.C., 1956, U.S. Government Printing Office, Chapter 7.

Wynn, P. C. B.: Rehabilitation of the hand, London, 1966, Butterworth's.

Zachary, R. B.: Results of nerve suture. In Seddon, H. J., editor: Peripheral nerve injuries, London, 1954, Her Majesty's Stationery Office.

Zalis, A. W., Rodriquez, A. A., Oester, Y. T., and Mains, D. B.: Evaluation of nerve regeneration by means of nerve evoked potentials, J. Bone Joint Surg. **54A**:1246, 1972.

bined value is determined by the formula A% + B% (100% − A%) = combined value of percent loss of joints A and B. The larger percentage loss is used as the A value. For example, a finger exhibits a permanent partial disability of 35% at the proximal interphalangeal joint and 25% at the distal joint. From the formula we obtain 35% + 25% (100% − 35%). This provides a combined permanent partial disability of 51%. Using these guidelines, the physician must state his opinion regarding the final rating of disability.

In some states, permanent partial disability is expressed for each joint of a finger. Since the tables are prepared for ratings based on the finger as a whole, the following is used to make a proper conversion. For example, an injury at the proximal

# Index